Antioxidants in Age-Related Diseases and Anti-Aging Strategies

Antioxidants in Age-Related Diseases and Anti-Aging Strategies

Editors

Daniela-Saveta Popa
Laurian Vlase
Marius Emil Rusu
Ionel Fizesan

MDPI • Basel • Beijing • Wuhan • Barcelona • Belgrade • Manchester • Tokyo • Cluj • Tianjin

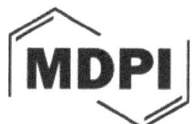

Editors

Daniela-Saveta Popa
Iuliu Hatieganu University of
Medicine and Pharmacy
Romania

Laurian Vlase
Iuliu Hatieganu University of
Medicine and Pharmacy
Romania

Marius Emil Rusu
Iuliu Hatieganu University of
Medicine and Pharmacy
Romania

Ionel Fizesan
Iuliu Hatieganu University of
Medicine and Pharmacy
Romania

Editorial Office
MDPI
St. Alban-Anlage 66
4052 Basel, Switzerland

This is a reprint of articles from the Special Issue published online in the open access journal *Antioxidants* (ISSN 2076-3921) (available at: https://www.mdpi.com/journal/antioxidants/special_issues/Antioxidants_Age).

For citation purposes, cite each article independently as indicated on the article page online and as indicated below:

LastName, A.A.; LastName, B.B.; LastName, C.C. Article Title. *Journal Name* **Year**, *Volume Number*, Page Range.

ISBN 978-3-0365-5589-8 (Hbk)
ISBN 978-3-0365-5590-4 (PDF)

© 2022 by the authors. Articles in this book are Open Access and distributed under the Creative Commons Attribution (CC BY) license, which allows users to download, copy and build upon published articles, as long as the author and publisher are properly credited, which ensures maximum dissemination and a wider impact of our publications.

The book as a whole is distributed by MDPI under the terms and conditions of the Creative Commons license CC BY-NC-ND.

Contents

Marius Emil Rusu, Ionel Fizeșan, Laurian Vlase and Daniela-Saveta Popa
Antioxidants in Age-Related Diseases and Anti-Aging Strategies
Reprinted from: *Antioxidants* **2022**, *11*, 1868, doi:10.3390/antiox11101868 1

Imen Ghzaiel, Amira Zarrouk, Thomas Nury, Michela Libergoli, Francesca Florio, Souha Hammouda, Franck Ménétrier, Laure Avoscan, Aline Yammine, Mohammad Samadi, Norbert Latruffe, Stefano Biressi, Débora Levy, Sérgio Paulo Bydlowski, Sonia Hammami, Anne Vejux, Mohamed Hammami and Gérard Lizard
Antioxidant Properties and Cytoprotective Effect of *Pistacia lentiscus* L. Seed Oil against 7β-Hydroxycholesterol-Induced Toxicity in C2C12 Myoblasts: Reduction in Oxidative Stress, Mitochondrial and Peroxisomal Dysfunctions and Attenuation of Cell Death
Reprinted from: *Antioxidants* **2021**, *10*, 1772, doi:10.3390/antiox10111772 7

Jae Won Ha and Yong Chool Boo
Siegesbeckiae Herba Extract and Chlorogenic Acid Ameliorate the Death of HaCaT Keratinocytes Exposed to Airborne Particulate Matter by Mitigating Oxidative Stress
Reprinted from: *Antioxidants* **2021**, *10*, 1762, doi:10.3390/antiox10111762 45

Seongin Jo, Young-Sung Jung, Ye-Ryeong Cho, Ji-Won Seo, Won-Chul Lim, Tae-Gyu Nam, Tae-Gyu Lim and Sanguine Byun
Oral Administration of *Rosa gallica* Prevents UVB–Induced Skin Aging through Targeting the c–Raf Signaling Axis
Reprinted from: *Antioxidants* **2021**, *10*, 1663, doi:10.3390/antiox10111663 65

Patrícia Correia, Paula Araújo, Carolina Ribeiro, Hélder Oliveira, Ana Rita Pereira, Nuno Mateus, Victor de Freitas, Natércia F. Brás, Paula Gameiro, Patrícia Coelho, Lucinda J. Bessa, Joana Oliveira and Iva Fernandes
Anthocyanin-Related Pigments: Natural Allies for Skin Health Maintenance and Protection
Reprinted from: *Antioxidants* **2021**, *10*, 1038, doi:10.3390/antiox10071038 79

Natalia A. Muraleva, Nataliya G. Kolosova and Natalia A. Stefanova
MEK1/2-ERK Pathway Alterations as a Therapeutic Target in Sporadic Alzheimer's Disease: A Study in Senescence-Accelerated OXYS Rats
Reprinted from: *Antioxidants* **2021**, *10*, 1058, doi:10.3390/antiox10071058 103

Andrila E. Collins, Tarek M. Saleh and Bettina E. Kalisch
Naturally Occurring Antioxidant Therapy in Alzheimer's Disease
Reprinted from: *Antioxidants* **2022**, *11*, 213, doi:10.3390/antiox11020213 115

Yong Chool Boo
Mechanistic Basis and Clinical Evidence for the Applications of Nicotinamide (Niacinamide) to Control Skin Aging and Pigmentation
Reprinted from: *Antioxidants* **2021**, *10*, 1315, doi:10.3390/antiox10081315 155

Daniela-Saveta Popa, Galya Bigman and Marius Emil Rusu
The Role of Vitamin K in Humans: Implication in Aging and Age-Associated Diseases
Reprinted from: *Antioxidants* **2021**, *10*, 566, doi:10.3390/antiox10040566 179

Sandra Maria Barbalho, Rosa Direito, Lucas Fornari Laurindo, Ledyane Taynara Marton, Elen Landgraf Guiguer, Ricardo de Alvares Goulart, Ricardo José Tofano, Antonely C. A. Carvalho, Uri Adrian Prync Flato, Viviane Alessandra Capelluppi Tofano, Cláudia Rucco Penteado Detregiachi, Patrícia C. Santos Bueno, Raul S. J. Girio and Adriano Cressoni Araújo
Ginkgo biloba in the Aging Process: A Narrative Review
Reprinted from: *Antioxidants* **2022**, *11*, 525, doi:10.3390/antiox11030525 . . . . **211**

Letiția Mateș, Daniela-Saveta Popa, Marius Emil Rusu, Ionel Fizeșan and Daniel Leucuța
Walnut Intake Interventions Targeting Biomarkers of Metabolic Syndrome and Inflammation in Middle-Aged and Older Adults: A Systematic Review and Meta-Analysis of Randomized Controlled Trials
Reprinted from: *Antioxidants* **2022**, *11*, 1412, doi:10.3390/antiox11071412 . . . . **239**

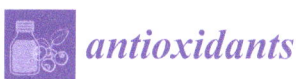

Editorial
Antioxidants in Age-Related Diseases and Anti-Aging Strategies

Marius Emil Rusu [1,*], Ionel Fizeșan [2], Laurian Vlase [1] and Daniela-Saveta Popa [2,*]

[1] Department of Pharmaceutical Technology and Biopharmaceutics, Faculty of Pharmacy, Iuliu Hatieganu University of Medicine and Pharmacy, 8 Victor Babes, 400012 Cluj-Napoca, Romania
[2] Department of Toxicology, Faculty of Pharmacy, Iuliu Hatieganu University of Medicine and Pharmacy, 8 Victor Babes, 400012 Cluj-Napoca, Romania
* Correspondence: rusu.marius@umfcluj.ro (M.E.R.); dpopa@umfcluj.ro (D.-S.P.); Tel.: +40-264-450-555 (D.-S.P.)

Aging is an intricate process and an important risk factor in the development and advancement of many disorders. As the world's population ages, chronic diseases associated with age will become increasingly common with a strong impact on quality of life. The pathogenesis of various diseases, including cardiometabolic disorders, neurodegenerative diseases, and cancer, consists of the accumulation of reactive oxygen species that leads to oxidative stress and inflammaging, which are major contributors to cellular senescence.

Different strategies have been suggested for healthy aging and for delaying or slowing aging. Plant matrices rich in antioxidant molecules, such as polyphenols, phytosterols, vitamins, and minerals, have been revealed to diminish the risk of age-associated syndromes in numerous in vitro studies [1,2]. Based on the fact that in vitro beneficial outcomes of any compound or extract should be confirmed through in vivo toxicological studies [3], the antioxidant and anti-inflammatory effects were replicated in animal model interventions revealing lower levels of reactive oxygen species (ROS), advanced glycation end products, or inflammatory biomarkers [4,5]. Moreover, clinical evidence supported the potential of bioactive compounds in the decrease in many risk factors related to aging and the likely prevention of age-related diseases [6].

This Special Issue "Antioxidants in Age-Related Diseases and Anti-Aging Strategies", which includes five research articles, four review reports, and one systematic review and meta-analysis, adds new contributions that describe the mechanisms by which oxidative stress and inflammatory factors cause the occurrence or progression of age-related chronic diseases, as well as new strategies to treat or prevent these pathological conditions.

The study by Ghzaiel et al. [7] assayed the chemical composition of *Pistacia lentiscus* L. seed oil (PLSO) in terms of polyphenols, flavonoids, phytosterols, α-tocopherol, β-carotene, and fatty acids and its antioxidant activity. This was followed by an in vitro evaluation of the potential of this plant to neutralize the cytotoxic effects induced by 7β-hydroxycholesterol (7β-OHC) in murine C2C12 myoblasts. 7β-OHC is an oxysterol that can activate oxidative stress and inflammation and contribute to age-related diseases, such as sarcopenia. The results showed that PLSO contains a combination of molecules capable of diminishing 7β-OHC-induced cytotoxic effects and activating cytoprotective properties, including the prevention of cell death and organelle dysfunction, attenuation of oxidative stress, and activity normalization of glutathione peroxidase (GPx) and superoxide dismutase (SOD), which are key antioxidant enzymes. Thus, PLSO can prevent age-related diseases, such as sarcopenia, an age-related gradual deterioration in skeletal muscle mass, strength, and function.

The skin is a barrier between the body and the environment, protecting the body from environmental pollutants and pathogens. One study [8] was conducted to discover a natural product that efficiently mitigates the cytotoxicity and oxidative stress induced by airborne particulate matter with a size of 10 μm or less (PM_{10}) in the skin. Data showed

Citation: Rusu, M.E.; Fizeșan, I.; Vlase, L.; Popa, D.-S. Antioxidants in Age-Related Diseases and Anti-Aging Strategies. *Antioxidants* **2022**, *11*, 1868. https://doi.org/10.3390/antiox11101868

Received: 10 September 2022
Accepted: 19 September 2022
Published: 21 September 2022

Publisher's Note: MDPI stays neutral with regard to jurisdictional claims in published maps and institutional affiliations.

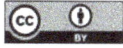

Copyright: © 2022 by the authors. Licensee MDPI, Basel, Switzerland. This article is an open access article distributed under the terms and conditions of the Creative Commons Attribution (CC BY) license (https://creativecommons.org/licenses/by/4.0/).

that Siegesbeckiae Herba extract (SHE), a hot water extract prepared from dried leaves of *Siegesbeckia pubescens* Makino, had the potential to relieve PM_{10}-induced cytotoxicity and increase the cellular antioxidant capacity in HaCaT cells, an immortalized human keratinocyte cell line. SHE mitigated PM_{10}-induced cell death, lactate dehydrogenase (LDH) release, and lipid peroxidation and lowered ROS production. Additionally, SHE activated the NRF2 system in cells by decreasing the expression of KEAP1, a negative regulator of NRF2, and increasing the expression of HMOX1 and NQO1, two main target genes of NRF2. Chlorogenic acid may be an active phytochemical in activating the NRF2 pathway. Moreover, SHE selectively induced the enzymes involved in the synthesis and regeneration of reduced glutathione (GSH) and increased the cellular content of GSH, preventing the oxidation of GSH to GSSG triggered by PM_{10} exposure. The findings of this experiment should be verified using normal human epidermal keratinocytes and animal models.

Another study [9] analyzed plant compounds that might mitigate skin wrinkle formation, inflammation, pigmentation, and dehydration caused by chronic irradiation with ultraviolet B (UVB) light. UVB can activate signaling pathways, leading to the upregulation of genes, including matrix metalloproteinases (MMPs), especially MMP-1, involved in collagen degradation and wrinkle formation, and cyclooxygenase 2 (COX-2), involved in skin inflammation and photoaging. *Rosa gallica*, one of the most commonly used Rosa species for culinary, medicinal, and cosmetic purposes, which showed in vitro potential to prevent biomarkers of skin aging, was used in this in vivo study. The gavage administration of *Rosa gallica* extract prevented UVB-mediated skin wrinkle development and collagen degradation in the dorsal skin of female mice by down-regulating UVB-induced COX-2 and MMP-1 expression. Gallic acid was the major molecule contributing to the anti-skin-aging effect by selectively inhibiting c-Raf/MEK/ERK/c-Fos signaling axis. Since molecules targeting the c-Raf pathway exert chemopreventive and chemotherapeutic effects against different cancer types, gallic acid could potentially suppress carcinogenesis. The study concluded that *Rosa gallica* and gallic acid could protect skin cells against free radicals and inflammatory reactions, leading to a reduction in skin aging.

The third study [10] exploring skin health examined the beneficial activities of cyanidin- and malvidin-3-*O*-glucosides, molecules belonging to the anthocyanin family, and some of their structurally related pigments. Most of the examined compounds were found to reduce biofilm production by *Staphylococcus aureus* and *Pseudomonas aeruginosa*, displayed UV-filter capacity, and also reduced the production of ROS in human skin epidermal keratinocytes and dermal fibroblast. Furthermore, the molecules revealed inhibitory activity of skin-degrading enzymes, hyaluronidase, collagenase, and elastase, the three main enzymes responsible for the regulation of the structural integrity of skin layers, showing no significant cytotoxicity. The stability issue of anthocyanin family compounds can be overcome by the use of anthocyanin's structural derivatives, such as carboxypyranocyanidin-3-*O*-glucoside, a molecule with great structural stability that could be included in topical formulations for cosmeceutical purposes.

In their study, Muraleva et al. [11] investigated the effects of mitochondria-targeted antioxidant plastoquinonyl-decyltriphenylphosphonium (SkQ1) in MEK1/2-ERK pathway alterations as a therapeutic target in Alzheimer's disease (AD). MEK1 and MEK2 are tyrosine/threonine protein kinases found in the Ras/Raf/MEK/ERK mitogen-activated protein kinase (MAPK) signaling pathway. The study included senescence-accelerated OXYS rats that develop neurodegenerative changes almost similar (>90% of cases) to the signs of sporadic AD in humans. The results showed that, compared to untreated control (Wistar) rats, SkQ1 eliminated differences in the expression of eight out of nine genes involved in the hippocampal extracellular regulated kinases' (ERK1 and -2) signaling pathways. Additionally, SkQ1 reduced the hyperphosphorylation of tau protein that is present in pathological aggregates in AD. Thus, SkQ1 alleviates AD pathology in the OXYS rat hippocampus by reducing MEK1/2-ERK1/2 phosphorylation and may be a promising drug for human AD.

Collins et al. [12] presented a thorough revision of antioxidant therapy in AD. Strong evidence supports the role of oxidative stress in the pathogenesis and progression of AD and aging. Oxidative stress appears when there is an imbalance among antioxidants and the production and buildup of ROS, related to an insufficient or dysfunctional antioxidant defense system with damaging effects to important cellular structures including proteins, lipids, and nucleic acids. Adequate cellular homeostasis, a balance between the production and depletion of ROS, occurs through the protective mechanisms of natural and synthetic antioxidants. Natural antioxidants can be further divided into enzymatic antioxidants, enzymes produced in the body with free-radical-scavenging abilities, such as SOD, catalase (CAT), GPx, glutathione reductase (GR), and glucose-6-phosphate dehydrogenase (G6PDH) and non-enzymatic antioxidants, including polyphenols, carotenoids, vitamins, and minerals.

Although available medications help with AD symptom management, there are no treatments to prevent or cure the disease, and furthermore, none of the currently existing treatments address oxidative stress. Thus, recent studies focused on the use of antioxidants to diminish the oxidative stress effects on the central nervous system. In preclinical in vitro and in vivo experiments, a combination of antioxidant compounds improved the overall antioxidant capacity of drug therapy, enhanced the bioavailability to various cellular locations, and increased the functionality of antioxidant molecules. The therapeutic potential of natural antioxidants in preventing and/or treating neurodegenerative conditions is presently assessed in human clinical trials.

The biological activities and cosmeceutical properties of nicotinamide were discussed in an interesting review [13]. Nicotinamide (niacinamide) is mostly used as a nutritional supplement for vitamin B3 (nicotinic acid, niacin), and vitamin B3 is further used in the synthesis of the NAD^+ family of coenzymes, related to cellular energy metabolism and defense systems. Nicotinamide supplementation restores mitochondrial energetics and cellular NAD^+ pool, prevents the skin pigmentation process, and diminishes oxidative stress and inflammatory response. This molecule has the potential to support skin homeostasis by regulating the cellular redox status. In clinical trials, topically applied nicotinamide was well tolerated by the skin and reduced hyperpigmentation and the progression of skin aging. Therefore, it may be useful as a cosmeceutical ingredient to attenuate skin aging, especially in the elderly or in patients with reduced NAD^+ pool in the skin.

Another review [14] examined vitamin K and its role as a vital cofactor in the activation of several proteins, which act against age-related diseases. It was shown that vitamin K carboxylates osteocalcin, a protein responsible for transporting and fixing calcium in bones, activates matrix Gla protein, an inhibitor of vascular calcification and cardiovascular incidents; carboxylates Gas6 protein, which is involved in the physiology of the brain and may inhibit cognitive decline and neurodegenerative disease; and improves insulin sensitivity, thus decreasing diabetes risk. Additionally, vitamin K presents antiproliferative, proapoptotic, and autophagic effects and is associated with reduced cancer risk. Recent evidence indicates that protein S, another vitamin K-dependent protein, might prevent the cytokine storm noticed in COVID-19 cases. The latest scientific documents emphasize the vitamin K role in preventing age-associated diseases and improving the efficiency of medical treatments in the elderly.

In a narrative review, Barbalho et al. [15] analyzed *Ginkgo biloba* (GB), a medicinal plant in the Ginkgoaceae family considered to be the oldest tree alive in the world. GB extracts account for some health benefits for memory and cognition, AD, Parkinson's disease (PD), and dementia, which are attributed to its antioxidant, anti-inflammatory, and antiapoptotic activities. In addition, GB can exert benefits in cardiovascular conditions, hypertension, insulin resistance, fasting serum glucose, glycated hemoglobin, and dyslipidemia. Moreover, it can improve cerebral blood flow supply, executive function, attention/concentration, and non-verbal memory and decrease stress. In many European states, GB extract is the only drug therapy for the treatment of mild cognitive impairment. The bioactive compounds, mainly polyphenols, flavonoids, terpenoids, and organic acids, are responsible for the beneficial effects. This review revealed that GB could be considered in the therapeutic and preventative methods for aging-associated conditions and the aging process. However, more studies are required to determine the doses, pharmaceutical form, and treatment time needed in aging conditions.

A systematic review and meta-analysis [16] investigated biomarkers of metabolic syndrome and inflammation as pathophysiological predictors of senescence and age-related diseases. Recent evidence confirmed that particular diets rich in antioxidant bioactive compounds and a balanced lipid profile, such as walnuts, could have beneficial results on human health. A systematic search in several databases was performed to find randomized controlled trials reporting on the outcomes of walnut consumption on metabolic syndrome and inflammatory markers in middle-aged and older adults. The investigation extracted 17 studies, including 11 crossover and 6 parallel trials. The analysis revealed that walnut-enriched diets had significant reducing effects on triglyceride, total cholesterol, LDL cholesterol levels, and some inflammatory markers, with no adverse effects on anthropometric and glycemic parameters. While further and better-designed reports are required, the outcomes stress the benefits of including walnuts in the dietary plans of middle-aged and older adults.

We would like to acknowledge all the authors who have contributed to this Special Issue and have provided a better understanding of the importance of antioxidants in the delaying of aging and prevention of diseases associated with aging, and the need to develop future therapeutic strategies targeting these diseases.

Funding: This research received no external funding.

Conflicts of Interest: The authors declare no conflict of interest.

References

1. Rusu, M.E.; Fizesan, I.; Pop, A.; Mocan, A.; Gheldiu, A.M.; Babota, M.; Vodnar, D.C.; Jurj, A.; Berindan-Neagoe, I.; Vlase, L.; et al. Walnut (*Juglans regia* L.) Septum: Assessment of Bioactive Molecules and in Vitro Biological Effects. *Molecules* **2020**, *25*, 2187. [CrossRef] [PubMed]
2. Pop, A.; Fizesan, I.; Vlase, L.; Rusu, M.E.; Cherfan, J.; Babota, M.; Gheldiu, A.-M.; Tomuta, I.; Popa, D.-S. Enhanced Recovery of Phenolic and Tocopherolic Compounds from Walnut (*Juglans regia* L.) Male Flowers Based on Process Optimization of Ultrasonic Assisted-Extraction: Phytochemical Profile and Biological Activities. *Antioxidants* **2021**, *10*, 607. [CrossRef] [PubMed]
3. Vedeanu, N.; Voica, C.; Magdas, D.A.; Kiss, B.; Stefan, M.G.; Simedrea, R.; Georgiu, C.; Berce, C.; Vostinaru, O.; Boros, R.; et al. Subacute Co-Exposure to Low Doses of Ruthenium(III) Changes the Distribution, Excretion and Biological Effects of Silver Ions in Rats. *Environ. Chem.* **2020**, *17*, 163–172. [CrossRef]
4. Rusu, M.E.; Georgiu, C.; Pop, A.; Mocan, A.; Kiss, B.; Vostinaru, O.; Fizesan, I.; Stefan, M.G.; Gheldiu, A.M.; Mates, L.; et al. Antioxidant Effects of Walnut (*Juglans regia* L.) Kernel and Walnut Septum Extract in a D-Galactose-Induced Aging Model and in Naturally Aged Rats. *Antioxidants* **2020**, *9*, 424. [CrossRef] [PubMed]
5. Fizeșan, I.; Rusu, M.E.; Georgiu, C.; Pop, A.; Ștefan, M.G.; Muntean, D.M.; Mirel, S.; Vostinaru, O.; Kiss, B.; Popa, D.S. Antitussive, Antioxidant, and Anti-Inflammatory Effects of a Walnut (*Juglans regia* L.) Septum Extract Rich in Bioactive Compounds. *Antioxidants* **2021**, *10*, 119. [CrossRef] [PubMed]
6. Rusu, M.E.; Mocan, A.; Ferreira, I.C.F.R.; Popa, D.S. Health Benefits of Nut Consumption in Middle-Aged and Elderly Population. *Antioxidants* **2019**, *8*, 302. [CrossRef] [PubMed]
7. Ghzaiel, I.; Zarrouk, A.; Nury, T.; Libergoli, M.; Florio, F.; Hammouda, S.; Ménétrier, F.; Avoscan, L.; Yammine, A.; Samadi, M.; et al. Antioxidant Properties and Cytoprotective Effect of Pistacia lentiscus L. Seed Oil against 7β-hydroxycholesterol-induced Toxicity in C2C12 Myoblasts: Reduction in Oxidative Stress, Mitochondrial and Peroxisomal Dysfunctions and Attenuation of Cell Death. *Antioxidants* **2021**, *10*, 1772. [CrossRef] [PubMed]
8. Ha, J.W.; Boo, Y.C. Siegesbeckiae Herba Extract and Chlorogenic Acid Ameliorate the Death of HaCaT Keratinocytes Exposed to Airborne Particulate Matter by Mitigating Oxidative Stress. *Antioxidants* **2021**, *10*, 1762. [CrossRef] [PubMed]
9. Jo, S.; Jung, Y.S.; Cho, Y.R.; Seo, J.W.; Lim, W.C.; Nam, T.G.; Lim, T.G.; Byun, S. Oral Administration of Rosa gallica Prevents UVB-induced Skin Aging through Targeting the c-Raf Signaling Axis. *Antioxidants* **2021**, *10*, 1663. [CrossRef] [PubMed]
10. Correia, P.; Araújo, P.; Ribeiro, C.; Oliveira, H.; Pereira, A.R.; Mateus, N.; de Freitas, V.; Brás, N.F.; Gameiro, P.; Coelho, P.; et al. Anthocyanin-Related Pigments: Natural Allies for Skin Health Maintenance and Protection. *Antioxidants* **2021**, *10*, 1038. [CrossRef] [PubMed]
11. Muraleva, N.A.; Kolosova, N.G.; Stefanova, N.A. MEK1/2-ERK Pathway Alterations as a Therapeutic Target in Sporadic Alzheimer's Disease: A Study in Senescence-Accelerated OXYS Rats. *Antioxidants* **2021**, *10*, 1058. [CrossRef] [PubMed]

12. Collins, A.E.; Saleh, T.M.; Kalisch, B.E. Naturally Occurring Antioxidant Therapy in Alzheimer's Disease. *Antioxidants* **2022**, *11*, 213. [CrossRef] [PubMed]
13. Boo, Y.C. Mechanistic Basis and Clinical Evidence for the Applications of Nicotinamide (Niacinamide) to Control Skin Aging and Pigmentation. *Antioxidants* **2021**, *10*, 1315. [CrossRef] [PubMed]
14. Popa, D.S.; Bigman, G.; Rusu, M.E. The Role of Vitamin K in Humans: Implication in Aging and Age-Associated Diseases. *Antioxidants* **2021**, *10*, 566. [CrossRef] [PubMed]
15. Barbalho, S.M.; Direito, R.; Laurindo, L.F.; Marton, L.T.; Guiguer, E.L.; de Alvares Goulart, R.; Tofano, R.J.; Carvalho, A.C.A.; Flato, U.A.P.; Tofano, V.A.C.; et al. Ginkgo biloba in the Aging Process: A Narrative Review. *Antioxidants* **2022**, *11*, 525. [CrossRef] [PubMed]
16. Mateș, L.; Popa, D.-S.; Rusu, M.E.; Fizeșan, I.; Leucuța, D. Walnut Intake Interventions Targeting Biomarkers of Metabolic Syndrome and Inflammation in Middle-Aged and Older Adults: A Systematic Review and Meta-Analysis of Randomized Controlled Trials. *Antioxidants* **2022**, *11*, 1412. [CrossRef] [PubMed]

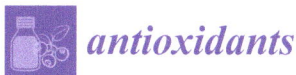

Article

Antioxidant Properties and Cytoprotective Effect of *Pistacia lentiscus* L. Seed Oil against 7β-Hydroxycholesterol-Induced Toxicity in C2C12 Myoblasts: Reduction in Oxidative Stress, Mitochondrial and Peroxisomal Dysfunctions and Attenuation of Cell Death

Imen Ghzaiel [1,2,3], Amira Zarrouk [2,4,*], Thomas Nury [1], Michela Libergoli [5], Francesca Florio [5], Souha Hammouda [2], Franck Ménétrier [6], Laure Avoscan [7], Aline Yammine [1], Mohammad Samadi [8], Norbert Latruffe [1], Stefano Biressi [5], Débora Levy [9], Sérgio Paulo Bydlowski [9,10], Sonia Hammami [2], Anne Vejux [1], Mohamed Hammami [2] and Gérard Lizard [1,*]

[1] Team 'Biochemistry of the Peroxisome, Inflammation and Lipid Metabolism' EA7270/Inserm, University Bourgogne Franche-Comté, 21000 Dijon, France; imenghzaiel93@gmail.com (I.G.); thomas.nury@u-bourgogne.fr (T.N.); alineyammine5@gmail.com (A.Y.); norbert.latruffe@u-bourgogne.fr (N.L.); anne.vejux@u-bourgogne.fr (A.V.)

[2] Lab-NAFS 'Nutrition—Functional Food & Vascular Health', Faculty of Medicine, University of Monastir, LR12ES05, Monastir 5000, Tunisia; souhahammouda51@gmail.com (S.H.); sonia.hammami@fmm.rnu.tn (S.H.); mohamed.hammami@fmm.rnu.tn (M.H.)

[3] Faculty of Sciences of Tunis, University Tunis-El Manar, Tunis 2092, Tunisia

[4] Faculty of Medicine, University of Sousse, Sousse 4000, Tunisia

[5] Department of Cellular, Computational and Integrative Biology (CIBio) and Dulbecco Telethon Institute, University of Trento, 38123 Trento, Italy; michela.libergoli@unitn.it (M.L.); francesca.florio@unitn.it (F.F.); stefano.biressi@unitn.it (S.B.)

[6] Centre des Sciences du Goût et de l'Alimentation, AgroSup Dijon, CNRS, INRAE, Université Bourgogne Franche-Comté, 21065 Dijon, France; franck.menetrier@inrae.fr

[7] Agroécologie, AgroSup Dijon, CNRS, INRAE, University Bourgogne Franche-Comté, Plateforme DimaCell, 21000 Dijon, France; laure.avoscan@inrae.fr

[8] LCPMC-A2, ICPM, Department of Chemistry, University Lorraine, Metz Technopôle, 57070 Metz, France; mohammad.samadi@univ-lorraine.fr

[9] Lipids, Oxidation and Cell Biology Team, Laboratory of Immunology (LIM19), Heart Institute (InCor), Faculdade de Medicina, Universidade de São Paulo, São Paulo 05403-900, Brazil; d.levy@hc.fm.usp.br (D.L.); spbydlow@usp.br (S.P.B.)

[10] National Institute of Science and Technology in Regenerative Medicine (INCT-Regenera), CNPq, Rio de Janeiro 21941-902, Brazil

* Correspondence: zarroukamira@gmail.com (A.Z.); gerard.lizard@u-bourgogne.fr (G.L.); Tel.: +216-94-837-999 or +1-212-241 9304 (A.Z.); +33-380-396-256 (G.L.)

Abstract: Aging is characterized by a progressive increase in oxidative stress, which favors lipid peroxidation and the formation of cholesterol oxide derivatives, including 7β-hydroxycholesterol (7β-OHC). This oxysterol, which is known to trigger oxidative stress, inflammation, and cell death, could contribute to the aging process and age-related diseases, such as sarcopenia. Identifying molecules or mixtures of molecules preventing the toxicity of 7β-OHC is therefore an important issue. This study consists of determining the chemical composition of Tunisian *Pistacia lentiscus* L. seed oil (PLSO) used in the Tunisian diet and evaluating its ability to counteract the cytotoxic effects induced by 7β-OHC in murine C2C12 myoblasts. The effects of 7β-OHC (50 µM; 24 h), associated or not with PLSO, were studied on cell viability, oxidative stress, and on mitochondrial and peroxisomal damages induction. α-Tocopherol (400 µM) was used as the positive control for cytoprotection. Our data show that PLSO is rich in bioactive compounds; it contains polyunsaturated fatty acids, and several nutrients with antioxidant properties: phytosterols, α-tocopherol, carotenoids, flavonoids, and phenolic compounds. When associated with PLSO (100 µg/mL), the 7β-OHC-induced cytotoxic effects were strongly attenuated. The cytoprotection was in the range of those observed with α-tocopherol. This cytoprotective effect was characterized by prevention of cell death and organelle dysfunction (restoration of cell adhesion, cell viability, and plasma membrane integrity; prevention of mitochondrial and peroxisomal damage) and attenuation of oxidative stress (reduction in reactive oxygen species overproduction in whole cells and at the mitochondrial level; decrease in lipid and protein oxidation products formation; and normalization of antioxidant enzyme activities: glutathione peroxidase (GPx) and superoxide dismutase (SOD)). These results provide evidence that PLSO has similar antioxidant properties than α-tocopherol used at high concentration and contains a mixture of molecules capable to attenuate 7β-OHC-induced cytotoxic effects in C2C12 myoblasts. These data reinforce the interest in edible oils associated with the Mediterranean diet, such as PLSO, in the prevention of age-related diseases, such as sarcopenia.

Keywords: aging; 7β-hydroxycholesterol; mitochondria; C2C12 myoblasts; oxidative stress; peroxisome; *Pistacia lentiscus* L. seed oil; sarcopenia

1. Introduction

Aging is characterized by a progressive loss of physiological functions, coupled with a reduction in the ability to maintain homeostasis [1]. One of the hallmark effects of aging is sarcopenia, which is widely defined as an age-related progressive decline in skeletal muscle mass, strength, and function [2,3]. From the age of 30, humans lose approximately 3–8% of muscle mass per decade with an accelerated rate of decline after the age of 60 [4–6]. This decline leads to limited functional mobility in older adults [7], but it may also aggravate their vulnerability [8]. Indeed, skeletal muscle is the largest organ in the human body. It accounts for 30–40% of total body weight [9,10] and plays a primordial role in locomotion [11], respiration [12], thermogenesis [13], and regulation of lipids (fatty acids, cholesterol) [14,15] and glucose metabolism [16]. The aging skeletal muscle is marked by the development of an alteration of energy substrates use. In fact, in response to insulin stimulation, mitochondria of elderly subjects are unable to move from lipid oxidation to carbohydrate oxidation as do mitochondria of young subjects, showing a loss of metabolic flexibility during aging [17]. These data suggest an alteration in metabolic dynamism and highlight the inability of muscle cells to adapt to environmental variations. It is therefore important to better understand the underlying mechanisms leading to sarcopenia but also to identify the chemical epigenetic factors that may promote it. In addition, during aging, to allow the maintenance of muscle mass, strength and quality, and to act on these parameters, it is important to identify natural or synthetic molecules, as well as mixtures of molecules that can be provided in the form of food supplements, or functional foods [18]. An adapted diet, as well as foods acting on the muscle, must also be considered. Several aging mechanisms have been identified, including telomere shortening, genomic instability, epigenetic alterations, and organelle dysfunction (mainly mitochondrial changes), which can trigger cellular senescence [18]. In addition, among the parameters that can affect the aging of skeletal muscle, oxidative stress is one of the major contributors that can favor skeletal muscle damage [19,20]. Skeletal muscle consumes large quantities of oxygen compared to other tissues, resulting in higher amounts of reactive oxygen species (ROS) [21]. This increase in ROS levels could be due to two main factors: (i) altered functions of the mitochondrial respiratory chain; and (ii) impairment in cellular antioxidant defense mechanisms [22]. These ROS contribute to increased uptake of both glucose and cholesterol into the cells [23]. Cholesterol is a major component of cellular membranes, including the sarcolemma of skeletal muscle [24]. In the presence of oxidative stress, glucose and cholesterol can undergo auto-oxidation by a free-radical mechanism. The cholesterol oxide derivatives (oxysterols) formed by cholesterol auto-oxidation in oxidative stress conditions mainly correspond to those that are oxidized at position C7 (7-ketocholesterol (7KC) and 7β-hydroxycholesterol (7β-OHC)) [25–28]. Interestingly, 7KC and 7β-OHC have similar cytotoxic effects (although the induction of cell death is faster with 7β-OHC) and these two oxysterols can be interconverted: the enzyme 11β-hydroxysteroid dehydrogenase-1

(11β-HSD1) converts 7KC into 7β-OHC, whereas 11β-hydroxysteroid dehydrogenase-2 (11β-HSD2) converts 7β-OHC into 7KC [29,30]. In addition, these oxysterols have been identified as key elements in the development of age-related diseases: cardiovascular diseases, neurodegenerative diseases (Alzheimer's and Parkinson's), and ocular diseases (cataract, age-related macular degeneration) [28,31–33]. On various cell lines from different species, 7KC and 7β-OHC but also 24S-hydroxycholesterol trigger a mode of cell death by oxiapoptophagy, which includes oxidative stress and mitochondrial, lysosomal, and peroxisomal dysfunction, leading to an apoptotic mode of cell death associated with autophagic criteria [30,34–36]. Oxysterols are also involved in many physiologic processes: regulation of cholesterol metabolism [37] and RedOx homeostasis [38]; control of inflammation, including cytokine production [39]; albumin synthesis [40]; and cell differentiation [41]. Despite the considerable interest in oxysterols in the aging process, the impact of these molecules on skeletal muscle cells has not yet been studied. On human promonocytic U937 cells, 7KC, 7β-OHC and 5β,6β-epoxicholesterol showed high cytotoxicity, characterized by a high percentage of dead cells, overproduction of ROS, and secretion of pro-inflammatory cytokines [42]. It has been shown that the most toxic oxysterol on U937 cells, but also on other cells, was 7β-OHC [30,42].

Therefore, to mimic an age-related pro-oxidant environment, C2C12 murine myoblasts cultured in the presence of 7β-OHC were used as a cellular model. The effects of 7β-OHC were characterized on C2C12 and cytoprotective agents were investigated. The effect of α-tocopherol that protects many cells from the toxicity induced by 7β-OHC and 7KC was also analyzed [28] as well as that of *Pistacia lentiscus* L. seed oil (PLSO), widely used in the Tunisian diet. It is well known that vegetable oils are a valuable source of natural antioxidants, playing a crucial role in the improvement of human health [43] and in delaying muscle atrophy [44]. One of the most well-known powerful medicinal plants is *Pistacia lentiscus* L. (PL). PL is one of the Mediterranean's most valuable and important aromatic bushes. Its application in traditional medicine has increased over time and it is used as a therapeutic agent in the treatment of scabies, rheumatism, the manufacture of anti-diarrheal medicine, and in minor burns [45–47]. Extracts of different parts of the plant show various activities, such as antioxidant, anti-inflammatory, anti-proliferative, and neuroprotective effects [48–51]. The fruits of PL give an edible oil with high nutritional value due to its richness in unsaturated fatty acids, such as oleic acid (C18:1 n−9) and linoleic acid (C18:2 n−6) [52]. PLSO also has a comparable carotenoid and total polyphenols content than olive oil [53,54], and it has been demonstrated that it has antioxidant and protective effects against various diseases associated with oxidative stress [55,56].

In the present study, the first objective was to determine the biochemical composition of PLSO in polyphenols, flavonoids, β-carotene, fatty acids, phytosterols, and α-tocopherol, and its antioxidant properties. Furthermore, among the sarcopenic patients studied, as the level of 7β-OHC (mainly formed by cholesterol auto-oxidation, considered as a marker of oxidative stress, and known for its important pro-oxidant properties) was significantly higher than in non-sarcopenic subjects, the second objective of the study was to evaluate the ability of PLSO, compared to α-tocopherol, to attenuate the cytotoxic effects induced by 7β-OHC on murine C2C12 myoblasts; specifically, the effects on cell proliferation and viability, plasma membrane integrity, oxidative stress, and mitochondrial and peroxisomal status.

2. Material and Methods
2.1. Chemical Profile of Pistacia lentiscus L. Seed Oil
2.1.1. Seed Material and Oil Extraction

The mature fruits of PL (lentisk-mastic tree) were collected in November 2019 from plants growing in the region of Tabarka (extreme north-west of Tunisia). After the harvest, fruits were ground using an ordinary grinder; the resulting paste was then manually mixed and let to stand overnight in a refrigerator. The next day, the paste was macerated in cold water. Subsequently, the mixture was placed in a water bath to prevent direct exposure of the ground material to the heat and thus degradation of the oil quality. After filtration, the oil was separated from the water by a decantation process. The procedure of *Pistacia lentiscus* L. seed oil is summarized in Supplementary Figure S1. The oils obtained were stored and maintained at 4 °C for further analyses.

2.1.2. Colorimetric Determination of Total Phenolics, Flavonoids, and Carotenoids Contents of *Pistacia lentiscus* L. Seed Oil

The quantification of total phenolics and flavonoids was preceded by an extraction performed as follows: 4 g of PLSO was mixed thoroughly with 2 mL of n-hexane followed by the addition of 4 mL of methanol/water (60:40, *v/v*). The mixture was vortexed vigorously and centrifuged at 1490× *g* for 3 min to separate the two phases. The hydroalcoholic phase was collected, and the hexanic phase was re-extracted two more times with 4 mL of methanol/water (60:40, *v/v*) solution. Finally, the hydroalcoholic fraction obtained was combined, washed with 4 mL of n-hexane, and stored at −20 °C until analysis.

Phenolic compounds: Total phenolic compounds content was assayed by the Folin–Ciocalteau's method [57]. Briefly, 200 µL of the combined hydroalcoholic fraction or standard gallic acid solutions was mixed thoroughly with 1 mL of freshly prepared Folin–Ciocalteau reagent and 0.8 mL of 7.5% sodium carbonate (Na_2CO_3). After incubation for 30 min in the dark at room temperature, the absorbance was measured at 765 nm and the results were expressed as mg of gallic acid equivalent per g of sample.

Flavonoids: Quantification of total flavonoids was determined using an aluminum chloride ($AlCl_3$) colorimetric assay [58]. A volume of 100 µL of the combined hydroalcoholic fraction or standard catechin solutions was combined with 400 µL of distilled water and subsequently with 30 µL of 5% sodium nitrite ($NaNO_2$) solution. After 5 min, 20 µL of a 10% $AlCl_3$ solution and 200 µL of 1 M Na_2CO_3 solution were added. The final volume was adjusted with distilled water and mixed thoroughly. The absorbance was recorded at 510 nm, and the concentrations were expressed as mg of catechin equivalent per g of the sample.

Carotenoids: Total carotenoids content was measured by a colorimetric assay according to the method previously described by Dhibi et al. [59], and was expressed using the following formula:

$$\text{Carotenoids} = A\max \times (10^5/2.65)$$

where $A\max$ is the maximum of absorption between 440 and 480 nm.

2.1.3. Polyphenols Analysis

In order to identify and quantify the polyphenolic compounds in PLSO, we analyzed them by high-performance liquid chromatography (HPLC). To this end, 1 g of oil was dissolved in 6 mL of petroleum ether and was then purified on a silica SPE cartridge (previously conditioned by 6 mL petroleum ether 40–60). The cartridge was then washed with 12 mL of petroleum ether and dried under nitrogen for 10 min. Polyphenolic compounds were eluted with 8 mL of a mixture of methanol/distilled water 80/20 (*v/v*), and then with 8 mL of acetonitrile. The eluate was evaporated to dryness under reduced pressure at 50 °C. The residue was taken up in 400 µL of methanol. The resulting extract was filtered through a 0.45 µm nylon membrane. Polyphenol analysis was performed by HPLC on a Perkin Elmer series 200 apparatus equipped with an automatic injector, a quaternary pump, a column oven to Peltier effect, and a DAD detector. HPLC analyses were carried out using RPHPLC with a licrospher 100 RP-18 column (150 × 4.6 mm internal diameter (i.d.), 5 µm particle size, Merck). A gradient elution was programmed using as a mobile phase A, distilled water with an adjusted pH of 2.2 using trifluoroacetic acid (TFA), and as a mobile phase B, acetonitrile. The samples were eluted according to the following gradient: 0 to 5 min with solvent A 100%, and 5 to 50 min with solvent A 100 to 45%. The flow rate was set at 1 mL/min throughout the gradient and the column temperature was maintained at 25 °C. The injection volume was 20 µL, and UV detection was carried out at a wavelength of 280 nm. The calibration curve was constructed using quercetin standard solution at different concentration levels (25 to 400 mg quercetin/L). Data were expressed in mg equivalents quercetin/100 g of oil. Polyphenols analysis was realized by the Lara-Spiral laboratory (Couternon, France). The available polyphenol spectra present in the database of the Lara-Spiral company are listed in Supplementary Table S1.

2.1.4. Fatty Acids Analysis

Total lipids were extracted from PLSO according to the method described by Moilanen and Nikkari [60]. C19:0 was used as the internal standard in the experiments realized in LR12ES05, Lab-NAFS 'Nutrition—Functional Food & Vascular Health', Monastir, Tunisia. Lipids were trans-methylated with 14% boron trifluoride in methanol (BF_3-MeOH) using the method of Morrison and Smith [61]. Subsequently, fatty acid methyl esters were analyzed by gas chromatography (GC) under the same conditions described by Zarrouk et al. [62]. Fatty acids were identified by comparison with synthetic standards. This experiment was performed in triplicate and the data expressed either as g/100 g of oil (C19:0 used as internal standard) or as percentages of total fatty acids.

2.1.5. Phytosterols Analysis

The analysis of phytosterols was realized as described by Zarrouk et al. [62]. Briefly, the quantification of phytosterols was based on an isolation of the unsaponifiable fraction and a silylation of the unsaponifiable fraction before direct injection in gas chromatography (GC). Then, GC separations were performed with a Hewlett-Packard (HP 5890D, Palo Alto, CA, USA) using a capillary column (30 m length × 0.25 mm i.d. film thickness 0.25 μm). Working conditions were as follow: carrier gas, helium; flow through the column, 1 mL/min; injector temperature, 290 °C; detector temperature, 290 °C; oven temperature, 260 °C; injection volume 1 μL. The phytosterols were characterized and quantified by gas chromatography–flame ionization detection (GC-FID). The spectra were compared with those of the internal library INRAE (Dijon, France). Likewise, they were confirmed with the NIST Mass Spectral Library and with the literature. The concentration of each PLSO sterol was expressed in mg/100 g of oil and obtained by three independent analyses.

2.1.6. α-Tocopherol Analysis

PLSO was diluted 10 folds (w/w) with hexane. An amount of 5 mg diluted solution was mixed for 1 min with 200 μL of saline solution, 200 μL of ethanol/butylated hydroxy toluene (BHT) (Sigma-Aldrich; 50 mg/L) containing Tocol used as internal standard (1 ng/μL), and 500 μL of hexane. The extract was centrifuged at 10,000× g for 5 min at 4 °C. The upper layer (100 μL) was collected into a new tube and evaporated to dryness with a nitrogen stream. The dried extract was suspended with 50 μL of methanol/BHT (50 mg/L) and further centrifuged at 10,000× g for 5 min at 4 °C. The supernatant (40 μL) was finally transferred to an injection vial. Extract (2 μL) was injected with an 1100 autosampler into a Poroshell 120 EC-C18 (3 × 50 mm, 2.7 μm) maintained at 35 °C. Separation was achieved with a 1260 HPLC pump (Agilent Technologies, Santa Clara, CA, USA) using a linear gradient of methanol (90% up to 100% in 5 min, and maintained at 100% for 3 min). Detection was realized with a Fluorescence Light Detector (Agilent Technologies, Craven Arms, England) at λ_{Exmax} = 292 nm and λ_{Emmax} = 325 nm. Authentic α-tocopherol standards (0, 50, 100, 200, 400, 600, and 800 ng) were extracted with the same protocol as the PLSO sample. Area ratios of α-tocopherol (room temperature (RT) = 5.4 min) to tocol (RT = 4.0 min) were calculated for PLSO and calibrations standards. A linear calibration curve was used for the calculations. The α-tocopherol analysis was realized by the lipidomic analytical platform (LAP, Dijon, France).

2.2. Antioxidant Activity of Pistacia lentiscus L. Seed Oil

The hydroalcoholic fraction of PLSO was also used for the quantification of antioxidants activities with DPPH, FRAP, and FIC assays.

2.2.1. Free Radical Scavenging Activity with DPPH Assay

The free radical scavenging activity was determined by the 1,1-diphenyl-2-picryl-hydrazyl (DPPH) assay as described by Molyneux et al. [63], with some modifications. To this end, 50 µL of a hydroalcoholic fraction of PLSO (from 0.016 mg/mL to 2 mg/mL) was mixed with 950 µL of a methanolic DPPH solution (10^{-4} M). After incubation for 30 min in the dark, the absorbance was measured at 517 nm. The antioxidant activity related to the DPPH radical scavenging effect was expressed as a percent of inhibition (PI) using the following equation:

$$PI = [(A0 - A1)/A0] \times 100$$

where A0 is the absorbance of the DPPH solution and A1 is the absorbance of the DPPH solution after the addition of the sample. The antioxidant activity was expressed as IC50. A low IC50 value corresponds to a high antiradical activity. Ascorbic acid was used as the positive control and all tests were carried in triplicate.

2.2.2. Ferric Reducing Antioxidant Power (FRAP) Assay

The ferric reducing antioxidant power (FRAP) was determined according to the method of Bassene et al. [64]. Briefly, 400 µL of a hydroalcoholic fraction of PLSO (from 0.016 mg/mL to 2 mg/mL) was mixed with 1 mL of phosphate buffer (0.2 M; pH 6.6) and 1 mL of 1% potassium hexacyanoferrate ($K_3Fe(CN)_6$). After incubation in a water bath at 50 °C for 30 min in the dark, 1 mL of 10% trichloroacetic acid was added, and the mixture was then centrifuged at $1750 \times g$ for 10 min. Then, 1 mL of the obtained supernatant was incubated with 200 µL of 0.1% (w/v) ferric chloride ($FeCl_3$) solution and allowed to stand for 30 min in dark. The absorbance of the reaction mixture was measured spectrophotometrically at 700 nm. Higher value absorbance of the reaction mixture indicated greater reducing power. Ascorbic acid was used as a positive control. The test was carried out in triplicate. The FRAP value of the hydroalcoholic fraction of PLSO was calculated as follows:

$$FRAP\ [\%] = [(Absorbance_{sample}/Absorbance_{blank}) \times 100/Absorbance_{sample}]$$

2.2.3. Ferrous-Ion Chelating (FIC) Assay

The ferrous ion chelating (FIC) activity of PLSO was determined according to the method of Dinis et al. [65], with minor modifications. In total, 100 µL of a hydroalcoholic fraction of PLSO (from 0.016 mg/mL to 2 mg/mL) was mixed with 50 µL of 2 mM $FeCl_2$, and 100 µL of 5 mM ferrozine. The mixture was allowed to stand for 10 min at room temperature. The ferrous iron–ferrozine complex formation was then monitored by measuring the absorbance at 562 nm against a blank. Ethylenediaminetetraacetic acid (EDTA) was used as positive control. The assays were performed in triplicate. The percentage of inhibition of ferrozine-Fe^{2+} complex formation was calculated as below:

$$FIC\ (\%) = [(Absorbance_{negative\ control} - Absorbance_{sample}) \times 100/Absorbance_{negative\ control}]$$

2.2.4. KRL Test

The overall antioxidant defense potential of the PLSO was measured with the KRL test (Kit Radicaux Libres) [62,66]. This test consists of submitting whole blood to free radical attack to mobilize the radical scavengers present in the blood and to neutralize the oxidation processes [66]. Diluted control blood samples in the presence or absence of PLSO, which was diluted in DMSO, were oxidized by molecular oxygen in an aqueous suspension using a 2.2′–azobis (2-amidinopropane) dihydrochloride (AAPH) solution. Hemolysis was recorded using a 96-well microplate reader (KRL Reader, Kirial International, Lara-Spiral, Couternon, France) by measuring the turbidimetric optical density decay at 620 nm. The antioxidant efficiency of the oil was expressed in Trolox equivalent. The same analysis was conducted with α-tocopherol (Sigma-Aldrich, St-Quentin-Fallavier, France) used as control. The KRL test was realized by the Lara-Spiral laboratory (Couternon, France).

2.3. In Vitro Study

2.3.1. Cell Culture and Treatments

Murine C2C12 myoblasts were grown in Dulbecco's modified Eagle's medium (DMEM) supplemented with 10% (v/v) of heat-inactivated fetal bovine serum (FBS) and 1% (v/v) of penicillin (100 U/mL)/streptomycin (100 mg/mL). The cells were maintained in a humidified atmosphere (5% CO_2, 95% air) at 37 °C. For subcultures, cells were trypsinized (0.05% trypsin − 0.02% EDTA solution) and passed twice a week. 7β-OHC was either from Sigma-Aldrich or provided by Mohammad Samadi (University of Lorraine, Metz, France); the purity was higher than 98%. The stock solutions of 7β-OHC was prepared at 800 µg/mL (2 mM), as previously described by Ragot et al. [67], and stored in the dark at 4 °C. A stock solution of PLSO was prepared at 80 mg/mL in dimethyl sulfoxide (DMSO; Sigma-Aldrich) and stored in the dark at 4 °C. An α-tocopherol (the major component of vitamin E; Sigma-Aldrich) solution was prepared to 80 mM in absolute ethanol, as previously described [60], and stored in the dark at 4 °C. For the different experiments, C2C12 myoblasts were used at 80% confluency; they were seeded either into Petri dishes of 10 cm in diameter (1.2×10^6 cells per Petri dish), in six-well plates (2×10^5 cells per well), or in 96-well plates (10×10^4 cells per well). After 12 h, the growth medium was removed and the C2C12 cells were incubated with 7β-OHC (20 µg/mL/50 µM) for 24 h with or without PLSO (100 µg/mL), or α-tocopherol (400 µM) (used as a positive control for cytoprotection) [28]. PLSO and α-tocopherol were introduced in the culture medium 2 h before 7β-OHC. The choice of the concentration of 7β-OHC (20 µg/mL/50 µM) and PLSO (100 µg/mL) was based on the dose-effect of 7β-OHC (5–80 µg/mL/12.5–200 µM) and PLSO (5–3200 µg/mL), which was realized with an MTT assay.

2.3.2. Evaluation of Cell Morphology by Phase-Contrast Microscopy

After 24 h of treatment with or without 7β-OHC (20 µg/mL/50 µM) in the presence or absence of PLSO (100 µg/mL), or of α-tocopherol (400 µM), the cell morphology and cell density of C2C12 myoblasts cells were observed and photographed using a phase-contrast microscope (Axiovert 40 CFL, Zeiss, Jena, Germany) equipped with a digital camera (Axiocam lCm1, Zeiss).

2.3.3. Evaluation of Cell Viability with the MTT Assay

Cell viability was measured using an MTT (3-(4, 5-dimethylthiazol-2-yl)-2, 5-diphenyltetrazolium bromide) assay. MTT salt is reduced to formazan in metabolically active cells by the mitochondrial enzyme succinate dehydrogenase [35]. C2C12 cells were seeded into 96-well flat-bottom culture plates. After 24 h of treatment as described above, an MTT solution (0.05 mg/mL, dissolved in culture medium) was added to each well and incubated for 3 h at 37 °C. The medium was removed and 100 µL of dimethyl sulfoxide (DMSO) was added to dissolve the formed formazan crystals. The percentage of viable cells was calculated based on a reduction of the MTT dye into formazan crystals at 570 nm using a microplate reader (Tecan Sunrise, Tecan, Lyon, France).

2.3.4. Measurement of Cell Viability with the Fluorescein Diacetate Assay

The fluorescein diacetate (FDA) assay evaluates the ability of living cells to transform the FDA to fluorescein after cleavage by plasma membrane esterases [68]. After 24 h of treatment with or without 7β-OHC (50 µM) in the presence or absence of PLSO (100 µg/mL), α-tocopherol (400 µM), or MitoQ (1 µM) [69,70], C2C12 cells were incubated for 5 min at 37 °C with 50 µM FDA (Sigma-Aldrich) and then lysed with 10 mM of a Tris-HCl solution containing 1% sodium dodecyl sulfate (SDS, Sigma-Aldrich). The fluorescence intensity of the fluorescein ($\lambda_{Ex\,max}$ = 485 nm, $\lambda_{Em\,max}$ = 528 nm) was measured with a Tecan fluorescence microplate reader (Tecan Infinite M200 Pro, Lyon, France) in order to quantify the living cells. The results were expressed as the % of control: (Fluorescence (assay)/Fluorescence (control)) $\times$ 100.

2.3.5. Measurement of Plasma Membrane Permeability with Propidium Iodide

Propidium iodide (PI) was used to evaluate the plasma membrane permeability and cell death. This dye penetrates cells with damaged plasma membranes considered as dead cells [71]. After 24 h of treatment with or without 7β-OHC (50 µM) in the presence or absence of PLSO (100 µg/mL) or α-tocopherol (400 µM), C2C12 cells (adherent and non-adherent cells) were stained with a PI solution (1 µg/mL of PBS) for 5 min at 37 °C, and then immediately analyzed on a BD Accuri™ C6 flow cytometer (BD Biosciences, San Jose, CA, USA). The red fluorescence was selected on a 630 nm band-pass filter and 10,000 cells were acquired for each sample. Data analyses were performed using FlowJo software (Carrboro, NC, USA).

2.3.6. Measurement of Oxidative Stress

Evaluation of Reactive Oxygen Species Production with Dihydroethidium

Dihydroethidium (DHE) was used to detect ROS, mainly superoxide anion ($O_2^{\bullet-}$) production. DHE, a dye that can freely diffuse across cell membranes, is rapidly oxidized under the action of ROS to fluorescent ethidium. This latter exhibits an orange/red fluorescence ($\lambda_{Ex\,max}$ = 488 nm; $\lambda_{Em\,max}$ = 575 nm) [72]. After 24 h of treatment, C2C12 cells (adherent and non-adherent cells) were stained with a 2 µM DHE solution for 15 min at 37 °C and then analyzed on a BD Accuri™ C6 flow cytometer (BD Biosciences). The fluorescent signals of the DHE-stained cells were collected through a 580 nm band-pass filter and 10,000 cells were acquired for each sample. Data analyses were performed using FlowJo software.

Quantification of Antioxidant Enzymes Activities: Glutathione Peroxidase (GPx) and Superoxide Dismutase (SOD)

Glutathione peroxidase (GPx) activity was evaluated according to the method described by Flohe and Günzler [73]. After 24 h of treatment, C2C12 cells were trypsinized, lysed by sonication, and centrifuged at $20,000\times g$ (30 min; 4 °C). The supernatant was incubated for 5 min at 25 °C with 0.1 mM of reduced glutathione (GSH) and phosphate buffer saline (50 mM, pH 7.8). The reaction was initiated by the addition of H_2O_2 and stopped by cell incubation with trichloroacetic acid, for 30 min on ice. After centrifugation at $1000\times g$ for 10 min, the supernatant was transferred into a new tube and 0.32 M of $Na_2HPO_4 \cdot 12H_2O$ and 1 mM of DTNB were added to the supernatant and the color developed was measured at 412 nm. GPx activity was expressed as the percentage of control cells.

Superoxide dismutase (SOD) activity was measured following the method of Beauchamp and Fridovich [74]. Cell lysates were incubated in the presence of 50 mM phosphate buffer, 0.1 mM EDTA, 13 mM L-methionine, 2 µM riboflavin, and 75 mM nitro bleu tetrazolium (NBT). The mixture was exposed to white light for 20 min. The developed blue color is proportional to SOD activity and was measured at 560 nm. Units of SOD activity are expressed as the amount of enzyme required to inhibit by 50% the reduction in NBT. SOD activity was expressed as a percentage of the controls. Antioxidant enzyme activity was expressed relative to the protein content, determined with a Bradford assay.

Measurement of Lipid Peroxidation Products: Malondialdehyde (MDA) and Conjugated Dienes (CDs)

Oxidation of polyunsaturated fatty acid was estimated by the measurement of the final lipid peroxidation products, such as malondialdehyde (MDA) and conjugated dienes (CDs).

Measurement of MDA level: The MDA level was measured using the method described by Yoshioka et al. [75]. Briefly, C2C12 cell lysates were mixed with 1.5 mL of a reactive mixture containing 20% trichloroacetic acid and 0.67% thiobarbituric acid. The samples were incubated for 30 min in a water bath at a temperature of 95 °C. After cooling, 4 mL of n-butanol was added, and the mixture was centrifuged ($1600\times g$ for 10 min) to remove undissolved materials. Then, the absorbance was measured at 532 nm. The concentration of MDA was expressed as nmol/mg of protein.

Measurement of CDs level: The CDs level was quantified as previously described by Esterbauer et al. [76]. Lipids were extracted from C2C12 cell lysates using a chloroform and methanol mixture (2:1; v/v). After vigorous agitation for 2 min, the material was subjected to centrifugation (1200× g; 3 min), and the lower layer was aspirated, transferred into a new test tube, and evaporated under a nitrogen atmosphere. The residue was reconstituted with 1 mL of hexane and measured spectrophotometrically at 243 nm. The results were expressed as nmoles hydroperoxide/mg of protein.

Measurement of Protein Oxidation Products: Carbonylated Proteins (CPs)

Carbonylated proteins (CPs) concentration was measured as described by Oliver et al. [77]. This assay is based on the reaction between 2,4-dinitrophenylhydrazine (DNPH) and CPs to form protein hydrazones. Briefly, C2C12 cell lysates were incubated with DNPH (10 mM in 2.5 N HCl) in the dark for 1 h at room temperature. Then, 20% trichloroacetic acid was added for a 10 min incubation time on ice and the tubes were centrifuged at 1600× g for 5 min. The protein pellets were washed with 10% trichloroacetic acid and ethanol-ethyl acetate (1:1; v/v) mixture to remove free DNPH. The final pellet was dissolved in a 6 M guanidine hydrochloride solution, and the absorbance was read at 370 nm. The concentration of CPs was expressed in nmol/mg of protein.

2.3.7. Evaluation of Mitochondrial Function

Measurement of Transmembrane Mitochondrial Potential with $DiOC_6(3)$

The variation in the mitochondrial transmembrane potential ($\Delta\Psi m$) was detected using 3,3′-dihexyloxacarbocyanine iodide ($DiOC_6(3)$) [67]. After 24 h of treatment, adherent and non-adherent C2C12 cells were pooled, stained with a solution of $DiOC_6(3)$ (Invitrogen/Thermo Fisher Scientific, Montigny le Bretonneux, France) at 40 nM (15 min; 37 °C), and then analyzed on a BD Accuri™ C6 flow cytometer (BD Biosciences). The loss of $\Delta\Psi m$ is indicated by a decrease in the green fluorescence intensity collected through a 520 ± 10 nm band-pass filter. For each sample, 10,000 cells were acquired, and data analyses were performed with FlowJo software.

Measurement of ATP Levels

The adenosine triphosphate (ATP) assay was performed using the ATP Bioluminescence Assay Kit CLS II (ref # 11699709001, Roche, Meylan, France), according to the manufacturer's procedure. At the end of the treatments, cells were collected by trypsinization, adherent and non-adherent cells were mixed, and the ATP level was determined after cell lysis. To this end, 100 µL of cell lysis reagent was added on the cell pellets. After 10 min of incubation at RT, a centrifugation was realized at 1000× g for 5 min. Then, 50 µL of luciferase was added to 50 µL of each cell lysate to measure the bioluminescence of the samples using a microplate reader (Tecan Infinite M200 Pro). A standard calibration curve was prepared from an ATP stock solution (10.5 mg/mL) using lyophilized ATP provided by the kit to determine the cellular ATP concentration.

Measurement of Mitochondrial Reactive Oxygen Species with MitoSOX-Red

Mitochondrial ROS production, including superoxide anion ($O_2^{\bullet-}$), was measured by flow cytometry after staining with MitoSOX-Red (Thermo Fisher Scientific, Asheville, NC, USA). Once in the mitochondria, this probe is oxidized and exhibits an orange/red fluorescence ($\lambda_{Ex\ max}$ = 510 nm; $\lambda_{Em\ max}$ = 580 nm) [78]. After 24 h of treatment, adherent and non-adherent C2C12 cells were polled and stained with a 5 mM MitoSOX-Red solution for 15 min at 37 °C and then analyzed on a BD Accuri™ C6 flow cytometer. The fluorescent signals were collected through a 580 ± 20 nm band pass filter. For each sample, 10,000 cells were acquired, and data analyses were performed using FlowJo software.

2.3.8. Determination of the Peroxisomal Status

Evaluation of the Level and Topography of Abcd3 Peroxisomal Transporter by Structured Illumination Microscopy (Apotome)

ATP binding cassette subfamily D member (Abcd3) peroxisomal transporter was detected by indirect immunofluorescence [79,80]. Cells were cultured on glass slides in six-well plates. At the end of the treatment, adherent and non-adherent C2C12 cells were collected, fixed with 2% (w/v) paraformaldehyde for 15 min at RT, and then rinsed twice with PBS. Cells were permeabilized for 30 min at RT with a PFS buffer (PBS/0.05% saponin/10% FCS). After washing in PBS, cells were incubated (1 h, RT) with an appropriate rabbit polyclonal antibody raised against Abcd3 (# 11523651, Pierce/Thermo Fisher Scientific, Asheville, NC, USA) diluted (1/500) in PFS buffer. Cells were washed and incubated in the dark (30 min, RT) with a goat anti-rabbit 488-Alexa antibody (Santa-Cruz Biotechnology, Santa Cruz, CA, USA) diluted at 1/500 in PFS buffer. After washing in PBS, cells were stained with Hoechst 33342 (1 µg/mL) and then mounted in Dako fluorescent mounting medium (Dako, Copenhagen, Denmark). The slides were stored in the dark at 4 °C and examined with structured illumination microscopy (Apotome). The images were realized with ZEN imaging software (Zeiss).

Flow Cytometric Quantification of Abcd3 Peroxisomal Transporter

For flow cytometric analyses, adherent and non-adherent C2C12 cells were collected, fixed with 2% (w/v) paraformaldehyde diluted in PBS for 15 min at RT and then rinsed twice with PBS. Cells were permeabilized for 30 min at RT with PFS buffer. After washing in PBS, cells were incubated (1 h, RT) with an appropriate rabbit polyclonal antibody raised against Abcd3 (# 11523651, Pierce/Thermo Fisher Scientific) diluted (1/500) in PFS buffer. Cells were washed and incubated in the dark (30 min, RT) with a goat anti-rabbit 488-Alexa antibody (Santa-Cruz Biotechnology, Santa Cruz, CA, USA) diluted at 1/500 in a PFS buffer. After washing in PBS, cells were resuspended in PBS and immediately analyzed on a BD Accuri™ C6 flow cytometer (BD Biosciences). The green fluorescence of 488-Alexa was collected with a 520 ± 20 nm band-pass filter. For each sample, 10,000 cells were acquired, and data analyses were performed using FlowJo software.

Gas Chromatography—Mass Spectrometry Analysis of Fatty Acids

Fatty acids, including very-long-chain fatty acids (VLCFA; $C \geq 22$) [81], were analyzed using gas chromatography coupled to mass spectrometry (GC-MS), as previously described by Blondelle et al. [82]. Total cellular lipids were extracted, according to the method of Folch et al. [83]. Fatty acids were quantitated by calculating the relative response ratios to their closest internal standard. Calibration curves were obtained with fatty acid authentic standards processed as cell pellets.

Transmission Electron Microscopy Analysis

At the ultrastructural level, transmission electron microscopy (TEM) is the most powerful tools to observe morphological changes caused by various physical or chemical agents [84]. TEM was used to visualize mitochondrial and peroxisomal changes [80] in C2C12 cells cultured for 24 h in the presence or absence of 7β-OHC (50 µM) without or with PLSO (100 µg/mL) or α-tocopherol (400 µM) [85]. The samples were fixed for 1 h at 4 °C in 2.5% (w/v) glutaraldehyde diluted in a cacodylate buffer (0.1 M, pH 7.4), washed twice in cacodylate buffer, incubated in the dark for 1 h at 21 °C in Tris–HCl (0.05 M, pH 9.0) containing diaminobenzidine (DAB: 2.5 mg/mL) and H_2O_2 (10 µL/mL of a 3% solution); washed in cacodylate buffer (0.1 M, pH 7.4) for 5 min at 21 °C; post-fixed in 1% (w/v) osmium tetroxide diluted in cacodylate sodium (0.1 M, pH 7.4) for 1 h at 21 °C in the dark; and rinsed in cacodylate buffer (0.1 M, pH 7.4). The preparations were dehydrated in graded ethanol solutions and then embedded in Epon. Ultrathin sections were cut with an ultramicrotome, contrasted with uranyl acetate and lead citrate, and examined using an HT7800 electron microscope (Hitachi, Tokyo, Japan) operating at 100 kV and equipped with two advanced microscopy technique (AMT) cameras (Woburn, MA, USA).

Analysis of Abcd3 Peroxisomal Transporter mRNA by Real-Time Quantitative Polymerase Chain Reaction

Total mRNA from C2C12 cells were extracted and purified using the RNeasy Mini Kit (Qiagen, Courtaboeuf, France). Total mRNA concentration was measured with TrayCell (Hellma, Paris, France) and the purity of the nucleic acids was controlled by the ratio of absorbance at 260 nm and 280 nm (ratios between 1.8 and 2.2 were considered satisfactory). One microgram of total mRNA from each sample was converted into single-stranded cDNA using the iScript cDNA Synthesis kit (BioRad, Marne la Coquette, France) according to the following procedure: 5 min at 25 °C, 20 min at 46 °C, and 5 min at 95 °C. cDNA was then amplified using the Takyon TM Rox SYBR Master Mix dTTP Blue (Eurogentec, Liège, Belgium) and 300 nM of forward and reverse mouse Abcd3 primer. The forward and reverse Abcd3 primer sequences were the following: Forward: 5′-ctgggcgtgaaatgactagattg-3′; Reverse 5′-cttctcctgttgtgacaccattg-3′.

Thermal cycling conditions were as follows: activation of DNA polymerase (95 °C, 10 min), followed by 40 cycles of amplification at 95 °C for 15 s, 60 °C for 30 s, and 72 °C for 30 s, followed by a melting curve analysis to control for the absence of non-specific products. Gene expression was quantified using cycle to threshold (Ct) values and normalized by the 36B4 reference gene (Forward: 5′-gcgacctggaagtccaacta-3′; Reverse: 5′-atctgcttggagcccacat-3′). Abcd3 level was determined as fold induction of the control.

2.4. Gas Chromatography—Mass Spectrometry Analysis of Cholesterol and Oxysterols Oxidized at C7 (7-Ketocholesterol, 7β-Hydroxycholesterol) in the Plasma of Sarcopenic Patients

Cholesterol and oxysterols levels (7KC, 7β-OHC) were determined by GC-MS on plasma samples from Tunisian subjects. All subjects gave their written consent before being enrolled in this preliminary study. In total, 45 adults of 65 years and older (23 men, 22 women) were recruited over a period of 1 month from January to February 2019. All participants were recruited from a nursing home (Sousse, Tunisia). The Timed Up and Go (TUG) test was used to classify patients as sarcopenic (22 subjects; age = 80 ± 4.16; female/male = 15/7) and non-sarcopenic (23 subjects; age = 70.84 ± 4.38; female/male = 7/16). Blood samples were collected in EDTA tubes after overnight fasting. The blood samples were centrifuged at $800 \times g$ (10 min; 4 °C), and the plasma was divided into several aliquots that were immediately frozen at -80 °C and stored for one year until GC-MS analysis. Oxysterols were quantified as follows: in a glass tube, 300 µL of plasma was suspended in absolute ethanol containing BHT (50 µg/mL). 7KC (d7) and 7β-OHC (d7) (Avanti Polar Lipids, 700 Industrial Park Drive Alabaster, AL, USA) were used as internal standards. Samples were subjected to alkaline hydrolysis with 10 M KOH (1 h; 37 °C). The reaction mixture was washed with water in order to adjust to pH 7 and sterols were extracted with hexane. After solvent evaporation, 100 µL of a mixture of pyridine/hexamethyldisilazane (HMDS)/trimethylchlorosilane (TMCS) (3:2:1; *v/v/v*) (Acros Organics, Fisher Scientific, Asheville, NC, USA) was added, and samples were incubated at 60 °C for 30 min to form trimethylsilyl ethers. After evaporation, the residue was dissolved in 100 µL hexane for GC-MS analysis. GC-MS was performed using an Agilent Technology 6890 GC equipped with an HP7683 injector and a 5973-mass selective detector (Agilent Technologies, Santa Clara, CA, USA). Chromatography was performed using an HP-5MS-fused silica capillary column (length: 25 m; i.d.: 0.25 mm; film thickness: 0.25 µm; Agilent Technologies, Santa Clara, CA, USA). GC-MS conditions were as follows: carrier gas, helium at a flow rate of 1.1 mL/min; injector temperature, 250 °C; oven temperature 180 °C, which increased at 10 °C/min to 260 °C, then at 1 °C/min to 280 °C and held for 5 min. The mass spectrometer was operated in the electron impact mode with electron energy of 70 eV. The ion source temperature and the quadrupole temperature were 230 °C and 150 °C, respectively. The ions used for analysis were 7β-OHC 456 *m/z*, 7β-OHC (d7) 463 *m/z*, and

7KC 472 *m/z*, 7KC (d7) 479 *m/z*. Calibration curves were obtained using authentic standards extracted with the method used for the samples.

2.5. Statistical Analysis

The experimental results were statistically analyzed with GraphPad Prism 8.0 software (GraphPad Software, San Diego, CA, USA). In vitro data were expressed as the mean ± standard deviation (SD) and compared with an ANOVA test followed by a Tukey's test, which allows multiple comparisons and permits to assess any interaction. Clinical data were compared with a Student's *t*-test. A *p*-value less than 0.05 was considered statistically significant. The heatmap representation was realized with GraphPad Prism 8.0 software.

3. Results

3.1. Biochemical Composition of Pistacia lentiscus L. Seed Oil

The profiles of polyphenols, flavonoids, and carotenoids contents in *Pistacia lentiscus* L. seed oil (PLSO) were measured using colorimetric methods and the results are shown in Table 1. The amounts of total phenols, flavonoids, and carotenoids in PLSO are 28.50 ± 0.77 gallic acid equivalents (mg GAE/g of extract), 51.36 ± 2.30 catechin equivalent (mg CE/g of extract), and 2083.59 ± 55.00 (mg/kg of extract), respectively.

Table 1. Total phenols, flavonoids, and carotenoids contents of *Pistacia lentiscus* seed oil (PLSO).

	Total Phenols (mg GAE/g of Extract)	Flavonoids (mg CE/g of Extract)	Carotenoids (mg/kg)
Pistacia lentiscus seed oil	28.50 ± 0.77	51.36 ± 2.30	2083.59 ± 55.00

GAE: gallic acid equivalent; CE: catechin equivalent. Each value represents the mean of three determinations ± standard deviation.

In PLSO, the polyphenols identified and characterized by HPLC coupled with UV analysis were protocatechuic acid, which is a dihydroxybenzoic acid and a type of phenolic acid, and coumarin, which belongs to a polyphenol subclass (hydroxycoumarins) (Table 2).

Table 2. *Pistacia lentiscus* seed oil polyphenol content (mg equivalents quercetin/100 g of oil).

Polyphenols	(mg Equivalents Quercetin/100 g of Oil)
Protocatechuic acid	0.140 ± 0.001
Coumarin	0.650 ± 0.003

Polyphenols chromatogram obtained by HPLC (Supplementary Figure S2). Each value represents the mean of three determinations ± standard deviation.

The fatty acid profile of PLSO, expressed as percentage of total fatty acids, was determined using GC and the results are presented in Table 3. The main fatty acids detected in PLSO were oleic acid (49.77 ± 0.12%), palmitic acid (27.20 ± 0.22%), and linoleic acid (17.19 ± 0.10%), followed by palmitoleic acid (2.25 ± 0.01%), vaccenic acid (1.51 ± 0.03%), and stearic acid (1.26 ± 0.01%). Likewise, PLSO also contains α-linolenic acid, gadoleic acid, and arachidic acid but in much smaller quantities (0.12–0.39%). Minor monounsaturated fatty acids, such as myristic acid, margaric acid, lignoceric acid, and behenic acid, were also detected, but in trace amounts (≤0.05%).

The sterol composition of PLSO was determined using GC and spectral analysis and the results are shown in Table 4. The most abundant detected phytosterols in PLSO were β-sitosterol (67.25 ± 3.24 mg/100 g oil), α-epoxysitostanol (33.36 ± 1.65 mg/100 g oil), and 24-methylene cycloartenol (16.10 ± 2.72 mg/100 g oil) followed by cycloartenol (9.35 ± 1.49 mg/100 g oil) and campestanol (4.48 ± 0.85 mg/100 g oil). All other phytosterols were present in small amounts.

Table 3. *Pistacia lentiscus* seed oil fatty acids profile (g/100 g of oil; % of total fatty acids).

Fatty Acids	g/100 g of Oil (*)	% (**)
∑SFA	32.333 ± 0.566	28.77 ± 0.24
Myristic acid (C14:0)	0.015 ± 0.000	0.05 ± 0.01
Palmitic acid (C16:0)	30.457 ± 0.355	27.20 ± 0.22
Margaric acid (C17:0)	0.022 ± 0.003	0.05 ± 0.00
Stearic acid (C18:0)	1.527 ± 0.124	1.26 ± 0.01
Arachidic acid (C20:0)	0.041 ± 0.012	0.12 ± 0.00
Behenic acid (C22:0)	0.271 ± 0.072	0.04 ± 0.00
Lignoceric acid (C24:0)	ND	0.05 ± 0.00
∑UFA	94.706 ± 2.910	71.25 ± 0.28
∑MUFA	64.736 ± 1.827	53.67 ± 0.17
Palmitoleic acid (C16:1 n−7)	2.623 ± 0.084	2.25 ± 0.01
Heptadecenoic acid (C17:1)	0.179 ± 0.058	ND
Oleic acid (C18:1 n−9)	60.183 ± 1.556	49.77 ± 0.12
Vaccenic acid (C18:1 n−7)	1.670 ± 0.073	1.51 ± 0.03
Gadoleic acid (C20:1 n−9)	0.081 ± 0.056	0.14 ± 0.01
∑PUFA	29.970 ± 1.083	17.58 ± 0.11
Linoleic acid (C18:2 n−6)	29.665 ± 0.990	17.19 ± 0.10
α-linolenic acid (C18:3 n−3)	0.305 ± 0.093	0.39 ± 0.01
∑SFA/∑UFA	0.34 ± 0.19	0.41 ± 0.86

SFA: saturated fatty acids; MUFA: monounsaturated fatty acids; PUFA: polyunsaturated fatty acids; ND: not detected. Each value represents the mean of three determinations ± standard deviation. (*): data obtained at the University of Monastir (Monastir, Tunisia) with (C19:0) used as internal standard; (**) data obtained at INRAE (Dijon, France) without an internal standard. Data were obtained with the same sample of PLSO. The corresponding chromatograms are shown in Supplementary Figure S3A,B.

Table 4. *Pistacia lentiscus* seed oil phytosterol profile (mg/100 g of oil).

Phytosterol	(mg/100 g of Oil)
Campesterol	4.48 ± 0.85
Stigmasterol	2.69 ± 0.23
β-Sitosterol	67.25 ± 3.24
Δ^5-Avenasterol	3.10 ± 0.90
β-Amyrine	1.81 ± 0.19
Cycloartenol	9.35 ± 1.49
24-Methylene cycloartenol	16.10 ± 2.72
α-Epoxysitostanol	33.36 ± 1.65
Other phytosterols	16.76 ± 2.83
Total	154.89 ± 5.40

The phytosterol chromatogram obtained by GC-FID is shown in Supplementary Figure S4. Each value represents the mean of three determinations ± standard deviation.

The α-tocopherol content of PLSO is given in Table 5. The results show that α-tocopherol represented 68.1 ± 3.41 mg/kg of oil.

Table 5. α-Tocopherol content (mg/kg) of *Pistacia lentiscus* seed oil (PLSO).

	α-Tocopherol (mg/kg)
Pistacia lentiscus seed oil	68.10 ± 3.41

Values are the mean ± SD of three determinations.

3.2. Evaluation of the Antioxidant Properties of Pistacia lentiscus L. Seed Oil

The antioxidant activities of PLSO were measured with different assays: DPPH, FRAP, FIC, and KRL. The results are shown in Table 6. PLSO exhibits free radical scavenging activity, as shown by the IC50 value (5.01 ± 0.095 mg/mL). The half-maximal inhibitory concentration (IC50) (volume of oil required to lower the initial DPPH concentration by

50%) was determined from the dose–response curve. This activity was less than those of ascorbic acid (AA) used as the standard.

Table 6. Antioxidant activity of *Pistacia lentiscus* seed oil (PLSO).

Samples	IC50 Values (mg/mL)			(Trolox Equivalent)
	DPPH	FRAP	Iron Chelating (FIC)	KRL
PLSO	5.010 ± 0.095	1.15 ± 0.23	5.61 ± 0.14	4440.00 ± 493.60
AO	–	–	–	360.80 ± 153.60
EDTA (standard)	–	–	0.60 ± 0.09	–
AA (standard)	0.810 ± 0.270	0.41 ± 0.16	–	–
α-tocopherol	–	–	–	0.94 ± 0.01

Each value represents the mean of three determinations ± standard deviation. IC50: half-maximal inhibitory concentration; PLSO: *Pistacia lentiscus* L. seed oil; AO: argan oil, EDTA: ethylenediaminetetraacetic acid; AA: ascorbic acid; DPPH: 2,2-diphenyl-1-picrylhydrazyl; FIC: Ferrous Iron Chelating FRAP: Ferric Reducing Antioxidant Power; KRL: Kit Radicaux Libres. For the KRL test, data are presented in Trolox equivalent: 1 mL of PLSO is equivalent to X moles of Trolox (value shown in the table).

The reducing power of PLSO measured by FRAP assay was investigated along with AA used as the standard reference. The IC50 value was 1.15 ± 0.23 mg/mL (Table 6). In addition, an iron-chelating activity evaluated with the FIC assay was observed in PLSO with an IC50 of 5.61 ± 0.14 mg/mL (Table 6).

The antioxidant properties of α-tocopherol, PLSO, and Argan Oil Roasted Agadir (AO) were evaluated with the KRL test. For the PLSO and AO, the antioxidant activities were expressed in Trolox equivalent (mole Trolox/mL of oil). For the KRL test, we used α-tocopherol as the positive control and AO stored for 5 years at 4 °C in the dark as the negative control (the corresponding AO freshly prepared has been previously characterized and described and was strongly antioxidant [86]). PLSO showed a higher KRL antioxidant status than the 5 years stored AO. KRL values were 4440.00 ± 493.60 and 360.8 ± 153.6 (Trolox equivalent) in PLSO and AO, respectively (Table 6), illustrating that after 5 years of storage, AO shows a notable decrease in antioxidant activity.

3.3. Evaluation of 7-Ketocholesterol and 7β-Hydroxycholesterol Plasma Levels in Sarcopenic and Non-Sarcopenic Subjects

As several studies support that 7KC and 7β-OHC, mainly resulting from cholesterol auto-oxidation, are involved in the development of major age-related diseases [31,87], these oxysterols as well as cholesterol were measured by GC-MS in the plasma of non-sarcopenic and sarcopenic subjects. In sarcopenic patients, the 7β-OHC level was significantly higher than in non-sarcopenic subjects whereas no significant difference in 7KC and cholesterol level was observed (Supplementary Figure S5). This plasma increase in 7β-OHC could favor the accumulation of this oxysterol in skeletal muscle. Indeed, in male Wistar rats in response to chronic alcohol feeding, there were significant increases in the soleus (type I fiber, glycolytic, aerobic activity) of 7α-OHC, 7β-OHC, and 7KC, whereas in the plantaris (type II fiber, anaerobic activity) only 7β-OHC was increased [88]. Furthermore, in zebra fish, 25-hydroxycholesterol alters muscle morphology and reduces mobility; a similar effect can be envisaged with 7β-OHC [89]. Based on this previous works, and knowing that lipotoxicity (defined as an abnormal accumulation of lipids in tissues such as skeletal muscles) leads to metabolic and functional dysfunctions [90], it is important to clarify whether 7β-OHC can have cytotoxic effects on skeletal muscle cells, and if so, to find treatments to counteract this toxicity. To evaluate this hypothesis, the C2C12 murine myoblast model cultured in the presence of 7β-OHC in the presence or absence of PLSO was used.

3.4. Evaluation of the Effects of Pistacia lentiscus L. Seed Oil on 7β-Hydroxycholesterol-Induced Morphological Changes and Cell Death

At first, initial experiments were performed on C2C12 cells to evaluate whether PLSO and 7β-OHC alone induce cell death on murine C2C12 myoblast cells. To this end, C2C12 were incubated with various concentrations of PLSO (5 to 3200 µg/mL) for 24 h and cell viability was determined using an MTT assay. As shown in Supplementary Figure S6A, no cytotoxic effects of PLSO (5–800 µg/mL) were observed compared to untreated cells; however, in the presence of PLSO used at 1600 µg/mL and 3200 µg/mL, the percentage of viable cells decreased from 50 to 70%, respectively.

To define whether 7β-OHC was able to influence C2C12 cell viability, C2C12 cells were exposed to various concentrations of 7β-OHC (12.5 to 200 µM) for 24 h. In the presence of 7β-OHC (50 µM), cell viability significantly decreased to 48.4% compared to untreated cells (Supplementary Figure S6B). Based on these results, PLSO (100 µg/mL) and 7β-OHC (50 µM) were selected to perform further experiments.

Thus, C2C12 cells were incubated for 24 h with or without 7β-OHC (50 µM) in the presence or absence of PLSO (100 µg/mL) or α-tocopherol (400 µM) used as positive control for cytoprotection. PLSO and α-tocopherol were added 2 h prior 7β-OHC. Based on the observations performed by phase-contrast microscopy, morphological changes in C2C12 cells were observed under treatment with 7β-OHC. In 7β-OHC-treated C2C12 cells, compared to untreated cells, an increased number of round cells floating in the culture medium were observed, reflecting a loss of cell adhesion and an induction of cell death; a reduced number of adherent cells was also observed This effect was remarkably corrected when the cells were simultaneously incubated with PLSO (100 µg/mL) or α-tocopherol (400 µM), indicating that PLSO and α-tocopherol provided protection against 7β-OHC-induced loss of cell adhesion and cell death (Supplementary Figure S7A). By phase-contrast microscopy, no effects on cell adhesion and cell growth of the different vehicles used were observed (Supplementary Figure S7B).

The cytoprotective effect of PLSO (100 µg/mL) was confirmed with the MTT assay. As shown in Figure 1A, the percentage of MTT-positive cells, reflecting metabolically active cells, was significantly decreased in the 7β-OHC (50 µM)-treated cells compared to the control. Noteworthy, when PLSO (100 µg/mL) was associated with 7β-OHC (50 µM), the percentage of MTT-positive cells was significantly increased: this demonstrates that PLSO attenuates 7β-OHC-induced cell death. Similar results were obtained with α-tocopherol.

To further investigate the effect of PLSO on plasma membrane permeability and/or cell death, staining with propidium iodide (PI) was used. As illustrated in Figure 1B, the percentage of PI-positive cells was significantly increased after exposure to 7β-OHC (50 µM), indicating that this oxysterol caused altered plasma membrane and/or cell death in C2C12 cells. In the presence of PLSO (100 µg/mL) or α-tocopherol (400 µM) associated with 7β-OHC (50 µM), the percentage of PI-positive cells was significantly decreased compared to 7β-OHC-treated cells. Comparatively to untreated cells, no effect of PLSO (100 µg/mL) or α-tocopherol (400 µM) alone was observed on plasma membrane permeability. Altogether, these data show that PLSO as well as α-tocopherol strongly attenuate 7β-OHC-induced C2C12 cell death.

3.5. Evaluation of the Effects of Pistacia lentiscus L. Seed Oil on 7β-Hydroxycholesterol-Induced Oxidative Stress

To study the effect of PLSO (100 µg/mL) against 7β-OHC (50 µM)-induced oxidative stress, we measured the production of reactive oxygen species (ROS), lipid peroxidation products (MDA, CDs), carbonylated proteins (CPs), and antioxidant enzyme activities (SOD, GPx) (Figure 2).

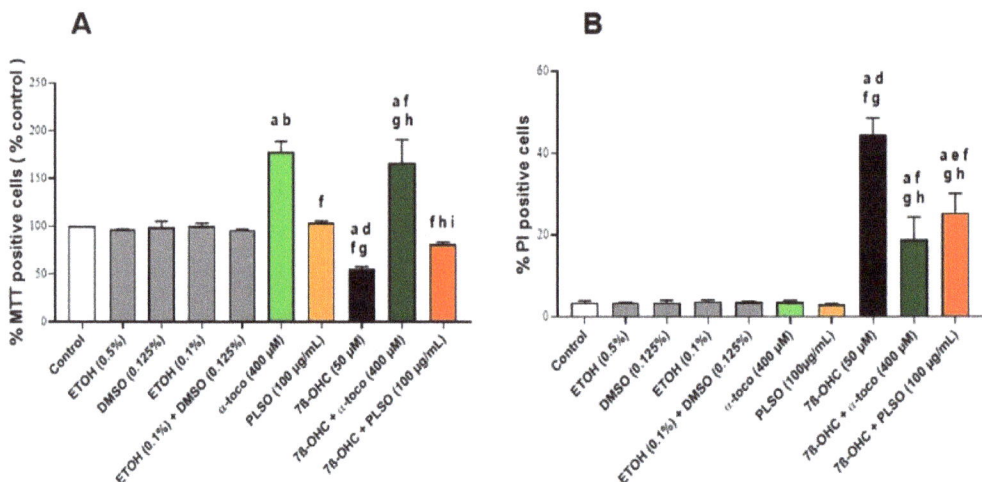

Figure 1. Effect of *Pistacia lentiscus* L. seed oil (PLSO) and 7β-hydroxycholesterol in C2C12 cell viability. C2C12 cells were incubated for 24 h with or without 7β-OHC (50 µM) in the presence or absence of PLSO (100 µg/mL) or α-tocopherol (400 µM). The protective effect of PLSO and α-tocopherol against 7β-OHC-induced cell death was evaluated with the MTT assay (**A**) and by flow cytometry after staining with propidium iodide (PI) (**B**). Data are the mean ± SD of two independent experiments performed in triplicate. A multiple comparative analysis between the groups, taking into account the interactions, was carried out using an ANOVA test followed by a Tukey's test. A p-value less than 0.05 was considered statistically significant. The statistically significant differences between the groups, which are indicated by different letters, take into account the vehicle used. a: comparison versus control; b: comparison versus ETOH (0.5%); c: comparison versus DMSO (0.125%); d: comparison versus ETOH (0.1%); e: comparison versus (ETOH (0.1%) + DMSO (0.125%)); f: comparison versus α-toco (400 µM); g: comparison versus PLSO (100 µg/mL); h: comparison versus 7β-OHC (50 µM); i: comparison versus 7β-OHC (50 µM) + α-toco (400 µM). No significant differences were observed between the untreated (control) and vehicle-treated cells: EtOH (0.5%), DMSO (0.125%), EtOH (0.1%), and EtOH (0.1%) +DMSO (0.125%).

ROS overproduction was quantified by flow cytometry with DHE. As shown in Figure 2A, treatment with 7β-OHC induced a significant increase in the percentage of DHE-positive cells compared to the untreated (control) and vehicle-treated (EtOH 0.1%) cells; this increase in ROS production was significantly attenuated when 7β-OHC was associated with PLSO or α-tocopherol.

In addition, the levels of MDA, CDs, and CPs, which are the main products of lipid and protein oxidation, respectively, were significantly higher in 7β-OHC-treated cells compared to untreated (control) or vehicle-treated (EtOH 0.1%) cells; these increases were significantly reduced when the cells were incubated with 7β-OHC in the presence of PLSO or α-tocopherol, comparatively to 7β-OHC (Figure 2B–D).

In another hand, superoxide dismutase (SOD) and glutathione peroxidase (GPx) activities were significantly decreased in 7β-OHC-treated C2C12 cells when compared with untreated (control) and vehicle-treated (EtOH 0.1%) cells; these decreases were also significantly attenuated when 7β-OHC was associated with PLSO or α–tocopherol (Figure 3).

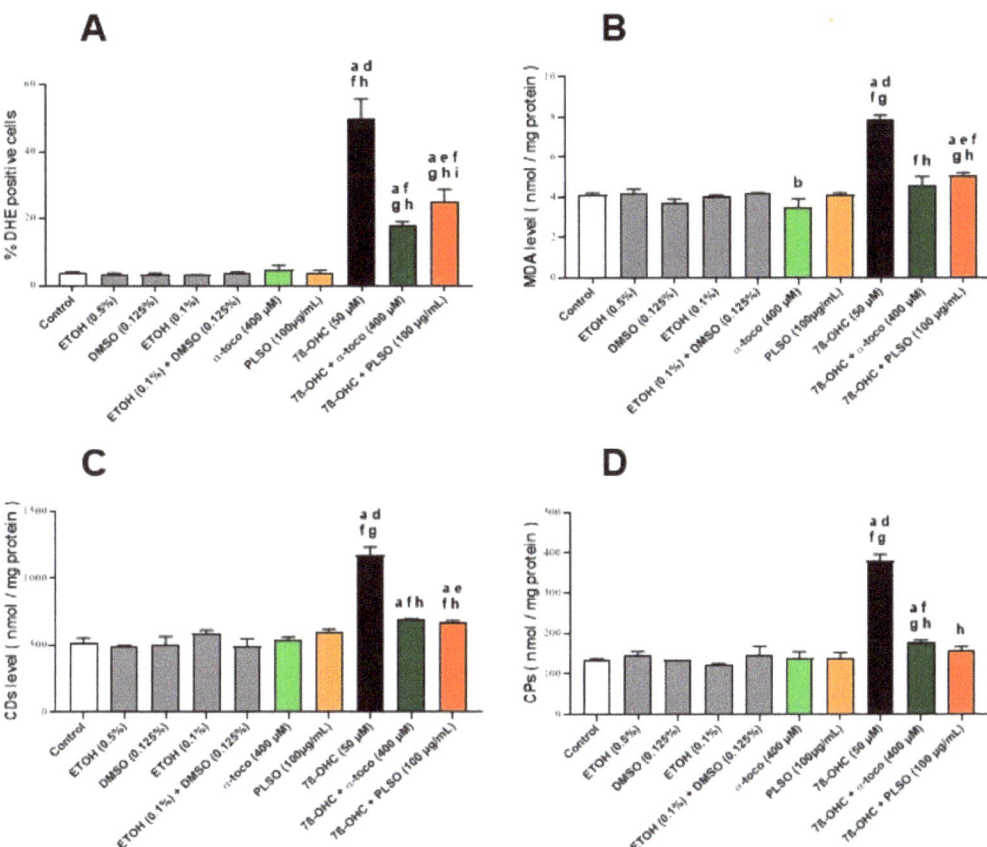

Figure 2. Effect of Pistacia lentiscus L. seed oil (PLSO) on 7β-hydroxycholesterol-induced overproduction of reactive oxygen species (ROS) and lipid and protein oxidation products in C2C12 cells. C2C12 cells were incubated for 24 h with or without 7β-OHC (50 μM) in the presence or absence of PLSO (100 μg/mL) or α-tocopherol (400 μM). ROS overproduction was measured by flow cytometry after staining with dihydroethidium (DHE) (**A**). Lipid and protein oxidation products were determined with malondialdehyde (MDA) (**B**), conjugated dienes (CDs) (**C**) and carbonylated proteins (CPs) levels (**D**). Data are presented as the mean ± SD of two independent experiments performed in triplicate. A multiple comparative analysis between the groups, taking into account the interactions, was carried out using an ANOVA test followed by a Tukey's test. A p-value less than 0.05 was considered statistically significant. The statistically significant differences between the groups, which are indicated by different letters, take into account the vehicle used. a: comparison versus control; b: comparison versus ETOH (0.5%); c: comparison versus DMSO (0.125%); d: comparison versus ETOH (0.1%); e: comparison versus (ETOH (0.1%) + DMSO (0.125%)); f: comparison versus α-toco (400 μM); g: comparison versus PLSO (100 μg/mL); h: comparison versus 7β-OHC (50 μM); i: comparison versus 7β-OHC (50 μM) + α-toco (400 μM). No significant differences were observed between the untreated (control) and vehicle-treated cells.

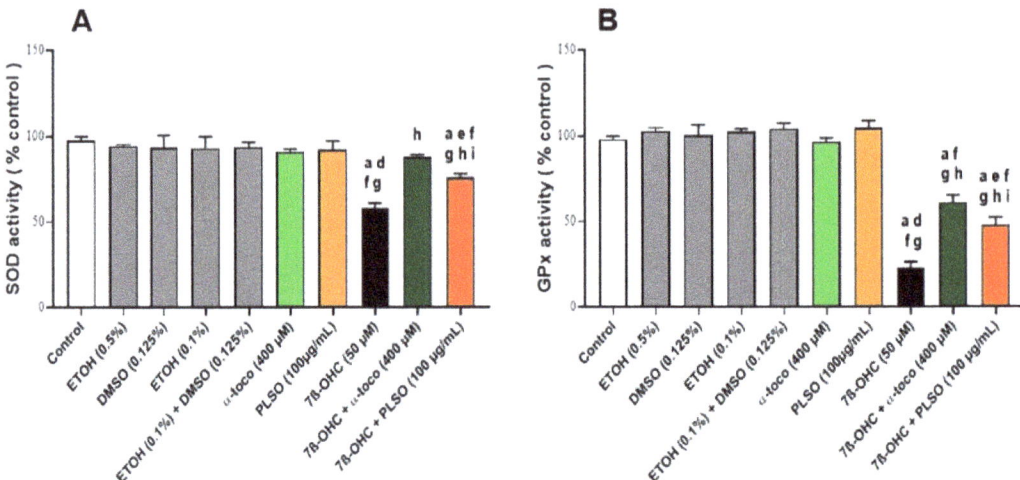

Figure 3. Effect of Pistacia lentiscus L. seed oil (PLSO) and 7β-hydroxycholesterol on antioxidant enzyme activities (SOD, GPx) in C2C12 cells. C2C12 cells were incubated for 24 h with or without 7β-OHC (50 μM) in the presence or absence of PLSO (100 μg/mL) or α-tocopherol (400 μM). The measurement of superoxide dismutase (SOD) activity (**A**) and glutathione peroxidase (GPx) activity (**B**) were realized. Data are presented as the mean ± SD of two independent experiments performed in triplicate. A multiple comparative analysis between the groups, taking into account the interactions, was carried out using an ANOVA test followed by a Tukey's test. A *p*-value less than 0.05 was considered statistically significant. The statistically significant differences between the groups, which are indicated by different letters, take into account the vehicle used. a: comparison versus control; b: comparison versus ETOH (0.5%); c: comparison versus DMSO (0.125%); d: comparison versus ETOH (0.1%); e: comparison versus (ETOH (0.1%) + DMSO (0.125%)); f: comparison versus α-toco (400 μM); g: comparison versus PLSO (100 μg/mL); h: comparison versus 7β-OHC (50 μM); i: comparison versus 7β-OHC (50 μM) + α-toco (400 μM). No significant differences were observed between the untreated (control) and vehicle-treated cells.

3.6. Evaluation of the Effects of Pistacia lentiscus L. Seed Oil on 7β-Hydroxycholesterol-Induced Mitochondrial Damages

To evaluate the effect of PLSO (100 μg/mL) against 7β-OHC (50 μM)-induced mitochondrial dysfunction, we measured the mitochondrial transmembrane potential (ΔΨm) after staining with $DiOC_6(3)$, the overproduction of ROS at the mitochondrial level after staining with MitoSOX-Red, as well as the ATP level by bioluminescence (Figure 4).

Under treatment with 7β-OHC, and comparatively to the untreated (control) and vehicle-treated (EtOH 0.1%) cells, a marked decrease in ΔΨm, revealed by an increase in the percentage of cells with depolarized mitochondria ($DiOC_6(3)$-negative cells), was observed (Figure 4A). In addition, a reduction in ATP production was observed under treatment with 7β-OHC (Figure 4B). With MitoSOX-Red, a marked increase in MitoSOX-Red-positive cells was revealed, confirming a disturbed oxidative phosphorylation and the induction of mitochondrial damage under treatment with 7β-OHC (Figure 4C). Interestingly, in the presence of PLSO or α-tocopherol, the loss of ΔΨm, decrease in ATP, as well as overproduction of mitochondrial ROS was strongly attenuated (Figure 4A–C). In the presence of MitoQ (1 μM), which blocks ROS overproduction at the mitochondrial level, a slight but not significant cytoprotective effect was observed with the FDA test whereas a significant and marked cytoprotection was found with PLSO and α-tocopherol (Supplementary Figure S8), supporting (i) that mitochondrial targeting with an antioxidant is not sufficient to prevent 7β-OHC-induced cell death; and (ii) that PLSO and α-tocopherol, which act at the mitochondrial levels, also have other cellular targets.

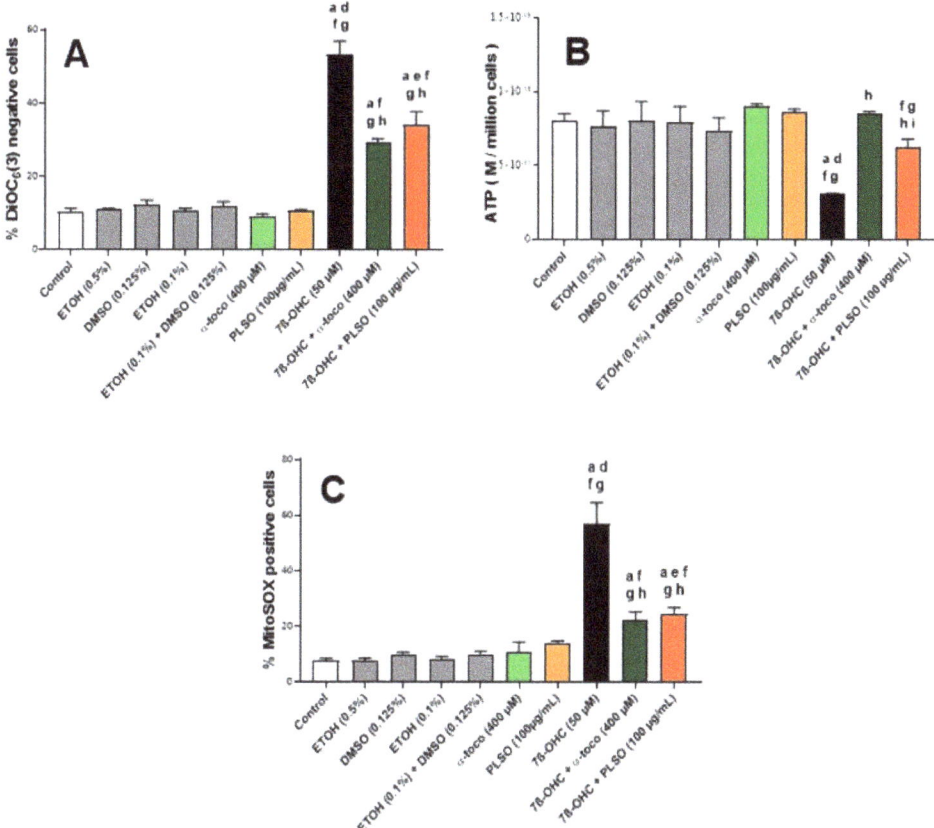

Figure 4. Effect of *Pistacia lentiscus* L. seed oil (PLSO) on 7β-hydroxycholesterol-induced mitochondrial damage in C2C12 cells. C2C12 cells were incubated for 24 h with or without 7β-OHC (50 μM) in the presence or absence of PLSO (100 μg/mL) or α-tocopherol (400 μM). Mitochondrial transmembrane potential (ΔΨm) (**A**), mitochondrial ATP production (**B**), and mitochondrial production of superoxide anion($O_2^{\bullet-}$) (**C**) were measured. The data are presented as the mean ± SD of two independent experiments performed in triplicate. A multiple comparative analysis between the groups, taking into account the interactions, was carried out using an ANOVA test followed by a Tukey's test. A *p*-value less than 0.05 was considered statistically significant. The statistically significant differences between the groups, which are indicated by different letters, take into account the vehicle used. a: comparison versus control; b: comparison versus ETOH (0.5%); c: comparison versus DMSO (0.125%); d: comparison versus ETOH (0.1%); e: comparison versus (ETOH (0.1%) + DMSO (0.125%)); f: comparison versus α-toco (400 μM); g: comparison versus PLSO (100 μg/mL); h: comparison versus 7β-OHC (50 μM); i: comparison versus 7β-OHC (50 μM) + α-toco (400 μM). No significant differences were observed between the untreated (control) and vehicle-treated cells.

3.7. Evaluation of the Effects of Pistacia lentiscus L. Seed Oil on 7β-Hydroxycholesterol-Induced Peroxisomal Damages

Abcd3 (ATP binding cassette subfamily D member) is a major component of the peroxisomal membrane and a common constituent of peroxisomes in different tissues [91,92] (Supplementary Figure S9). This peroxisomal transporter is frequently used to evaluate the peroxisomal mass, thus providing information on peroxisome biogenesis [79]. The effect of 7β-OHC (50 μM) with and without PLSO (100 μg/mL) and α-tocopherol (400 μM) was determined on the topography and expression of Abcd3 revealed by indirect immunofluorescence using structured illumination microscopy (Apotome) and flow cytometry (Figure 5).

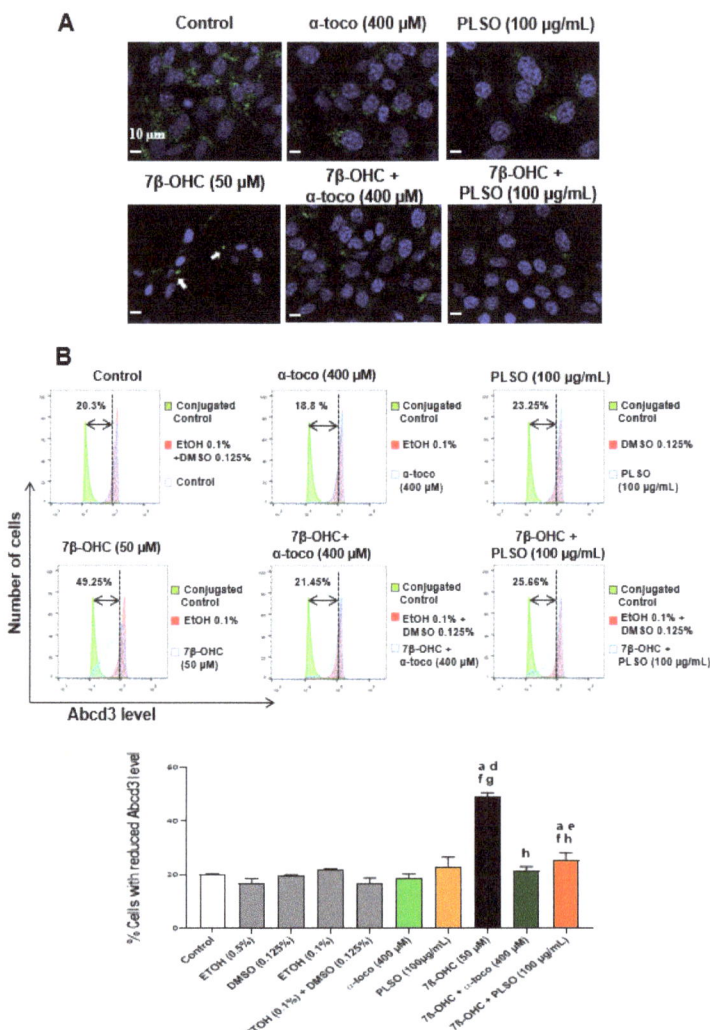

Figure 5. Effect of *Pistacia lentiscus* L. seed oil (PLSO) and 7β-hydroxycholesterol on the expression of the major peroxisomal membrane transporter (Abcd3) used to evaluate the peroxisomal topography and mass. C2C12 cells were incubated for 24 h with or without 7β-OHC (50 μM) in the presence or absence of PLSO (100 μg/mL) or α-tocopherol (400 μM). The protective effect of PLSO and α-tocopherol (400 μM) against 7β-OHC were analyzed by structured illumination microscopy (apotome) (**A**) and flow cytometry (**B**). The white arrows point towards cells with an accumulation of peroxisomes in a particular area of the cytoplasm. The data are presented as the mean ± SD of two independent experiments performed in triplicate. A multiple comparative analysis between the groups, taking into account the interactions, was carried out using an ANOVA test followed by a Tukey's test. A p-value less than 0.05 was considered statistically significant. The statistically significant differences between the groups, which are indicated by different letters, take into account the vehicle used. a: comparison versus control; b: comparison versus ETOH (0.5%); c: comparison versus DMSO (0.125%); d: comparison versus ETOH (0.1%); e: comparison versus (ETOH (0.1%) + DMSO (0.125%)); f: comparison versus α-toco (400 μM); g: comparison versus PLSO (100 μg/mL); h: comparison versus 7β-OHC (50 μM); i: comparison versus 7β-OHC (50 μM) + α-toco (400 μM). In addition, no significant differences were observed between the untreated (control) and vehicle-treated cells.

Using structure illumination microscopy (Figure 5A), a high density of peroxisomes was observed in the cytoplasm of untreated (control) cells, PLSO-, and α-tocopherol-treated cells. An important decrease in peroxisomal density was revealed under treatment with 7β-OHC. In addition, the peroxisomes were homogeneously distributed in the cytoplasm of the control and vehicle-treated cells as well as of PLSO- and α-tocopherol-treated cells, whereas they were preferentially amassed in a particular area of the cytoplasm in 7β-OHC-treated cells. When the cells were cultured in the presence of 7β-OHC associated with PLSO or α-tocopherol, the aspect of the peroxisome in the cytoplasm evocate those of untreated (control) and vehicle-treated cells, although the peroxisomal density remains lower.

Under treatment with 7β-OHC, the decrease in peroxisomal density observed by microscopy suggests a decrease in peroxisomal biogenesis. To confirm this hypothesis, flow cytometric analyses were performed (Figure 5B). The analysis of Abcd3 levels in C2C12 cells did not reveal any difference between untreated (control) and α-tocopherol-treated cells; a slight increase was observed in the presence of PLSO. Under treatment with 7β-OHC, a significant increase in the percentage of cells with a reduced Abcd3 level was observed. Interestingly, this decreased expression of Abcd3 was significantly inhibited when 7β-OHC was combined with PLSO or α-tocopherol.

With regard to peroxisome function, peroxisomal damages (alteration of peroxisomal β-oxidation) (Supplementary Figure S9) can favor the accumulation of very-long-chain fatty acids (VLCFA; $C \geq 22$) [81], which can contribute to amplify cell dysfunctions [93]. Therefore, we determined the effect of 7β-OHC (50 μM) associated or not with PLSO (100 μg/mL) or α-tocopherol (400 μM) on VLCFA levels in C2C12 cells. In untreated cells (control) and the vehicle, no significant differences were found; similar levels of VLCFA (C22:0, C24:0, C24:1 n−9, C26:0, and C26:1 n−9) were observed (Figure 6). When C2C12 cells were exposed to 7β-OHC, a significant increase in VLCFA was detected, and the latter was significantly reduced when 7β-OHC was associated with PLSO or α-tocopherol (Figure 6).

However, enhanced ELOVL1 activity could also be involved in the increased level of VLCFA. At the moment, seven enzymes termed ELOVL 1–7 (Elongation of Very-Long-Chain Fatty Acid), which are localized in the endoplasmic reticulum, have been identified. ELOVL1 is suggested to control VLCA synthesis up to C26:0. This is the most potent elongase for C24:0 and C26:0, whereas, depending on the cell type considered, similar elongase activity have been reported with ELOVL3 and ELOVL6 [94,95]. Our results also support an increase in the elongase activity index (which could correspond to ELOVL1, 3, and 6 activity; ratio (C24:0/C22:0), and ratio (C26:0/C22:0)) under treatment with 7β-OHC; these different elongase activity indexes were also strongly attenuated when 7β-OHC was associated with PLSO or α-tocopherol (Figure 7).

In addition, as shown by qRT-PCR, the important decreases in the Abcd3 mRNA levels, observed under treatment with 7β-OHC (50 μM), were prevented by treatment with PLSO (100 μg/mL), as well as α-tocopherol (400 μM) (Figure 8).

3.8. Evaluation by Transmission Electron Microscopy of the Effects of Pistacia lentiscus L. Seed Oil on 7β-Hydroxycholesterol-Induced Cellular, Mitochondrial, and Peroxisomal Changes

Transmission electron microscopy analysis was realized to study the morphological changes in C2C12 myoblasts (Figures 9 and 10).

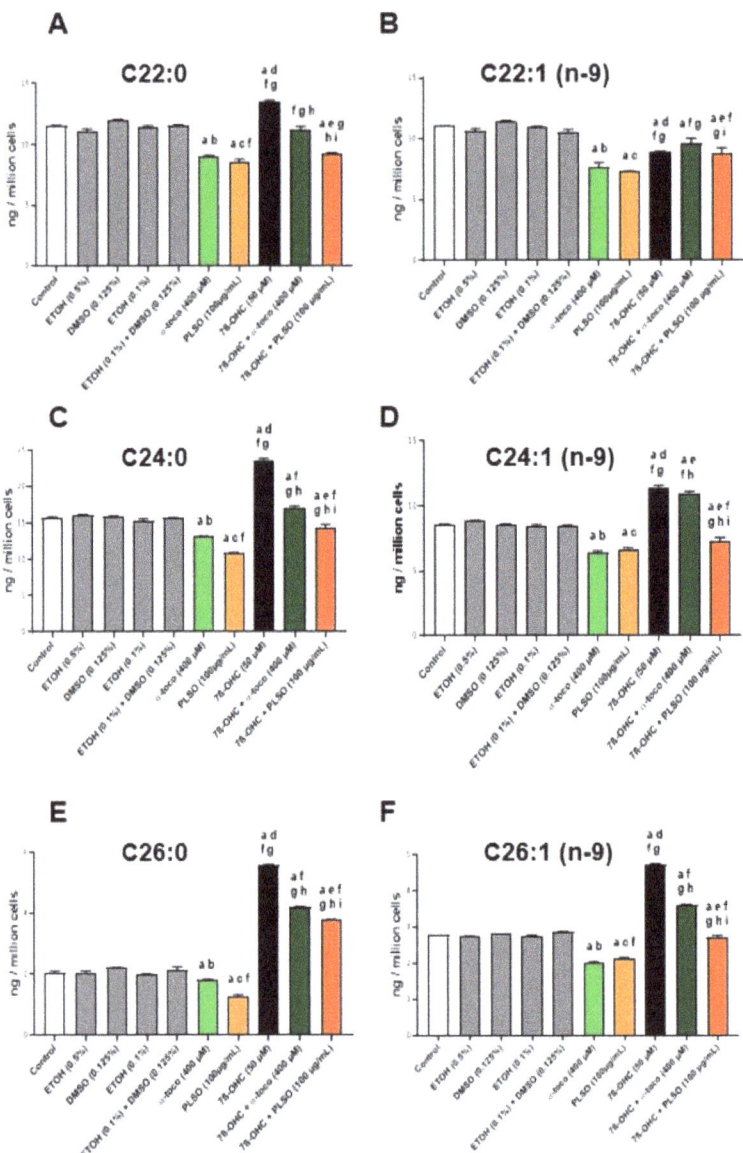

Figure 6. Effect of 7β-hydroxycholesterol with and without *Pistacia lentiscus* L. seed oil (PLSO) on very-long-chain fatty acid (VLCFA) levels. C2C12 cells were incubated for 24 h with or without 7β-OHC (50 μM) in the presence or absence of PLSO (100 μg/mL) or α-tocopherol (400 μM). The level of VLCFA (C ≥ 22) was determined by GC-MS: C22:0 (**A**), C22:1 n−9 (**B**), C24:0 (**C**), C24:1 n−9 (**D**), C26:0 (**E**) and C26:1 n−9 (**F**). Data are the mean ± SD of two independent experiments. A multiple comparative analysis between the groups, taking into account the interactions, was carried out using an ANOVA test followed by a Tukey's test. A p-value less than 0.05 was considered statistically significant. The statistically significant differences between the groups, which are indicated by different letters, take into account the vehicle used. a: comparison versus control; b: comparison versus ETOH (0.5%); c: comparison versus DMSO (0.125%); d: comparison versus ETOH (0.1%); e: comparison versus (ETOH (0.1%) + DMSO (0.125%)); f: comparison versus α-toco (400 μM); g: comparison versus PLSO (100 μg/mL) ; h: comparison versus 7β-OHC (50 μM); i: comparison versus 7β-OHC (50 μM) + α-toco (400 μM). No significant differences were observed between the untreated (control) and vehicle-treated cells.

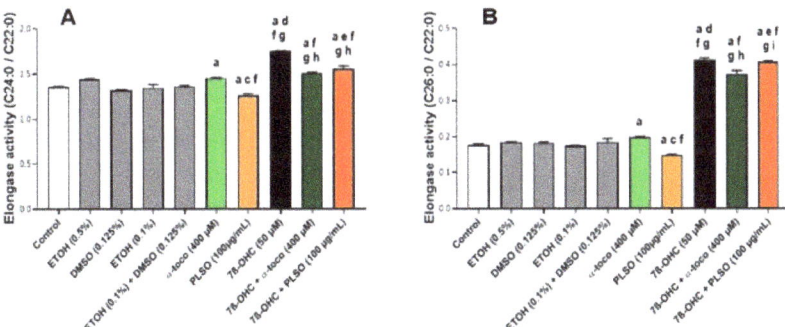

Figure 7. Effect of *Pistacia lentiscus* L. seed oil (PLSO) and 7β-hydroxycholesterol on elongase activities. C2C12 cells were incubated for 24 h with or without 7β-OHC (50 μM) in the presence or absence of PLSO (100 μg/mL) or α-tocopherol (400 μM). The levels of C22:0, C24:0, and C26:0 were determined by GC-MS, and the corresponding elongase activity index, which could correspond to ELOVL1, 3, and 6 activity (ratio (C24:0/C22:0) (**A**) and ratio (C26:0/C22:0) (**B**)) were calculated. Data are the mean ± SD of two independent experiments. A multiple comparative analysis between the groups, taking into account the interactions, was carried out using an ANOVA test followed by a Tukey's test. A *p*-value less than 0.05 was considered statistically significant. The statistically significant differences between the groups, which are indicated by different letters, take into account the vehicle used. a: comparison versus control; b: comparison versus ETOH (0.5%); c: comparison versus DMSO (0.125%); d: comparison versus ETOH (0.1%); e: comparison versus (ETOH (0.1%) + DMSO (0.125%)); f: comparison versus α-toco (400 μM); g: comparison versus PLSO (100 μg/mL); h: comparison versus 7β-OHC (50 μM); i: comparison versus 7β-OHC (50 μM) + α-toco (400 μM). No significant differences were observed between the untreated (control) and vehicle-treated cells.

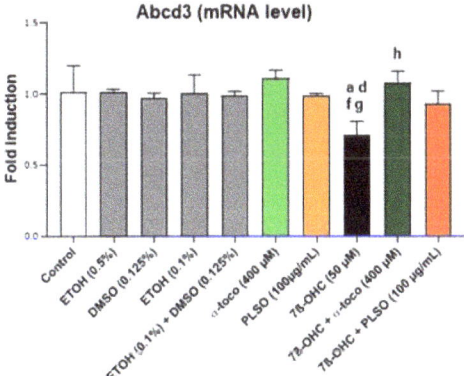

Figure 8. Effects of 7β-hydroxycholesterol with and without *Pistacia lentiscus* L. on Abcd3 gene expression. C2C12 cells were incubated for 24 h with or without 7β-OHC (50 μM) in the presence or absence of PLSO (100 μg/mL) or α-tocopherol (400 μM). The mRNA expression of Abcd3 was evaluated by qRT-PCR. Data shown are representative of three independent experiments. A multiple comparative analysis between the groups, taking into account the interactions, was carried out using an ANOVA test followed by a Tukey's test. A *p*-value less than 0.05 was considered statistically significant. The statistically significant differences between the groups, which are indicated by different letters, take into account the vehicle used. a: comparison versus control; b: comparison versus ETOH (0.5%); c: comparison versus DMSO (0.125%); d: comparison versus ETOH (0.1%); e: comparison versus (ETOH (0.1%) + DMSO (0.125%)); f: comparison versus α-toco (400 μM); g: comparison versus PLSO (100 μg/mL); h: comparison versus 7β-OHC (50 μM); i: comparison versus 7β-OHC (50 μM) + α-toco (400 μM). No significant differences were observed between the untreated (control) and vehicle-treated cells.

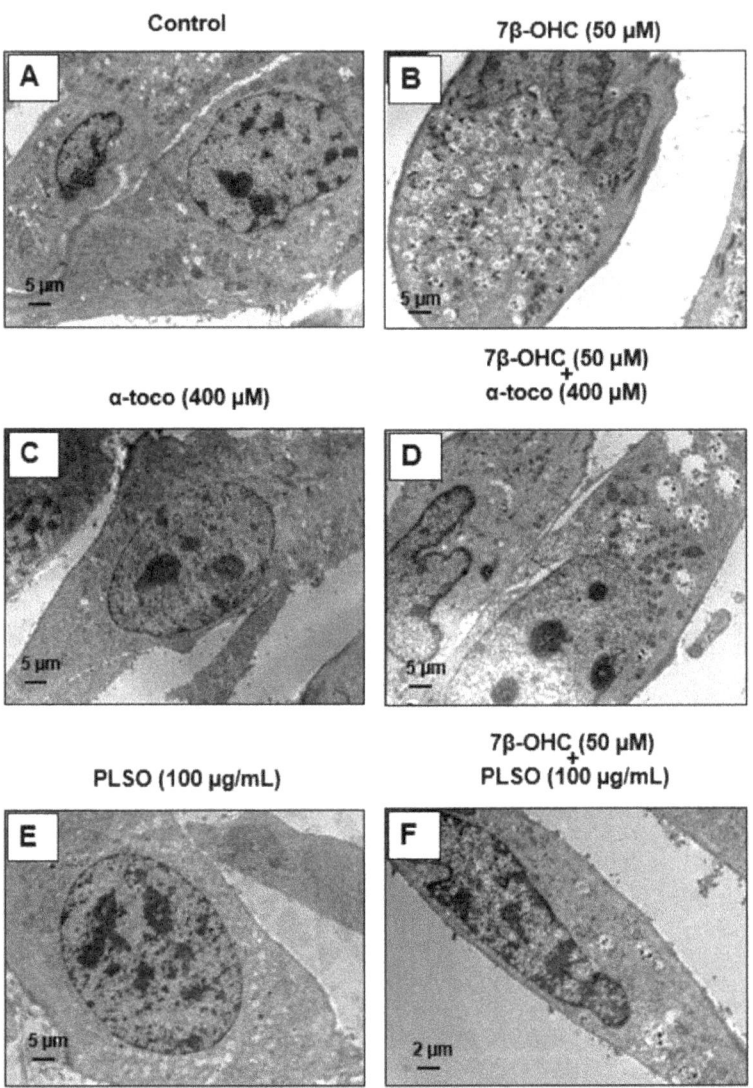

Figure 9. Analysis of morphological changes in C2C12 myoblasts using transmission electron microscopy. C2C12 cells were incubated for 24 h with or without 7β-OHC (50 μM) in the presence or absence of PLSO (100 μg/mL) or α-tocopherol (400 μM). In untreated cells (control) (**A**), α-tocopherol (400 μM)-treated cells (**C**), and PLSO (100 μg/mL)-treated cells (**E**), cells have a fusiform shape, with large round central nuclei containing several nucleoli; they have several small empty vacuoles and morphologically normal mitochondria and peroxisomes. In the 7β-OHC (50 μM)-treated cells (**B**), cells have an abnormal morphology: they have a round shape, irregular nuclei, and a lot of cytoplasmic vacuoles containing cell debris, as well as altered mitochondria and peroxisomes. In (7β-OHC + α-tocopherol and 7β-OHC+ PLSO)-treated cells, mainly morphologically normal cells were observed; they contain empty vacuoles and have mainly mitochondria and peroxisomes resembling those present in the control cells (**D–F**). No differences were observed between the control (**A**), α-tocopherol-treated (**C**), and PLSO-treated cells (**E**). Representative TEM images of the C2C12 myoblasts cultured in the presence of the vehicles are shown in Supplementary Figure S10.

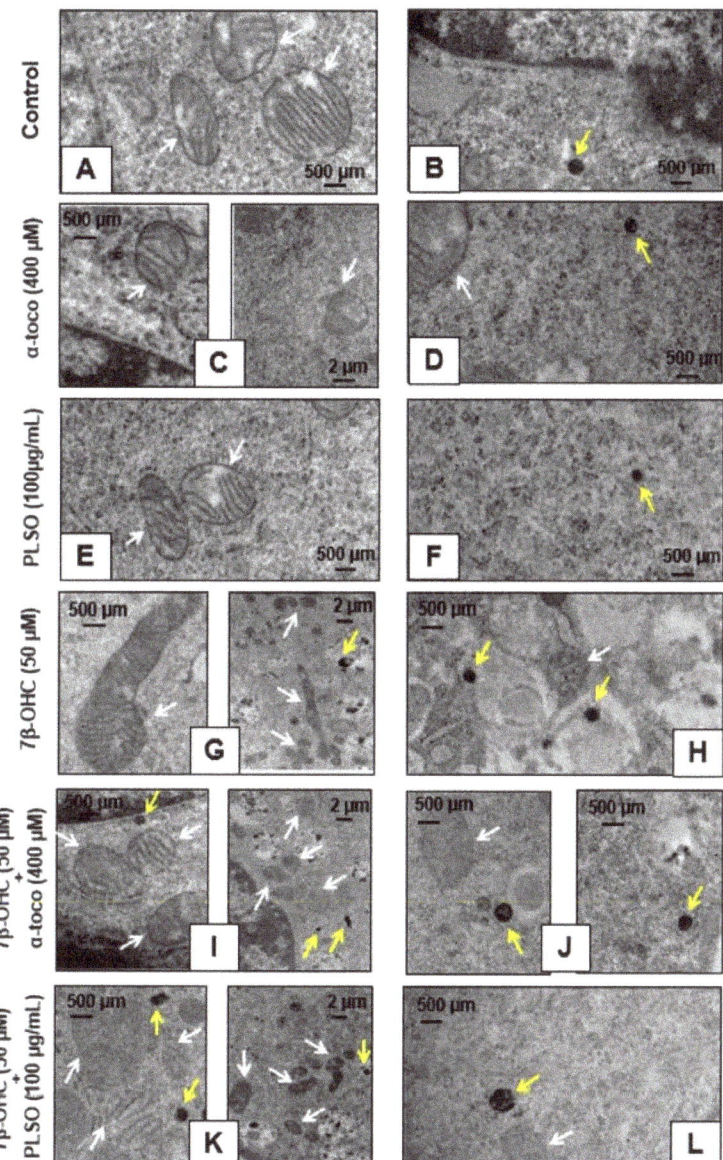

Figure 10. Visualization of the mitochondria and peroxisomes in C2C12 myoblasts by transmission electron microscopy. C2C12 cells were incubated for 24 h with or without 7β-OHC (50 µM) in the presence or absence of PLSO (100 µg/mL) or α-tocopherol (400 µM). In untreated cells (control) (A,B), α-tocopherol (400 mM)-treated cells (C,D), and PLSO (100 µg/mL)-treated cells (E,F), numerous mitochondria with clear cristae as well as round and regular peroxisomes were detected. In 7β-OHC (50 µM)-treated cells (G,H), irregular mitochondria with an increased size, reduced matrix density, and disrupted cristae, as well as peroxisomes with abnormal sizes and shapes were visualized. In (7β-OHC + α-tocopherol)-treated (I,J) and (7β-OHC+ PLSO) (K,L)-treated cells, mainly mitochondria and peroxisomes morphologically similar than those present in the control cells were observed. The white arrows point towards mitochondria and the yellow arrows point towards peroxisomes.

Control cells (Figure 9A), α-tocopherol (400 mM)-treated cells (Figure 9C), and PLSO (100 µg/mL)-treated cells (Figure 9E) have a well-preserved cell morphology with a fusiform shape and a large central round nucleus containing some nucleoli; in the cytoplasm, they have small empty vacuoles and morphologically normal mitochondria and peroxisomes. Compared to C2C12 control cells, 7β-OHC (50 µM)-treated cells showed significant alterations in cell morphology: most often round cells with irregular nuclei were observed, they contained several cytoplasmic vacuoles associated with a lot of cell debris as well as altered mitochondria and peroxisomes (Figure 9B). This disturbed morphology was attenuated by α-tocopherol (400 mM) and PLSO (100 µg/mL) treatment (Figure 9D,F). α-Tocopherol- and PLSO-treated cells (Figure 9C,E) have a similar morphology than control cells (Figure 9A). No morphological differences were observed between the control (Supplementary Figure S10A) and vehicle-treated cells (Supplementary Figures S10B,D).

Moreover, TEM observation of the C2C12 cells allowed us to highlight the essential cellular constituents, namely, mitochondria and peroxisomes. Control cells, α-tocopherol (400 mM)-treated cells, and PLSO (100 µg/mL)-treated cells have morphologically normal mitochondria with numerous cristae as well as round peroxisomes that are homogeneous in size in the range of 0.4 ± 0.1 µm (Figure 10A,F). However, major changes in the size and shape of these organelles were observed when C2C12 cells were treated with 7β-OHC; thus, several mitochondria with abnormal sizes and shapes were observed: larger size, reduced matrix density, and disrupted cristae (Figure 10G). In addition, several peroxisomes were detected in numerous cytoplasmic vacuoles, evoking a pexophagy process (Figure 10G,H). It is noteworthy that these changes in mitochondrial and peroxisomal topography and/or morphology were attenuated when 7β-OHC was combined with α-tocopherol (400 µM) or PLSO (100 µg/mL) (Figure 10I,L).

Indeed, we note that the mitochondria returned to their rounded shapes and the peroxisomes present in the vacuoles were rarely detected. Altogether, our data by TEM confirm that 7β-OHC induced several mitochondrial and peroxisomal changes, and that α-tocopherol and PLSO have strong cytoprotective effects on these organelles.

4. Discussion

Aging is characterized by the variable decline in many biological functions, which can seriously alter the life quality of elderly people. Among the major alterations occurring during the aging process is sarcopenia, which corresponds to a loss of mass, quality, and strength of skeletal muscles [2,3]. Sarcopenia is generally accompanied by an impairment in muscle regeneration and a rupture of RedOx homeostasis, leading to ROS overproduction, which may, in turn, lead to the loss of muscle function [96]. ROS overproduction can favor lipid peroxidation, and increased levels of cholesterol auto-oxidation products, such as 7KC and 7β-OHC, are known to contribute to the development of several age-related diseases [31,81]. Interestingly, low physiological levels of ROS help maintain and heal skeletal muscle [97]; yet, tissue repair delay is caused by an excessive amount of ROS in the muscles, resulting in worsening the injury and creating atrophy [98]. Among the factors known to increase antioxidant defense and protect muscle from harmful effects of oxidative stress is nutrition. In that regard, in the current study, PLSO has been shown to contain a lot of compounds with antioxidant properties and this edible Mediterranean oil has a protective and antioxidant activity against 7β-OHC-induced cytotoxicity in C2C12 skeletal muscle cells. The data obtained are summarized in a heatmap (Figure 11).

Plants are an important source of bioactive molecules with therapeutic potential [99]. The genus *Pistacia* is a particular genus of the Anacardiaceae family due to its dioeciousness and naked flowers [100]. The species *Pistacia lentiscus* L. is a medicinal plant that grow wild in forests, low mountains, and in all types of soil [101]. Despite its limited distribution in the world, *Pistacia lentiscus* L. is known worldwide for several therapeutic properties, such as antioxidant, anti-inflammatory, anti-proliferative, and neuro-protective effects [48–51].

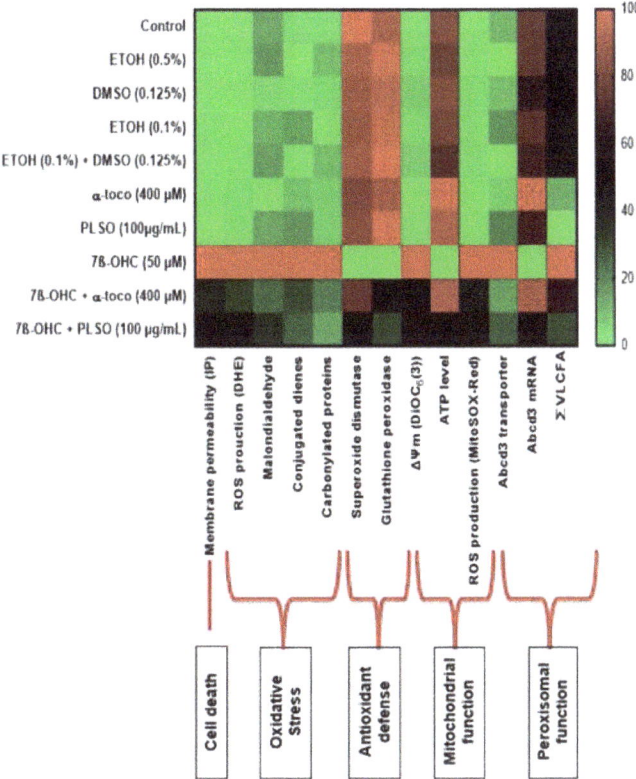

Figure 11. Heatmap representation of the toxicity of 7β-hydroxycholesterol and of the cytoprotective effects of PLSO and α-tocopherol on C2C12 cells. Heatmap graded from green (little or no effect: 0) to red (maximum effect: 100).

Using C2C12 cells cultured in the presence of 7β-OHC associated with many age-related diseases [31], our results show why there is interest in PLSO to prevent skeletal muscle cell dysfunction in a pro-oxidant environment. The results obtained establish that PLSO strongly attenuates the toxicity of 7β-OHC against which few cytoprotective molecules or mixtures of molecules have been identified [28]. Noteworthy, PLSO, which has a high nutritional value based on its biochemical profile established in this study, has a cytoprotective effects against 7β-OHC, which is of the same order of magnitude as that observed with α-tocopherol used at high concentration.

In the present study, we report that PLSO from Tunisia (area of Tabarka) has comparable amounts of total phenolics than PLSO from Algeria and Morocco (28.50 ± 0.77 mg/GAE/g vs. 25.15 ± 1.01 mg/GAE/g and 22.61 ± 1.42 mg/GAE/g, respectively) [102,103]. This similarity may be due to the fact that these three regions are in the same bioclimatic area. However, the flavonoids content of the PLSO used in this study was higher than the PLSO from Morocco [103].

The PLSO from Tunisia also showed a notable quantity of carotenoids. Thus, we could consider that PLSO is a great natural source for these pigments when compared to virgin olive oil (1.58–2.84 mg/kg of oil) [53]. These pigments, mainly β-carotene, are precursors of vitamin A. Dietary carotenoids are antioxidants thought to provide health benefits in the prevention of cardiovascular diseases and cancer [104,105]. In addition, β-carotene given to 8-week-old male mice by oral gavage for 7 or 14 days was able to maintain and enhance skeletal muscle mass by increasing the expression level of insulin-like growth factor-1 (IGF-1) [106]. In addition, fatty acids are considered a genetic code of oils; they are major components of most naturally occurring lipids in plants. The analysis of the fatty acid profile of PLSO from Tunisia is in accordance with the finding of Brahmi et al., (fatty acid profile expressed in g/100 g of PLSO) [102] and Dhifi et al., (fatty acid profile expressed in %) [107]. It has been reported that the most abundant unsaturated fatty acids present in PLSO were oleic acid (OA; C18:1 n−9) and linoleic acid (LA; C18:2 n−6). OA is reputed for its effect on oils oxidative stability and its nutritional value [108]. OA also has strong antioxidant activities against 7-KC-induced cell death on murine microglial BV-2 cells [55,109]. LA is also an essential fatty acid and a precursor of polyunsaturated fatty acids with longer chains, which enhances the nutritional value of the vegetable shortening [110]. Lee et al., (2009) indicated that unsaturated fatty acids, especially OA and LA, enhanced the proliferation of C2C12 skeletal muscle cells [111]. In the current study, palmitic acid (C16:0) was the predominant saturated fatty acid found in PLSO, which is consistent with previous studies [107,112]. According to the literature, PLSO presents a higher palmitic acid content than olive oil (9.85–20.30%) and other vegetable oils, such as milk thistle seed oil (6.25–13.06%) and argan oil (12.11–13.05%) [62]. This saturated fatty acid has been thought to increase the total cholesterol, and specifically the LDL cholesterol levels, although a previous study demonstrated that high consumption of palmitic acid in healthy volunteers does not increase the cholesterol if it is combined with LA, as is the case in PLSO [113]. Noteworthy, the low saturated/unsaturated fatty acids ratio (0.404%) indicates that PLSO contains a huge amount of unsaturated fatty acids, which gives it valuable nutritional and dietetic value as well as curative properties [107].

The PLSO sterol profile also showed that β-sitosterol is the most abundant phytosterol (67.25 ± 3.24 mg/100 g of oil) followed by α-epoxysitostanol and 24-methylene cycloartenol. β-sitosterol was also the most representative sterol in the PLSO harvested from different Tunisian locations but the amount of this sterol changed according to geographic origin (99.61 mg/100 g of oil in Korbousand; 389.50 mg/100 g of oil in Rimel) [52]. A lower amount of β-sitosterol was found in Algerian PLSO (58.79 ± 1.19 mg/100 g of oil) [102]. β-sitosterol is one of the most abundant dietary phytosterols that have potential health benefits. Several experimental studies demonstrated that β-sitosterol could regulate the glucose and lipid metabolism [114] and inhibit inflammation and oxidative stress [115,116]. In addition, an in vitro study showed that C2C12 skeletal muscle cells treatment by β-sitosterol improves mitochondrial biogenesis and function via increasing mitochondrial electron transport and energy demand and by activating protein kinase/PGC-1 [117]; these observations give the PLSO a great nutritional and therapeutic value.

In addition, tocopherols are also major ingredients in the oils since they have high antioxidant activity [118]. They could protect polyunsaturated fatty acids (PUFA) from oxidation by scavenging lipid peroxyl radicals (ROO$^\bullet$) [119]. In PLSO, α-tocopherol is present in the highest quantity and contributes to the natural conservation of PLSO. It is important to highlight that PLSO is an excellent source of vitamin E, which is constituted of four tocopherols and four tocotrienols [120].

In another hand, the antioxidant potential of PLSO, evaluated by DPPH, FRAP, and FIC assays, demonstrated an important antioxidant potential of this oil, reinforcing our interest to study the cytoprotective properties of this oil in vitro. Consequently, in the context of sarcopenia, we evaluated the protective properties of PLSO against 7β-OHC-induced cytotoxicity on a model of murine C2C12 myoblast cells.

Indeed, several oxysterols, including 7β-OHC, are present at increased levels and high amounts in the plasma and tissues of patients with age-related diseases [31,121], and our preliminary data obtained by GC-MS on the plasma from subjects with and without sarcopenia have revealed significant higher plasma levels of 7β-OHC in sarcopenic patients. It has been shown that 7β-OHC, which is a potent inducer of oxidative stress by stimulating at least in part NAD(P)H activity [122], was among the most cytotoxic oxysterol on different cell types from different species [42]. Oxidative damage is supposed to be the main responsible factor for cellular aging. A potential oxidative alteration of satellite cells could induce problems in muscle regeneration, as is the case in aging [123]. Therefore, in age-related diseases, including sarcopenia, the identification of molecules or mixture of molecules capable to attenuate 7β-OHC-induced cell death, defined as oxiapoptophagy [124], has a crucial interest to prevent and/or treat these diseases.

In the present study, 7β-OHC (50 µM, 24 h) showed cytotoxic effects on C2C12 myoblasts cells, which are characterized by an induction of cell death associated with ROS overproduction as well as mitochondrial and peroxisomal dysfunction. Some of these effects were previously obtained on vascular cells, hematopoietic and immune cells, retinal cells, and nerve cells exposed to 7β-OHC [30,109,125,126]. As previously reported on numerous adherent cells, 7β-OHC induces a loss of cell adhesion on C2C12 cells, which is characterized by an increase in round and floating cells, suggesting an alteration of membrane constituents associated with cell death. These alterations could be triggered by a RedOx imbalance and an induction of oxidative stress, which could modify the structure and the physical properties of plasma membranes, favoring the degradation of adhesion molecules and cell junctions by mechanisms involving the ROS-dependent activation of matrix metalloproteinases [127]. In addition, 7β-OHC-induced plasma membrane modifications, revealed in the present study by an increased permeability to PI, could modify the ionic homeostasis (Ca^{2+}, N^+, K^+) with important consequences on numerous signaling pathways, especially those involved in the activation of apoptosis [30,128] or the transmission of nerve influx [129]. In sarcopenic patients, the alteration in nerve influx could also amplify muscle dysfunction at the neuro–muscular junction. In support of the key role of oxidative stress in 7β-OHC-induced cell death [124], our results obtained in C2C12 cells showed that 7β-OHC also induced an overproduction of mitochondrial ROS, associated with an accumulation of lipid and protein oxidation products, such as MDA, CDs, and CPs, as well as a decrease in the major antioxidant enzymes activities (superoxide dismutase (SOD) and glutathione peroxidase (GPx)). These results evocate the cytotoxic effects observed with 7KC on different types of neuronal cells (158 N murine oligodendrocytes, BV-2 murine microglial cells, and N2a murine neuronal cells) on which the activation of the oxidative stress is at the origin of the toxicity of this oxysterol [126,130].

On C2C12 cells as well as on other cell types, under treatment with 7β-OHC, it can be considered that ROS overproduction results from the activation of different NADPH oxidase isoforms [35] and from mitochondrial dysfunctions. As ROS overproduction and mitochondrial dysfunction are considered as major phenomena involved in senescence and aging [131], our data support the hypothesis that 7β-OHC could contribute to the aging process in skeletal muscle cells. 7β-OHC induces ROS overproduction probably also contributes to the alterations in mitochondrial structures and of mitochondrial proteins present in the mitochondrial complexes contributing to oxidative phosphorylation. This could favor not only a loss of transmembrane mitochondrial potential (Δψm) but also a disruption of the respiratory chain function and a limitation in energy production, leading to the decreased ATP production observed in the present study. Consequently, in tissues with a low cell turnover, such as the skeletal muscle, alteration of the mitochondria under the action of 7β-OHC may have important detrimental effects on the muscular function.

Like mitochondria, the peroxisomes, which are metabolically tightly connected to the mitochondria [132], represent another important source of intracellular ROS (mainly H_2O_2), and it is now well established that peroxisomal dysfunctions increase ROS overproduction and disturb mitochondrial activity [80,133]. It has been shown on 158 N murine oligodendrocytes that the inactivation of the peroxisomal transporters ABCD1 and 2 associated with peroxisomal β-oxidation, as well as of ACOX1, which is the main limiting enzyme of peroxisomal β-oxidation, favor oxidative stress and increase ROS production in whole cells and at the mitochondrial level [134]. The peroxisome, in addition to its implication in the regulation of RedOx homeostasis, is implicated in the control of lipid metabolism and non-cytokinic inflammation [135]. It has also been suggested that the peroxisome may also play a crucial role in cellular aging [136]. However, still little is known about the contribution of the peroxisome in the aging process but an involvement of this organelle in the amplification of mitochondrial dysfunction is quite well documented [93]. The present study realized on C2C12 cells clearly shows peroxisomal alterations in the presence of 7β-OHC, which is characterized by a reduced peroxisomal density and a lower level of Abcd3 peroxisomal transporter. As 7β-OHC could affect and reduce the peroxisomal transport and degradation of VLCFA (C24:0, C24:1, C26:0, and C26:1), whose intracellular accumulation can have toxic consequences [137], the levels of VLCFA have been measured by GC-MS and the elongase activity index of the enzyme ELOVL1 associated with VLCFA metabolism has been determined [138]. Measuring the level of some VLCFA in sarcopenia could be of interest since some fatty acids behave as metabolic inhibitors, uncouplers of oxidative phosphorylation, and membrane permeability transition (MPT) inducers; it is thus hypothesized that these pathophysiological mechanisms could contribute to the muscular symptoms in sarcopenia [139].

Based on the results obtained on C2C12, preventing the toxicity of 7β-OHC, which is essentially formed by auto-oxidation of cholesterol and is increased in many age-related diseases, remains a major challenge [28]. For this purpose, it is still necessary to identify the molecules or mixtures of molecules allowing to prevent or reduce its toxicity. Indeed, at the moment only few natural and synthetic molecules as well as mixtures of molecules capable to inhibit 7β-OHC-induced cytotoxicity have been identified [28]. Noteworthy, we reported that PLSO is an edible oil with high nutritional value containing several antioxidant nutrients known for their protective effects against various diseases associated with oxidative stress, and our data indicate that PLSO exhibits strong cytoprotective activities against 7β-OHC on C2C12 mouse skeletal muscle cells. The effects observed with PLSO were in the range of order of those obtained with α-tocopherol known to strongly counteract 7β-OHC-induced oxidative stress and cell death induction on several cell types [30]. In accordance with these findings, it has been reported that PLSO was able to inhibit H_2O_2-induced oxidative stress in human skin culture [140]. Besides PLSO, other oils and natural bioactive compounds, such as Schisandrae semen essential oil [141], isorhamnetin [142], resveratrol [143], and phloretin [144], were described as antioxidant molecules in C2C12 murine skeletal muscle cells. Our data clearly show that PLSO attenuates both mitochondrial and peroxisomal dysfunctions induced by 7β-OHC through the restoration of succinate dehydrogenase activity and $\Delta\psi m$, a reduction in mitochondrial ROS production, normalization of Abcd3 expression, and VLCFA levels. Thus, PLSO acts on the major targets involved in aging—those contributing to the development of major age-related diseases—namely, oxidative stress, mitochondria, and peroxisome. The cytoprotective results obtained with LPSO evocate those obtained with several other oils associated with the Mediterranean diet (olive oil, milk thistle seed oil, and argan oil) [86,109]. Thus, the value of the lipid mixtures is underscored by these different data to restrain cell death and oxidative stress induced by oxysterols.

5. Conclusions

This study demonstrates that 7β-OHC triggers oxidative stress, mitochondrial and peroxisomal dysfunction, and cell death on C2C12 myoblast cells. Noteworthy, in the presence of PLSO as well as of α-tocopherol, these different cytotoxic effects were strongly attenuated and PLSO was as efficient as α-tocopherol used at a high concentration. Noteworthy, as MitoQ, which selectively accumulates in the mitochondria, did not attenuate 7β-OHC-induced cell death, our data suggest that attenuation of mitochondrial dysfunction is not sufficient to counteract 7β-OHC-induced cell death, and that PLSO, which strongly reduces mitochondrial dysfunction, also act on other cellular targets. On the basis of the biochemical composition of PLSO (fatty acids, tocopherols, and polyphenols), of its antioxidant properties, and of its cytoprotective effects, it is suggested that a diet associated with this oil could contribute to the prevention of skeletal muscle dysfunctions. In a therapeutic context, the bioavailability and the efficiency of the biological compounds present in PLSO could be improved using a number of approaches. These later could include micro- and nano-encapsulation strategies, chimeric tractable molecules, and targeted-specific cell compartments and organelles (mitochondria, peroxisomes), such as Targeted Organelle Nano-therapy (TORN-therapy) [145,146] as well as functional foods.

Supplementary Materials: The following are available online at https://www.mdpi.com/article/10.3390/antiox10111772/s1. Supplementary Figure S1: Different stages of preparation of the Pistachia lentiscus L. seed oil (PLSO) with seeds collected in Tunisia (area of Tabarka); Supplementary Figure S2: polyphenols chromatogram obtained by HPLC (protocatechuic acid and coumarin were identified based on their UV spectra (280 nm)); Supplementary Figure S3: Fatty acid chromatogram obtained by GC; Supplementary Figure S4: Phytosterol chromatogram obtained by GC-FID; Supplementary Figure S5: Plasma levels of cholesterol, 7β-hydroxycholesterol (7β-OHC) and 7-ketocholesterol in sarcopenic patients and non-sarcopenic patients; Supplementary Figure S6: Evaluation with the MTT assay of the effects of Pistacia lentiscus L. seed oil (PLSO) and 7β-hydroxycholesterol on C2C12 cell viability; Supplementary Figure S7A: Effect of 7β-hydroxycholesterol and Pistacia lentiscus L. seed oil (PLSO) on C2C12 cell morphology; Supplementary Figure S7B: Absence of effect of vehicles (EtOH 0.5%; DMSO 1.125%; EtOH 0.1%; EtOH 0.1%+ DMSO 0.125%) on C2C12 cell morphology; Supplementary Figure S8: Evaluation with the fluorescein diacetate (FDA) assay of the effect of MitoQ on 7β-hydroxycholesterol-induced cell death; Supplementary Figure S9: Biochemical pathway of the peroxisomal β-oxidation of very-long-chain fatty acids; Supplementary Figure S10: Comparison by transmission electron microscopy of cell morphology in control C2C12 myoblasts and vehicles-treated C2C12 myoblasts. Supplementary Table S1: List of available polyphenols spectra present in the database of LARA-Spiral company (Couternon, France).

Author Contributions: Conceptualization, A.Z. and G.L.; study management: G.L. and A.Z.; investigation/experimental work: I.G., A.Z., T.N., A.V. and S.H. (Souha Hammouda), S.B., M.L., F.F., D.L. amd A.Y. (molecular and cell biology); F.M., L.A., I.G. and G.L. (transmission electron microscopy); M.S. (organic chemistry); funding: G.L., M.H., S.B., S.P.B., N.L. and S.H. (Sonia Hammami); writing—original draft: I.G., A.Z. and G.L.; discussion: I.G., A.Z. and G.L.; proofreading: all authors (mainly I.G. and G.L.). All authors have read and agreed to the published version of the manuscript.

Funding: This work was funded by Université de Bourgogne (Dijon, France) and Université Tunis El Manar (Tunis, Tunisia); University of Trento (Italy); Telethon and Provincia autonoma di Trento (Italy) (grant No. TCP13007 to SB); AFM-Téléthon (France) (grant No. #23758 to SB); Muscular Dystrophy Association (USA) (grant No. 874294 to SB).

Institutional Review Board Statement: The clinical study (quantification of oxysterols in the plasma of non-sarcopenic subjects and sarcopenic patients) was conducted according to the guidelines of the Declaration of Helsinki and approved by the Research Ethic Committee of the "University of Monastir, Faculty of Medicine, Monastir, Tunisia"; protocol code: IORG 0009738 n°79/OMB 0990-0279 (The pdf file of the original document has been provided to the Journal).

Informed Consent Statement: All subjects included in the clinical study gave their written informed consent (The anonymized pdf files have been provided to the Journal).

Data Availability Statement: Data from the in vitro study are available in the laboratory notebooks and on the computers from the Université de Bourgogne (EA7270) (Dijon, France) and from the University of Monastir (Monastir and Sousse, Tunisia). Data related to biochemical analysis and electron microscopy are stored on the computers from the Université de Bourgogne, INRAE (Dijon, France) and Lara-Spiral (Couternon, France).

Acknowledgments: The authors would like to thank the association "Mediterranean Nutrition and Health (NMS: Nutrition Méditerranéenne & Santé)". Emmanuelle Prost-Camus, Philippe Durand, and Michel Prost (PLSO polyphenols analysis and KRL assay; Laboratoire LARA-Spiral, Couternon, France), Lucy Martine and Niyazi Acar (PLSO fatty acids and phytosterols analysis; Centre des Sciences du Goût et de l'Alimentation, AgroSup Dijon, CNRS, INRAE, Université Bourgogne Franche-Comté, Dijon, France), Imed Cheraief (PLSO fatty acids analysis; University of Monastir, Faculty of Medicine, LR12ES05, Lab-NAFS, Monastir, Tunisia), Valerio Leoni and Claudio Caccia (analysis of very-long-chain fatty acids; laboratory of Clinical Chemistry, Hospitals of Desio, ASST-Brianza and the Department of Medicine and Surgery, University of Milano-Bicocca, Monza, Italy) and Jean-Paul Pais de Barros (α-tocopherol analysis in PLSO; plasma oxysterols analysis; Lipidomic Facility, Université de Bourgogne Franche-Comté (UBFC), 21078 Dijon, France) are warmly thanked for their technical support. Imen Ghzaiel received financial support from NMS and was awarded the NMS prize (Romanée-Conti) in 2021. The present work was presented as part of the 'Forum des Jeunes Chercheurs UBFC' (web meeting, 2021). Part of the cytotoxic effects of 7β-OHC was presented in an oral communication during the 10th ENOR symposium (web meeting, 16–17 September 2021) (https://www.oxysterols.net/). Imen Ghzaiel also received financial support from ABASIM (Association Bourguignonne pour les Applications des Sciences de l'Information en Médecine; Dijon, France).

Conflicts of Interest: The authors declare no conflict of interest.

References

1. Knapowski, J.; Wieczorowska-Tobis, K.; Witowski, J. Pathophysiology of ageing. *J. Physiol. Pharmacol.* **2002**, *53*, 135–146. [PubMed]
2. Rosenberg, I.H.; Roubenoff, R. Stalking sarcopenia. *Ann. Intern. Med.* **1995**, *123*, 727–728. [CrossRef] [PubMed]
3. Mankhong, S.; Kim, S.; Moon, S.; Kwak, H.B.; Park, D.H.; Kang, J.H. Experimental Models of Sarcopenia: Bridging molecular mechanism and therapeutic strategy. *Cells* **2020**, *9*, 1385. [CrossRef] [PubMed]
4. Troen, B.R. The biology of aging. *Mt. Sinai J. Med.* **2003**, *70*, 3–22. [PubMed]
5. Melton, L.J.; Khosla, S.; Crowson, C.S.; O'Connor, M.K.; O'Fallon, W.M.; Riggs, B.L. Epidemiology of sarcopenia. *J. Am. Geriatr. Soc.* **2000**, *48*, 625–630. [CrossRef]
6. Pereira, A.F.; Silva, A.J.; Matos Costa, A.; Monteiro, A.M.; Bastos, E.M.; Cardoso Marques, M. Muscle tissue changes with aging. *Acta Med. Port.* **2013**, *26*, 51–55.
7. Marquez, D.X.; Hoyem, R.; Fogg, L.; Bustamante, E.E.; Staffileno, B.; Wilbur, J. Physical activity of urban community-dwelling older latino adults. *J. Phys. Act. Health* **2011**, *8*, S161–S170. [CrossRef]
8. Kirchengast, S.; Huber, J. Gender and age differences in lean soft tissue mass and sarcopenia among healthy elderly. *Anthropol. Anz.* **2009**, *67*, 139–151. [CrossRef]
9. Goodpaster, B.H.; Park, S.W.; Harris, T.B.; Kritchevsky, S.B.; Nevitt, M.; Schwartz, A.V.; Simonsick, E.M.; Tylavsky, F.A.; Visser, M.; Newman, A.B. The loss of skeletal muscle strength, mass, and quality in older adults: The health, aging and body composition study. *J. Gerontol. Med. Sci.* **2006**, *61*, 1059–1064. [CrossRef]
10. Rathnayake, N.; Alwis, G.; Lenora, J.; Lekamwasam, S. Concordance between appendicular skeletal muscle mass measured with DXA and estimated with mathematical models in middle-aged women. *J. Physiol. Anthropol.* **2018**, *37*, 19. [CrossRef]
11. Deshmukh, A.S. Proteomics of skeletal muscle: Focus on insulin resistance and exercise biology. *Proteomes* **2016**, *4*, 6. [CrossRef]
12. Gransee, H.M.; Mantilla, C.B.; Sieck, G.C. Respiratory muscle plasticity. *Compr. Physiol.* **2012**, *2*, 1441–1462.
13. Periasamy, M.; Herrera, J.L.; Reis, F.C.G. Skeletal muscle thermogenesis and its role in whole body energy metabolism. *Diabetes Metab. J.* **2017**, *41*, 327–336. [CrossRef]
14. Thomson, D.M.; Winder, W.W. AMPK control of fat metabolism in skeletal muscle. *Acta Physiol.* **2009**, *196*, 147–154. [CrossRef]
15. Muscat, G.E.; Wagner, B.L.; Hou, J.; Tangirala, R.K.; Bischoff, E.D.; Rohde, P.; Petrowski, M.; Li, J.; Shao, G.; Macondray, G.; et al. Regulation of cholesterol homeostasis and lipid metabolism in skeletal muscle by liver X receptors. *J. Biol. Chem.* **2002**, *25*, 40722–40728. [CrossRef]
16. Evans, P.L.; McMillin, S.L.; Weyrauch, L.A.; Witczak, C.A. Regulation of skeletal muscle glucose transport and glucose metabolism by exercise training. *Nutrients* **2019**, *11*, 2432. [CrossRef]
17. Kelley, D.E.; Mandarino, L.J. Hyperglycemia normalizes insulin-stimulated skeletal-muscle glucose-oxidation and storage in noninsulin-dependent diabetes-mellitus. *J. Clin. Investig.* **1990**, *86*, 1999–2007. [CrossRef]
18. Li, Z.; Zhang, Z.; Ren, Y.; Wang, Y.; Fang, J.; Yue, H.; Ma, S.; Guan, F. Aging and age-related diseases: From mechanisms to therapeutic strategies. *Biogerontology* **2021**, *22*, 165–187. [CrossRef]
19. Crowe, A.V.; McArdle, A.; McArdle, F.; Pattwell, D.M.; Bell, G.M.; Kemp, G.J.; Bone, J.M.; Griffiths, R.D.; Jackson, M.J. Markers of oxidative stress in the skeletal muscle of patients on haemodialysis. *Nephrol. Dial. Transplant.* **2007**, *22*, 1177–1183. [CrossRef]
20. Gustafsson, T.; Ulfhake, B. Sarcopenia: What is the origin of this aging-induced disorder? *Front. Genet.* **2021**, *12*, 686526. [CrossRef]

21. Gomes, M.J.; Martinez, P.F.; Pagan, L.U.; Damatto, R.L.; Cezar, M.D.M.; Lima, A.R.R.; Okoshi, K.; Okoshi, M.P. Skeletal muscle aging: Influence of oxidative stress and physical exercise. *Oncotarget* **2017**, *8*, 20428–20440. [CrossRef]
22. Fulle, S.; Protasi, F.; Di Tano, G.; Pietrangelo, T.; Beltramin, A.; Boncompagni, S.; Vecchiet, L.; Fano, G. The contribution of reactive oxygen species to sarcopenia and muscle ageing. *Exp. Gerontol.* **2004**, *39*, 17–24. [CrossRef]
23. Seo, E.; Kang, H.; Choi, H.; Choi, W.; Jun, H.S. Reactive oxygen species-induced changes in glucose and lipid metabolism contribute to the accumulation of cholesterol in the liver during aging. *Aging Cell* **2019**, *18*, e12895. [CrossRef]
24. Simons, K.; Ikonen, E. How cells handle cholesterol. *Science* **2000**, *290*, 1721–1726. [CrossRef]
25. Iuliano, L. Pathways of cholesterol oxidation via non-enzymatic mechanisms. *Chem. Phys. Lipids* **2011**, *164*, 457–468. [CrossRef]
26. Zerbinati, C.; Iuliano, L. Cholesterol and related sterols autoxidation. *Free Radic. Biol. Med.* **2017**, *111*, 151–155. [CrossRef]
27. Anderson, A.; Campo, A.; Fulton, E.; Corwin, A.; Jerome III, W.G.; O'Connor, M.S. 7-Ketocholesterol in disease and aging. *Redox Biol.* **2020**, *29*, 101380. [CrossRef]
28. Nury, T.; Yammine, A.; Ghzaiel, I.; Sassi, K.; Zarrouk, A.; Brahmi, F.; Samadi, M.; Rup-Jacques, S.; Vervandier-Fasseur, D.; de Barros, J.P.; et al. Attenuation of 7-ketocholesterol- and 7β-hydroxycholesterol-induced oxiapoptophagy by nutrients, synthetic molecules and oils: Potential for the prevention of age-related diseases. *Ageing Res. Rev.* **2021**, *68*, 101324. [CrossRef]
29. Mitic, T.; Andrew, R.; Walker, B.R.; Hadoke, P.W.F. 11b-Hydroxysteroid dehydrogenase type 1 contributes to the regulation of 7-oxysterol levels in the arterial wall through the inter-conversion of 7-ketocholesterol and 7b-hydroxycholesterol. *Biochimie* **2013**, *95*, 548–555. [CrossRef]
30. Vejux, A.; Abed-Vieillard, D.; Hajji, K.; Zarrouk, A.; Mackrill, J.J.; Ghosh, S.; Nury, T.; Yammine, A.; Zaibi, M.; Mihoubi, W.; et al. 7-Ketocholesterol and 7β-hydroxycholesterol: In vitro and animal models used to characterize their activities and to identify molecules preventing their toxicity. *Biochem. Pharmacol.* **2020**, *173*, 113648. [CrossRef]
31. Zarrouk, A.; Vejux, A.; Mackrill, J.; O'Callaghan, Y.; Hammami, M.; O'Brien, N.; Lizard, G. Involvement of oxysterols in age-related diseases and ageing processes. *Ageing Res. Rev.* **2014**, *18*, 148–162. [CrossRef] [PubMed]
32. Mutemberezi, V.; Guillemot-Legris, O.; Muccioli, G.G. Oxysterols: From cholesterol metabolites to key mediators. *Prog. Lipid Res.* **2016**, *64*, 152–169. [CrossRef] [PubMed]
33. Samadi, A.; Sabuncuoglu, S.; Samadi, M.; Isikhan, S.Y.; Chirumbolo, S.; Peana, M.; Lay, I.; Yalcinkaya, A.; Bjorklund, G. A Comprehensive Review on Oxysterols and Related Diseases. *Curr. Med. Chem.* **2021**, *28*, 110–136. [CrossRef] [PubMed]
34. Nury, T.; Zarrouk, A.; Vejux, A.; Doria, M.; Riedinger, J.M.; Delage-Mourroux, R.; Lizard, G. Induction of oxiapoptophagy, a mixed mode of cell death associated with oxidative stress, apoptosis and autophagy, on 7-ketocholesterol-treated 158N murine oligodendrocytes: Impairment by α-tocopherol. *Biochem. Biophys. Res. Commun.* **2014**, *446*, 714–719. [CrossRef] [PubMed]
35. Nury, T.; Zarrouk, A.; Mackrill, J.J.; Samadi, M.; Durand, P.; Riedinger, J.M.; Doria, M.; Vejux, A.; Limagne, E.; Delmas, D.; et al. Induction of oxiapoptophagy on 158N murine oligodendrocytes treated by 7-ketocholesterol-, 7β-hydroxycholesterol-, or 24 (S)-hydroxycholesterol: Protective effects of α-tocopherol and docosahexaenoic acid (DHA; C22: 6 n-3). *Steroids* **2015**, *99*, 194–203. [CrossRef] [PubMed]
36. Klionsky, D.J.; Arcbdelmohsen, K.; Arobe, A.; Arbediasn, E.M.J.; Arbelimotovich, H.; Arioszena, A.R.A.; Armstrongdachi, J.L.H.; Arnouldams, T.C.M.; Adams, P.D.; Adeli, K.; et al. Guidelines for the use and interpretation of assays for monitoring autophagy. *Autophagy* **2016**, *12*, 1–222. [CrossRef] [PubMed]
37. Accad, M.; Farese, R.V. Cholesterol homeostasis: A role for oxysterols. *Curr. Biol.* **1998**, *8*, R601–R604. [CrossRef]
38. Samadi, A.; Gurlek, A.; Sendur, S.N.; Karahan, S.; Akbiyik, F.; Lay, I. Oxysterol species: Reliable markers of oxidative stress in diabetes mellitus. *J. Endocrinol. Investig.* **2019**, *42*, 7–17. [CrossRef]
39. Liu, Y.; Hulten, L.M.; Wiklund, O. Macrophages isolated from human atherosclerotic plaques produce IL-8, and oxysterols may have a regulatory function for IL-8 production. *Arterioscler. Thromb. Vasc. Biol.* **1997**, *17*, 317–323. [CrossRef]
40. Bourdon, E.; Loreau, N.; Davignon, J.; Bernier, L.; Blache, D. Involvement of oxysterols and lysophosphatidylcholine in the oxidized LDL-induced impairment of serum albumin synthesis by HEPG2 cells. *Arterioscler. Thromb. Vasc. Biol.* **2000**, *20*, 2643–2650. [CrossRef]
41. Hanley, K.; Ng, D.C.; He, S.S.; Lau, P.; Min, K.; Elias, P.M.; Bikle, D.D.; Mangelsdorf, D.J.; Williams, M.L.; Feingold, K.R. Oxysterols induce differentiation in human keratinocytes and increase Ap-1-dependent involucrin transcription. *J. Investig. Dermatol.* **2000**, *114*, 545–553. [CrossRef]
42. Lemaire-Ewing, S.; Prunet, C.; Montange, T.; Vejux, A.; Berthier, A.; Besseède, G.; Corcos, L.; Gambert, P.; Neel, D.; Lizalrd, G. Comparison of the cytotoxic, pro-oxidant and pro-inflammatory characteristics of different oxysterols. *Cell Biol. Toxicol.* **2005**, *21*, 97–114. [CrossRef]
43. Vergallo, C. Nutraceutical Vegetable Oil Nanoformulations for Prevention and Management of Diseases. *Nanomaterials* **2020**, *10*, 1232. [CrossRef]
44. Kang, P.; Wang, Y.; Li, X.G.; Wan, Z.C.; Wang, X.Y.; Zhu, H.L.; Wang, C.W.; Zhao, S.J.; Chen, H.F.; Liu, Y.L. Effect of flaxseed oil on muscle protein loss and carbohydrate oxidation impairment in a pig model after lipopolysaccharide challenge. *Br. J. Nutr.* **2020**, *123*, 859–869. [CrossRef]
45. Daoued, K.B.; Chouaibi, M.; Gaout, N.; Haj, O.B.; Hamdi, S. Chemical composition and antioxidant activities of cold pressed lentisc (*Pistacialentiscus* L.) seed oil. *Riv. Grasse* **2016**, *93*, 31–38.
46. Le Floc'h, E. *Contribution à une étude Ethnobotanique de la Flore Tunisienne*; Imprimerie Officielle de la République Tunisienne: Radès, Tunisia, 1983.

47. Ben Khedir, S.; Bardaa, S.; Chabchoub, N.; Moalla, D.; Sahnoun, Z.; Rebai, T. The healing effect of Pistacialentiscus fruit oil on laser burn. *Pharm. Biol.* **2017**, *55*, 1407–1414. [CrossRef]
48. Saidi, S.A.; Ncir, M.; Chaaben, R.; Jamoussi, K.; van Pelt, J.; Elfeki, A. Liver injury following small intestinal ischemia reperfusion in rats is attenuated by Pistacia lentiscus oil: Antioxidant and anti-inflammatory effects. *Arch. Physiol. Biochem.* **2017**, *123*, 199–205. [CrossRef]
49. Milia, E.; Bullitta, S.M.; Mastandrea, G.; Szotáková, B.; Schoubben, A.; Langhansová, L.; Quartu, M.; Bortonet, A.; Eick, S. Leaves and Fruits Preparations of *Pistacialentiscus* L.: A Review on the Ethnopharmacological Uses and Implications in Inflammation and Infection. *Antibiotics* **2021**, *10*, 425.
50. Mezni, F.; Shili, S.; Ben Ali, N.; Khouja, M.L.; Khaldi, A.; Maaroufi, A. Evaluation of Pistacialentiscus seed oil and phenolic compounds for in vitro antiproliferative effects against BHK21 cells. *Pharm. Biol.* **2016**, *54*, 747–751. [CrossRef]
51. Ammari, M.; Othman, H.; Hajri, A.; Sakly, M.; Abdelmelek, H. Pistacia lentiscus oil attenuates memory dysfunction and decreases levels of biomarkers of oxidative stress induced by lipopolysaccharide in rats. *Brain Res. Bull.* **2018**, *140*, 140–147. [CrossRef]
52. Trabelsi, H.; Sakouhi, F.; Renaud, J.; Villeneuve, P.; Khouja, M.L.; Mayer, P.; Boukhchina, S. Fatty acids, 4-desmethylsterols, and triterpene alcohols from Tunisian lentisc (Pistacialentiscus) fruits. *Eur. J. Lipid Sci. Technol.* **2012**, *114*, 968–973. [CrossRef]
53. Gimeno, E.; Castellote, A.I.; Lamuela-Raventós, R.M.; De la Torre, M.C.; López-Sabater, M.C. The effects of harvest and extraction methods on the antioxidant content (phenolics, α-tocopherol, and β-carotene) in virgin olive oil. *Food Chem.* **2002**, *78*, 207–211. [CrossRef]
54. Matos, L.C.; Pereira, J.A.; Andrade, P.B.; Seabra, R.M.; Oliveira, M.B.P. Evaluation of a numerical method to predict the polyphenols content in monovarietal olive oils. *Food Chem.* **2007**, *102*, 976–983. [CrossRef]
55. Debbabi, M.; Zarrouk, A.; Bezine, M.; Meddeb, W.; Nury, T.; Badreddine, A.; Sghaier, R.; Bretillon, L.; Guyot, S.; Samadi, M.; et al. Comparison of the effects of major fatty acids present in the Mediterranean diet (oleic acid, docosahexaenoic acid) and in hydrogenated oils (elaidic acid) on 7-ketocholesterol-induced oxiapoptophagy in microglial BV-2 cells. *Chem. Phys. Lipids* **2017**, *207*, 151–170. [CrossRef]
56. Yammine, A.; Nury, T.; Vejux, A.; Latruffe, N.; Vervandier-Fasseur, D.; Samadi, M.; Gretige-Gerges, H.; Auezova, L.; Lizard, G. Prevention of 7-Ketocholesterol-Induced Overproduction of Reactive Oxygen Species, Mitochondrial Dysfunction and Cell Death with Major Nutrients (Polyphenols, ω3 and ω9 Unsaturated Fatty Acids) of the Mediterranean Diet on N2a Neuronal Cells. *Molecules* **2020**, *25*, 2296. [CrossRef]
57. Singleton, V.L.; Rossi, J.A. Colorimetry of total phenolics with phosphomolybdic-phosphotungstic acid reagents. *Am. J. Enol. Vitic.* **1965**, *16*, 144–158.
58. Kim, D.O.; Chun, O.K.; Kim, Y.J.; Moon, H.Y.; Lee, C.Y. Quantification of polyphenolics and their antioxidant capacity in fresh plums. *J. Agric. Food Chem.* **2003**, *51*, 6509–6515. [CrossRef]
59. Dhibi, M.; Issaoui, M.; Brahmi, F.; Mechri, B.; Mnari, A.; Cheraif, I.; etSkhiri, F.; Galzzah, N.; Hammami, M. Nutritional quality of fresh and heated Aleppo pine (*Pinus halepensis* Mill.) seed oil: Trans-fatty acid isomers profiles and antioxidant properties. *J. Food Sci. Technol.* **2014**, *51*, 1442–1452. [CrossRef]
60. Moilanen, T.; Nikkari, T. The effect of storage on the fatty acid composition of human serum. *Clin. Chim. Acta* **1981**, *114*, 111–116. [CrossRef]
61. Morrison, W.R.; Smith, L.M. Preparation of fatty acid methyl esters and dimethylacetals from lipids with boron fluoride–methanol. *J. Lipid Res.* **1964**, *5*, 600–608. [CrossRef]
62. Zarrouk, A.; Martine, L.; Grégoire, S.; Nury, T.; Meddeb, W.; Camus, E.; Badreddine, A.; Durand, P.; Namsi, A.; Yammine, A.; et al. Profile of fatty acids, tocopherols, phytosterols and polyphenols in mediterranean oils (argan oils, olive oils, milk thistle seed oils and nigella seed oil) and evaluation of their antioxidant and cytoprotective activities. *Curr. Pharm. Des.* **2019**, *25*, 1791–1805. [CrossRef] [PubMed]
63. Molyneux, P. The use of the stable free radical diphenylpicrylhydrazyl (DPPH) for estimating antioxidant activity. Songklanakarin. *J. Sci. Technol.* **2004**, *26*, 211–219.
64. Bassene, E. *Initiation à la Recherche sur les Substances Naturelles: Extraction-Analyse-Essais Biologiques*; Presses Universitaires de Dakar: Dakar, Sénégal, 2012.
65. Dinis, T.C.; Madeira, V.M.; Almeida, L.M. Action of phenolic derivatives (acetaminophen, salicylate, and 5-aminosalicylate) as inhibitors of membrane lipid peroxidation and as peroxyl radical scavengers. *Arch. Biochem. Biophys.* **1994**, *315*, 161–169. [CrossRef] [PubMed]
66. Rossi, R.; Pastorelli, G.; Corino, C. Application of KRL test to assess total antioxidant activity in pigs: Sensitivity to dietary antioxidants. *Res. Vet. Sci.* **2013**, *94*, 372–377. [CrossRef]
67. Ragot, K.; Mackrill, J.J.; Zarrouk, A.; Nury, T.; Aires, V.; Jacquin, A.; Athias, A.; de Barros, J.-P.P.; Vejux, A.; Riedinger, J.-M.; et al. Absence of correlation between oxysterol accumulation in lipid raft microdomains, calcium increase, and apoptosis induction on 158N murine oligodendrocytes. *Biochem. Pharm.* **2013**, *86*, 67–79. [CrossRef]
68. Jones, K.H.; Senft, J.A. An improved method to determine cell viability by simultaneous staining with fluorescein diacetate-propidium iodide. *J. Histochem. Cytochem.* **1985**, *33*, 77–79. [CrossRef]
69. Patková, J.; Anděl, M.; Trnka, J. Palmitate-induced cell death and mitochondrial respiratory dysfunction in myoblasts are not prevented by mitochondria-targeted antioxidants. *Cell Physiol. Biochem.* **2014**, *33*, 1439–1451. [CrossRef]

70. Cui, L.; Zhou, Q.; Zheng, X.; Sun, B.; Zhao, S. Mitoquinone attenuates vascular calcification by suppressing oxidative stress and reducing apoptosis of vascular smooth muscle cells via the Keap1/Nrf2 pathway. *Free Radic. Biol. Med.* **2020**, *161*, 23–31. [CrossRef]
71. Yeh, C.J.; His, B.L.; Faulk, W.P. Propidium iodide as a nuclear marker in immunofluorescence. II. Use with cellular identification and viability studies. *J. Immunol Methods* **1981**, *43*, 269–275. [CrossRef]
72. Rothe, G.; Valet, G. Flow cytometric analysis of respiratory burst activity in phagocytes with hydroethidine and 2′, 7′-dichlorofluorescin. *J. Leukoc. Biol.* **1990**, *47*, 440–448. [CrossRef]
73. Flohe, L.; Günzler, W.A. Assays of glutathione peroxidase. *Methods Enzym.* **1984**, *105*, 114–120.
74. Beauchamp, C.; Fridovich, I. Superoxide dismutase: Improved assays and an assay applicable to acrylamide gels. *Anal. Biochem.* **1971**, *44*, 276–287. [CrossRef]
75. Yoshioka, T.; Kawada, K.; Shimada, T.; Mori, M. Lipid peroxidation in maternal and cord blood and protective mechanism against activated-oxygen toxicity in the blood. *Am. J. Obstet. Gynecol.* **1979**, *135*, 372–376. [CrossRef]
76. Esterbauer, H.; Striegl, G.; Puhl, H.; Rotheneder, M. Continuous monitoring of in vitro oxidation of human low density lipoprotein. *Free Radic. Res. Commun.* **1989**, *6*, 67–75. [CrossRef]
77. Oliver, C.N.; Ahn, B.W.; Moerman, E.J.; Goldstein, S.; Stadtman, E.R. Age-related changes in oxidized proteins. *J. Biol. Chem.* **1987**, *262*, 5488–5491. [CrossRef]
78. Zarrouk, A.; Vejux, A.; Nury, T.; El Hajj, H.I.; Haddad, M.; Cherkaoui-Malki, M.; Rietdinger, J.-M.; Hammami, M.; Lizard, G. Induction of mitochondrial changes associated with oxidative stress on very long chain fatty acids (C22: 0, C24: 0, or C26: 0)-treated human neuronal cells (SK-NB-E). *Oxidative Med. Cell Longev.* **2012**, *2012*, 623257. [CrossRef]
79. Gray, E.; Rice, C.; Hares, K.; Redondo, J.; Kemp, K.; Williams, M.; etBrown, A.; Scolding, N.; Wilkins, A. Reductions in neuronal peroxisomes in multiple sclerosis grey matter. *Mult. Scler. J.* **2014**, *20*, 651–659. [CrossRef]
80. Nury, T.; Sghaier, R.; Zarrouk, A.; Ménétrier, F.; Uzun, T.; Leoni, V.; Caccia, C.; Meddeb, W.; Namsi, A.; Sassi, K.; et al. Induction of peroxisomal changes in oligodendrocytes treated with 7-ketocholesterol: Attenuation by α-tocopherol. *Biochimie* **2018**, *153*, 181–202. [CrossRef]
81. Savary, S.; Trompier, D.; Andréoletti, P.; Le Borgne, F.; Demarquoy, J.; Lizard, G. Fatty acids-induced lipotoxicity and inflammation. *Curr. Drug Metab.* **2012**, *13*, 1358–1370. [CrossRef]
82. Blondelle, J.; de Barros, J.P.P.; Pilot-Storck, F.; Tiret, L. Targeted lipidomic analysis of myoblasts by GC-MS and LC-MS/MS. In *Skeletal Muscle Development*; Humana Press: New York, NY, USA, 2017; pp. 39–60.
83. Folch, J.; Lees, M.; Stanley, G.S. A simple method for the isolation and purification of total lipides from animal tissues. *J. Biol. Chem.* **1957**, *226*, 497–509. [CrossRef]
84. Lizard, G.; Fournel, S.; Genestier, L.; Dhedin, N.; Chaput, C.; Flacher, M.; Mutin, M.; Panayet, G.; Revillalrd, J.-P. Kinetics of plasma membrane and mitochondrial alterations in cells undergoing apoptosis. *Cytom. J. Int. Soc. Anal. Cytol.* **1995**, *21*, 275–283. [CrossRef] [PubMed]
85. Baarine, M.; Ragot, K.; Genin, E.C.; El Hajj, H.; Trompier, D.; Andreoletti, P.; Ghandour, S.; Menetrier, F.; Cherkaoui-Malki, M.; Savary, S.; et al. Peroxisomal and mitochondrial status of two murine oligodendrocytic cell lines (158N, 158JP): Potential models for the study of peroxisomal disorders associated with dysmyelination processes. *J. Neurochem.* **2009**, *111*, 119–131. [CrossRef] [PubMed]
86. Badreddine, A.; Zarrouk, A.; Karym, E.M.; Debbabi, M.; Nury, T.; Meddeb, W.; Sghaier, R.; Bezine, M.; Vejux, A.; Martine, L.; et al. Argan oil-mediated attenuation of organelle dysfunction, oxidative stress and cell death induced by 7-ketocholesterol in murine oligodendrocytes 158N. *Int. J. Mol. Sci.* **2017**, *18*, 2220. [CrossRef] [PubMed]
87. Sottero, B.; Rossin, D.; Staurenghi, E.; Gamba, P.; Poli, G.; Testa, G. Omics analysis of oxysterols to better understand their pathophysiological role. *Free Radic. Biol. Med.* **2019**, *144*, 55–71. [CrossRef]
88. Fujita, T.; Adachi, J.; Ueno, Y.; Peters, T.J.; Preedy, V.R. Chronic ethanol feeding increases 7-hydroperoxycholesterol and oxysterols in rat skeletal muscle. *Metab. -Clin. Exp.* **2002**, *51*, 737–742. [CrossRef]
89. Jamadagni, P.; Patten, S.A. 25-hydroxycholesterol impairs neuronal and muscular development in zebrafish. *Neurotoxicology* **2019**, *75*, 14–23. [CrossRef]
90. Nishi, H.; Higashihara, T.; Inagi, R. Lipotoxicity in kidney, heart, and skeletal muscle dysfunction. *Nutrients* **2019**, *11*, 1664. [CrossRef]
91. Kemp, S.; Theodoulou, F.L.; Wanders, R.J. Mammalian peroxisomal ABC transporters: From endogenous substrates to pathology and clinical significance. *Br. J. Pharmacol.* **2011**, *164*, 1753–1766. [CrossRef]
92. Tawbeh, A.; Gondcaille, C.; Trompier, D.; Savary, S. Peroxisomal ABC Transporters: An Update. *Int. J. Mol. Sci.* **2021**, *22*, 6093. [CrossRef]
93. Trompier, D.; Vejux, A.; Zarrouk, A.; Gondcaille, C.; Geillon, F.; Nury, T.; etSavary, S.; Lizalrd, G. Brain peroxisomes. *Biochimie* **2014**, *98*, 102–110. [CrossRef]
94. Jakobsson, A.; Westerberg, R.; Jacobsson, A. Fatty acid elongases in mammals: Their regulation and roles in metabolism. *Prog. Lipid Res.* **2006**, *45*, 237–249. [CrossRef]
95. Kihara, A. Very long-chain fatty acids: Elongation, physiology and related disorders. *J. Biochem.* **2021**, *152*, 387–395. [CrossRef]
96. Musaro, A.; Fulle, S.; Fano, G. Oxidative stress and muscle homeostasis. *Curr. Opin. Clin. Nutr. Metab. Care* **2010**, *13*, 236–242. [CrossRef]

97. Powers, S.K.; Talbert, E.E.; Adhihetty, P.J. Reactive oxygen and nitrogen species as intracellular signals in skeletal muscle. *J. Physiol.* **2011**, *589*, 2129–2138. [CrossRef]
98. Valko, M.; Leibfritz, D.; Moncol, J.; Cronin, M.T.; Mazur, M.; Telser, J. Free radicals and antioxidants in normal physiological functions and human disease. *Int. J. Biochem. Cell Biol.* **2007**, *39*, 44–84. [CrossRef]
99. Pistollato, F.; Giampieri, F.; Battino, M. The use of plant-derived bioactive compounds to target cancer stem cells and modulate tumor microenvironment. *Food Chem. Toxicol.* **2015**, *75*, 58–70. [CrossRef]
100. Gaussen, H.; Leroy, J.F.; Ozenda, P. *Précis de Botanique. 2- Végétaux Supérieurs*, 2nd ed.; Editions Masson: Paris, France, 1982; pp. 307–308.
101. Fazeli-nasab, B.; Fooladvand, Z. Classification and Evaluation of medicinal plant and medicinal properties of mastic. *Int. J. Adv. Biol. Biomed. Res.* **2014**, *2*, 2155–2161.
102. Brahmi, F.; Haddad, S.; Bouamara, K.; Yalaoui-Guellal, D.; Prost-Camus, E.; De Barros, J.P.P.; Prost, M.; Atanasov, A.G.; Madani, K.; Boulekbache-Makhlouf, L.; et al. Comparison of chemical composition and biological activities of Algerian seed oils of *Pistacialentiscus* L., *Opuntia ficusindica* (L.) mill. and Argania spinosa L. Skeels. *Ind. Crop. Products* **2020**, *151*, 112456. [CrossRef]
103. Bouyahya, A.; Dakka, N.; Talbaoui, A.; El Moussaoui, N.; Abrini, J.; Bakri, Y. Phenolic contents and antiradical capacity of vegetable oil from *Pistacialentiscus* (L). *J. Mater. Environ. Sci.* **2018**, *9*, 1518–1524.
104. Maria, A.G.; Graziano, R.; Nicolantonio, D.O. Carotenoids: Potential allies of cardiovascular health? *Food Nutr. Res.* **2015**, *59*, 26762. [CrossRef]
105. Smith, T.A. Carotenoids and cancer: Prevention and potential therapy. *Br. J. Biomed. Sci.* **1998**, *55*, 268.
106. Kitakaze, T.; Harada, N.; Imagita, H.; Yamaji, R. β-Carotene increases muscle mass and hypertrophy in the soleus muscle in mice. *J. Nutr. Sci. Vitaminol.* **2015**, *61*, 481–487. [CrossRef]
107. Dhifi, W.; Jelali, N.; Chaabani, E.; Beji, M.; Fatnassi, S.; Omri, S.; Mnif, W. Chemical composition of Lentisk (*Pistacialentiscus* L.) seed oil. *Afr. J. Agric. Res.* **2013**, *8*, 1395–1400.
108. Aguilera, C.M.; Ramírez-Tortosa, M.C.; Mesa, M.D.; Gil, A. Do MUFA and PUFA have beneficial effects on the development of cardiovascular disease? *Recent Res. Dev. Lipids* **2000**, *4*, 369–390.
109. Debbabi, M.; Nury, T.; Zarrouk, A.; Mekahli, N.; Bezine, M.; Sghaier, R.; Grégoire, S.; Martine, L.; Durand, P.; Prost, E.; et al. Protective effects of α-tocopherol, γ-tocopherol and oleic acid, three compounds of olive oils, and no effect of trolox, on 7-ketocholesterol-induced mitochondrial and peroxisomal dysfunction in microglial BV-2 cells. *Int. J. Mol. Sci.* **2016**, *17*, 1973. [CrossRef]
110. Jandacek, R.J. Linoleic Acid: A Nutritional Quandary. *Healthcare* **2017**, *5*, 25. [CrossRef]
111. Lee, J.H.; Tachibana, H.; Morinaga, Y.; Fujimura, Y.; Yamada, K. Modulation of proliferation and differentiation of C2C12 skeletal muscle cells by fatty acids. *Life Sci.* **2009**, *84*, 415–420. [CrossRef] [PubMed]
112. Charef, M.; Yousfi, M.; Saidi, M.; Stocker, P. Determination of the fatty acid composition of acorn (Quercus), Pistacialentiscus seeds growing in Algeria. *J. Am. Oil Chem. Soc.* **2008**, *85*, 921–924. [CrossRef]
113. French, M.A.; Sundram, K.; Clandinin, M.T. Cholesterolaemic effect of palmitic acid in relation to other dietary fatty acids. *Asia Pac. J. Clin. Nutr.* **2002**, *11*, S401–S407. [CrossRef] [PubMed]
114. Hwang, S.-L.; Kim, H.-N.; Jung, H.-H.; Kim, J.-E.; Choi, D.-K.; Hur, J.-M.; Lee, J.-Y.; Song, H.; Song, K.-S.; Huh, T.-L. Beneficial effects of β-sitosterol on glucose and lipid metabolism in L6 myotube cells are mediated by AMP-activated protein kinase. *Biochem. Biophys. Res. Commun.* **2008**, *377*, 1253–1258. [CrossRef] [PubMed]
115. Liao, P.-C.; Lai, M.-H.; Hsu, K.-P.; Kuo, Y.-H.; Chen, J.; Tsai, M.-C.; Li, C.-X.; Yin, X.-J.; Jetyashoke, N.; Chao, L.K.-P. Identification of β-sitosterol as in vitro anti-inflammatory constituent in Moringa oleifera. *J. Agric. Food Chem.* **2018**, *66*, 10748–10759. [CrossRef]
116. Gupta, R.; Sharma, A.K.; Dobhal, M.P.; Sharma, M.C.; Gupta, R.S. Antidiabetic and antioxidant potential of β-sitosterol in streptozotocin-induced experimental hyperglycemia. *J. Diabetes* **2011**, *3*, 29–37. [CrossRef]
117. Wong, H.S.; Leong, P.K.; Chen, J.; Leung, H.Y.; Chan, W.M.; Ko, K.M. β-Sitosterol increases mitochondrial electron transport by fluidizing mitochondrial membranes and enhances mitochondrial responsiveness to increasing energy demand by the induction of uncoupling in C2C12 myotubes. *J. Funct. Foods* **2016**, *23*, 253–260. [CrossRef]
118. Chen, Y. Endogenous Phenolics from Expeller-Pressed Canola Oil Refining Byproducts: Evaluation of Antioxidant Activities in Cell Culture and Deep-Fat Frying Models. Master's Thesis, University of Manitoba, Winnipeg, MB, Canada, 2014.
119. Zingg, J.M.; Meydani, M. Interaction between vitamin E and polyunsaturated fatty acids. In *Vitamin E in Human Health*; Humana Press: Cham, Switzerland, 2019; pp. 141–159.
120. Rimbach, G.; Minihane, A.M.; Majewicz, J.; Fischer, A.; Pallauf, J.; Virgli, F.; Weinberg, P.D. Regulation of cell signalling by vitamin E. *Proc. Nutr. Soc.* **2002**, *61*, 415–425. [CrossRef]
121. Testa, G.; Rossin, D.; Poli, G.; Biasi, F.; Leonarduzzi, G. Implication of oxysterols in chronic inflammatory human diseases. *Biochimie* **2018**, *153*, 220–231. [CrossRef]
122. Pedruzzi, E.; Guichard, C.; Ollivier, V.; Driss, F.; Fay, M.; Prunet, C.; Marie, J.-C.; Pouzet, C.; Samadi, M.; Elbim, C.; et al. NAD (P) H oxidase Nox-4 mediates 7-ketocholesterol-induced endoplasmic reticulum stress and apoptosis in human aortic smooth muscle cells. *Mol. Cell. Biol.* **2004**, *24*, 10703–10717. [CrossRef]
123. Szentesi, P.; Csernoch, L.; Dux, L.; Keller-Pintér, A. Changes in redox signaling in the skeletal muscle with aging. *Oxidative Med. Cell Longev.* **2019**, *2019*. [CrossRef]

124. Nury, T.; Zarrouk, A.; Yammine, A.; Mackrill, J.J.; Vejux, A.; Lizard, G. Oxiapoptophagy: A type of cell death induced by some oxysterols. *Br. J. Pharmacol.* **2021**, *178*, 3115–3123. [CrossRef]
125. Sghaier, R.; Nury, T.; Leoni, V.; Caccia, C.; De Barros, J.-P.P.; Cherif, A.; Vejux, A.; Moreau, T.; Limem, K.; Samadi, M.; et al. Dimethyl fumarate and monomethyl fumarate attenuate oxidative stress and mitochondrial alterations leading to oxiapoptophagy in 158N murine oligodendrocytes treated with 7β-hydroxycholesterol. *J. Steroidbiochemistry Mol.* **2019**, *194*, 105432. [CrossRef]
126. Yammine, A.; Zarrouk, A.; Nury, T.; Vejux, A.; Latruffe, N.; Vervandier-Fasseur, D.; Samadi, M.; Mackrill, J.J.; Greige-Gerges, H.; Auezova, L.; et al. Prevention by dietary polyphenols (resveratrol, quercetin, apigenin) against 7-ketocholesterol-induced oxiapoptophagy in neuronal N2a cells: Potential interest for the treatment of neurodegenerative and age-related diseases. *Cells* **2020**, *9*, 2346. [CrossRef]
127. Poli, G.; Biasi, F.; Leonarduzzi, G. Oxysterols in the pathogenesis of major chronic diseases. *Redox Biol.* **2013**, *1*, 125–130. [CrossRef]
128. Kunzelmann, K. Ion channels in regulated cell death. *Cell Mol. Life Sci.* **2016**, *73*, 2387–2403. [CrossRef]
129. Bezine, M.; Namsi, A.; Sghaier, R.; Ben Khalifa, R.B.; Hamdouni, H.; Brahmi, F.; Badreddine, I.; Mihoubi, W.; Nury, T.; Vejux, A.; et al. The effect of oxysterols on nerve impulses. *Biochimie* **2018**, *153*, 46–51. [CrossRef]
130. Zarrouk, A.; Ben Salem, Y.B.; Hafsa, J.; Sghaier, R.; Charfeddine, B.; Limem, K.; etHammami, M.; Maljdoub, H. 7β-hydroxycholesterol-induced cell death, oxidative stress, and fatty acid metabolism dysfunctions attenuated with sea urchin egg oil. *Biochimie* **2018**, *153*, 210–219. [CrossRef]
131. Rufini, A.; Tucci, P.; Celardo, I.; Melino, G. Senescence and aging: The critical roles of p53. *Oncogene* **2013**, *32*, 5129–5143. [CrossRef]
132. Lismont, C.; Nordgren, M.; Van Veldhoven, P.P.; Fransen, M. Redox interplay between mitochondria and peroxisomes. *Front. Cell Dev. Biol.* **2015**, *3*, 35. [CrossRef]
133. Pascual-Ahuir, A.; Manzanares-Estreder, S.; Proft, M. Pro-and antioxidant functions of the peroxisome-mitochondria connection and its impact on aging and disease. *Oxidative Med. Cell Longev.* **2017**, *2017*, 9860841. [CrossRef]
134. Baarine, M.; Andreoletti, P.; Athias, A.; Nury, T.; Zarrouk, A.; Ragot, K. Evidence of oxidative stress in very long chain fatty acid–treated oligodendrocytes and potentialization of ROS production using RNA interference-directed knockdown of ABCD1 and ACOX1 peroxisomal proteins. *Neuroscience* **2012**, *213*, 1–18. [CrossRef] [PubMed]
135. Wanders, R.J. Metabolic functions of peroxisomes in health and disease. *Biochimie* **2014**, *98*, 36–44. [CrossRef]
136. Titorenko, V.I.; Terlecky, S.R. Peroxisome metabolism and cellular aging. *Traffic* **2011**, *12*, 252–259. [CrossRef]
137. Unger, R.H.; Orci, L. Lipoapoptosis: Its mechanism and its diseases. *Biochim. Et Biophys. Acta -Mol. Cell Biol. Lipids* **2002**, *1585*, 202–212. [CrossRef]
138. Amery, L.; Fransen, M.; De Nys, K.; Mannaerts, G.P.; Van Veldhoven, P.P. Mitochondrial and peroxisomal targeting of 2-methylacyl-CoA racemase in humans. *J. Lipid Res.* **2000**, *41*, 1752–1759. [CrossRef]
139. Cecatto, C.; Amaral, A.U.; Roginski, A.C.; Castilho, R.F.; Wajner, M. Impairment of mitochondrial bioenergetics and permeability transition induction caused by major long-chain fatty acids accumulating in VLCAD deficiency in skeletal muscle as potential pathomechanisms of myopathy. *Toxicol. Vitr.* **2020**, *62*, 104665. [CrossRef] [PubMed]
140. Ben Khedir, S.; Moalla, D.; Jardak, N.; Mzid, M.; Sahnoun, Z.; Rebai, T. Pistacia lentiscus fruit oil reduces oxidative stress in human skin explants caused by hydrogen peroxide. *Biotech. Histochem.* **2016**, *91*, 480–491. [CrossRef]
141. Kang, J.S.; Han, M.H.; Kim, G.-Y.; Kim, C.M.; Chung, H.Y.; Hwang, H.J.; Kim, B.W.; Choi, Y.H. Schisandrae semen essential oil attenuates oxidative stress-induced cell damage in C2C12 murine skeletal muscle cells through Nrf2-mediated upregulation of HO-1. *Int. J. Mol.* **2015**, *35*, 453–459. [CrossRef]
142. Choi, Y.H. Protective effects of isorhamnetin against hydrogen peroxide-induced apoptosis in c2c12 murine myoblasts. *J. Korean Med. Obes. Res.* **2015**, *15*, 93–103. [CrossRef]
143. Leporini, L.; Giampietro, L.; Amoroso, R.; Ammazzalorso, A.; Fantacuzzi, M.; Menghini, L.; Maccallini, C.; Ferrante, C.; Brunetti, L.; Orlando, G.; et al. In vitro protective effects of resveratrol and stilbene alkanoic derivatives on induced oxidative stress on C2C12 and MCF7 cells. *J. Biol. Regul. Homeost. Agents* **2017**, *31*, 589–601.
144. Li, J.; Yang, Q.; Han, L.; Pan, C.; Lei, C.; Chen, H.; Lan, X. C2C12 mouse myoblasts damage induced by oxidative stress is alleviated by the antioxidant capacity of the active substance phloretin. *Front. Cell Dev. Biol.* **2020**, *8*, 953. [CrossRef]
145. Badreddine, A.; Zarrouk, A.; Meddeb, W.; Nury, T.; Rezig, L.; Debbabi, M.; Bessam, F.Z.; Brahmi, F.; Vejux, A.; Mejri, M.; et al. Antioxidant and neuroprotective properties of Mediterranean Oils: Argan Oil, Olive Oil, and Milk Thistle Seed Oil. In *Oxidative Stress and Dietary Antioxidants in Neurological Diseases*; Elsevier: Amsterdam, The Netherlands, 2020; pp. 143–154.
146. Brahmi, F.; Vejux, A.; Sghaier, R.; Zarrouk, A.; Nury, T.; Meddeb, W.; Rezig, L.; Namsi, A.; Sassi, K.; Yammine, A.; et al. Prevention of 7-ketocholesterol-induced side effects by natural compounds. *Crit. Rev. Food Sci. Nutr.* **2019**, *59*, 3179–3198. [CrossRef]

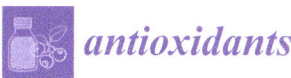

Article

Siegesbeckiae Herba Extract and Chlorogenic Acid Ameliorate the Death of HaCaT Keratinocytes Exposed to Airborne Particulate Matter by Mitigating Oxidative Stress

Jae Won Ha and Yong Chool Boo *

Department of Molecular Medicine, School of Medicine, BK21 Plus KNU Biomedical Convergence Program, Cell and Matrix Research Institute, Kyungpook National University, 680 Gukchaebosang-ro, Jung-gu, Daegu 41944, Korea; jaewon1226@knu.ac.kr
* Correspondence: ycboo@knu.ac.kr; Tel.: +82-53-420-4946

Citation: Ha, J.W.; Boo, Y.C. Siegesbeckiae Herba Extract and Chlorogenic Acid Ameliorate the Death of HaCaT Keratinocytes Exposed to Airborne Particulate Matter by Mitigating Oxidative Stress. *Antioxidants* **2021**, *10*, 1762. https://doi.org/10.3390/antiox10111762

Academic Editors: Daniela-Saveta Popa, Laurian Vlase, Marius Emil Rusu and Ionel Fizesan

Received: 3 October 2021
Accepted: 2 November 2021
Published: 4 November 2021

Publisher's Note: MDPI stays neutral with regard to jurisdictional claims in published maps and institutional affiliations.

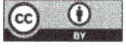

Copyright: © 2021 by the authors. Licensee MDPI, Basel, Switzerland. This article is an open access article distributed under the terms and conditions of the Creative Commons Attribution (CC BY) license (https://creativecommons.org/licenses/by/4.0/).

Abstract: Airborne particulate matter with a size of 10 μm or less (PM_{10}) can cause oxidative damages and inflammatory reactions in the skin. This study was conducted to discover natural products that are potentially useful in protecting the skin from PM_{10}. Among the hot water extracts of a total of 23 medicinal plants, Siegesbeckiae Herba extract (SHE), which showed the strongest protective effect against PM_{10} cytotoxicity, was selected, and its mechanism of action and active constituents were explored. SHE ameliorated PM_{10}-induced cell death, lactate dehydrogenase (LDH) release, lipid peroxidation, and reactive oxygen species (ROS) production in HaCaT cells. SHE decreased the expression of KEAP1, a negative regulator of NRF2, and increased the expression of NRF2 target genes, such as HMOX1 and NQO1. SHE selectively induced the enzymes involved in the synthesis of GSH (GCL-c and GCL-m), the regeneration of GSH (GSR and G6PDH), and GSH conjugation of xenobiotics (GSTκ1), rather than the enzymes that directly scavenge ROS (SOD1, CAT, and GPX1). SHE increased the cellular content of GSH and mitigated the oxidation of GSH to GSSG caused by PM_{10} exposure. Of the solvent fractions of SHE, the n-butyl alcohol (BA) fraction ameliorated cell death in both the absence and presence of PM_{10}. The BA fraction contained a high amount of chlorogenic acid. Chlorogenic acid reduced PM_{10}-induced cell death, LDH release, and ROS production. This study suggests that SHE protects cells from PM_{10} toxicity by increasing the cellular antioxidant capacity and that chlorogenic acid may be an active phytochemical of SHE.

Keywords: Siegesbeckiae Herba; *Siegesbeckia pubescens* Makino; airborne particulate matter; PM_{10}; glutamate-cysteine ligase; nuclear factor erythroid 2-related factor 2; glutathione; chlorogenic acid; caffeic acid

1. Introduction

Air pollution, exacerbated by rapid climate change and industrial development, poses a major environmental factor that threatens human health [1]. Particulate matter (PM) suspended in the atmosphere is a complex material that contains various organic compounds and heavy metals [2]. Continued exposure to high concentrations of PM increases the incidence of various diseases, including respiratory and cardiovascular diseases, and mortality [3]. PM with an approximate diameter of less than 10 or 2.5 μm is called PM_{10} and $PM_{2.5}$, respectively [4].

As the interface between the body and the environment, the skin acts as a barrier to protect our body from environmental pollutants, but it is an organ directly exposed to environmental pollutants. The pores of the skin are large enough for PM to penetrate [5], and children with immature skin or patients with compromised skin barriers are relatively vulnerable to the percutaneous absorption and damage of PM compared to healthy adults [6–8]. PM exacerbates inflammatory skin diseases, such as atopic dermatitis, acne, and psoriasis by various mechanisms [3,9].

PM exposure stimulates Ca^{2+} signaling and increases the production of reactive oxygen species (ROS), such as superoxide radical (O$_2^{\bullet -}$), hydrogen peroxide (H$_2$O$_2$), and hydroxyl radical ($^{\bullet}$OH) [10]. Aryl hydrocarbons contained in PM increase the production of ROS in the process of metabolism [11]. Transition metal components also catalyze chemical reactions that generate ROS [12]. PM stimulates the NADPH oxidase family to increase ROS production [13]. Among the NADPH oxidase family, dual oxidase 2 has been reported to mediate the generation of ROS stimulated by PM$_{10}$ or house dust mites [14,15].

PM enhances the expression of cyclooxygenase 2 and increases the production of the eicosanoid mediator prostaglandin E$_2$ [16,17]. In addition, it stimulates the cell signaling system to increase the secretion of inflammatory cytokines, such as tumor necrosis factor-α, interleukin (IL)-1β, IL-6, and IL-8 [18]. PM also stimulates the expression of matrix metalloproteinases (MMPs), leading to increased degradation of the extracellular matrix, such as collagen [19]. Thus, there is a need for antioxidative countermeasures against skin inflammation and aging due to PM.

Plants are a good source of natural products with biological activities that are potentially useful for maintaining skin health and beauty [20–23]. It should be noted that certain phytochemicals can act as either antioxidants or prooxidants and have a positive or negative effect on cell survival depending on their type and concentration [24–27]. Phytochemicals that can reduce cellular oxidative stress directly or indirectly are expected to provide a useful strategy to reduce PM-induced skin inflammation and aging [28]. They can directly scavenge ROS or enhance cellular antioxidant capacity by inducing nuclear factor erythroid 2-related factor (NRF) 2-mediated gene expression [29]. In a previous study, our research team found that several phenolic compounds derived from terrestrial and marine plants, such as punicalagin, (−)-epigallocatechin-3-gallate, and dieckol relieve oxidative damage and reduce ROS production in HaCaT cells stimulated by PM$_{10}$ and inhibit the subsequent cell signaling process and inflammatory responses [17,18,26].

This study aimed to discover a natural product that effectively relieves PM$_{10}$-induced cytotoxicity and oxidative stress. To this end, the effects of several medicinal plant extracts on the viability of HaCaT keratinocytes exposed to PM$_{10}$ were compared. As a result, Siegesbeckiae Herba extract (SHE) among the extracts of 23 medicinal plants, most effectively defended against PM$_{10}$ cytotoxicity. Siegesbeckiae Herba generally refers to the dried aerial parts of *Siegesbeckia orientalis* L, *Siegesbeckia pubescens* Makino, and *Siegesbeckia glabrescens* Makino, and has been used as a traditional medicine in Korea, Japan, China, and Vietnam [30]. Studies on the phytochemicals and biological efficacy of SHE have been increasing recently [31,32]. However, studies on the protective action of SHE against PM cytotoxicity have not yet been reported. In the present study, the antioxidant properties of SHE prepared from the dried leaves of *Siegesbeckia pubescens* Makino were investigated in HaCaT cells exposed to PM$_{10}$, with a special focus on the mechanism of action and active constituents. The results of this study suggest that SHE increases cell defense gene expression and thereby mitigates cell death and oxidative damage caused by PM$_{10}$. It was also suggested that chlorogenic acid rather than caffeic acid may be the active constituent providing the cell protection effect.

2. Materials and Methods

2.1. Reagents

Standardized fine dust (PM$_{10}$-like) (European Reference Material ERM-CZ120), chlorogenic acid (Cat. C3878), and caffeic acid (Cat. C0625) were purchased from Sigma-Aldrich (St. Louis, MO, USA).

2.2. Extracts of Medicinal Plants

Medicinal plant extracts were obtained from the Plant Extract Bank of Korea (https://portal.kribb.re.kr/kpeb) (Cheongju, Korea). The plant sources and catalog numbers of the extracts used in this study are as follow; Castaneae Semen, CW01-011; Eucomiae Folium, CW01-052; Peucedani Japonici Radix, CW01-065; Melonis Calyx, CW02-003; Arisaematis

Rhizoma, CW02-006; Eucomiae Ramulus, CW02-011; Dioscoreae Rhizoma, CW02-051; Mori Ramulus, CW02-060; Pruni Humilidis Semen, CW02-085; Angelicae tenuissimae Radix, CW03-008; Fagopyri Semen, CW03-011; Aconiti Jaluencis Tuber, CW03-082; Biotae Orientalis Folium, CW03-084; Gardeniae Fructus, CW03-087; Vitis Viniferae Caulis, CW03-100; Benincasae Semen, CW04-004; Akebiae Caulis, CW04-006; Pini Ramulus, CW04-021; Pini Pollen, CW04-022; Machili Thunbergi Cortex, CW04-056; Cyperi Rhizoma, CW04-069; Glycine Semen nigra, CW04-098; Siegesbeckiae Herba, CW04-100.

2.3. Siegesbeckiae Herba Extract and Its Solvent Fractions

Dried Siegesbeckiae Herba (*Siegesbeckia pubescens* Makino) was purchased from Sinsun Herb (http://sinsunherb.co.kr) (Seoul, Korea) and its extract was prepared in this laboratory. Dried leaves (140 g) were ground and extracted with 0.9 L water at 90 °C for 1 h. The extracted solution was evaporated under reduced pressure to obtain the crude extract (9 g). The SHE was dispersed in 150 mL water and partitioned sequentially with an equal volume of methylene chloride (MC), ethyl acetate (EA), and n-butyl alcohol (BA). Evaporation of the organic solvents yielded MC fraction (0.27 g), EA fraction (0.16 g), and BA fraction (0.46 g). The aqueous layer was filtered to remove insoluble material (1.15 g) and then evaporated to obtain a water (WT) fraction (6.64 g).

2.4. High-Performance Liquid Chromatography with Photodiode Array Detection (HPLC-DAD)

HPLC-DAD analysis was carried out using a Waters Alliance HPLC system (Waters, Milford, MA, USA) consisting of an e2695 separation module and a 2996 photodiode array detector. The stationary phase was a Hector-M C_{18} column (4.6 mm × 250 mm, 5 m) (RS Tech Co., Daejeon, Korea). The mobile phase was a mixture of 0.1% phosphoric acid (A) and acetonitrile (B) with the following composition: 0–30 min, a linear gradient from 0 to 100% B; 30–40 min, 100% B. The solvent gradient program was as follows: 0–30 min, a linear gradient from 0 to 100% B; 30–40 min, 100% B; 40–45 min, a linear gradient from 100 to 0% B. The flow rate of the mobile phase was 0.6 mL min^{-1}. The sample injection volume was 10 µL.

2.5. Cell Culture and PM_{10} Treatment

HaCaT cells, an immortalized human keratinocyte cell line originally established by Dr. Fusenig [33], were obtained from Dr. In-San Kim (Kyungpook National University, Daegu, Korea) and cultured in a closed incubator at 37 °C in humidified air containing 5% CO_2. Cells were administered DMEM/F-12 medium (GIBCO-BRL, Grand Island, NY, USA) containing 10% fetal bovine serum, 100 U mL^{-1} penicillin, 100 µg mL^{-1} streptomycin, 0.25 µg mL^{-1} amphotericin B, and 10 µg mL^{-1} hydrocortisone every three days. Cells were cultured on 96-well, 12-well, or 6-well culture plates (SPL Life Sciences, Pocheon, Korea) for at least 24 h and then treated with either test materials, PM_{10}, or both, at the specified concentrations for up to 48 h.

2.6. Cell Viability and Lactate Dehydrogenase (LDH) Release Assays

Cell viability was assessed by a method using 3-(4,5-dimethylthiazol-2-yl)-2,5-diphenyl tetrazolium bromide (MTT) [34]. Cells were plated onto 96-well culture plates at 4×10^3 cells/well and maintained in a 200 µL culture medium for 24 h. The cells were treated with a vehicle or a test material and cultured in the absence or presence of PM_{10} (200 µg mL^{-1}) for 48 h. After discarding or saving the conditioned medium, adherent cells were incubated in a 100 µL growth medium containing 1 mg mL^{-1} MTT (Amresco, Solon, OH, USA) for 2 h in an incubator. After removing the medium and washing the cells with phosphate-buffered saline (PBS), the dye was extracted from the cells with 100 µL dimethyl sulfoxide, and the absorbance of the extracts was measured at 570 nm with a SPECTROstar nano microplate reader (BMG LABTECH GmbH, Ortenberg, Germany).

The saved medium was used in the assay for LDH release using the TaKaRa LDH cytotoxicity detection kit (TaKaRa Bio Inc., Shiga, Japan). Briefly, 50 µL aliquot of the medium diluted 2-times with PBS was mixed with 50 µL of the reaction mixture prepared according to manufacturer protocol (this mixture contains sodium lactate, diaphorase, NAD$^+$, and iodotetrazolium chloride). The final reaction mixture was incubated for 30 min at 25 °C and the absorbance was measured at 490 nm with a SPECTROstar nano microplate reader.

2.7. Cellular Lipid Peroxidation Assay

Cellular lipid peroxidation was assessed using a 2-thiobarbituric acid (TBA) method [35]. The cells were plated onto 6-well culture plates at 2×10^5 cells/well and maintained in a 2 mL culture medium for 24 h. The cells were treated with vehicle or test material and cultured in the absence or presence of PM_{10} (200 µg mL^{-1}) for 48 h. After discarding the medium and washing the cells with PBS, the adherent cells were lysed using the lysis buffer A (20 mM Tris-Cl, 2.5 mM ethylenediamine-N,N,N',N'-tetraacetic acid, 1.0% sodium dodecyl sulfate, pH 7.5). The assay mixture consisted of 100 µL cell lysate, 50 µL 1.0% meta-phosphoric acid, and 350 µL 0.9% TBA (Sigma-Aldrich), which was then heated in a boiling water bath for 45 min. After cooling, 500 µL N-butyl alcohol (BA) was added to the mixture, which was then vortex-mixed and centrifuged at 13,000 rpm for 15 min to produce two separate layers. The fluorescence intensity of the BA layer (excitation at 544 nm and emission at 590 nm) was measured by using a Gemini EM fluorescence microplate reader (Molecular Devices, Sunnyvale, CA, USA). Data are presented as thiobarbituric acid-reactive substance (TBARS) levels corrected for protein contents. A standard curve was prepared using 1,1,3,3-tetramethoxypropane (Sigma-Aldrich) as a donor of malondialdehyde.

2.8. Cellular ROS Production Assay

Cellular ROS production was assessed by using 2′,7′-dichlorodihydrofluorescein diacetate (DCFH-DA), a cell-permeable fluorescent dye sensitive to changes in the redox state of a cell [36]. The cells were plated onto 12-well culture plates at 8×10^4 cells/well for 24 h. Cells were pre-labeled with 10 µM DCFH-DA (Sigma-Aldrich) for 60 min and treated with 200 µg mL^{-1} PM_{10} alone or in combination with a test material at different concentrations for 60 min. Cells were washed twice with PBS and the images of cells fluorescing due to the oxidation of DCFH-DA were obtained with a LEICA DMI3000 B microscope (Leica Microsystems GmbH, Wetzlar, Germany). The dye was extracted from cells using the lysis buffer A (150 µL/well). The extracted solution was centrifuged at 13,000 rpm for 15 min and the supernatant was used for the measurement of fluorescence intensity (excitation at 485 nm and emission at 538 nm) with a Gemini EM fluorescence microplate reader.

2.9. Glutathione (GSH) and Glutathione Disulfide (GSSG) Assay

GSH and GSSG contents were measured in a recycling assay using 5,5′-dithio-bis-2-nitrobenzoic acid (DTNB) [37]. Cells were plated onto 6-well culture plates at 2×10^5 cells/well and maintained in a 2 mL culture medium for 24 h. The cells were treated with vehicle or test material and cultured in the absence or presence of PM_{10} (200 µg mL^{-1}) for 24 h. Cells were extracted using 5% meta-phosphoric acid (150 µL per well). The extracted solution was centrifuged at 13,000 rpm for 15 min and the supernatant was used for the measurement of GSH/GSSG, using a GSH/GSSG assay kit (product number GT40) from Oxford Biomedical Research (Oxford, UK). Total GSH plus GSSG content was measured using the extract as it is, and the GSSG content was quantified after pre-scavenging GSH in the extract with a pyridine derivative. Absorbance change due to reduction of DTNB was measured at 412 nm, and a calibration curve was prepared using a GSSG standard. The GSH content was calculated by subtracting the GSSG content from the total GSH plus GSSG content.

2.10. Quantitative Reverse Transcriptase-Polymerase Chain Reaction (qRT-PCR)

The mRNA levels of catalase (CAT), glucose 6-phosphate dehydrogenase (G6PDH), glutamate-cysteine ligase catalytic subunits (GCL-c), glutamate-cysteine ligase modifier subunit (GCL-m), glutathione disulfide reductase (GSR), glutathione peroxidase (GPX) 1, glutathione S-transferase (GST) κ1, heme oxygenase (HMOX) 1, kelch-like ECH-associated protein (KEAP) 1, NRF2, NAD(P)H quinone oxidoreductase (NQO) 1, and superoxide dismutase (SOD) 1 and were determined by qRT-PCR using a StepOnePlus Real-Time PCR System (Applied Biosystems, Foster City, CA, USA). The cells were plated onto 6-well culture plates at 2×10^5 cells/well and maintained in a 2 mL culture medium for 24 h. The cells were treated with vehicle or test material and cultured in the absence or presence of PM_{10} (200 µg mL^{-1}) for 24 h. Total cellular RNA was extracted from cells with an RNeasy kit (Qiagen, Valencia, CA, USA), and this RNA was used as a template for the synthesis of complementary DNA with a high-capacity cDNA archive kit (Applied Biosystems). Gene-specific primers for qRT-PCR were purchased from Macrogen (Seoul, Korea), and their nucleotide sequences are shown in Table 1. The qRT-PCR reaction mixture (20 µL) consisted of SYBR Green PCR Master Mix (Applied Biosystems), complementary DNA (60 ng), and gene-specific primer sets (2 picomole). Thermal cycling parameters were set as follows: 50 °C for 2 min, 95 °C for 10 min, 40 amplification cycles of 95 °C for 15 s and 60 °C for 1 min, and a dissociation step. In each run, the melting curve analysis confirmed the homogeneity of the PCR product. The mRNA levels of each gene were calculated relative to that of the internal reference, glyceraldehyde 3-phosphate dehydrogenase (GAPDH), using the comparative Ct method [37]. Ct is defined as the number of cycles required for the PCR signal to exceed the threshold level. Fold changes in the test group compared to the control group were calculated as $2^{-\Delta\Delta Ct}$, where $\Delta\Delta Ct = \Delta Ct_{(test)} - \Delta Ct_{(control)} = (Ct_{(gene, test)} - Ct_{(reference, test)}) - (Ct_{(gene, control)} - Ct_{(reference, control)})$.

Table 1. Sequences of primers used for the quantitative reverse transcriptase-polymerase chain reaction (qRT-PCR) of gene transcripts.

Gene Name	GenBank Accession #	Forward (F) and Reverse (R) Primer Sequences	Reference
Catalase (CAT)	NM_001752.4	F: 5′-CATCGCCACATGAATGGATA-3′ R: 5′-CCAACTGGGATGAGAGGGTA-3′	[38]
Glucose 6-phosphate dehydrogenase (G6PDH)	NM_001042351.3	F: 5′-GACATCCGCAAACAGAGTGA-3′ R: 5′-GGAGGCTGCATCATCGTACT-3′	[39]
Glutamate-cysteine ligase-catalytic subunit (GCL-c)	NM_001197115.2	F: 5′-CTGGGAGTGATTTCTGCAT-3′ R: 5′-AGGAGGGGGCTTAAATCTCA-3′	[40]
Glutamate-cysteine ligase-modifier subunit (GCL-m)	NM_002061.4	F: 5′-TTTGGTCAGGGAGTTTCCAG-3′ R: 5′-TGGTTTTACCTGTGCCCACT-3′	[40]
Glutathione disulfide reductase (GSR)	NM_000637.5	F: 5′-CCAGCTTAGGAATAACCAGCGATGG-3′ R: 5′-GTCTTTTTAACCTCCTTGACCTGGGAGAAC-3′	[41]
Glutathione peroxidase (GPX) 1	NM_001329503.2	F: 5′-TTCCCGTGCAACCAGTTTG-3′ R: 5′-GGACGTACTTGAGGGAATTCAGA-3′	[42]
Glutathione S-transferase (GST) κ1	NM_001143679.2	F: 5′-TCTCCAGATTCCCATCCACTTCCC-3′ R: 5′-CTGCGGCTCGGTGATGTCTTC-3′	[43]
Glyceraldehyde 3-phosphate dehydrogenase (GAPDH)	NM_001357943.2	F: 5′-ATGGGGAAGGTGAAGGTCG-3′ R: 5′-GGGGTCATTGATGGCAACAA-3′	[17]
Heme oxygenase (HMOX) 1	NM_002133.3	F: 5′-CGGGCCAGCAACAAAGTG-3′ R: 5′-ACTGTCGCCACCAGAAAGCT-3′	[44]
Kelch-like ECH-associated protein (KEAP) 1	NM_012289.4	F: 5′-CAGAGGTGGTGGTGTTGCTTAT-3′ R: 5′-AGCTCGTTCATGATGCCAAAG-3′	[45]
NAD(P)H quinone oxidoreductase (NQO) 1	NM_001025434.2	F: 5′-GCACTGATCGTACTGGCTCACT-3′ R: 5′-CCACCACCTCCCATCCTTT-3′	This study
Nuclear factor erythroid 2-related factor (NRF) 2	NM_006164.5	F: 5′-GAGAGCCCAGTCTTCATTGC-3′ R: 5′-ACTCGTTGGGGTCTTGTGTG-3′	This study
Superoxide dismutase (SOD) 1	NM_000454.5	F: 5′-AGGGCATCATCAATTTCGAG-3′ R: 5′-ACATTGCCCAAGTCTCCAAC-3′	[46]

2.11. Western Blotting

Western blotting was performed as previously described [47]. Primary antibodies for GCL-c (#390811), GCL-m (#55586), G6PDH (#373886), and β-actin (#47778) were purchased from Santa Cruz Biotechnology (Santa Cruz, CA, USA). Anti-rabbit IgG (#2357) and anti-goat IgG (#2020) secondary antibodies were purchased from Santa Cruz Biotechnology, and anti-mouse IgG (#7076) secondary antibody was purchased from Cell Signaling Technology (Danvers, MA, USA). Antibodies were diluted in TBST (137 mM sodium chloride, 20 mM Tris, 0.1% Tween 20, pH 7.6.) containing 5% skim milk. Proteins in cell lysate samples were denatured by adding Laemmli 5× sample buffer and heating at 95 °C for 5 min. Proteins (40 μg) were resolved with 10% SDS-polyacrylamide gel electrophoresis at 80 V and electrically transferred to a polyvinylidene difluoride membrane (Amersham Pharmacia, Little Chalfont, UK) at 4 °C overnight. After blocking incubation with TBST containing 5% skim milk, the membrane was incubated with the primary antibody at 4 °C overnight, followed by incubation with the secondary antibody at room temperature for 1 h. The target protein bands were visualized with a chemiluminescence method using the picoEPD Western Reagent kit (ELPIS-Biotech, Daejeon, Korea). The captured blot images were analyzed using the Image J program from U.S. National Institutes of Health (Bethesda, MD, USA).

2.12. Statistical Analysis

Data are expressed as mean ± standard deviation (SD) of three or more independent experiments. Experimental results were statistically analyzed using SigmaStat v.3.11 software (Systat Software Inc., San Jose, CA, USA). The presence of significantly different group means was determined using a one-way analysis of variance (ANOVA) at $p < 0.05$ level. Dunnett's test was then used to compare each experimental group with the control group. Alternatively, Duncan's multiple range test was used to compare all groups to each other.

3. Results

3.1. Effects of Medicinal Plant Extracts on the PM_{10}-Induced Toxicity in HaCaT Keratinocytes

A preliminary experiment was performed to select plant extracts that alleviate the cytotoxicity of PM_{10}. HaCaT cells were treated with each plant extract at 50 μg mL^{-1} and exposed to 200 μg mL^{-1} PM_{10} for 48 h. As shown in Figure 1, in the case of the vehicle control group, the cell viability decreased by about 40% by PM_{10} exposure. Of the 23 plant extracts tested, seven plant extracts showed their own toxicity, significantly reducing cell viability in the absence of PM_{10}; they are the extracts derived from Eucomiae Folium, Eucomiae Ramulus, Mori Ramulus, Angelicae tenuissimae Radix, Gardeniae Fructus, Akebiae Caulis, and Pini Pollen. On the other hand, the nine plant extracts had no effect on cell viability by themselves, and also mitigated the decrease in cell viability caused by PM_{10}; they are the extracts derived from Castaneae Semen, Peucedani Japonici Radix, Arisaematis Rhizoma, Dioscoreae Rhizoma, Biotae Orientalis Folium, Vitis Viniferae Caulis, Machili Thunbergi Cortex, Cyperi Rhizoma, and Siegesbeckiae Herba. Among them, Siegesbeckiae Herba extract (SHE) most effectively restored the viability of PM_{10}-exposed cells, so this extract was selected for subsequent experiments.

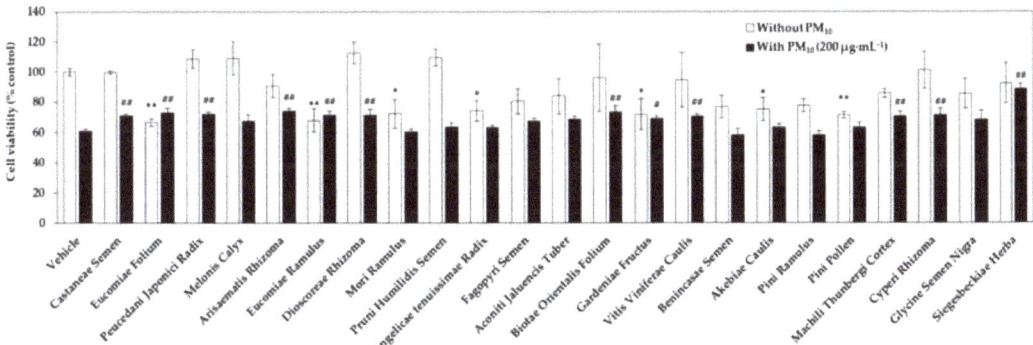

Figure 1. Effects of medicinal plant extracts on the viability of HaCaT keratinocytes cultured in the absence and presence of particulate matter with an approximate diameter of less than 10 μm (PM_{10}). Cells were pretreated with vehicle or each extract (50 μg mL^{-1}) and cultured in the absence or presence of PM_{10} (200 μg mL^{-1}) for 48 h. Cell viability was determined by the 3-(4,5-dimethylthiazol-2-yl)-2,5-diphenyl tetrazolium bromide (MTT) assay. Data are presented as mean ± SD ($n = 3$). Statistical significance of intergroup differences was determined using one-way ANOVA followed by Dunnett's test. * $p < 0.05$ and ** $p < 0.01$ versus vehicle control; # $p < 0.05$ and ## $p < 0.01$ versus PM_{10} only control.

3.2. Effects of SHE on the Viability, LDH Release, Lipid Peroxidation, and ROS Production in HaCaT Cells Exposed to PM_{10}

SHE used in the preliminary experiment was purchased from an external plant extract bank. We also manufactured SHE from the dried leaves of *Siegesbeckia pubescens* Makino in our laboratory. Figure 2A,B shows the HPLC patterns of SHE purchased from an external plant extract bank and SHE prepared in our laboratory. The two extracts appeared to share several peaks with the same retention times, while the heights of these peaks were somewhat different. The effects of the two extracts on the viability of HaCaT cells in the presence or absence of PM_{10} exposure were compared in Figure 2C,D. Both extracts did not affect cell viability by themselves at the concentrations tested, and significantly increased the viability of cells exposed to PM_{10} to some degree. These results indicate that the phytochemical composition and biological activity of the two extracts are similar to each other. In subsequent experiments, SHE manufactured in our laboratory was used.

Figure 3A,B shows the dose curves of PM_{10} and SHE on HaCaT cell viability. PM_{10} showed a gradual increase in toxicity up to 300 μg mL^{-1}. In this study, PM_{10} was treated at 200 μg mL^{-1} as this concentration induced consistent and substantial cytotoxicity. SHE had no effect on the cell viability up to 100 μg mL^{-1} but reduced it at 200 μg·mL^{-1}. We selected the PM_{10} treatment concentration (200 μg·mL^{-1}) that showed sufficient toxicity for the experimental purpose, and the SHE treatment concentrations (50 μg mL^{-1} and 100 μg mL^{-1}) were selected in the concentration range that did not reduce the cell viability. In Figure 3C–E, SHE treatment at 50 μg mL^{-1} and 100 μg mL^{-1} inhibited the decrease in cell viability, the increase in LDH release, and the increase in lipid peroxidation induced by PM_{10} treatment at 200 μg mL^{-1}.

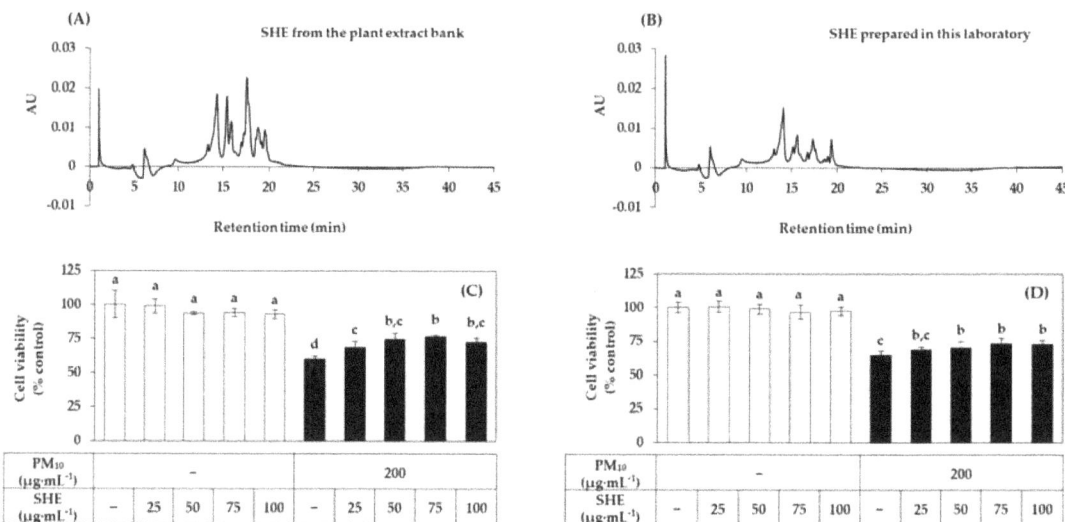

Figure 2. Comparison of Siegesbeckiae Herba extracts (SHEs) purchased from the plant extract bank and prepared in this laboratory. For the comparison of phytochemical composition, high-performance liquid chromatography (HPLC) profiles of the SHEs from the plant extract bank (**A**) and prepared in this laboratory (**B**) are shown (concentration 0.1%). For the comparison of bioactivity, HaCaT keratinocytes were treated with SHEs from the plant extract bank (**C**) and prepared in this laboratory (**D**) at different concentrations and cultured in the absence or presence of PM_{10} (200 μg mL^{-1}) for 48 h. Cell viability was determined by the MTT assay. Data are presented as mean ± SD (n = 4). Duncan's multiple range test was performed to compare all group means to each other. Groups that share the same letters (a–d) do not have significantly different means at the $p < 0.05$ level.

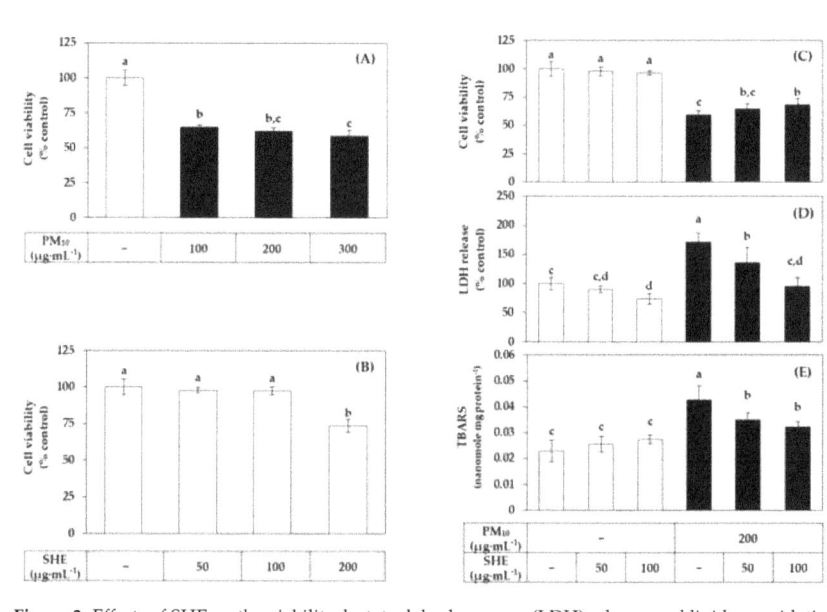

Figure 3. Effects of SHE on the viability, lactate dehydrogenase (LDH) release, and lipid peroxidation in HaCaT keratinocytes exposed to PM_{10}. In (**A**,**B**), cells were treated with PM_{10} (**A**) or SHE (**B**) at different concentrations for 48 h. In (**C**–**E**), cells were treated with SHE at different concentrations and cultured in the absence or presence of PM_{10} (200 μg mL^{-1}) for 48 h. Cell viability was determined by

the MTT assay (**A–C**). LDH release was assessed using the conditioned medium (**D**). Lipid peroxidation of cell lysates was determined by the 2-thiobarbituric acid assay and data are presented as 2-thiobarbituric acid-reactive substance (TBARS) levels corrected for protein contents (**E**). Data are presented as mean ± SD (n = 5 for (**A–D**); n = 4 for (**E**)). Duncan's multiple range test was performed to compare all group means to each other. Groups that share the same letters (a–d) do not have significantly different means at the $p < 0.05$ level.

Figure 4A shows the PM_{10} dose and time-dependency of ROS production in HaCaT cells. In the following experiments, PM_{10} was treated at 200 μg mL^{-1} for 60 min as this condition induced ROS production at a substantial level. ROS production was detected using DCFH-DA, a redox-sensitive dye that fluoresces after being oxidized by ROS. As shown in Figure 4B, SHE treatment at 50 μg mL^{-1} and 100 μg mL^{-1} inhibited the increase in ROS production induced by PM_{10} treatment at 200 μg mL^{-1} for 60 min. Typical fluorescence pictures of cells treated differently are shown in Figure 4C. The fluorescence due to the oxidation of DCFH-DA was increased by PM_{10} and the change was reduced by SHE.

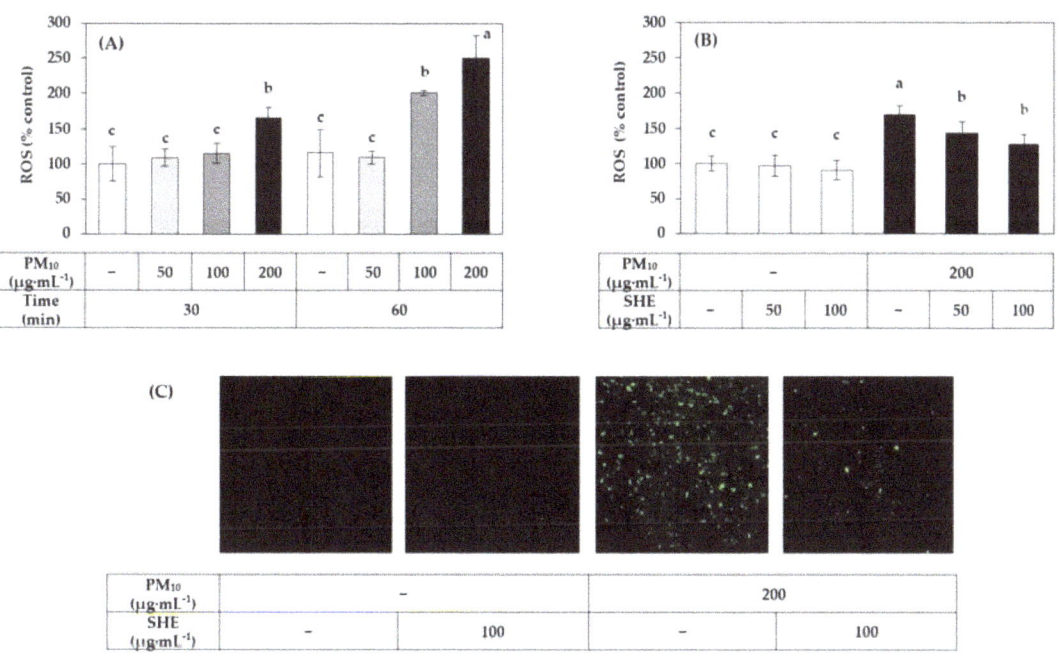

Figure 4. Effects of SHE on the reactive oxygen species (ROS) production in HaCaT keratinocytes exposed to PM_{10}. In (**A**), cells were labeled with 2′,7′-dichlorofluorescin diacetate (DCFH-DA) and exposed to PM_{10} at the indicated concentrations for 30 min or 60 min. In (**B**,**C**), cells were labeled with DCFH-DA, treated with SHE at the indicated concentrations, and exposed to PM_{10} (200 μg mL^{-1}) for 60 min or not. Typical images of cells fluorescing due to the oxidation of DCFH-DA by ROS are shown in (**C**). The fluorescence of the cell extracts was measured to determine ROS levels (**A**,**B**). Data are presented as mean ± SD (n = 5 for (**A**) and n = 6 for (**B**)). Duncan's multiple range test was performed to compare all group means to each other. Groups that share the same letters (a–c) do not have significantly different means at the $p < 0.05$ level.

3.3. Effects of SHE on the Expression of the Defense Genes in HaCaT Cells under Basal and PM_{10}-Exposed Conditions

To gain insight into the mechanism of action of SHE to alleviate cellular oxidative damage, we examined the effect of SHE on the mRNA expression of several defense enzymes in HaCaT cells in the absence or presence of PM_{10} exposure, and the results are shown in Figure 5. SHE did not have a remarkable effect on the expression of NRF2, a master transcription factor that induces the expression of various genes in the body's antioxidant defense system, but decreased the expression of its negative regulator, KEAP1, both in the absence and presence of PM_{10} exposure. SHE further increased the mRNA expression of HMOX1 and NQO1, the main target genes of NRF2.

The mRNA expression of SOD1, which scavenges superoxide radicals, and CAT, which decomposes hydrogen peroxide, was not significantly affected by SHE. The mRNA expression of GPX1, which decomposes hydrogen peroxide or lipid peroxide, tended to be decreased by SHE, and that of GSTκ1, which catalyzes GSH conjugation of xenobiotics, showed a tendency to slightly increase. The mRNA expression of GSR, which catalyzes the reduction of GSSG coupled with NADPH oxidation, was increased by SHE, and the mRNA expression of G6PDH, which supplies NADPH, was also significantly increased. In addition, the mRNA expressions of GCL-m and GCL-c acting at the rate-regulating step of GSH biosynthesis were increased by SHE. These results suggest that SHE enhances cellular antioxidant capacity, including synthesis and regeneration of GSH.

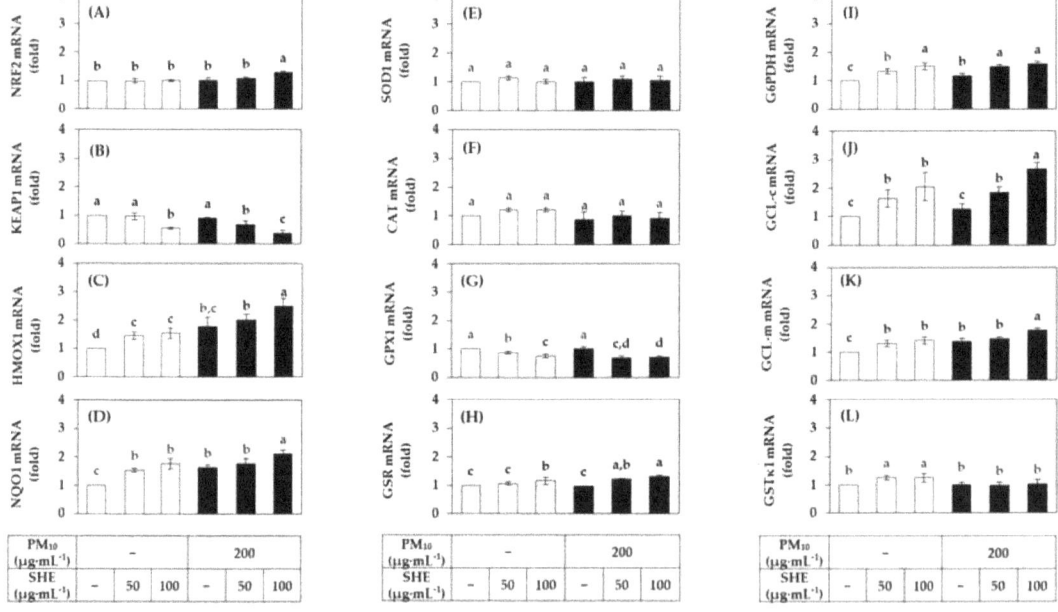

Figure 5. Effects of SHE on the mRNA expression levels of the defense genes in HaCaT keratinocytes under basal and PM_{10}-exposed conditions. Cells were treated with SHE at different concentrations and cultured in the absence or presence of PM_{10} (200 μg mL^{-1}) for 24 h. The mRNA levels of nuclear factor erythroid 2-related factor (NRF) 2 (**A**), kelch-like ECH-associated protein (KEAP) 1 (**B**), heme oxygenase (HMOX) 1 (**C**), NAD(P)H quinone oxidoreductase (NQO) 1 (**D**), superoxide dismutase (SOD) 1 (**E**), catalase (CAT) (**F**), glutathione peroxidase (GPX) 1 (**G**), glutathione disulfide reductase (GSR) (**H**), glucose 6-phosphate dehydrogenase (G6PDH) (**I**), glutamate-cysteine ligase catalytic subunit (GCL-c) (**J**), glutamate-cysteine ligase modifier subunit (GCL-m) (**K**), and glutathione S-transferase (GST) κ1 (**L**) were determined by quantitative real time-polymerase chain reaction (qRT-PCR) and normalized to that of glyceraldehyde 3-phosphate dehydrogenase (GAPDH). Data are presented as mean ± SD ($n = 3$). Duncan's multiple range test was performed to compare all group means to each other. Groups that share the same letters (a, b, c, or d) do not have significantly different means at the $p < 0.05$ level.

Western blot was performed to analyze the protein level of GCL-c, GCL-m and G6PDH as the representative proteins, and β-actin as a reference protein. As shown in Figure 6, SHE increased the protein levels of GCL-c and G6PDH in both the absence and presence of PM_{10}. It also tended to increase the protein level of GCL-m although the differences were not statistically significant. The changes in the protein levels of these proteins were consistent with those in the mRNA levels observed above.

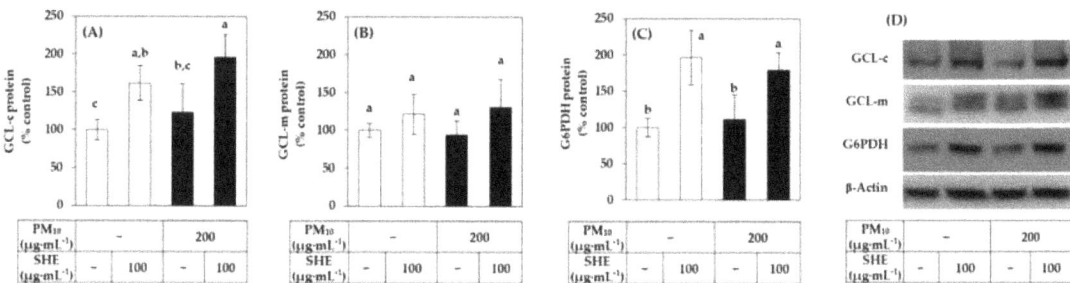

Figure 6. Effects of SHE on the protein levels of GCL-c, GCL-m, and G6PDH in HaCaT keratinocytes under basal and PM_{10}-exposed conditions. Cells were treated with SHE (100 μg mL^{-1}) and cultured in the absence or presence of PM_{10} (200 μg mL^{-1}) for 24 h. The protein levels of GCL-c (**A**), GCL-m (**B**), and G6PDH (**C**) were determined by the Western blotting and normalized to that of β-actin. Representative blots are shown in (**D**). Data are presented as percentages of the control (mean ± SD, n = 3). Duncan's multiple range test was performed to compare all group means to each other. Groups that share the same letters (a–c) do not have significantly different means at the $p < 0.05$ level.

3.4. Effects of SHE on the GSH and GSSG Levels in HaCaT Cells Exposed to PM_{10}

The effect of SHE on the contents of GSH and its oxidized form, GSSG, in cells was investigated. As shown in Figure 7, SHE increased the GSH content in both the absence and presence of PM_{10}. PM_{10} did not significantly affect the level of GSH, but significantly increased the level of GSSG. As a result, the total GSH plus GSSG content increased by SHE in a concentration-dependent manner. Interestingly, the proportion of GSSG in the total GSH and GSSG content was greatly increased by PM_{10} and this change was attenuated by SHE. This suggests that SHE enhances cell resistance to PM_{10}-induced oxidative stress by increasing the synthesis of GSH in cells.

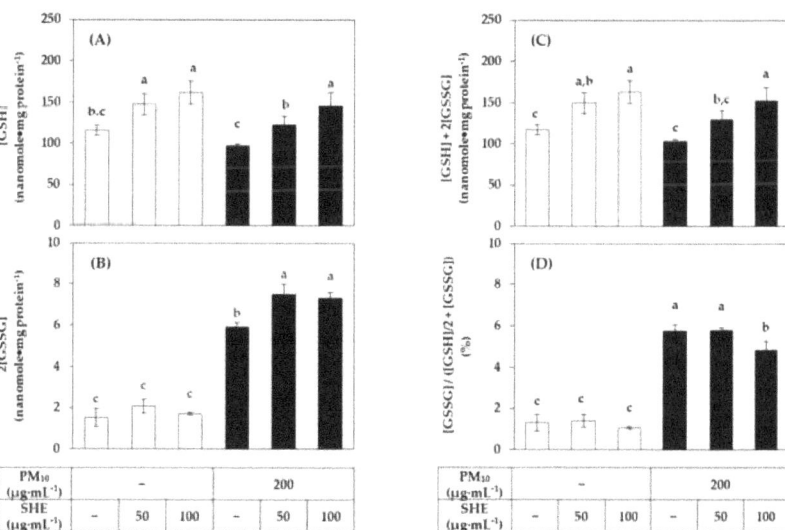

Figure 7. Effects of SHE on the contents of reduced glutathione (GSH) and its oxidized form, glutathione disulfide (GSSG) in HaCaT keratinocytes exposed to PM_{10}. Cells were treated with SHE

at different concentrations and cultured in the absence or presence of PM_{10} (200 μg mL^{-1}) for 24 h. The GSH contents (**A**) were calculated by subtracting the GSSG contents (**B**) from the total GSH plus GSSG contents (**C**). The relative ratios of GSSG contents to the total GSH plus GSSG contents were presented in (**D**). Data are presented as mean ± SD (n = 3). Duncan's multiple range test was performed to compare all group means to each other. Groups that share the same letters (a–c) do not have significantly different means at the p < 0.05 level.

3.5. Effects of Solvent Fractions of SHE on the Viability of HaCaT Cells Exposed to PM_{10}

To investigate which phytochemicals contained in SHE alleviate the cytotoxicity of PM_{10}, this extract was divided into several solvent fractions, namely, MC, EA, BA, and WT fractions according to the method illustrated in Figure 8A. Additionally, the effect of each fraction on the viability of HaCaT cells under PM_{10} exposure or non-exposure conditions was comparatively evaluated. As shown in Figure 8B, the MC fraction itself showed severe cytotoxicity. Although the EA fraction and WT fraction had weaker cytotoxicity, they did not alleviate PM_{10} cytotoxicity. Notably, the BA fraction increased the cell viability compared to the vehicle control in both the absence and presence of PM_{10}.

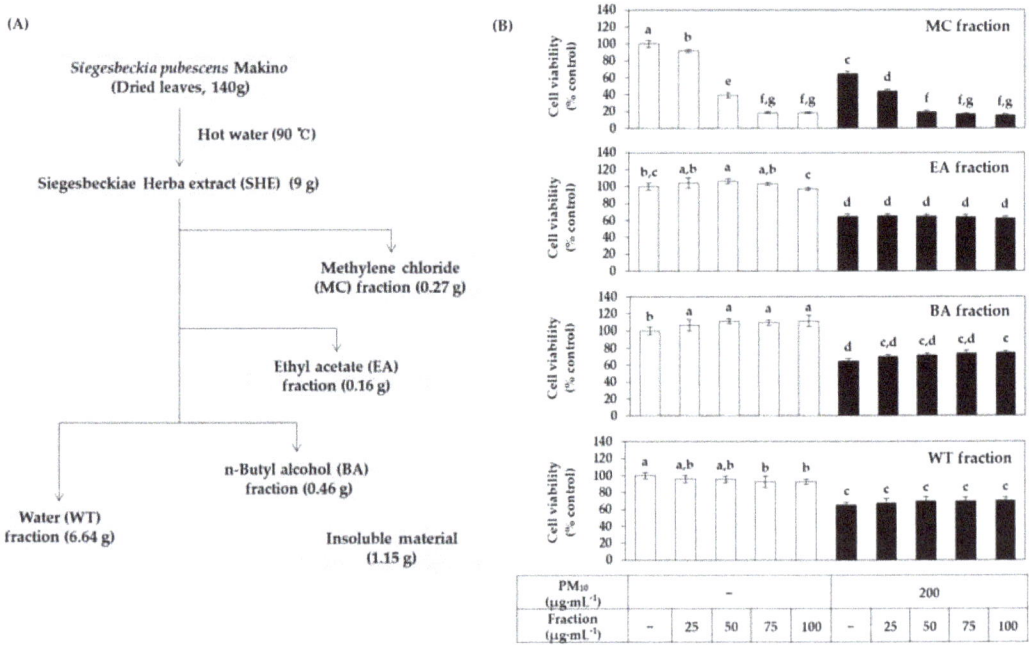

Figure 8. Effects of various solvent fractions of SHE on the viability in HaCaT keratinocytes exposed to PM_{10}. (**A**) SHE was separated into methylene chloride (MC), ethyl acetate (EA), n-butyl alcohol (BA), and water (WT) fractions. (**B**) Cells were treated with each solvent fraction at different concentrations and cultured in the absence or presence of PM_{10} (200 μg mL^{-1}) for 48 h. Cell viability was determined by the MTT assay. Data are presented as mean ± SD (n = 4). Duncan's multiple range test was performed to compare all group means to each other. Groups that share the same letters (a–g) do not have significantly different means at the p < 0.05 level.

3.6. HPLC-DAD Analysis of Solvent Fractions of SHE

HPLC-DAD analysis was performed on SHE and its MC, EA, BA, and WT fractions. As shown in Figure 9, it was shown that the BA fraction contained chlorogenic acid and the EA fraction contained caffeic acid. This was based on a comparison of retention times and absorption spectra of the specified peaks with standard materials.

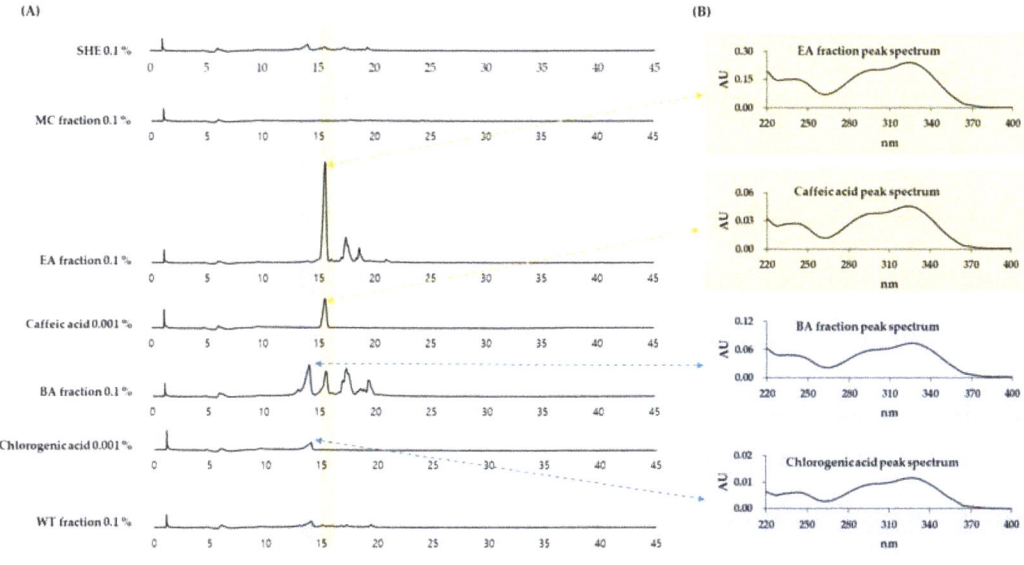

Figure 9. High-performance liquid chromatography-photodiode array detection (HPLC-DAD) analysis of SHE and its solvent fractions. SHE was separated into MC, EA, BA, and WT fractions. HPLC-DAD analysis conditions are described in Materials and Methods. Authentic chlorogenic acid and caffeic acid were used to identify the major peaks by comparing retention times and spectra. Chromatograms detected at 330 nm are shown in (**A**). UV absorption spectra of the indicated peaks are shown in (**B**).

3.7. Effects of Chlorogenic Acid vs. Caffeic Acid on the Viability, LDH Release, and ROS Production of HaCaT Cells Exposed to PM_{10}

Chlorogenic acid is a compound of caffeic acid and quinic acid (Figure 10A,B). In the following experiments, we comparatively evaluated the effects of these two phytochemicals on the viability and ROS production of HaCaT cells under PM_{10} exposure or non-exposure conditions. As shown in Figure 10C, chlorogenic acid increased the cell viability compared to the vehicle control in both the presence and absence of PM_{10}. However, this action was not observed with caffeic acid (Figure 10D).

The activity of inhibiting PM_{10}-induced LDH release was found to be relatively superior with chlorogenic acid compared to caffeic acid (Figure 10E,F).

Figure 11A,B shows the inhibitory effects of chlorogenic acid and caffeic acid on the ROS production induced by PM_{10}. Among these two compounds, chlorogenic acid showed a stronger inhibitory effect against PM_{10}-induced ROS production. Typical fluorescence pictures of cells are shown in Figure 11C. The fluorescence due to the oxidation of DCFH-DA by ROS was increased by PM_{10} and the change was reduced by chlorogenic acid more effectively than caffeic acid.

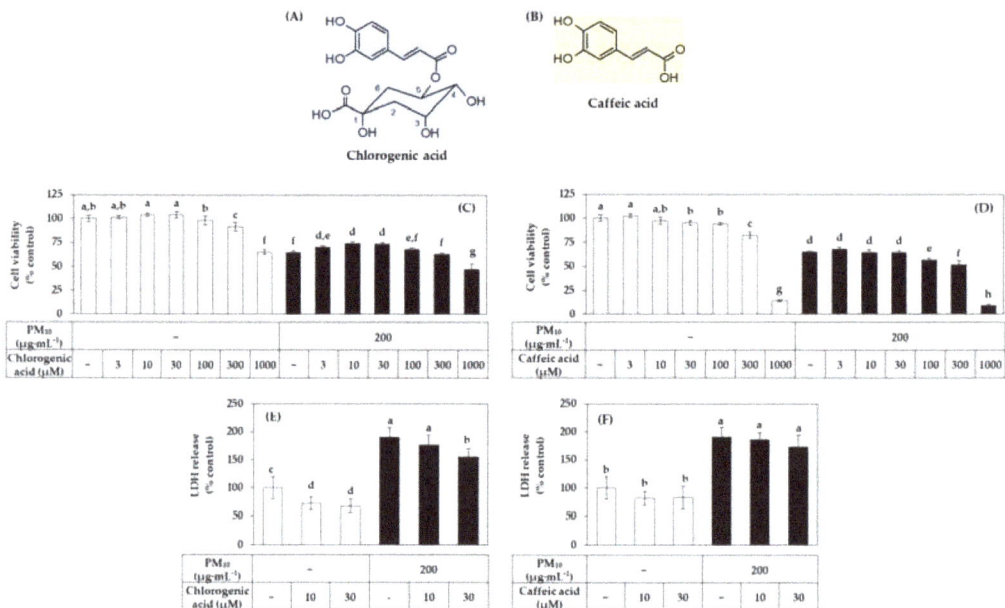

Figure 10. Effects of chlorogenic acid versus caffeic acid on the viability and LDH release of HaCaT keratinocytes exposed to PM_{10}. The chemical structures of chlorogenic acid and caffeic acid are shown in (**A**,**B**). In (**C**–**F**), cells were treated with chlorogenic acid (**C**) or caffeic acid (**D**) at the specified concentrations and incubated in the absence or presence of PM_{10} (200 μg mL^{-1}) for 48 h. Cell viability was determined by the MTT assay (**C**,**D**). LDH release was assessed using the conditioned medium (**E**,**F**). Data are presented as mean ± SD (n = 4 for (**C**,**D**); n = 5 for (**E**,**F**)). Duncan's multiple range test was performed to compare all group means to each other. Groups that share the same letters (a–h) do not have significantly different means at the $p < 0.05$ level.

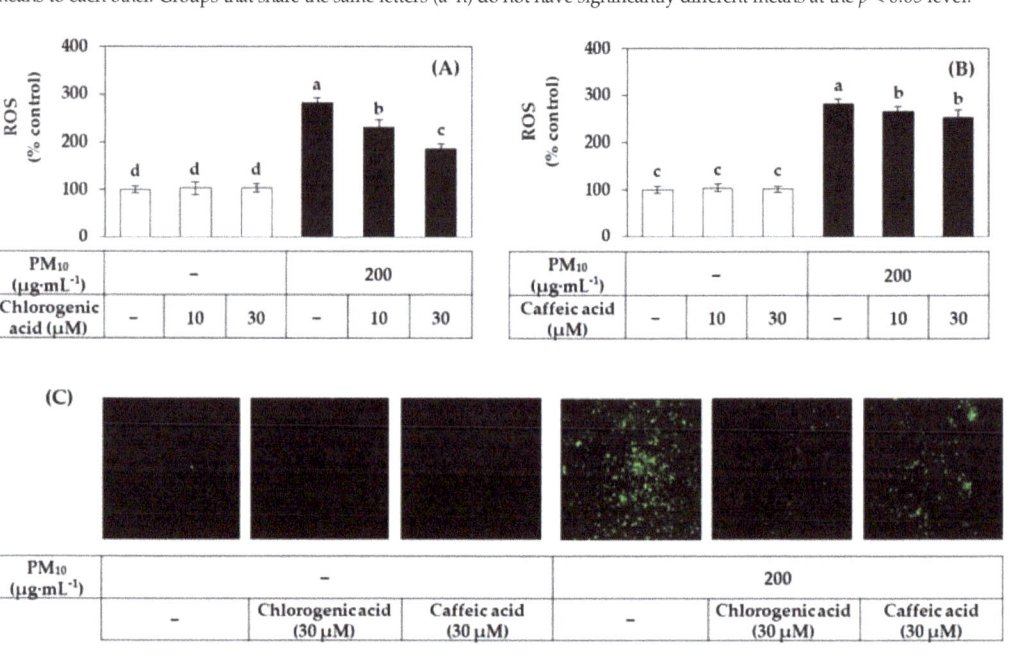

Figure 11. Effects of chlorogenic acid versus caffeic acid on the ROS production in HaCaT keratinocytes exposed to PM_{10}.

Cells were labeled with DCFH-DA, treated with SHE at different concentrations, and exposed to PM_{10} (200 μg mL^{-1}) for 60 min or not. Typical images of cells fluorescing due to the oxidation of DCFH-DA by ROS are shown in (**C**). The fluorescence of the cell extracts was measured to determine ROS levels (**A**,**B**). Data are presented as mean ± SD (n = 4). Duncan's multiple range test was performed to compare all group means to each other. Groups that share the same letters (a–d) do not have significantly different means at the $p < 0.05$ level.

4. Discussion

This study demonstrated that SHE is a useful plant extract to alleviate PM_{10}-induced death of HaCaT cells. PM_{10} increased ROS production and lipid peroxidation in HaCaT cells, and these changes were moderated by SHE in a dose-dependent manner. It is suggested that SHE enhances antioxidant capacity by increasing the expression of defense genes in cells (Figure 12).

Enzymes such as SOD1, CAT, and GPX1 expressed in cells have the activity to directly remove $O_2^{\bullet-}$, H_2O_2, and lipid peroxide [48]. GSH is a tripeptide that plays an important role in maintaining the redox balance of cells, which is used as a substrate in enzymatic reactions mediated by GPX1 and GSTκ1 and acts as a direct antioxidant [49]. GSR and G6PDH expressed in cells are involved in the regeneration of GSH [50,51], and GCL-c and GCL-m are involved in the synthesis of GSH [49,52]. The results of this study showed that SHE increased the expression of GSTκ1, GSR, G6PDH, GCL-c, and GCL-m rather than the expression of SOD1, CAT, and GPX1. This suggests that SHE selectively induces enzymes involved in the synthesis of GSH through glutamate-cysteine, the regeneration of GSH from GSSG, and GSH conjugation of xenobiotics, rather than enzymes involved in direct scavenging of ROS. Consistently, SHE increased the content of GSH and mitigated the increase in GSSG caused by PM_{10}.

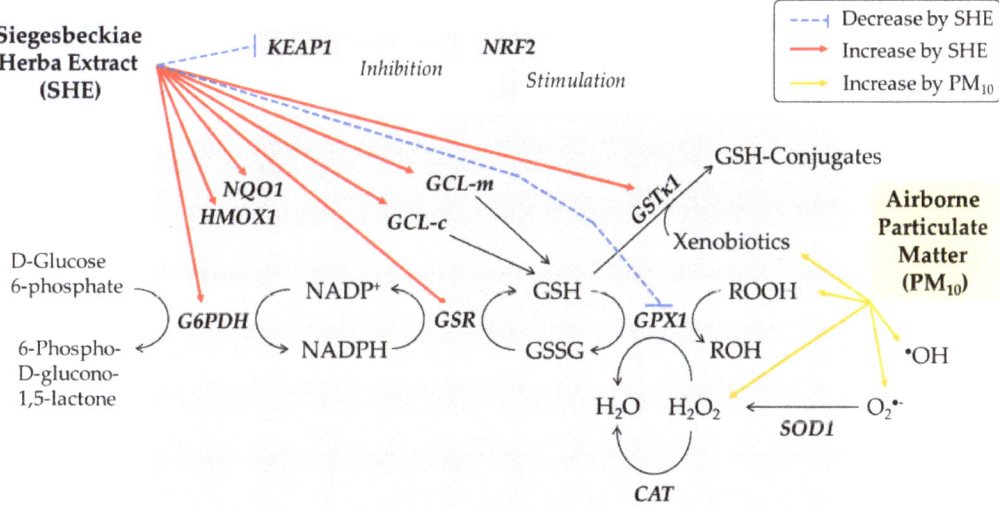

Figure 12. Working model for the protective effects of SHE against PM_{10}-induced oxidative stress in HaCaT keratinocytes. PM_{10} increases ROS, such as superoxide radical ($O_2^{\bullet-}$), hydrogen peroxide (H_2O_2), and hydroxyl radical ($^{\bullet}OH$), and lipid peroxide (ROOH), causing oxidative stress and death of HaCaT cells. SHE does not change the mRNA expression of NRF2, but decreases that of KEAP1, a negative regulator of NRF2, leading to the activation of NRF2 to induce the expression of target genes, such as HMOX1 and NQO1. SHE selectively induces the enzymes involved in the synthesis of GSH (GCL-c and GCL-m), the regeneration of GSH (GSR and G6PDH), and GSH conjugation of xenobiotics (GSTκ1), rather than the enzymes that directly scavenge ROS (SOD1, CAT, and GPX1). SHE increases the cellular content of GSH and mitigates the oxidation of GSH to GSSG caused by PM_{10}.

NRF2 is a transcription factor that induces the expression of phase II metabolism/antioxidant enzymes and plays an important function in regulating the body's defense mechanisms [53,54]. Activation of this transcription factor is regulated by various mechanisms, and KEAP1 is one of its negative regulators [55]. Upon binding to KEAP1, NRF2 is excluded from the nucleus and degraded in the proteasome. On the other hand, when NRF2 is separated from KEAP1 by a certain stimulus, the free NRF2 enters the nucleus and can bind to the antioxidant response element (ARE) of the promoter of the target gene together with various other factors. This transactivates the expression of several genes, such as HMOX1, NQO1, GCL-c, GCL-m, and GSTκ1. In this study, SHE did not change the expression of NRF2 but decreased the expression of KEAP1. SHE increased the expression of target genes, such as HMOX1 and NQO1. This suggests that SHE activated the NRF2 system in cells.

As plant-derived substances can have positive or negative effects on cell physiology [24–27], it is important to select safe and effective types and to select their optimal concentration for use. The plant extracts tested in this study showed different or opposite effects on cell viability in the absence and presence of PM_{10}. Among them, SHE was selected as a plant extract that safely and effectively alleviates the cytotoxicity of PM_{10}. SHE is a mixture of various substances, and therefore the observed results are the combined effects of several components. Interesting results were obtained by comparing the effects of different solvent fractions of SHE. That is, among the solvent fractions of SHE, the BA fraction increased the cell viability whereas the MC fraction decreased the cell viability, and the other two fractions had no significant effect. The BA fraction contained a high amount of chlorogenic acid whereas the EA fraction contained a high amount of caffeic acid. Thus, we could predict that chlorogenic acid contained in the BA fraction might be an active ingredient that provided cytoprotective effects against PM_{10} toxicity. Consistently with this notion, chlorogenic acid ameliorated the death of HaCaT cells exposed to PM_{10} and reduced PM_{10}-induced cellular ROS production more effectively than caffeic acid. In this study, about 100 μg mL^{-1} of SHE and 30 μM (10.6 μg·mL^{-1}) of chlorogenic acid were selected as the optimal concentrations to use with high safety and cell protection efficacy.

It was previously reported that chlorogenic acid reduced oxidative stress by activating the NRF2 pathway in various in vitro and in vivo models [56–58]. Therefore, when combined with the results of our current study, SHE containing chlorogenic acid is suggested to mitigate PM_{10} cytotoxicity by activating the NRF2 pathway.

SHE derived from *Siegesbeckia pubescens* exhibits anti-inflammatory and wound healing properties in various in vitro and in vivo models [59–61]. Several terpenoids and phenolic compounds have been proposed as active ingredients that provide anti-inflammatory action [62–64]. Furthermore, 5,3'-dihydroxy-3,7,4'-trimethoxyflavone isolated from *Siegesbeckia pubescens* was shown to exert cytoprotective and neuroinflammatory activities in cells by involving HMOX1 induction [65]. However, there was no previous study on the cytoprotective effect of SHE derived from *Siegesbeckia pubescens* against PM toxicity. Meanwhile, an extract of tart cherry (*Prunus cerasus* L.) containing chlorogenic acid, quercetin, and kaempferol was reported to inhibit the production of ROS and the expression of apoptosis-related genes in HaCaT keratinocytes exposed to PM_{10} [66]. However, no specific experimental results were provided for chlorogenic acid itself. Therefore, our present study is the first to report the protective effect of SHE and chlorogenic acid against PM_{10}.

In this study, the MTT assay was used to measure cell viability. Since particles and redox-sensitive substances can interfere with the MTT assay [67–69], the cells had been carefully washed with PBS to remove interfering materials before the assay. In addition, cell damage was also evaluated using the LDH release assay.

DCFH-DA was used as a fluorescent probe for measuring intracellular ROS production. Because the black pigment of PM_{10} interferes with the accurate measurement of low levels of fluorescence generated from the cells, we used a method of collecting cells from 12-well culture plates, extracting with a small volume (150 μL) of lysis buffer, centrifuging to remove the insoluble precipitate, and measuring the fluorescence of the extract, instead of directly measuring the fluorescence of the attached cells. For complementary purposes, fluorescence images of cells were additionally presented.

Immortalized HaCaT keratinocytes were used in this study and it is necessary to confirm the main findings of this study using normal human epidermal keratinocytes, 3-dimensional skin models, and in vivo animal models. It is also important to examine whether the phytochemicals have the same or different outcomes in transformed and normal cells in future studies.

5. Conclusions

In conclusion, the results of this study suggest that SHE derived from *Siegesbeckia pubescens* can increase the cellular antioxidant capacity through induction of defense genes, such as GCL-c, GCL-m, and G6PDH, and mitigate oxidative stress and enhance cell viability under PM_{10}-exposed conditions. It is also suggested that chlorogenic acid enriched in the BA fraction of SHE may be the active phytochemical of SHE providing such antioxidant and cytoprotective effects.

Author Contributions: Investigation, J.W.H. and Y.C.B.; writing, J.W.H. and Y.C.B.; conceptualization, supervision and funding acquisition, Y.C.B. All authors have read and agreed to the published version of the manuscript.

Funding: This research was supported by a grant of the Korea Health Technology R&D Project through the Korea Health Industry Development Institute (KHIDI), funded by the Ministry of Health and Welfare, Republic of Korea (grant number: HP20C0004).

Institutional Review Board Statement: Not applicable.

Informed Consent Statement: Not applicable.

Data Availability Statement: The data presented in this study are available in this manuscript.

Conflicts of Interest: The authors declare no conflict of interest.

Abbreviations

ARE	antioxidant response element
BA	n-butyl alcohol
CAT	catalase
DCFH-DA	2′,7′-dichlorodihydrofluorescein diacetate
DTNB	5,5-dithio-bis-2-nitrobenzoic acid
EA	ethyl acetate
G6PDH	glucose 6-phosphate dehydrogenase
GAPDH	glyceraldehyde 3-phosphate dehydrogenase
GCL-c	glutamate-cysteine ligase catalytic subunit
GCL-m	glutamate-cysteine ligase modifier subunit
GPX	glutathione peroxidase
GSH	glutathione
GSR	glutathione disulfide reductase
GSSG	glutathione disulfide
GST	glutathione S-transferase
HMOX	heme oxygenase
HPLC-DAD	high-performance liquid chromatography-photodiode array detection
IL	interleukin
KEAP	kelch-like ECH-associated protein
LDH	lactate dehydrogenase
MC	methylene chloride
MMP	matrix metalloproteinase
MTT	3-[4,5-dimethylthiazol-2-yl]-2,5-diphenyl tetrazolium bromide
NQO	NAD(P)H quinone oxidoreductase
NRF	nuclear factor erythroid 2-related factor

PBS	phosphate-buffered saline
PM	particulate matter
qRT-PCR	quantitative reverse transcriptase-polymerase chain reaction
ROS	reactive oxygen species
SHE	Siegesbeckiae Herba extract
SOD	superoxide dismutase
TBA	2-thiobarbituric acid
TBARS	2-thiobarbituric acid-reactive substance
WT	water

References

1. Mukherjee, A.; Agrawal, M. World air particulate matter: Sources, distribution and health effects. *Environ. Chem. Lett.* **2017**, *15*, 283–309. [CrossRef]
2. Fuzzi, S.; Baltensperger, U.; Carslaw, K.; Decesari, S.; Van Der Gon, H.D.; Facchini, M.C.; Fowler, D.; Koren, I.; Langford, B.; Lohmann, U.; et al. Particulate matter, air quality and climate: Lessons learned and future needs. *Atmos. Chem. Phys. Discuss.* **2015**, *15*, 8217–8299. [CrossRef]
3. Ngoc, L.T.N.; Park, D.; Lee, Y.; Lee, Y.-C. Systematic Review and Meta-Analysis of Human Skin Diseases Due to Particulate Matter. *Int. J. Environ. Res. Public Health* **2017**, *14*, 1458. [CrossRef] [PubMed]
4. Zhu, X.; Qiu, H.; Wang, L.; Duan, Z.; Yu, H.; Deng, R.; Zhang, Y.; Zhou, L. Risks of hospital admissions from a spectrum of causes associated with particulate matter pollution. *Sci. Total Environ.* **2019**, *656*, 90–100. [CrossRef] [PubMed]
5. Lademann, J.; Schaefer, H.; Otberg, N.; Teichmann, A.; Blume-Peytavi, U.; Sterry, W. Penetration von Mikropartikeln in die menschliche Haut. *Der Hautarzt* **2004**, *55*, 1117–1119. [CrossRef] [PubMed]
6. Song, S.; Lee, K.; Lee, Y.-M.; Lee, J.-H.; Lee, S.I.; Yu, S.-D.; Paek, D. Acute health effects of urban fine and ultrafine particles on children with atopic dermatitis. *Environ. Res.* **2011**, *111*, 394–399. [CrossRef] [PubMed]
7. Ahn, K. The role of air pollutants in atopic dermatitis. *J. Allergy Clin. Immunol.* **2014**, *134*, 993–999. [CrossRef]
8. Jin, S.-P.; Li, Z.; Choi, E.K.; Lee, S.; Kim, Y.K.; Seo, E.Y.; Chung, J.H.; Cho, S. Urban particulate matter in air pollution penetrates into the barrier-disrupted skin and produces ROS-dependent cutaneous inflammatory response in vivo. *J. Dermatol. Sci.* **2018**, *91*, 175–183. [CrossRef] [PubMed]
9. Kim, K.E.; Cho, D.; Park, H.J. Air pollution and skin diseases: Adverse effects of airborne particulate matter on various skin diseases. *Life Sci.* **2016**, *152*, 126–134. [CrossRef] [PubMed]
10. Lee, D.U.; Ji, M.J.; Kang, J.Y.; Kyung, S.Y.; Hong, J.H. Dust particles-induced intracellular Ca2+ signaling and reactive oxygen species in lung fibroblast cell line MRC5. *Korean J. Physiol. Pharmacol.* **2017**, *21*, 327–334. [CrossRef] [PubMed]
11. Tsuji, G.; Takahara, M.; Uchi, H.; Takeuchi, S.; Mitoma, C.; Moroi, Y.; Furue, M. An environmental contaminant, benzo(a)pyrene, induces oxidative stress-mediated interleukin-8 production in human keratinocytes via the aryl hydrocarbon receptor signaling pathway. *J. Dermatol. Sci.* **2011**, *62*, 42–49. [CrossRef] [PubMed]
12. Verma, V.; Shafer, M.M.; Schauer, J.J.; Sioutas, C. Contribution of transition metals in the reactive oxygen species activity of PM emissions from retrofitted heavy-duty vehicles. *Atmos. Environ.* **2010**, *44*, 5165–5173. [CrossRef]
13. Ryu, Y.S.; Kang, K.A.; Piao, M.J.; Ahn, M.J.; Yi, J.M.; Hyun, Y.-M.; Kim, S.H.; Ko, M.K.; Park, C.O.; Hyun, J.W. Particulate matter induces inflammatory cytokine production via activation of NFκB by TLR5-NOX4-ROS signaling in human skin keratinocyte and mouse skin. *Redox Biol.* **2019**, *21*, 101080. [CrossRef] [PubMed]
14. Seok, J.K.; Cho, M.A.; Ha, J.W.; Boo, Y.C. Role of Dual Oxidase 2 in Reactive Oxygen Species Production Induced by Airborne Particulate Matter PM10 in Human Epidermal Keratinocytes. *J. Soc. Cosmet. Sci. Korea* **2018**, *45*, 57–67. [CrossRef]
15. Ko, E.; Choi, H.; Park, K.-N.; Park, J.-Y.; Lee, T.R.; Shin, N.W.; Bae, Y.S. Dual oxidase 2 is essential for house dust mite-induced pro-inflammatory cytokine production in human keratinocytes. *Exp. Dermatol.* **2015**, *24*, 936–941. [CrossRef] [PubMed]
16. Lee, C.-W.; Lin, Z.-C.; Hsu, L.-F.; Fang, J.-Y.; Chiang, Y.-C.; Tsai, M.-H.; Lee, M.-H.; Li, S.-Y.; Hu, S.C.-S.; Lee, I.-T.; et al. Eupafolin ameliorates COX-2 expression and PGE2 production in particulate pollutants-exposed human keratinocytes through ROS/MAPKs pathways. *J. Ethnopharmacol.* **2016**, *189*, 300–309. [CrossRef]
17. Ha, J.W.; Song, H.; Hong, S.S.; Boo, Y.C. Marine Alga Ecklonia cava Extract and Dieckol Attenuate Prostaglandin E2 Production in HaCaT Keratinocytes Exposed to Airborne Particulate Matter. *Antioxidants* **2019**, *8*, 190. [CrossRef] [PubMed]
18. Seok, J.K.; Lee, J.-W.; Kim, Y.M.; Boo, Y.C. Punicalagin and (−)-Epigallocatechin-3-Gallate Rescue Cell Viability and Attenuate Inflammatory Responses of Human Epidermal Keratinocytes Exposed to Airborne Particulate Matter PM10. *Ski. Pharmacol. Physiol.* **2018**, *31*, 134–143. [CrossRef] [PubMed]
19. Kim, M.; Kim, J.H.; Jeong, G.J.; Park, K.Y.; Lee, M.; Seo, S.J. Particulate matter induces pro-inflammatory cytokines via phosphorylation of p38 MAPK possibly leading to dermal inflammaging. *Exp. Dermatol.* **2019**, *28*, 809–815. [CrossRef] [PubMed]
20. Boo, Y.C. p-Coumaric Acid as An Active Ingredient in Cosmetics: A Review Focusing on its Antimelanogenic Effects. *Antioxidants* **2019**, *8*, 275. [CrossRef]

21. Boo, Y.C. Human Skin Lightening Efficacy of Resveratrol and Its Analogs: From In Vitro Studies to Cosmetic Applications. *Antioxidants* **2019**, *8*, 332. [CrossRef] [PubMed]
22. Boo, Y.C. Emerging Strategies to Protect the Skin from Ultraviolet Rays Using Plant-Derived Materials. *Antioxidants* **2020**, *9*, 637. [CrossRef] [PubMed]
23. Boo, Y. Arbutin as a Skin Depigmenting Agent with Antimelanogenic and Antioxidant Properties. *Antioxidants* **2021**, *10*, 1129. [CrossRef] [PubMed]
24. Pasciu, V.; Posadino, A.M.; Cossu, A.; Sanna, B.; Tadolini, B.; Gaspa, L.; Marchisio, A.; Dessole, S.; Capobianco, G.; Pintus, G. Akt Downregulation by Flavin Oxidase–Induced ROS Generation Mediates Dose-Dependent Endothelial Cell Damage Elicited by Natural Antioxidants. *Toxicol. Sci.* **2010**, *114*, 101–112. [CrossRef]
25. Posadino, A.M.; Cossu, A.; Giordo, R.; Zinellu, A.; Sotgia, S.; Vardeu, A.; Hoa, P.T.; Deiana, L.; Carru, C.; Pintus, G. Coumaric Acid Induces Mitochondrial Damage and Oxidative-Mediated Cell Death of Human Endothelial Cells. *Cardiovasc. Toxicol.* **2013**, *13*, 301–306. [CrossRef]
26. Giordo, R.; Cossu, A.; Pasciu, V.; Hoa, P.T.; Posadino, A.M.; Pintus, G. Different Redox Response Elicited by Naturally Occurring Antioxidants in Human Endothelial Cells. *Open Biochem. J.* **2013**, *7*, 44–53. [CrossRef] [PubMed]
27. Bouayed, J.; Bohn, T. Exogenous Antioxidants—Double-Edged Swords in Cellular Redox State: Health Beneficial Effects at Physiologic Doses versus Deleterious Effects at High Doses. *Oxidative Med. Cell. Longev.* **2010**, *3*, 228–237. [CrossRef] [PubMed]
28. Boo, Y.C. Can Plant Phenolic Compounds Protect the Skin from Airborne Particulate Matter? *Antioxidants* **2019**, *8*, 379. [CrossRef] [PubMed]
29. Boo, Y.C. Natural Nrf2 Modulators for Skin Protection. *Antioxidants* **2020**, *9*, 812. [CrossRef]
30. Wang, Q.; Liang, Y.-Y.; Li, K.-W.; Li, Y.; Niu, F.-J.; Zhou, S.-J.; Wei, H.-C.; Zhou, C.-Z. Herba Siegesbeckiae: A review on its traditional uses, chemical constituents, pharmacological activities and clinical studies. *J. Ethnopharmacol.* **2021**, *275*, 114117. [CrossRef] [PubMed]
31. Tao, H.-X.; Xiong, W.; Zhao, G.-D.; Peng, Y.; Zhong, Z.-F.; Xu, L.; Duan, R.; Tsim, K.W.; Yu, H.; Wang, Y.-T. Discrimination of three *Siegesbeckiae* Herba species using UPLC-QTOF/MS-based metabolomics approach. *Food Chem. Toxicol.* **2018**, *119*, 400–406. [CrossRef]
32. Guo, H.; Zhang, Y.; Cheng, B.C.-Y.; Lau, M.-Y.; Fu, X.-Q.; Li, T.; Su, T.; Zhu, P.-L.; Chan, Y.-C.; Tse, A.K.-W.; et al. Comparison of the chemical profiles and inflammatory mediator-inhibitory effects of three *Siegesbeckia* herbs used as Herba *Siegesbeckiae* (Xixiancao). *BMC Complement. Altern. Med.* **2018**, *18*, 141. [CrossRef]
33. Boukamp, P.; Petrussevska, R.T.; Breitkreutz, D.; Hornung, J.; Markham, A.; Fusenig, N.E. Normal keratinization in a spontaneously immortalized aneuploid human keratinocyte cell line. *J. Cell Biol.* **1988**, *106*, 761–771. [CrossRef]
34. Denizot, F.; Lang, R. Rapid colorimetric assay for cell growth and survival. Modifications to the tetrazolium dye procedure giving improved sensitivity and reliability. *J. Immunol. Methods* **1986**, *89*, 271–277. [CrossRef]
35. Lee, J.-W.; Seok, J.K.; Boo, Y.C. Ecklonia cava Extract and Dieckol Attenuate Cellular Lipid Peroxidation in Keratinocytes Exposed to PM10. *Evid.-Based Complement. Altern. Med.* **2018**, *2018*, 8248323. [CrossRef]
36. Eruslanov, E.; Kusmartsev, S. Identification of ROS Using Oxidized DCFDA and Flow-Cytometry. *Methods Mol. Biol.* **2010**, *594*, 57–72. [CrossRef] [PubMed]
37. Tietze, F. Enzymic method for quantitative determination of nanogram amounts of total and oxidized glutathione: Applications to mammalian blood and other tissues. *Anal. Biochem.* **1969**, *27*, 502–522. [CrossRef]
38. Sun, X.; Li, B.; Li, X.; Wang, Y.; Xu, Y.; Jin, Y.; Piao, F.; Sun, G. Effects of sodium arsenite on catalase activity, gene and protein expression in HaCaT cells. *Toxicol. Vitr.* **2006**, *20*, 1139–1144. [CrossRef] [PubMed]
39. Rolfs, F.; Huber, M.; Kuehne, A.; Kramer, S.; Haertel, E.; Muzumdar, S.; Wagner, J.; Tanner, Y.; Böhm, F.; Smola, S.; et al. Nrf2 Activation Promotes Keratinocyte Survival during Early Skin Carcinogenesis via Metabolic Alterations. *Cancer Res.* **2015**, *75*, 4817–4829. [CrossRef]
40. Kanno, T.; Tanaka, K.; Yanagisawa, Y.; Yasutake, K.; Hadano, S.; Yoshii, F.; Hirayama, N.; Ikeda, J.-E. A novel small molecule, N-(4-(2-pyridyl)(1,3-thiazol-2-yl))-2-(2,4,6-trimethylphenoxy) acetamide, selectively protects against oxidative stress-induced cell death by activating the Nrf2–ARE pathway: Therapeutic implications for ALS. *Free. Radic. Biol. Med.* **2012**, *53*, 2028–2042. [CrossRef]
41. Priftis, A.; Angeli-Terzidou, A.; Veskoukis, A.S.; Spandidos, D.; Kouretas, D. Cell-specific and roasting-dependent regulation of the Keap1/Nrf2 pathway by coffee extracts. *Mol. Med. Rep.* **2018**, *17*, 8325–8331. [CrossRef] [PubMed]
42. Lim, K.H.; Ku, J.-E.; Rhie, S.-J.; Ryu, J.Y.; Bae, S.; Kim, Y.-S. Anti-oxidant and Anti-inflammatory Effects of Sinapic Acid in UVB Irradiation-Damaged HaCaT Keratinocytes. *Asian J. Beauty Cosmetol.* **2017**, *15*, 513–522. [CrossRef]
43. Lou, D.; Wei, X.; Xiao, P.; Huo, Q.; Hong, X.; Sun, J.; Shuai, Y.; Tao, G. Demethylation of the NRF2 Promoter Protects against Carcinogenesis Induced by Nano-SiO2. *Front. Genet.* **2020**, *11*, 818. [CrossRef]
44. Warabi, E.; Wada, Y.; Kajiwara, H.; Kobayashi, M.; Koshiba, N.; Hisada, T.; Shibata, M.; Ando, J.; Tsuchiya, M.; Kodama, T.; et al. Effect on Endothelial Cell Gene Expression of Shear Stress, Oxygen Concentration, and Low-Density Lipoprotein as Studied by a Novel Flow Cell Culture System. *Free. Radic. Biol. Med.* **2004**, *37*, 682–694. [CrossRef] [PubMed]
45. Zhao, R.; Hou, Y.; Zhang, Q.; Woods, C.G.; Xue, P.; Fu, J.; Yarborough, K.; Guan, D.; Andersen, M.; Pi, J. Cross-Regulations among NRFs and KEAP1 and Effects of their Silencing on Arsenic-Induced Antioxidant Response and Cytotoxicity in Human Keratinocytes. *Environ. Health Perspect.* **2012**, *120*, 583–589. [CrossRef] [PubMed]

46. Jeong, S.-H. Anti-oxidant Activities of Phytol on Keratinocytes. *Asian J. Beauty Cosmetol.* **2017**, *15*, 457–465. [CrossRef]
47. An, S.-M.; Koh, J.-S.; Boo, Y.-C. Inhibition of melanogenesis by tyrosinase siRNA in human melanocytes. *BMB Rep.* **2009**, *42*, 178–183. [CrossRef]
48. Limón-Pacheco, J.; Gonsebatt, M.E. The role of antioxidants and antioxidant-related enzymes in protective responses to environmentally induced oxidative stress. *Mutat. Res. Toxicol. Environ. Mutagen.* **2009**, *674*, 137–147. [CrossRef]
49. Kalinina, E.V.; Chernov, N.N.; Novichkova, M.D. Role of glutathione, glutathione transferase, and glutaredoxin in regulation of redox-dependent processes. *Biochemistry* **2014**, *79*, 1562–1583. [CrossRef]
50. Gong, Z.-H.; Tian, G.-L.; Huang, Q.-W.; Wang, Y.-M.; Xu, H.-P. Reduced glutathione and glutathione disulfide in the blood of glucose-6-phosphate dehydrogenase-deficient newborns. *BMC Pediatr.* **2017**, *17*, 172. [CrossRef]
51. Hoffmann, C.; Dietrich, M.; Herrmann, A.-K.; Schacht, T.; Albrecht, P.; Methner, A. Dimethyl Fumarate Induces Glutathione Recycling by Upregulation of Glutathione Reductase. *Oxidative Med. Cell. Longev.* **2017**, *2017*, 6093903. [CrossRef]
52. Föller, M.; Harris, I.S.; Elia, A.; John, R.; Lang, F.; Kavanagh, T.J.; Mak, T.W. Functional significance of glutamate–cysteine ligase modifier for erythrocyte survival in vitro and in vivo. *Cell Death Differ.* **2013**, *20*, 1350–1358. [CrossRef]
53. Beyer, T.A.; Keller, U.A.D.; Braun, S.; Schäfer, M.; Werner, S. Roles and mechanisms of action of the Nrf2 transcription factor in skin morphogenesis, wound repair and skin cancer. *Cell Death Differ.* **2007**, *14*, 1250–1254. [CrossRef] [PubMed]
54. He, F.; Ru, X.; Wen, T. NRF2, a Transcription Factor for Stress Response and Beyond. *Int. J. Mol. Sci.* **2020**, *21*, 4777. [CrossRef]
55. Yamamoto, M.; Kensler, T.W.; Motohashi, H. The KEAP1-NRF2 System: A Thiol-Based Sensor-Effector Apparatus for Maintaining Redox Homeostasis. *Physiol. Rev.* **2018**, *98*, 1169–1203. [CrossRef]
56. Wang, D.; Hou, J.; Wan, J.; Yang, Y.; Liu, S.; Li, X.; Li, W.; Dai, X.; Zhou, P.; Liu, W.; et al. Dietary chlorogenic acid ameliorates oxidative stress and improves endothelial function in diabetic mice via Nrf2 activation. *J. Int. Med. Res.* **2021**, *49*, 300060520985363. [CrossRef]
57. Han, D.; Chen, W.; Gu, X.; Shan, R.; Zou, J.; Liu, G.; Shahid, M.; Gao, J.; Han, B. Cytoprotective effect of chlorogenic acid against hydrogen peroxide-induced oxidative stress in MC3T3-E1 cells through PI3K/Akt-mediated Nrf2/HO-1 signaling pathway. *Oncotarget* **2017**, *8*, 14680–14692. [CrossRef] [PubMed]
58. Bao, L.; Li, J.; Zha, D.; Zhang, L.; Gao, P.; Yao, T.; Wu, X. Chlorogenic acid prevents diabetic nephropathy by inhibiting oxidative stress and inflammation through modulation of the Nrf2/HO-1 and NF-kB pathways. *Int. Immunopharmacol.* **2018**, *54*, 245–253. [CrossRef]
59. Wang, J.-P.; Ruan, J.-L.; Cai, Y.-L.; Luo, Q.; Xu, H.-X.; Wu, Y.-X. In vitro and in vivo evaluation of the wound healing properties of *Siegesbeckia pubescens*. *J. Ethnopharmacol.* **2011**, *134*, 1033–1038. [CrossRef] [PubMed]
60. Wang, J.; Cai, Y.; Wu, Y. Antiinflammatory and analgesic activity of topical administration of *Siegesbeckia pubescens*. *Pak. J. Pharm. Sci.* **2008**, *21*, 89–91. [PubMed]
61. Sang, W.; Zhong, Z.; Linghu, K.; Xiong, W.; Tse, A.K.W.; Cheang, W.S.; Yu, H.; Wang, Y. *Siegesbeckia pubescens* Makino inhibits Pam3CSK4-induced inflammation in RAW 264.7 macrophages through suppressing TLR1/TLR2-mediated NF-κB activation. *Chin. Med.* **2018**, *13*, 37. [CrossRef] [PubMed]
62. Li, Y.-S.; Zhang, J.; Tian, G.-H.; Shang, H.-C.; Tang, H.-B. Kirenol, darutoside and hesperidin contribute to the anti-inflammatory and analgesic activities of *Siegesbeckia pubescens* makino by inhibiting COX-2 expression and inflammatory cell infiltration. *J. Ethnopharmacol.* **2021**, *268*, 113547. [CrossRef] [PubMed]
63. Lee, S.-G.; Kim, M.; Kim, C.E.; Kang, J.; Yoo, H.; Sung, S.H.; Lee, M. Quercetin 3,7-O-dimethyl ether from *Siegesbeckia pubescens* suppress the production of inflammatory mediators in lipopolysaccharide-induced macrophages and colon epithelial cells. *Biosci. Biotechnol. Biochem.* **2016**, *80*, 2080–2086. [CrossRef] [PubMed]
64. Lee, M.; Kim, S.H.; Lee, H.K.; Cho, Y.; Kang, J.; Sung, S.H. ent-Kaurane and ent-Pimarane Diterpenes from *Siegesbeckia pubescens* Inhibit Lipopolysaccharide-Induced Nitric Oxide Production in BV2 Microglia. *Biol. Pharm. Bull.* **2014**, *37*, 152–157. [CrossRef] [PubMed]
65. Lee, D.-S.; Lee, M.; Sung, S.H.; Jeong, G.S. Involvement of heme oxygenase-1 induction in the cytoprotective and neuroinflammatory activities of *Siegesbeckia pubescens* isolated from 5,3′-dihydroxy-3,7,4′-trimethoxyflavone in HT22 cells and BV2 cells. *Int. Immunopharmacol.* **2016**, *40*, 65–72. [CrossRef] [PubMed]
66. Kim, D.-W.; Jung, D.-H.; Sung, J.; Min, I.; Lee, S.-J. Tart Cherry Extract Containing Chlorogenic Acid, Quercetin, and Kaempferol Inhibits the Mitochondrial Apoptotic Cell Death Elicited by Airborne PM_{10} in Human Epidermal Keratinocytes. *Antioxidants* **2021**, *10*, 443. [CrossRef] [PubMed]
67. Peng, L.; Wang, B.; Ren, P. Reduction of MTT by flavonoids in the absence of cells. *Colloids Surf. B Biointerfaces* **2005**, *45*, 108–111. [CrossRef] [PubMed]
68. Holder, A.; Goth-Goldstein, R.; Lucas, D.; Koshland, C.P. Particle-Induced Artifacts in the MTT and LDH Viability Assays. *Chem. Res. Toxicol.* **2012**, *25*, 1885–1892. [CrossRef] [PubMed]
69. Habtemariam, S. Catechols and quercetin reduce MTT through iron ions: A possible artefact in cell viability assays. *Phytother. Res.* **1995**, *9*, 603–605. [CrossRef]

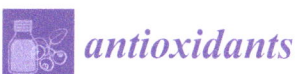

Article

Oral Administration of *Rosa gallica* Prevents UVB−Induced Skin Aging through Targeting the c−Raf Signaling Axis

Seongin Jo [1], Young-Sung Jung [2], Ye-Ryeong Cho [1], Ji-Won Seo [3], Won-Chul Lim [2], Tae-Gyu Nam [4], Tae-Gyu Lim [2,5,*] and Sanguine Byun [1,*]

[1] Department of Biotechnology, Yonsei University, Seoul 03722, Korea; sinnis25@naver.com (S.J.); choo9707@yonsei.ac.kr (Y.-R.C.)
[2] Korea Food Research Institute, Wanju-gun 55365, Korea; chembio@khu.ac.kr (Y.-S.J.); godqhr1105@naver.com (W.-C.L.)
[3] Department of Agricultural Biotechnology and Research, Institute of Agriculture and Life Sciences, Seoul National University, Seoul 08826, Korea; thinkbreaker@naver.com
[4] Major of Food Science and Biotechnology, Division of Bio-Convergence, Kyonggi University, Suwon 16227, Korea; tgzoo0706@kyonggi.ac.kr
[5] Department of Food Science & Biotechnology, Sejong University, Seoul 05006, Korea
* Correspondence: tglim@sejong.ac.kr (T.-G.L.); sanguine@yonsei.ac.kr (S.B.); Tel.: +82-2-3408-3260 (T.-G.L.); +82-2-2123-5896 (S.B.)

Abstract: *Rosa gallica* is a widely used Rosa species for medicinal and culinary purposes. *Rosa gallica* has been reported to display antioxidant, anti−inflammatory, and antibacterial activities. However, the effect of *Rosa gallica* against skin aging in vivo is unknown and its active components have not been fully understood. Oral administration of *Rosa gallica* prevented UVB−mediated skin wrinkle formation and loss of collagen/keratin fibers in the dorsal skin of mice. Examination of biomarkers at the molecular level showed that *Rosa gallica* downregulates UVB−induced COX−2 and MMP−1 expression in the skin. Through a direct comparison of major compounds identified using the UHPLC−MS/MS system, we discovered gallic acid as the primary component contributing to the anti-skin aging effect exhibited by *Rosa gallica*. Examination of the molecular mechanism revealed that gallic acid can potently and selectively target the c−Raf/MEK/ERK/c−Fos signaling axis. In addition, both gallic acid and MEK inhibitor blocked UVB−induced MMP−1 expression and restored collagen levels in a reconstructed 3D human skin model. Collectively, *Rosa gallica* could be used as a functional ingredient in the development of nutraceuticals against skin aging.

Keywords: *Rosa gallica*; skin aging; gallic acid; c−Raf; UHPLC−MS/MS

1. Introduction

Chronic irradiation of ultraviolet B (UVB) light causes skin wrinkle formation, inflammation, pigmentation, and dehydration [1,2]. UVB triggers signaling pathways leading to upregulation of genes involved in collagen degradation and inflammation [1,3]. Among these, matrix metalloproteinases (MMPs), especially MMP−1, play a key role in promoting collagen degradation and in turn, wrinkle formation [4]. In addition, cyclooxygenase 2 (COX−2), which can be induced by UVB light, mediates skin inflammation and photoaging [5]. Thus, food compounds that can inhibit the expression of MMP−1 or/and COX−2 have the potential to possess anti-skin aging effects [6,7].

Activator protein 1 (AP−1) and its upstream regulatory pathways have been known to be major contributing factors to MMP−1 expression and skin aging [8]. AP−1 is a dimeric transcription factor formed by Fos (c−Fos, FosB, Fra1, and Fra2) and Jun (c−Jun, JunB, and JunD) families. Activation of AP−1 induces transcription of genes involved in skin aging, cell proliferation, angiogenesis, and inflammation [8–10]. Especially as AP−1 directly induces MMP−1 expression leading to collagen degradation in the skin, downregulation of AP−1 components have been suggested as a promising strategy to block skin aging [11]. UV causes the activation of mitogen–activated protein kinases (MAPKs), including ERK1/2, p38, and JNK1/2, which act as key upstream regulators of AP−1 activity [8,12]. Hence, studies have demonstrated that inhibiting upstream regulatory pathways of AP−1, such as the MAPKs, MAP2Ks, or c−Raf can suppress skin aging [13–17].

Rosa species have been used as a cooking ingredient as well as a medicinal plant. Various types of roses, including *Rosa canina*, *Rosa damascene*, *Rosa centifolia*, and *Rosa gallica* have been reported to display antioxidant, antibacterial, anti−depressant, and anti−inflammatory properties [18,19]. Additionally, the Rosa species is known for its functional effects on the skin [20,21]. In particular, *Rosa gallica* is one of the most commonly used Rosa species for cosmetic, medicinal, and culinary purposes [22,23]. Although the potential of the *Rosa gallica* extract to prevent biomarkers of skin aging in vitro has been reported [24], there has been no study demonstrating the anti−skin aging effect of *Rosa gallica* in vivo. Moreover, active ingredients responsible for the bioactivity of *Rosa gallica* and Rosa species are poorly understood. Herein, we have orally administered the *Rosa gallica* extract to mice and evaluated its anti−skin aging effect to assess its potential as a functional food/nutraceutical agent. Moreover, we have identified the active ingredient of *Rosa gallica* by ultra−high performance liquid chromatography (UHPLC) with mass spectrometry (MS) and examined its molecular mechanism.

2. Materials and Methods

2.1. Materials

Gallic acid, quercetin, catechin, kaempferol, rutin, quercitrin, U0126, dimethyl sulfoxide (DMSO), and formic acid were purchased from Sigma−Aldrich (St. Louis, MO, USA). Antibody to detect COX−2 was purchased from Cayman Chemical (Ann Arbor, MI, USA), and the antibodies to detect MMP−1 and collagen I were obtained from Abcam (Cambridge, United Kingdom). Antibodies against c−Jun, p38, JNK, c−Raf, MKK4, vinculin, and GAPDH was provided by Santa Cruz Biotechnology, Inc. (Dallas, TX, USA). Antibody to detect c−Fos, phospho−c−Jun, phospho−ERK, ERK, phospho−p38, phospho−JNK, phospho−c−Raf, phospho−MEK, MEK, phospho−MKK4, phospho−MKK3, and MKK3 were purchased from Cell Signaling Technology (Danvers, MA, USA). *Rosa gallica* petals were imported from Turkey through GN Bio (Hanam, Korea). Analytical grade water and acetonitrile (ACN) were purchased from Thermo Fisher Scientific (Waltham, MA, USA).

2.2. Rosa gallica Extract Preparation

Rose petals were ground in a blender to obtain a powder. Dried powder (10 g) of rose petal was mixed with 1000 mL of 70% (v/v) ethanol and extracted at 70 °C for 3 h using reflux condenser. And then the extract was filtered through No. 2 filter paper (Whatman, Maidstone, UK). The solvent was subsequently evaporated, and the product was freeze-dried.

2.3. Experimental Animals and Treatments

Female SKH−1 hairless mice were obtained from Orient Bio (Seongnam, Korea). Mice had free access to food and water for 15 weeks. Seven mice were allocated into each group. The Institutional Animal Care and Use Committee (SEMI1−19−02) approved all experimental protocols. *Rosa gallica* extract was dissolved in distilled water at the indicated concentration and treated to mice every day by oral gavage. UVB was applied to the mice by UV−3000 (Dong Seo Science Co., Ltd., Seoul, Korea) starting at week 5 of the experiment. UVB irradiation was gradually increased from 1 MED to 4 MED (1 MED = 1 minimal erythema dose = 50 mJ/cm^2) with no injury.

2.4. Wrinkle Measurement

Skin replicas of mouse dorsal skin were made with the SILFLO (Amique Group Co. Ltd., Tokyo, Japan) at the end of the experiments. The skin replicas were photographed using

Nikon E600 (Nikon, Tokyo, Japan). Depth of the wrinkle was measured by Visioline® VL 650 (Courage&Khazaka GmbH, Koln, Germany).

2.5. Masson's Trichrome Staining

Tissue specimens were fixed with 4% (v/v) formalin solution. Tissue was embedded in paraffin. Approximately 4 μm–thick sections were subjected to stained with Masson's Trichrome for collagen and keratin fibers analysis. After tissue staining, slides were examined at 200 X magnification by Nikon DS–Fi3 (Nikon).

2.6. Immunoblot

Skin tissues or cell were lysed with RIPA buffer. Immunoblot was performed as previously described [25]. Briefly, lysates were centrifuged at 4 °C, 12,000× g for 10–20 min. Protein concentration of lysate was measured using BCA assay (Thermo Fisher Scientific). The proteins were separated using SDS−PAGE and transferred to a nitrocellulose (NC) membrane (PALL® Corporation, Port Washington, NY, USA). The NC membrane was blocked in the 5% skim milk in Tris−Buffered Saline in 0.1% Tween 20 for 1 hr. Membrane was incubated with a primary antibody at 4 °C overnight. Bands were detected with Western Lightning Plus−ECL (PerkinElmer, Waltham, MA, USA) after incubated with an HRP−conjugated secondary antibody. All blots presented in the manuscript are from a film scan generated from an automatic X−ray film processor (JPI Healthcare, Seoul, Korea).

2.7. UHPLC–LTQ–Orbitrap/MS/MS Conditions

The molecular weights of the peaks were displayed from high−resolution MS using LTQ Orbitrap XL (Thermo Fisher Scientific) coupled with Accelar UHPLC (Thermo Fisher Scientific). Mobile phase A was water containing 0.1% (v/v) formic acid, and mobile phase B was ACN containing 0.1% (v/v) formic acid. Separation of compounds was performed using a C_{18} column (Acquity UPLC® BEH; 2.1 mm × 100 mm, 1.7 μm; Waters Corp., Milford, MA, USA) at a flow rate of 0.4 mL/min using the following gradient 3–10% mobile phase B for 3 min; 10–40% B for 16 min; 40–80% B for 17 min; 80–3% B for 19 min; 3% B for 20 min. The UHPLC−MS/MS was operated with a Z−spray ion source in the positive ion, negative ion mode using the following conditions: capillary voltage of 20 V, capillary temperature of 350 °C, spray voltage 3.5 kV. Spectra were scanned in the range between 150 and 1500 m/z.

2.8. Cell Culture and UVB Irradiation

Human Dermal fibroblasts (HDFs) were kindly provided by Dr. Jin Ho Chung (Department of Dermatology, Seoul National University College of Medicine, Seoul, Korea). HDFs were cultured in Dulbecco's Modified Eagle's Media (DMEM, Corning Inc., Somerville, MA, USA) containing 10% fetal bovine serum (FBS, Thermo Fisher Scientific) with penicillin/streptomycin (Corning Inc.). Cells were irradiated with UVB using Bio−link−BLX (Vilber Lourmat, Paris, France), with the peak emission wavelength is 312 nm. The energy of UV was 0.03 J/cm^2.

2.9. SRB Staining

HDFs were seeded into a 6−well plate. After 24 h, the medium was replaced with serum–free DMEM. The next day, chemicals were treated at the indicated concentrations and incubated for 48 h. After fixing the cells, the living cells were stained with sulforhodamine B (SRB, Sigma−Aldrich). SRB was dissolved with 10 mM Tris and absorbance was measured at 554 nm.

2.10. Enzyme-Linked Immunosorbent Assay (ELISA)

HDFs were seeded in 12−well plates at a density of 1.8×10^5 cells/well. Cells were incubated for 24 h, after which the medium was replaced with serum−free media and incubated for another 24 h. Cells were treated with compounds at the indicated concentrations and then irradiated with UVB. Following 48 h of incubation, the culture supernatants were collected and centrifuged at 13,000× g to remove cell debris. The concentration of MMP−1 in the cell culture media was determined by corresponding ELISA kits (R&D Systems Inc., Minneapolis, MN, USA). These assays were performed as manufacturer's instructions.

2.11. Reconstructed 3D Human Skin Model

Reconstructed 3D human skin (Neoderm−ED) was obtained from Tegoscience (Seoul, Korea). The reconstructed 3D human skin model was treated with indicated chemicals for 1 h prior to UVB irradiation. The skin tissue was irradiated with UVB twice a day for 8 days, and the medium was changed every two days. The skin tissue was incubated at 37 °C under 5% CO_2 atmosphere.

2.12. Collagen Staining in Reconstructed 3D Human Skin Model

Skin sections from reconstructed 3D human skin model were fixed with 4% formalin solution. Paraffin−embedded sections were cut on glass slides. Slides were deparaffinized three times with xylene and hydrated through a grade alcohol bath. The deparaffinized sections were stained with Sirius Red/Fast Green solution (Chondrex, Inc. Woodinville, WA, USA). After tissue staining, slides were washed with 0.5% (v/v) acetic acid solution. Finally, slides were dehydrated through a reverse grade alcohol bath and mounted. Pictures of collagen−stained slides were taken using the Nikon eclipse Ts2 (Nikon).

2.13. Statistical Analysis

Statistical analyses were used one−way analysis of variance followed by GraphPad Prism 5 software (San Diego, CA, USA). All data are presented as means ± standard deviation (SD). A $p < 0.05$ was considered statistically significant.

3. Results

3.1. Oral Consumption of Rosa gallica Petal Extract (RPE) Suppresses UVB−Mediated Skin Wrinkle In Vivo

Mice were administered with *Rosa gallica* petal extract (RPE) and exposed to UVB for 10 weeks (Figure 1A). Continuous exposure to UVB induced skin wrinkle formation (Figure 1B). Interestingly, oral administration of RPE at 5 and 10 mg/kg B.W. led to a reduction in UVB−mediated wrinkle formation in the dorsal skin of mice (Figure 1B). Quantification of skin wrinkle demonstrated that RPE administration could block UVB−induced mean wrinkle depth and max wrinkle depth to near control levels (Figure 1C). These results clearly show that oral intake of RPE can suppress UVB−mediated skin aging in vivo.

3.2. RPE Does Not Show Side Effects In Vivo

To assess the safety of RPE in vivo, we evaluated several parameters after RPE administration. RPE did not display noticeable effects on body weight of mice (Figure 2A). In addition, RPE did not affect the amount of food and water intake (Figure 2B,C). Additionally, RPE did not cause any change to the weight of liver in the mice (Figure 2D). Collectively, these results demonstrate that oral consumption of RPE does not generate side effects in vivo at the treated concentrations.

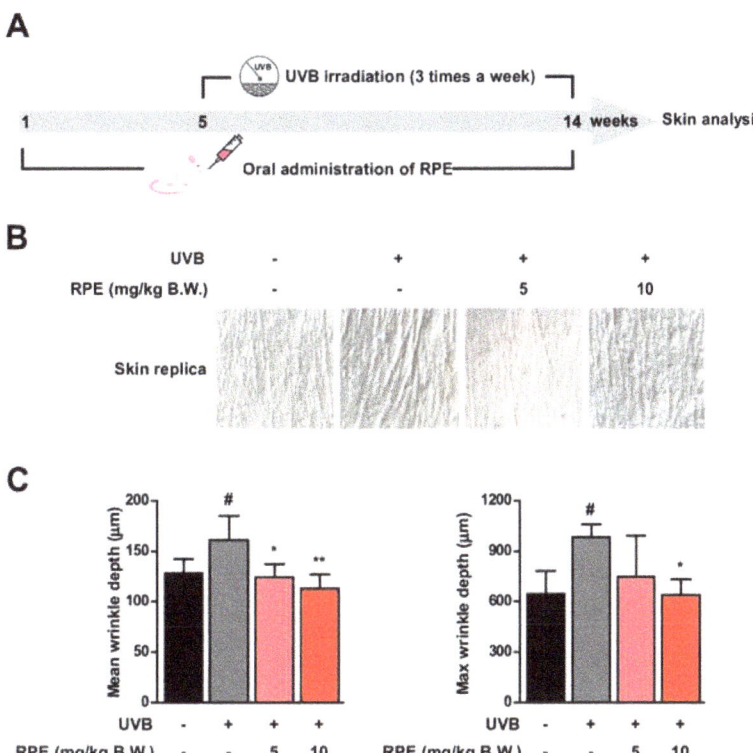

Figure 1. Rose petal extract (RPE) suppresses UVB−induced skin wrinkle formation. (**A**) RPE was orally administered to mice every day. UVB was irradiated three times a week as indicated in the experimental scheme. (**B**) Representative pictures of skin replica. (**C**) Mean wrinkle depth and max wrinkle depth were quantified. Data represent the means ± SD (n = 4). Significant differences between un−treated control and UVB−only treatment group (# p < 0.05) and significant differences between UVB and UVB + RPE administrated group (* p < 0.05, ** p < 0.01).

3.3. RPE Inhibits Collagen Degradation and Blocks UVB−Mediated Biomarker of Skin Aging

To further examine the anti−skin aging effect of RPE, we analyzed key biomarkers of skin aging. Collagen and keratin are major structural proteins constituting the skin and reduction of these proteins has been known to be responsible for skin wrinkle formation [26,27]. Results from Masson's trichrome staining of the skin demonstrate that RPE can prevent UVB−mediated decrease in collagen and keratin levels in the skin (Figure 3A). We also found that RPE suppresses UVB−induced COX−2 and MMP−1 expression in the skin (Figure 3B), suggesting that RPE can block major mediators of inflammation and collagen degradation. While there has been a previous report that RPE can attenuate MMP−1 in cells, this is the first time to show that RPE can suppress MMP−1 expression as well as collagen degradation and wrinkle formation in vivo.

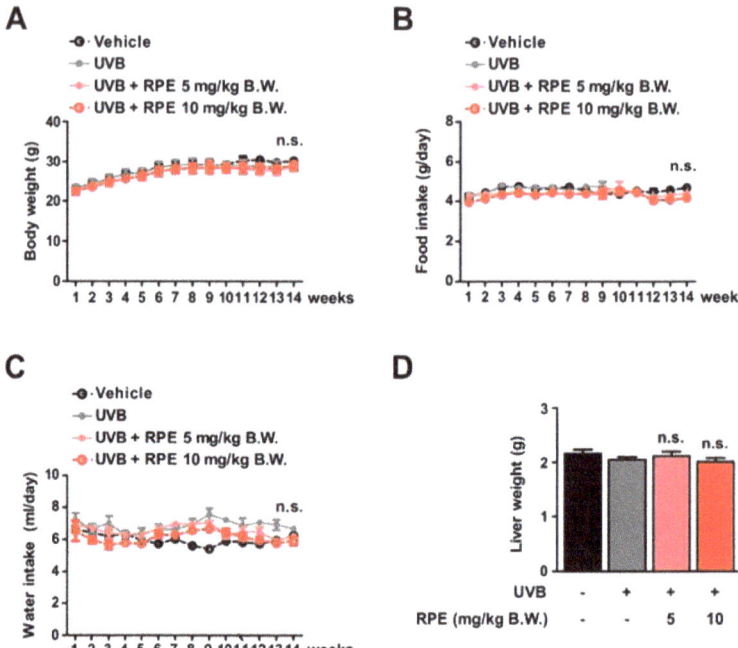

Figure 2. RPE does not show toxicity at the tested concentrations. (**A–C**) Body weight (n = 7), food intake (n = 4), and water intake (n = 4) were measured twice a week. (**D**) Liver weight was measured after sacrificing the mice at the end of the experiment (n = 7). Data represent the means ± SD. There was no significant difference (n.s.) among all groups.

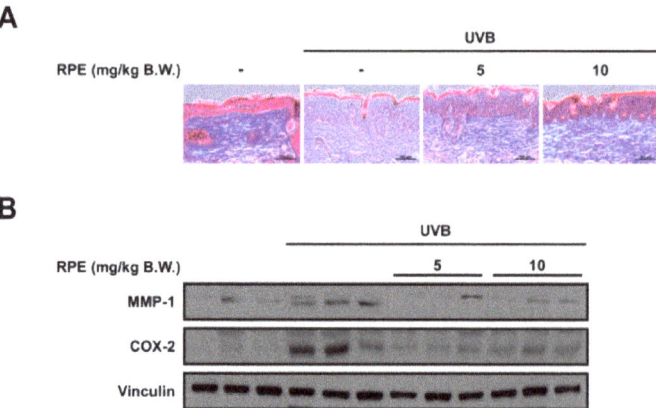

Figure 3. RPE inhibits collagen degradation and reverses biomarkers of skin aging. (**A**) Masson's trichrome staining for the visualization of collagen and keratin fibers in mouse skin tissue. Collagen fibers appear blue and keratin fibers appear red. The scale bar indicates 100 μm. (**B**) Protein expression of MMP−1, COX−2, and vinculin were determined in mouse tissue lysates using the corresponding antibody. Tissue lysates from three mice per group were used. Vinculin was used as a loading control.

3.4. Identification of Compounds in Rosa gallica

Main fragment ions of RPE obtained by UHPLC–LTQ–Orbitrap/MS/MS are shown in Figure 4. A total of 17 peaks excluding solvent peak were identified (Table 1). Tentative identification was performed using the obtained precursor ion and their fragment ions. Gallic acid (1) and catechin (2), which are relatively polar compounds, were detected rapidly with short retention times under reverse−phase condition. Compounds in which two glycosides are bound to quercetin (such as rutin, fragment ion value of 303.05 m/z) were identified at relatively short retention times, followed by a monoglycoside (quercetin of 303.05 m/z and kaempferol of 287.05 m/z) and an aglycone (dihydrokaempferol) type. In this study, since the binding structures of the glycoside moiety is unclear, it was expressed as a diglycoside. Among the identified compounds, 11 peaks were identified as quercetin (peaks no. 5, 6, 7, 8, 11, 14, and 15) or kaempferol (peaks no. 9, 10, 13, and 17) derivatives, which is in accordance with previous reports where the glycosides of quercetin and kaempferol are the most abundant flavonoids in roses among the reported compounds [28–30].

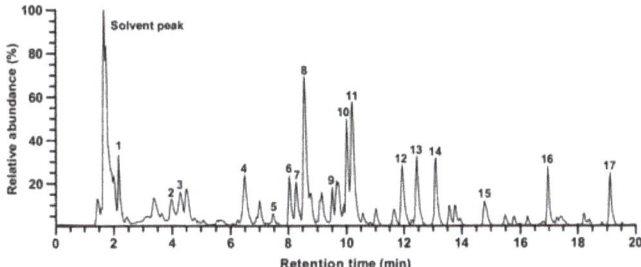

Figure 4. The peak intensity chromatogram of UHPLC−LTQ−Orbitrap/MS/MS of RPE. Peaks are indicated in Table 1.

Table 1. Identification of major chemical constituents in RPE by UHPLC−LTQ−Orbitrap/MS/MS.

Peak	t_R (min)	Molecular Weight	Ion Mode	Precursor Ion (m/z)	Fragment Ions (m/z)	Tentative Identification	Reference
1	2.16	170.1195	$[M - H]^-$	169.0000	N.D.	Gallic acid	[30]
2	4.04	290.2681	$[M + H]^+$	291.0864	N.D.	Catechin	[29]
3	4.28	954.7038	$[M + H]^+$	955.1054	N.D.	Rugosin B	[28]
4	6.50	936.6454	$[M + H]^+$	937.0934	N.D.	Casuarictin	[31]
5	7.45	616.4806	$[M + H]^+$	617.1137	303.0499	Quercetin-3-O-gallate-glucoside	[32]
6	8.00	610.5175	$[M + H]^+$	611.1607	465.1029, 303.0500	Rutin	[30]
7	8.28	464.3763	$[M + H]^+$	465.1028	303.0499	Quercetin-3-O-galactoside	[28,33]
8	8.56	464.3763	$[M + H]^+$	465.1026	303.0498	Quercetin-3-O-glucoside	[30,33]
9	9.51	448.3769	$[M + H]^+$	449.1078	287.0549	Kaempferol-3-O-galactoside	[28,33]
10	10.00	448.3769	$[M + H]^+$	449.1080	287.0550	Kaempferol-3-O-glucoside	[30,33]
11	10.20	448.3769	$[M + H]^+$	449.1078	303.0498	Quercitrin	[30]
12	11.94	438.5128	$[M - H]^-$	437.1445	N.D.	unknown	
13	12.44	432.3775	$[M + H]^+$	433.1130	287.0550	Kaempferol-3-O-rhamnoside	[30]
14	13.10	652.5542	$[M + H]^+$	653.1712	303.0500	Quercetin diglycoside	[30]
15	14.78	636.5548	$[M + H]^+$	637.1764	303.0500	Quercetin diglycoside	[30]
16	16.96	583.6741	$[M + H]^+$	584.2754	438.2387	Tricoumaroyl spermidine	[34]
17	19.12	288.2522	$[M + H]^+$	289.2373	271.2268	Dihydrokaempferol	[35]

RPE, rose petal extract; UHPLC-LTQ-Orbitrap/MS/MS, ultra-high performance liquid chromatography and tandem mass spectrometry; t_R, retention time; N.D., not detected.

3.5. Gallic Acid Is a Major Active Compound of Rosa gallica in Preventing Skin Aging

Based on the results from the chemical analysis (Figure 4 and Table 1), we selected gallic acid, quercetin, catechin, kaempferol, rutin, and quercitrin for further evaluation. The inhibitory activity against MMP−1 was measured using the six compounds. Treatment of gallic acid displayed the strongest reduction in UVB−induced MMP−1 levels among the tested compounds without any apparent cytotoxicity (Figure 5A,B). In addition, gallic acid was able to suppress MMP−1 levels in a dose−dependent manner (Figure 5C), suggesting gallic acid as a major contributing factor to the anti−skin aging effect exhibited by RPE.

3.6. Gallic Acid Targets the c−Raf Signaling Pathway

To understand the molecular mechanism of gallic acid, we investigated the effect of gallic acid on UVB−mediated signaling. As AP−1 is a crucial transcription factor controlling the expression of MMP−1 [4], we sought the test the effect of gallic acid on individual factors constituting the AP−1 dimer. Gallic acid downregulated c−Fos, whereas phosphorylation of c−Jun was not affected (Figure 6A). Since the expression of c−Fos has been known to be primarily regulated by MAPK family members (i.e., ERK1/2, p38, and JNK1/2) [8], we examined the effect of gallic acid against MAPK activation. We discovered that gallic acid can potently and selectively suppress ERK1/2 phosphorylation, while displaying no noticeable effects on JNK1/2 and p38 phosphorylations (Figure 6B). Gallic acid also attenuated phosphorylation of MEK1/2 which is the direct upstream regulator of ERK1/2 (Figure 6C). c−Raf is activated by UV and acts as an upstream regulator of the MEK/ERK pathway [36]. Results show that gallic acid can markedly reduce the activation of c−Raf (Figure 6C). In addition, gallic acid did not affect the phosphorylations of MKK4 and MKK3/6, further suggesting that gallic acid preferentially inhibits the c−Raf/MEK pathway (Figure 6C). Overall, these results show that gallic acid can selectively target the c−Raf/MEK/ERK/c−Fos pathway.

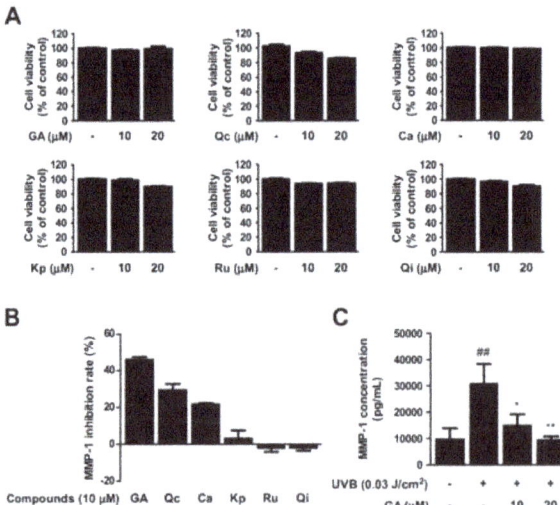

Figure 5. Effect of single compounds in RPE on UVB−induced MMP−1. (**A**) Cell viability was measured after cells were treated with gallic acid (GA), quercetin (Qc), catechin (Ca), kaempferol (Kp), rutin (Ru), Quercitrin (Qi) for 48 h (n = 5). (**B**) Human dermal fibroblasts (HDFs) were pre−treated with compounds at the indicated concentrations for 1 h before being exposed to UVB. After 48 h, MMP−1 production in cultured media was measured using ELISA (n = 3). Data represent MMP−1 inhibition rate compared to UVB−only treatment group. (**C**) HDFs were pre−treated with gallic acid (GA). MMP−1 concentration was measured using ELISA (n = 3). Data represent the means ± SD. Significant differences between un−treated control and UVB−only treatment group (## p < 0.01) and significant differences between UVB and UVB + GA treatment group (* p < 0.05, ** p < 0.01).

3.7. MEK Inhibition and Gallic Acid Blocks UVB−Induced MMP−1 Expression and Collagen Reduction in Reconstructed 3D Human Skin Model

As gallic acid selectively inhibited the c−Raf/MER/ERK signaling axis, we used a selective MEK inhibitor (i.e., U0126) to confirm the involvement of this signaling pathway in MMP−1 and collagen expression. U0126 suppressed UVB−induced MMP−1 in HDFs, demonstrating that activation of c−Raf/MER/ERK signaling is necessary for MMP−1 production (Figure 7A). We further utilized a reconstructed 3D human skin model to investigate the impact of U0126 and gallic acid on controlling MMP−1 and collagen levels. Reconstructed 3D human skin tissues were treated with U0126, gallic acid, or both and irradiated with UVB for 8 days. Both gallic acid and U0126 downregulated UVB−induced MMP−1 expression and prevented UVB−induced decrease in collagen (Figure 7B,C).

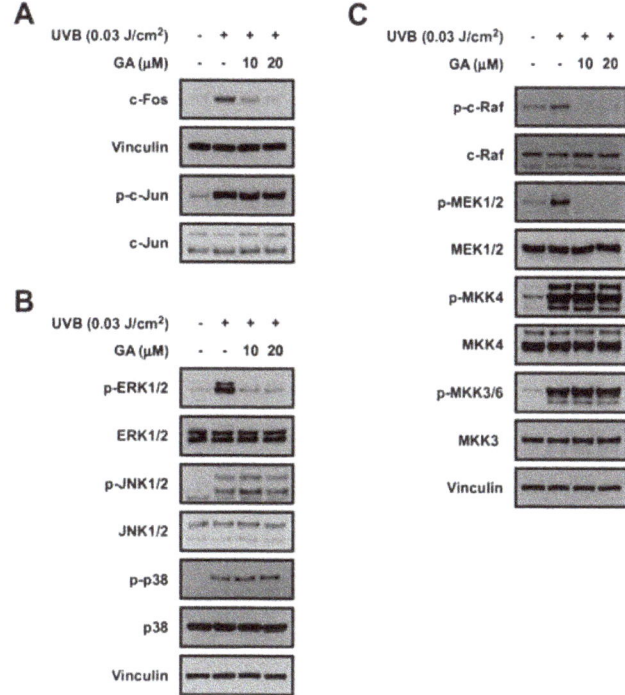

Figure 6. Effect of gallic acid (GA) on UVB−induced signaling pathways. (**A**) Protein expression of c−Fos, vinculin, p−c−Jun, and c−Jun were determined in human fibroblast cell lysates using the corresponding antibody. Vinculin was used as a loading control. (**B**) Effect of GA on MAPKs pathway in HDFs. Protein expression levels of phosphorylated and total ERK, JNK, p38, and vinculin were determined in cell lysates using the corresponding antibody by immunoblotting. Vinculin was used as a loading control. (**C**) Effect of GA on c−Raf and MAP2Ks pathway in HDFs. Protein expression levels of phosphorylated and total c−Raf, MEK1/2, MKK4, and MKK3, and vinculin were determined in cell lysates using the corresponding antibody by immunoblotting. Vinculin was used as a loading control.

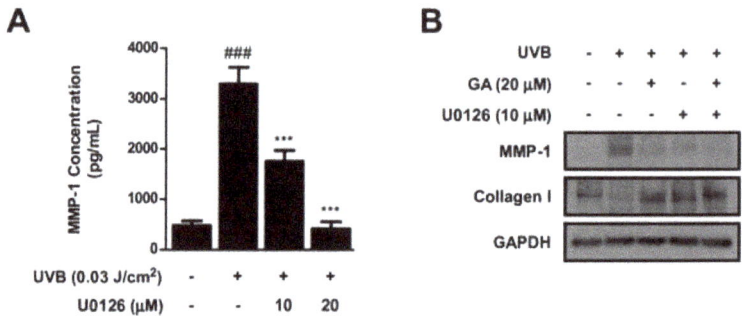

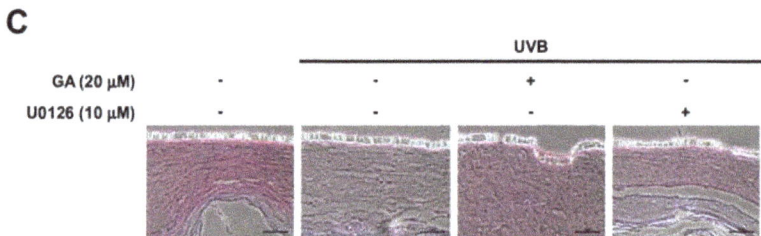

Figure 7. Effect of U0126 and gallic acid on MMP−1 and collagen expression in reconstructed 3D human skin model. (**A**) HDFs were pre−treated with U0126. MMP−1 concentration was measured using ELISA (n = 3). Data represent the means ± SD. Significant differences between un−treated control and UVB−only treatment group (### p < 0.001) and significant differences between UVB and UVB + U0126 treatment group (*** p < 0.001). (**B**) Effect of GA and U0126 on MMP−1 and collagen in a reconstructed 3D human skin model. GAPDH was used as a loading control. (**C**) Collagen was stained in sections from a reconstructed 3D human skin model using Sirius Red/Fast Green solution. The scale bar indicates 50 μm.

4. Discussion

In the current study, RPE was orally administered to mice and its protective effect against skin aging was examined. While a previous study reported the effect of RPE against UVB−induced skin aging under in vitro conditions [24,37], the efficacy of RPE in vivo was unknown. This is the first report to demonstrate that oral administration of *Rosa gallica* can block UVB−mediated skin aging in vivo without any noticeable toxicity. These results suggest that RPE can be a promising nutraceutical agent for the prevention of skin aging.

While previous studies reported bioactivities of *Rosa gallica*, the active components remained elusive. The identification of active compounds is a crucial step in understanding the mechanism of natural agents as well as developing it for practical applications. The active compound can be used as a marker for quality control or for optimizing processing conditions of the natural agent. Through combining UHPLC−MS/MS−based chemical analysis and activity evaluation, we have identified gallic acid as an active compound that can at least partially recapitulate the anti−skin aging effect exerted by RPE. Gallic acid was chosen as the major active compound because it showed the strongest inhibitory effect against MMP−1 expression compared to other compounds from RPE. Although weaker than gallic acid, quercetin and catechin also displayed inhibitory activity against MMP−1 expression (Figure 5B). This is consistent with previous studies which have also reported the anti-skin aging potential of quercetin and catechin [38,39]. Thus, the protective effect of RPE against skin aging may be attributed to a combination of several components. Based on our results gallic acid was chosen as a major active component, yet further studies to evaluate the activity of other compounds could aid in fully understanding the function of *Rosa gallica*.

When we examined the components of RPE, glycosidic derivatives of quercetin and kaempferol constituted a large portion among the identified compounds (Table 1). Rutin and quercitrin showed significantly weaker bioactivity compared to their aglycon compound, quercetin (Figure 5B), which is in accordance with previous reports where removal of the sugar moieties generally increases the bioactivity of the compound [40–43]. In line with this, while we were not able to test all the compounds found in the extract, considering that kaempferol generated minor effects in the tested condition (Figure 5B), it is likely that other glycosidic derivatives of kaempferol found in RPE would also produce relatively insignificant effects towards MMP−1 expression. However, there is a possibility that other compounds with distinct structures found in RPE could contribute to the anti-skin aging effect of *Rosa gallica*.

We have examined the molecular mechanism of gallic acid and discovered that gallic acid can selectively inhibit c−Raf, MEK, ERK, and c−Fos, while displaying no noticeable effects towards other MAPK and MAP2K family members. Gallic acid was previously reported to exert anti−skin aging effects; however, the responsible mode of action was largely unknown [44,45]. We report that gallic acid can inhibit UVB−induced c−Raf/MEK/ERK/c−Fos signaling axis in HDFs, and this may be the major mechanism to explain the gallic acid−driven downregulation of MMP−1. In addition, the c−Raf/MEK/ERK signaling pathway has been known to play a critical role in the development of various cancers, including melanoma, non−melanoma skin cancers, pancreatic cancer, and non−small cell lung cancer [46–48]. Considering that agents targeting the c−Raf pathway exert chemopreventive/chemotherapeutic effects against these types of cancers [47,49], gallic acid may also potentially suppress carcinogenesis.

At high concentrations phytochemicals may display toxicity, however, at low concentrations, they can modulate various physiological pathways, potentially providing health benefits. The concept of hormesis has been applied to understand the mechanism for the therapeutic effects reported by natural products [50,51]. Among these, the activation of cellular stress response pathways has been suggested as one of the potential modes of action for phytochemicals [51]. Indeed, many phytochemicals have been implicated to control cellular antioxidant systems as well as the signal transduction pathways [51,52]. In addition to targeting the c−Raf/MEK/ERK/c−Fos signaling axis, *Rosa gallica* and gallic acid may have exerted anti-skin aging activity through affecting regulators of oxidative stress. Gallic acid has been reported to modulate Keap1/Nrf2/ARE pathway [53,54] and Roses have been known to show antioxidant effects in cell models [37,55]. These attributes of *Rosa gallica* and gallic acid could have provided cellular protection through regulating the concentration of free radicals and subsequent inflammatory responses in the skin, leading to attenuation of skin aging.

5. Conclusions

Rosa gallica is an edible flower which has been used as an ingredient in traditional medicine and culinary practices. We have found that *Rosa gallica* can provide a protective function against skin aging in vivo. Gallic acid appears to function as an active compound of *Rosa gallica* through inhibiting the c−Raf signaling pathway (Figure 8). Discovering the possibility of *Rosa gallica* as an anti−skin aging food agent opens new opportunities to utilize rose petals as a nutraceutical.

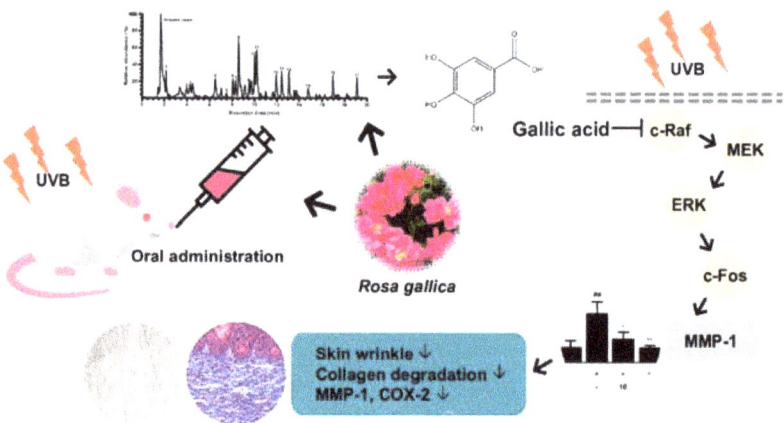

Figure 8. Schematic diagram summarizing the anti—skin aging effect of *Rosa gallica* and its mechanism.

Author Contributions: Conceptualization, S.J., T.-G.N., T.-G.L., S.B.; formal analysis, S.J., Y.-S.J., Y.-R.C., J.-W.S., W.-C.L.; investigation, S.J., Y.-S.J., Y.-R.C., J.-W.S., W.-C.L.; data curation, S.J., Y.-S.J., T.-G.L., S.B.; writing—original draft preparation, S.J., Y.-S.J., S.B.; writing—review and editing, T.-G.N., T.-G.L., S.B.; visualization, S.J.; supervision, T.-G.L., S.B.; project administration, T.-G.L., S.B.; funding acquisition, T.-G.L., S.B. All authors have read and agreed to the published version of the manuscript.

Funding: This research was funded by the Ministry of Science and ICT and by the National Research Foundation of Korea (NRF) grant funded by the Korea government (MSIT), grant number 2020R1C1C100467011 to T.L. and National Research Foundation of Korea (NRF) grant funded by the Korean government (Ministry of Science, ICT and Future Planning), grant number 2020R1A2C1010703 to S.B.

Institutional Review Board Statement: The study was approved by the Institutional Review Board (or Ethics Committee) of Institutional Animal Care and Use committee (protocol code SEMI1–19–02).

Informed Consent Statement: Not applicable.

Data Availability Statement: Data is contained within the article.

Conflicts of Interest: The authors declare no conflict of interest.

References

1. Yaar, M.; Gilchrest, B.A. Photoageing: Mechanism, prevention and therapy. *Br. J. Derm.* **2007**, *157*, 874–887. [CrossRef]
2. Perez-Sanchez, A.; Barrajon-Catalan, E.; Herranz-Lopez, M.; Micol, V. Nutraceuticals for Skin Care: A Comprehensive Review of Human Clinical Studies. *Nutrients* **2018**, *10*, 403. [CrossRef]
3. Rittie, L.; Fisher, G.J. Natural and sun-induced aging of human skin. *Cold Spring Harb. Perspect. Med.* **2015**, *5*, a015370. [CrossRef]
4. Fisher, G.J.; Kang, S.; Varani, J.; Bata-Csorgo, Z.; Wan, Y.; Datta, S.; Voorhees, J.J. Mechanisms of photoaging and chronological skin aging. *Arch. Derm.* **2002**, *138*, 1462–1470. [CrossRef]
5. Surowiak, P.; Gansukh, T.; Donizy, P.; Halon, A.; Rybak, Z. Increase in cyclooxygenase-2 (COX-2) expression in keratinocytes and dermal fibroblasts in photoaged skin. *J. Cosmet Derm.* **2014**, *13*, 195–201. [CrossRef] [PubMed]
6. Philips, N.; Auler, S.; Hugo, R.; Gonzalez, S. Beneficial regulation of matrix metalloproteinases for skin health. *Enzym. Res.* **2011**, *2011*, 427285. [CrossRef] [PubMed]
7. Habib, M.A.; Salem, S.A.; Hakim, S.A.; Shalan, Y.A. Comparative immunohistochemical assessment of cutaneous cyclooxygenase-2 enzyme expression in chronological aging and photoaging. *Photodermatol. Photoimmunol. Photomed.* **2014**, *30*, 43–51. [CrossRef]
8. Rittie, L.; Fisher, G.J. UV-light-induced signal cascades and skin aging. *Ageing Res. Rev.* **2002**, *1*, 705–720. [CrossRef]
9. Angel, P.; Szabowski, A.; Schorpp-Kistner, M. Function and regulation of AP-1 subunits in skin physiology and pathology. *Oncogene* **2001**, *20*, 2413–2423. [CrossRef] [PubMed]
10. Li, Y.; Alhendi, A.M.N.; Yeh, M.C.; Elahy, M.; Santiago, F.S.; Deshpande, N.P.; Wu, B.; Chan, E.; Inam, S.; Prado-Lourenco, L.; et al. Thermostable small-molecule inhibitor of angiogenesis and vascular permeability that suppresses a pERK-FosB/DeltaFosB-VCAM-1 axis. *Sci Adv.* **2020**, *6*, eaaz7815. [CrossRef]

11. Pittayapruek, P.; Meephansan, J.; Prapapan, O.; Komine, M.; Ohtsuki, M. Role of Matrix Metalloproteinases in Photoaging and Photocarcinogenesis. *Int. J. Mol. Sci.* **2016**, *17*, 868. [CrossRef] [PubMed]
12. Price, M.A.; Cruzalegui, F.H.; Treisman, R. The p38 and ERK MAP kinase pathways cooperate to activate Ternary Complex Factors and c-fos transcription in response to UV light. *EMBO J.* **1996**, *15*, 6552–6563. [CrossRef] [PubMed]
13. De Araujo, R.; Lobo, M.; Trindade, K.; Silva, D.F.; Pereira, N. Fibroblast Growth Factors: A Controlling Mechanism of Skin Aging. *Ski. Pharm. Physiol* **2019**, *32*, 275–282. [CrossRef] [PubMed]
14. Radler-Pohl, A.; Sachsenmaier, C.; Gebel, S.; Auer, H.P.; Bruder, J.T.; Rapp, U.; Angel, P.; Rahmsdorf, H.J.; Herrlich, P. UV-induced activation of AP-1 involves obligatory extranuclear steps including Raf-1 kinase. *EMBO J.* **1993**, *12*, 1005–1012. [CrossRef]
15. Bode, A.M.; Dong, Z. Mitogen-activated protein kinase activation in UV-induced signal transduction. *Sci. STKE* **2003**, *2003*, RE2. [CrossRef] [PubMed]
16. Lopez-Camarillo, C.; Ocampo, E.A.; Casamichana, M.L.; Perez-Plasencia, C.; Alvarez-Sanchez, E.; Marchat, L.A. Protein kinases and transcription factors activation in response to UV-radiation of skin: Implications for carcinogenesis. *Int. J. Mol. Sci.* **2012**, *13*, 142–172. [CrossRef]
17. Fisher, G.J.; Voorhees, J.J. Molecular Mechanisms of Photoaging and its Prevention by Retinoic Acid: Ultraviolet Irradiation Induces MAP Kinase Signal Transduction Cascades that Induce Ap-1-Regulated Matrix Metalloproteinases that Degrade Human Skin In Vivo. *J. Investig. Dermatol. Symp. Proc.* **1998**, *3*, 61–68. [CrossRef] [PubMed]
18. Chrubasik, C.; Roufogalis, B.D.; Muller-Ladner, U.; Chrubasik, S. A systematic review on the *Rosa canina* effect and efficacy profiles. *Phytother. Res.* **2008**, *22*, 725–733. [CrossRef]
19. Boskabady, M.H.; Shafei, M.N.; Saberi, Z.; Amini, S. Pharmacological effects of *Rosa Damascena*. *Iran. J. Basic Med. Sci.* **2011**, *14*, 295–307. [CrossRef]
20. Fujii, T.; Ikeda, K.; Saito, M. Inhibitory effect of rose hip (*Rosa canina* L.) on melanogenesis in mouse melanoma cells and on pigmentation in brown guinea pigs. *Biosci. Biotechnol. Biochem.* **2011**, *75*, 489–495. [CrossRef]
21. Jeon, H.; Kim, D.H.; Nho, Y.H.; Park, J.E.; Kim, S.N.; Choi, E.H. A Mixture of Extracts of *Kochia scoparia* and *Rosa multiflora* with PPAR α/γ Dual Agonistic Effects Prevents Photoaging in Hairless Mice. *Int. J. Mol. Sci.* **2016**, *17*, 1919. [CrossRef]
22. Pires, T.C.S.P.; Dias, M.I.; Barros, L.; Calhelha, R.C.; Alves, M.J.; Oliveira, M.B.P.P.; Santos-Buelga, C.; Ferreira, I.C.F.R. Edible flowers as sources of phenolic compounds with bioactive potential. *Food Res. Int.* **2018**, *105*, 580–588. [CrossRef]
23. Koczka, N.; Stefanovits-Banyai, E.; Ombodi, A. Total Polyphenol Content and Antioxidant Capacity of Rosehips of Some *Rosa* Species. *Medicines* **2018**, *5*, 84. [CrossRef] [PubMed]
24. Shin, E.J.; Han, A.R.; Lee, M.H.; Song, Y.R.; Lee, K.M.; Nam, T.G.; Lee, P.; Lee, S.Y.; Lim, T.G. Extraction conditions for *Rosa gallica* petal extracts with anti-skin aging activities. *Food Sci. Biotechnol.* **2019**, *28*, 1439–1446. [CrossRef]
25. Shin, S.H.; Lee, J.S.; Zhang, J.M.; Choi, S.; Boskovic, Z.V.; Zhao, R.; Song, M.; Wang, R.; Tian, J.; Lee, M.H.; et al. Synthetic lethality by targeting the RUVBL1/2-TTT complex in mTORC1-hyperactive cancer cells. *Sci. Adv.* **2020**, *6*, eaay9131. [CrossRef] [PubMed]
26. Sano, T.; Kume, T.; Fujimura, T.; Kawada, H.; Moriwaki, T.; Takema, Y. The formation of wrinkles caused by transition of keratin intermediate filaments after repetitive UVB exposure. *Arch. Derm. Res.* **2005**, *296*, 359–365. [CrossRef] [PubMed]
27. Yamaba, H.; Haba, M.; Kunita, M.; Sakaida, T.; Tanaka, H.; Yashiro, Y.; Nakata, S. Morphological change of skin fibroblasts induced by UV Irradiation is involved in photoaging. *Exp. Derm.* **2016**, *25* (Suppl. S3), 45–51. [CrossRef]
28. Cai, Y.Z.; Xing, J.; Sun, M.; Zhan, Z.Q.; Corke, H. Phenolic Antioxidants (Hydrolyzable Tannins, Flavonols, and Anthocyanins) Identified by LC-ESI-MS and MALDI-QIT-TOF MS from *Rosa chinensis* flowers. *J. Agric. Food Chem.* **2005**, *53*, 9940–9948. [CrossRef]
29. Barros, L.; Alves, C.T.; Duenas, M.; Silva, S.; Oliveira, R.; Carvalho, A.M.; Henriques, M.; Santos-Buelga, C.; Ferreira, I.C.F.R. Characterization of phenolic compounds in wild medicinal flowers from Portugal by HPLC-DAD-ESI/MS and evaluation of antifungal properties. *Ind. Crop. Prod.* **2013**, *44*, 104–110. [CrossRef]
30. Kumar, N.; Bhandari, P.; Singh, B.; Bari, S.S. Antioxidant activity and ultra-performance LC-electrospray ionization-quadrupole time-of-flight mass spectrometry for phenolics-based fingerprinting of Rose species: *Rosa damascena*, *Rosa bourboniana* and *Rosa brunonii*. *Food Chem. Toxicol.* **2009**, *47*, 361–367. [CrossRef]
31. Ochir, S.; Nishizawa, M.; Park, B.J.; Ishii, K.; Kanazawa, T.; Funaki, M.; Yamagishi, T. Inhibitory effects of *Rosa gallica* on the digestive enzymes. *J. Nat. Med.* **2010**, *64*, 275–280. [CrossRef]
32. Qing, L.S.; Xue, Y.; Zhang, J.G.; Zhang, Z.F.; Liang, J.; Jiang, Y.; Liu, Y.M.; Liao, X. Identification of flavonoid glycosides in *Rosa chinensis* flowers by liquid chromatography-tandem mass spectrometry in combination with ^{13}C nuclear magnetic resonance. *J. Chromatogr. A* **2012**, *1249*, 130–137. [CrossRef] [PubMed]
33. Ozga, J.A.; Saeed, A.; Wismer, W.; Reinecke, D.M. Characterization of cyanidin- and quercetin-derived flavonoids and other phenolics in mature saskatoon fruits (*Amelanchier alnifolia* Nutt.). *J. Agric. Food Chem.* **2007**, *55*, 10414–10424. [CrossRef] [PubMed]
34. Elejalde-Palmett, C.; de Bernonville, T.D.; Glevarec, G.; Pichon, O.; Papon, N.; Courdavault, V.; St-Pierre, B.; Giglioli-Guivarc'h, N.; Lanoue, A.; Besseau, S. Characterization of a spermidine hydroxycinnamoyltransferase in Malus domestica highlights the evolutionary conservation of trihydroxycinnamoyl spermidines in pollen coat of core Eudicotyledons. *J. Exp. Bot.* **2015**, *66*, 7271–7285. [CrossRef] [PubMed]
35. Tsimogiannis, D.; Samiotaki, M.; Panayotou, G.; Oreopoulou, V. Characterization of flavonoid subgroups and hydroxy substitution by HPLC-MS/MS. *Molecules* **2007**, *12*, 593–606. [CrossRef]

36. Hoyos, B.; Imam, A.; Korichneva, I.; Levi, E.; Chua, R.; Hammerling, U. Activation of c-Raf kinase by ultraviolet light. Regulation by retinoids. *J. Biol. Chem.* **2002**, *277*, 23949–23957. [CrossRef] [PubMed]
37. Lee, M.H.; Nam, T.G.; Lee, I.; Shin, E.J.; Han, A.R.; Lee, P.; Lee, S.Y.; Lim, T.G. Skin anti-inflammatory activity of rose petal extract (*Rosa gallica*) through reduction of MAPK signaling pathway. *Food Sci. Nutr.* **2018**, *6*, 2560–2567. [CrossRef]
38. Shin, H.-J.; Kim, S.-N.; Kim, J.-K.; Lee, B.-G.; Chang, I.-S. Effect of Green Tea Catechins on the Expression and Activity of MMPs and Type I Procollagen Synthesis in Human Dermal Fibroblasts. *J. Soc. Cosmet. Sci. Korea* **2006**, *32*, 117–121.
39. Shin, E.J.; Lee, J.S.; Hong, S.; Lim, T.G.; Byun, S. Quercetin Directly Targets JAK2 and PKCδ and Prevents UV-Induced Photoaging in Human Skin. *Int. J. Mol. Sci.* **2019**, *20*, 5262. [CrossRef]
40. Sudhakaran, M.; Parra, M.R.; Stoub, H.; Gallo, K.A.; Doseff, A.I. Apigenin by targeting hnRNPA2 sensitizes triple-negative breast cancer spheroids to doxorubicin-induced apoptosis and regulates expression of ABCC4 and ABCG2 drug efflux transporters. *Biochem. Pharm.* **2020**, *182*, 114259. [CrossRef]
41. Lin, C.F.; Leu, Y.L.; Al-Suwayeh, S.A.; Ku, M.C.; Hwang, T.L.; Fang, J.Y. Anti-inflammatory activity and percutaneous absorption of quercetin and its polymethoxylated compound and glycosides: The relationships to chemical structures. *Eur. J. Pharm. Sci.* **2012**, *47*, 857–864. [CrossRef] [PubMed]
42. Vijayaraj, P.; Nakagawa, H.; Yamaki, K. Cyanidin and cyanidin-3-glucoside derived from Vigna unguiculata act as noncompetitive inhibitors of pancreatic lipase. *J. Food Biochem.* **2019**, *43*, e12774. [CrossRef] [PubMed]
43. Hou, L.; Zhou, B.; Yang, L.; Liu, Z.L. Inhibition of human low density lipoprotein oxidation by flavonols and their glycosides. *Chem. Phys. Lipids* **2004**, *129*, 209–219. [CrossRef] [PubMed]
44. Zhao, P.; Alam, M.B.; Lee, S.H. Protection of UVB-Induced Photoaging by Fuzhuan-Brick Tea Aqueous Extract via MAPKs/*Nrf2*-Mediated Down-Regulation of MMP-1. *Nutrients* **2018**, *11*, 60. [CrossRef] [PubMed]
45. Hwang, E.; Park, S.Y.; Lee, H.J.; Lee, T.Y.; Sun, Z.W.; Yi, T.H. Gallic acid regulates skin photoaging in UVB-exposed fibroblast and hairless mice. *Phytother. Res.* **2014**, *28*, 1778–1788. [CrossRef]
46. Green, C.L.; Khavari, P.A. Targets for molecular therapy of skin cancer. *Semin. Cancer Biol.* **2004**, *14*, 63–69. [CrossRef]
47. Khazak, V.; Astsaturov, I.; Serebriiskii, I.G.; Golemis, E.A. Selective Raf inhibition in cancer therapy. *Expert Opin. Ther. Targets* **2007**, *11*, 1587–1609. [CrossRef]
48. Assi, M.; Achouri, Y.; Loriot, A.; Dauguet, N.; Dahou, H.; Baldan, J.; Libert, M.; Fain, J.S.; Guerra, C.; Bouwens, L.; et al. Dynamic Regulation of Expression of KRAS and Its Effectors Determines the Ability to Initiate Tumorigenesis in Pancreatic Acinar Cells. *Cancer Res.* **2021**, *81*, 2679–2689. [CrossRef]
49. Farrand, L.; Byun, S. Induction of Synthetic Lethality by Natural Compounds Targeting Cancer Signaling. *Curr. Pharm. Des.* **2017**, *23*, 4311–4320. [CrossRef]
50. Brunetti, G.; Di Rosa, G.; Scuto, M.; Leri, M.; Stefani, M.; Schmitz-Linneweber, C.; Calabrese, V.; Saul, N. Healthspan Maintenance and Prevention of Parkinson's-like Phenotypes with Hydroxytyrosol and Oleuropein Aglycone in *C. elegans*. *Int. J. Mol. Sci.* **2020**, *21*, 2588. [CrossRef]
51. Calabrese, V.; Cornelius, C.; Dinkova-Kostova, A.T.; Calabrese, E.J.; Mattson, M.P. Cellular stress responses, the hormesis paradigm, and vitagenes: Novel targets for therapeutic intervention in neurodegenerative disorders. *Antioxid. Redox Signal.* **2010**, *13*, 1763–1811. [CrossRef]
52. Miquel, S.; Champ, C.; Day, J.; Aarts, E.; Bahr, B.A.; Bakker, M.; Banati, D.; Calabrese, V.; Cederholm, T.; Cryan, J.; et al. Poor cognitive ageing: Vulnerabilities, mechanisms and the impact of nutritional interventions. *Ageing Res. Rev.* **2018**, *42*, 40–55. [CrossRef]
53. Sun, Z.; Du, J.; Hwang, E.; Yi, T.H. Paeonol extracted from *Paeonia suffruticosa* Andr. ameliorated UVB-induced skin photoaging via DLD/Nrf2/ARE and MAPK/AP-1 pathway. *Phytother. Res.* **2018**, *32*, 1741–1749. [CrossRef]
54. Feng, R.B.; Wang, Y.; He, C.; Yang, Y.; Wan, J.B. Gallic acid, a natural polyphenol, protects against tert-butyl hydroperoxide-induced hepatotoxicity by activating ERK-Nrf2-Keap1-mediated antioxidative response. *Food Chem. Toxicol.* **2018**, *119*, 479–488. [CrossRef]
55. Jimenez, S.; Gascon, S.; Luquin, A.; Laguna, M.; Ancin-Azpilicueta, C.; Rodriguez-Yoldi, M.J. *Rosa canina* Extracts Have Antiproliferative and Antioxidant Effects on Caco-2 Human Colon Cancer. *PLoS ONE* **2016**, *11*, e0159136. [CrossRef]

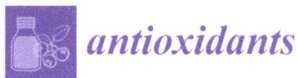

Article

Anthocyanin-Related Pigments: Natural Allies for Skin Health Maintenance and Protection

Patrícia Correia, Paula Araújo, Carolina Ribeiro, Hélder Oliveira, Ana Rita Pereira, Nuno Mateus, Victor de Freitas, Natércia F. Brás, Paula Gameiro, Patrícia Coelho, Lucinda J. Bessa, Joana Oliveira * and Iva Fernandes *

LAQV-REQUIMTE, Department of Chemistry and Biochemistry, Faculty of Sciences, University of Porto, 4169-007 Porto, Portugal; patricia.correia@fc.up.pt (P.C.); paula.araujo@fc.up.pt (P.A.); up201503157@fc.up.pt (C.R.); helder.oliveira@fc.up.pt (H.O.); anarita@fc.up.pt (A.R.P.); nbmateus@fc.up.pt (N.M.); vfreitas@fc.up.pt (V.d.F.); nbras@fc.up.pt (N.F.B.); agsantos@fc.up.pt (P.G.); patriciaines20@gmail.com (P.C.); lucindabessa12@gmail.com (L.J.B.)
* Correspondence: jsoliveira@fc.up.pt (J.O.); iva.fernandes@fc.up.pt (I.F.)

Citation: Correia, P.; Araújo, P.; Ribeiro, C.; Oliveira, H.; Pereira, A.R.; Mateus, N.; de Freitas, V.; Brás, N.F.; Gameiro, P.; Coelho, P.; et al. Anthocyanin-Related Pigments: Natural Allies for Skin Health Maintenance and Protection. *Antioxidants* 2021, *10*, 1038. https://doi.org/10.3390/antiox10071038

Academic Editors: Daniela-Saveta Popa, Laurian Vlase, Marius Emil Rusu and Ionel Fizesan

Received: 16 June 2021
Accepted: 21 June 2021
Published: 28 June 2021

Publisher's Note: MDPI stays neutral with regard to jurisdictional claims in published maps and institutional affiliations.

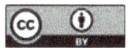

Copyright: © 2021 by the authors. Licensee MDPI, Basel, Switzerland. This article is an open access article distributed under the terms and conditions of the Creative Commons Attribution (CC BY) license (https://creativecommons.org/licenses/by/4.0/).

Abstract: Human skin is commonly described as a particularly dynamic and complex environment, with a physiological balance continuously orchestrated by numerous internal and external factors. Intrinsic aging, exposure to UV radiation and skin pathogens are some of the key players that account for dermatological alterations and ailments. In this regard, this study intended to explore the potential skin-health beneficial properties of a group of molecules belonging to the anthocyanin family: cyanidin- and malvidin-3-*O*-glucosides and some of their structurally related pigments, resulting in a library of compounds with different structural properties and color hues. The inclusion of both purified compounds and crude extracts provided some insights into their distinctive effects when tested as individual agents or as part of multicomponent mixtures. Overall, most of the compounds were found to reduce biofilm production by *S. aureus* and *P. aeruginosa* reference strains, exhibit UV-filter capacity, attenuate the production of reactive oxygen species in human skin keratinocytes and fibroblasts and also showed inhibitory activity of skin-degrading enzymes, in the absence of cytotoxic effects. Carboxypyranocyanidin-3-*O*-glucoside stood out for its global performance which, combined with its greater structural stability, makes this a particular interesting compound for potential incorporation in topical formulations. Results provide strong evidence of the skin protective effects of these pigments, supporting their further application for cosmeceutical purposes.

Keywords: natural bioactives; anthocyanins; photoprotection; UV-filter; oxidative stress; antimicrobial; skin aging; ECM; topical formulations; cosmeceuticals

1. Introduction

The importance of human skin goes way beyond its physical protective barrier role between body and surroundings, as it serves other crucial functions, including prevention of percutaneous water loss and immune surveillance [1]. Maintaining a good skin appearance is important, not only from a health standpoint but also for self-esteem and well-being since its appearance is inevitably linked to the visual perception of vitality. From a holistic perspective, skin can be deemed as a highly dynamic environment, whose overall condition is modulated by a complex network of cellular and molecular events that result from the interplay of a multitude of external (e.g., sun-light exposure and tobacco smoke) and internal factors (e.g., genetics and endocrine metabolism) [2]. The decay of its function and structural integrity naturally arises with intrinsic aging, in a sequence of events that affects both the epidermal and dermal layers of the skin, with the most prominent changes occurring in the latter, where the levels of essential components of the extracellular matrix (ECM), namely collagen and elastin, along with hyaluronic acid, gradually decline [3]. These changes are mostly driven by the continuous age-dependent accumulation of reactive oxygen species (ROS) in the skin, which activate specific cell signaling cascades that simultaneously up-regulate the expression of ECM degrading enzymes and down-regulate the synthesis of ECM constituents [4]. As a result, the levels of mechanical resistance of the ECM decrease, and so does the mechanical tension within dermal fibroblasts, disturbing their normal shape, size and function. Cells respond by increasing their intracellular levels of ROS, creating a self-perpetuating detrimental cycle, culminating in the appearance of wrinkles, skin dryness, roughness and laxity [1,5,6]. Solar ultraviolet radiation (UVR) cumulative exposure is one of the main culprits of overproduction of ROS in the skin, and also promotes inflammation, two processes that feed into one another and exacerbate the above-mentioned cell signaling pathways. Continuous UV-induced oxidative damage to cellular proteins, membranes and DNA contributes to the deep structural and functional changes inflicted on the skin, characteristic of so-called photoaging [7,8].

Cutaneous microbiota, mostly made up of bacteria, also plays a crucial role in the maintenance of dermatological health and commensal bacteria are important in the mediation of skin physiological processes. However, in situations where the integrity of the epidermal barrier is compromised or in dysbiotic conditions, the skin becomes susceptible to bacterial colonization, infection and the possible onset of serious and difficult to irradicate skin disorders [9].

Given the increasing awareness of the importance of skin health, there is a growing demand for efficient solutions for preventing and treating skin related damage and disorders. Within this context, the use of compounds derived from natural sources for dermatological applications has gone through an exponential growth in popularity [10]. There seems to be a clear trend shift in consumer preference for these types of natural ingredients, which has boosted the research for innovative combinations of these bioactives. Amongst the existing classes of phytochemicals, anthocyanins represent one of the most attractive, owing to their simultaneous acknowledged bioactivity repertoire and visually attractive colors [11]. The growing and compelling evidence of the biological relevance of these polyphenolic compounds for skin-related applications has raised the interest in their use as cosmeceuticals [12–15].

The purpose of this study was to assess the potential protective and health promoting skin effects of a group of molecules belonging to the same anthocyanin family, including their antimicrobial activity, UV-filter capacity and inhibitory action on ROS production and skin-degrading enzymes. Cyanidin- and malvidin-3-O-glucosides and their corresponding deoxyanthocyanins (which lack the substitution at the C-3 position, making these pigments much less sensitive to water addition at C2) were included in this study, along with some pyranoanthocyanins structures (commonly found in wine matrices during the aging process and known for their higher structural and color stability in a wider pH range), which were obtained by further chemical modifications of the two native anthocyanins, giving rise to a library of compounds with distinct structural and chromatic properties [16,17] (Figure 1). Purified compounds were used to understand the full potential of each and to establish some structure–activity relationships, while extracts were also included in some of the analyses to investigate possible existing synergy or antagonism effects in complex multicomponent mixtures.

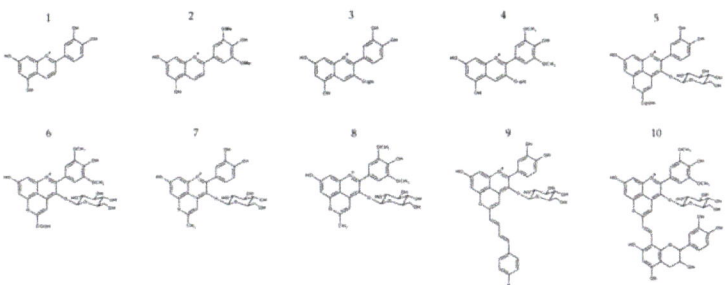

Figure 1. Chemical structure compounds (deoxyanthocyanins, anthocyanins and its related structures) selected for this study: 1—Luteolinidin (Lut); 2—Deoxymalvidin (DeoxyMv); 3—Cyanidin-3-O-glucoside (Cy-3-glc); 4—Malvidin-3-O-glucoside (Mv-3-glc); 5—Carboxypyranocyanidin-3-O-glucoside (CarboxypyCy-3-glc); 6—Carboxypyranomalvidin-3-O-glucoside (CarboxypyMv-3-glc); 7—Methylpyranocyanidin-3-O-glucoside (MethylpyCy-3-glc); 8—Methylpyranomalvidin-3-O-glucoside (MethylpyMv-3-glc); 9—4-(Dimethylamino)-cinnamyl-10-butadienylidene-pyranocyanidin-3-O-glucoside (Dimethylamino-cin-but-pyCy-3-glc); 10—Vinylpyranomalvidin-3-O-glucoside-catechin (VinylpyMv-3-glc-catechin).

2. Materials and Methods

2.1. Isolation and Synthesis of the Different Compounds

Deoxyanthocyanins were synthesized by acidic aldol condensation and consisted of the mixture of 2,4,6–trihydroxybenzaldehyde with 3,4-dihydroxyacetophenone and 3′,5′-dimethoxy-4′-hydroxyacetophenone (for luteolinidin and deoxymalvidin synthesis, respectively) [18]. Cyanidin- and malvidin-3-O-glucosides were obtained by the fractionation of blackberries and young red wine extract, and their further reaction with pyruvic acid (molar ratio of 1:100) and acetone (10% v/v aqueous solution) resulted in the formation of the carboxy and methylpyrano extracts, respectively, as described previously [19,20]. The obtained carboxypyranoanthocyanin extracts were tested as a complex mixture and also as a means of purifying carboxypyranocyanidin-3-O-glucoside and carboxypyranomalvidin-3-O-glucoside. The characterization of the extracts in terms of protein, lipids, sugar and total phenolic content and antioxidant activity is available in Supplementary Material (Table S1).

Amino-derived pyranocyanidin-3-O-glucoside was obtained from the reaction of methylpyranocy-3-glc with 4-(dimethylamino)-cinnamaldehyde as reported elsewhere [21]. The formation of vinylpyranomalvidin-3-O-glucoside-catechin resulted from the mixture of the carboxypyranomalvidin-3-O-glc with (+)-catechin, in the presence of acetaldehyde [22].

Synthesis reactions and the purity of the compounds were monitored by HPLC-DAD.

2.2. Antimicrobial and Antibiofilm Assays

2.2.1. Bacterial Strains and Growth Conditions

Compounds/extracts were tested against the following bacterial strains: *Pseudomonas aeruginosa* ATCC 27853, *Staphylococcus aureus* ATCC 29213, *Staphylococcus epidermidis* ATCC 14990, *Streptococcus pyogenes* ATCC 19615, and *Micrococcus luteus* ATCC 4698. Prior to each in vitro bioassay, fresh cultures were obtained for each strain using the appropriate medium and incubation conditions as follows. *Staphylococcus* spp. and *P. aeruginosa* were grown on Mueller–Hinton (MH) agar (Liofilchem srl, Roseto degli Abruzzi, Italy) for 24 h at 37 °C, while *M. luteus* was grown in Tryptic Soy agar (TSA, Liofilchem srl, Italy) for 24 h at 30 °C and *S. pyogenes* on TSA supplemented with 5% defibrinated sheep blood (Thermo Fisher Scientific, Waltham, MA, USA) for 24 h at 37 °C in an atmosphere of 5% CO_2.

2.2.2. Determination of Minimum Inhibitory and Minimum Bactericidal Concentrations

Minimum inhibitory concentrations (MICs) of compounds/extracts were determined using a broth microdilution technique, following the recommendations of the Clinical and Laboratory Standards Institute [23]. Briefly, fresh colonies of each strain were used to prepare the respective inocula with an optical density of 600 nm (OD_{600}) equal to 0.1 (approximately 1×10^8 CFU/mL). For all strains, cation-adjusted Mueller–Hinton broth (MHB2, Sigma-Aldrich, St. Louis, MO, USA) was used, but in the case of *S. pyogenes*, MBH2 was previously supplemented with 2.5% lysed horse blood (Thermo Fisher Scientific, USA). In 96-well, U-bottom microplates, each compound was serially diluted in the respective medium from stock solutions (10 mg/mL in DMSO) to achieve in-test concentrations ranging from 0.5 to 512 µg/mL. Wells were inoculated so that the final concentration in each was 5×10^5 CFU/mL. The plates were then incubated at 37 °C for 24 h. MIC was defined as the lowest concentration of compound inhibiting the bacterial growth visible to the naked eye. The concentration of DMSO in the highest in-test concentration did not affect the bacterial growth of the tested strains. Minimum bactericidal concentration (MBC) was determined by spreading 10 µL on MH agar (or blood agar in the case of *S. pyogenes*) from each well showing no visible growth, with further incubation for 24 h at 37 °C; the lowest concentration at which no growth occurred on MH plates was defined as the MBC.

2.2.3. Biofilm Formation Inhibition Assay

The capacity of all compounds/extracts to interfere with the biofilm formation by *P. aeruginosa* ATCC 27853 and *S. aureus* ATCC 29213 was assessed, using the crystal violet assay as previously reported [24]. TSB was used for *P. aeruginosa* ATCC 27853, whereas TSB supplemented with 1% glucose (TSBG) was used for *S. aureus* ATCC 29213. All compounds and extracts were used at three concentrations (256, 64 and 16 µg/mL), which were necessarily sub-inhibitory concentrations (below the MIC).

2.3. Determination of Solar Protection Factor (SPF)

To determine the in vitro solar protection factor (SPF), a relative measure of UVB protection, 1.0 mg of each compound/extract was weighed and diluted in ethanol (0.2 mg/mL), followed by ultra-sonication for 5 min. The absorption spectrum of each sample was collected in the range of 290 to 320 nm (every 5 nm), with 3 measurements for each point, using a 1 mm quartz cell and ethanol as blank. Additionally, SPF values were also determined in the presence of a conventional chemical UV filter, oxybenzone (Sigma-Aldrich, Spain), at a concentration of 0.1 mg/mL. Values were calculated according to Mansur equation:

$$SPF_{spectrophotometric} = CF \times \sum_{290}^{320} EE(\lambda) \times I(\lambda) \times Abs(\lambda)$$

where the *CF* (correction factor) is 10, *EE* (λ) represents the erythmogenic effect of radiation with wavelength λ, and *Abs* refers to spectrophotometric absorbance values at each wavelength λ. $EE(\lambda) \times I(\lambda)$ values are constant and are presented in Table 1.

Table 1. Normalized product function used for the calculation of SPF.

λ (nm)	EE × I (Normalized)
290	0.0150
295	0.0817
300	0.2874
305	0.3278
310	0.1864
315	0.0839
320	0.0180
Total	1

EE—erythemal effect spectrum; I—solar intensity spectrum.

2.4. Cell Culture Assays

2.4.1. Cell Lines and Growth Conditions

Primary Normal Human Epidermal Keratinocytes (HeKa) (ATCC® PCS200011™) were grown in Dermal Cell Basal Media (ATCC® PCS200030) supplemented with Keratinocyte Growth Kit components (ATCC® PCS200040) and 0.1% antibiotic/antimycotic solution (10 units/mL of penicillin, 10 µg/mL of streptomycin and 25 ng/mL of amphotericin B, from Sigma-Aldrich) at 37 °C in a humidified atmosphere with 5% CO_2. Cells were harvested using Trypsin-EDTA for Primary Cells (ATCC PCS999003) once a week, at 80% confluence.

Spontaneously transformed aneuploid immortal keratinocyte cell lines from adult human skin (HaCat) and human foreskin fibroblasts (HFF-1) were cultured in 22.1 cm^2 plates and maintained in Dulbecco's Modified Eagle Medium (DMEM, Cell Lines Service), supplemented with 10% or 15% fetal bovine serum (FBS, CLS) and 1% of antibiotic/antimycotic solution (100 units/mL of penicillin, 10 mg/mL of streptomycin and 0.25 mg/mL of amphotericin B, Sigma-Aldrich, St. Louis, MO, USA), at 37 °C in an atmosphere of 5% CO_2. Medium was renewed every two days and cells were harvested every two weeks.

2.4.2. Cytotoxicity Evaluation

Possible cytotoxic effects of the compounds towards HaCat and HFF-1 cells were evaluated using the standard MTT assay. Briefly, cells were seeded at a density of 5×10^4 (HaCat) and 1.4×10^4 cells/mL (HFF-1) onto 96-well plate and incubated for 24 h to allow cell attachment. Then, serially diluted compound solutions (0.78–100 µM) were added to the wells. Following a period of incubation of 48 h at 37 °C, wells were washed once with phosphate buffered saline (PBS, Sigma-Aldrich) and MTT solution (0.45 mg/mL) was added to each well. After 1.5 h of incubation, medium was discarded, and the formed formazan crystals were dissolved with dimethylsulfoxide (DMSO, Sigma-Aldrich). Absorbance was read at 570 nm (Biotek PowerWave XS, Winooski, VT, USA).

2.4.3. ROS Formation Assay

Reactive oxygen species production in HFF-1 and HaCat cells was evaluated following the standard method. Cells were seeded at a density of 5×10^4 cells/well onto 96-well plates and allowed to reach confluency. At this point, cells were washed twice with phosphate buffered saline solution (PBS, Sigma-Aldrich, St. Louis, MO, United States) and compounds were added at a concentration of 50 µM, followed by 24 h of incubation at 37 °C in a 5% CO_2 atmosphere. After that, cells were washed twice in Hank's Buffered Saline Solution (HBSS) and incubated with 100 µL of 50 µM DCFDA for 30 min in the same previous conditions. Afterwards, cells were washed twice with HBSS and incubated with fresh medium for 24 h, and the fluorescence intensity (498 nm excitation/522 nm emission) was then registered on a FlexStation 3 Multi-Mode Microplate Reader (Molecular Devices).

2.4.4. Transport Assay

HeKa cells were plated at a cell density of 2.6×10^5 cells/mL on 12-well transwell inserts with a 0.4 µm pore size (Corning Costar, Corning, NY, USA). The culture medium was changed every two days and cells were allowed to grow and differentiate to confluent monolayers for 8 days after the initial seeding. Cells were kept for 4 days in low calcium medium (0.06 mM) to allow them to form a monolayer. For differentiation, in the last 4 days medium was changed to high calcium (1.8 mM). Only HeKa monolayers with an integrity equivalent to a transepithelial electrical resistance (TEER) higher than 450 $\Omega.cm^2$ were used for the transport studies. Compound solutions at different concentrations were added to the apical compartment of the cell monolayers. The chamber was incubated at 37 °C for 1, 2, 3 or 24 h, after which both apical and basolateral aliquots were taken for HPLC-MS analysis. Transport rates were calculated as follows:

$$Transport\ rate\ \% = \frac{C_{BL}}{C_{AP}} \times 100$$

where C_{BL} represents the compound concentration at the basolateral side at a given time and C_{AP} represents the initial compound concentration at the apical side.

2.5. Enzymatic Inhibition Assays

2.5.1. Collagenase

A stock solution of *Clostridium histolyticum* collagenase (C0130, Sigma-Aldrich) was prepared in 100 mM of Phosphate Buffer pH 7.4 at a concentration of a 125 U/mL. Substrate N-[3-(2-furyl)-acryloyl]-Leu-Gly-Pro-Ala (FALGPA) and the different compounds were prepared in the same buffer at 6 mM and 200 µM, respectively. Compounds (75 µL) were incubated with the substrate (30 µL) for 10 min, followed by enzyme addition (40 µL) to start the reaction, which was followed by 35 min at 324 nm and 37 °C on a FlexStation 3 Multi-Mode Microplate Reader (Molecular Devices). Inhibition percentage was calculated using the following formula:

$$\text{Collagenase inhibition \%} = (1 - \frac{A - B}{C - D}) \times 100$$

where A and B represent the initial and final optical densities of the reaction in the presence of compounds, while C and D represent the initial and final optical densities of the reaction in the absence of compounds, respectively. Epigallocatechin-gallate (EGCG) was used as positive control at 50 µM.

2.5.2. Elastase

Experiments were conducted according to Sigma-Aldrich guidelines, with minor modifications. Briefly, 75 µL of each compound solution (200 µM), 30 µL of a freshly prepared working solution of porcine pancreatic elastase (0.3 U/mL) (Sigma-Aldrich, E1250), and 175 µL of Tris-HCl buffer pH 6.80 at 25 °C were mixed in a 96-well plate and incubated for 15 min. A reaction was initiated with the addition of 20 µL of N-Succinyl-Ala-Ala-Ala-p-nitroanilide (Bachem) (4.4 mM) and the release of p-nitroanilide (p-NA) was monitored spectrophotometrically at 405 nm for 40 min at 25 °C on a FlexStation 3 Multi-Mode Microplate Reader (Molecular Devices). The inhibition rate was calculated as follows:

$$\text{Elastase inhibition \%} = (1 - \frac{B - A}{D - C}) \times 100$$

where A and B represent the initial and final optical densities of the reaction in the presence of compounds, while C and D represent the initial and final optical densities of the reaction in the absence of compounds, respectively. N-Methoxysuccinyl-Ala-Ala-Ala-Val-chloromethyl ketone (MAAPVCK) (M0398, Sigma-Aldrich) was used as a positive control at 10 µM.

2.5.3. Hyaluronidase

30 µL from a stock solution of type I-S hyaluronidase from bovine testes (20 U/mL in 0.02 M phosphate buffer, pH 7, containing 50 mM NaCl) (H3506, Sigma-Aldrich) were mixed with 37.5 µL of a stock solution of each compound (200 µM) and then pre incubated for 10 min at 37 °C. Hyaluronic acid sodium salt from rooster comb (H5388, Sigma-Aldrich) was dissolved in sodium phosphate aqueous solution (0.03% in 300 mM sodium phosphate, pH 5.35) and heated at 60–70 °C for 20 min to ensure complete dissolution. After that, 30 µL of hyaluronic acid were added to the mixture and the 96-well plate was incubated at 37 °C for 60 min. Residual undigested hyaluronic acid was precipitated with 150 µL of 'stop reaction' solution (2.5% *w/v* CTAB in 2% *w/v* NaOH). The plate was left at room temperature for 10 min and the absorbance was measured at 400 nm on a FlexStation 3 Multi-Mode Microplate Reader (Molecular Devices, San Jose, California, USA). The percentage of inhibition was calculated as follows:

$$\text{Hyaluronidase inhibition \%} = \left(1 - \frac{A}{B}\right) \times 100$$

where A and B represent the enzymatic activity in the presence and absence of the compound, respectively. Quercetin at 50 µM was used as the positive control.

2.6. Molecular Docking

The X-ray structure of hyaluronidase of bee venom was obtained from Protein Data Bank (PDBID 1FCV at 2.65 Å resolution) [25]. This structure was chosen because it has an active site similar to the human enzyme and it has been used successfully in similar studies [25,26]. In this study, the binding of the pseudobase carbinol and chalcone forms of cyanidin-3-O-glucoside (Cy-3-glc), luteolinidin (Lut), malvidin-3-O-glucoside (Mv-3-glc) and deoxymalvidin (DeoxyMv), as well as the carboxypyranocyanidin-3-O-glucoside (CarboxypyCy-3-glc), methylpyranocyanidin-3-O-glucoside (MethylpyCy-3-glc), carboxypyranomalvidin-3-O-glucoside (CarboxypyMv-3-glc) and methylpyranomalvidin-3-O-glucoside (MethylpyMv-3-glc) were assessed. Quercetin (Que) and quercetin-3-glucoside (Que-3-glc) were used as positive controls. Ligand structures were built using the Avogadro software [27] and the molecular docking procedure was performed using the Autodock 4.2 software [28]. The docking process was validated by the re-docking of the crystallographic tetrasaccharide, consisting of two units of glucuronic acid and N-acetylglucosamine, and then the same molecular docking protocol was applied to the ligands under study. Crystallographic water molecules were removed and the hydrogen atoms were added to the enzyme, considering the protonation state of all protein residues in their physiological state (the exception was the protonated Glu219 residue). The PROPKA program [29] was used to check the pK_a values of all ionizable residues. Two disulfide bridges (Cys22-Cys313 and Cys189-Cys201) were also defined. The grid center was: X—2.606; Y—31.694; Z—−8.535 and comprised $60 \times 60 \times 60$ points with a spacing of 0.375. The Lamarckian genetic algorithm with a total of 50 solutions was used. The population size was 150, the maximum number of evaluations was 250,000 and the number of generations was 27,000. All solutions were ranked by the $\Delta G_{binding}$ values. The best docking solutions for each ligand were analyzed using the Visual Molecular Dynamics (VMD) program [30].

2.7. Statistical Analysis

Results were expressed as the mean ± standard error mean (SEM) of at least 3 independent experiments. Statistical analysis was performed with GraphPad Prism 8.2.1. software, using one-way analysis of variance (one-way ANOVA) with Turkey's test to estimate significant differences between the means of different experimental groups. Significance was set at $p < 0.05$.

3. Results and Discussion

3.1. Antimicrobial and Antibiofilm Activities

3.1.1. Antibacterial Activity

Overall, the compounds and extracts tested did not show antibacterial activity (Table 2). MIC values could only be determined for Lut and dimethylamino-cin-but-pyCy-3-glc against *M. luteus* and for Lut against *S. epidermidis*, but the values presented were relatively high.

Table 2. Minimum inhibitory concentration (MIC) and minimum bactericidal concentration (MBC) values, in μg/mL and in mM, of compounds and extracts against *P. aeruginosa* ATCC 27853, *S. aureus* ATCC 29213, *M. luteus* ATCC 4698, *S. epidermidis* ATCC 14990 and *S. pyogenes* ATCC 19615.

Extract/Compound	*P. aeruginosa* ATCC 27853	*S. aureus* ATCC 29213	*M. luteus* ATCC 4698	*S. epidermidis* ATCC 14990	*S. pyogenes* ATCC 19615
	MIC—μg/mL (mM)				
Lut	>512 (>1.67)	>512 (>1.67)	128 (0.42) *	128 (0.42) *	>512 (>1.67)
DeoxyMv	>512 (>1.46)	>512 (>1.46)	>512 (>1.46)	>512 (>1.46)	>512 (>1.46)
Cy-3-glc	>512 (>1.06)	>512 (>1.06)	>512 (>1.06)	512 (1.06) *	>512 (>1.06)
CarboxypyCy-3-glc	>512 (>0.93)	>512 (>0.93)	>512 (>0.93)	>512 (>0.93)	>512 (>0.93)
Elderberry carboxypyranoanthocyanin extract (Elderberry extract)	>512	>512	512 *	>512	>512
MethylpyCy-3-glc	>512 (>0.98)	>512 (>0.98)	>512 (>0.98)	>512 (>0.98)	>512 (>0.98)
Dimethylamino-cin-but-pyCy-3-glc	>512 (>0.75)	>512 (>0.75)	64 (0.09) *	>512 (>0.75)	512 (0.75) *
Mv-3-glc	>512 (>0.97)	>512 (>0.97)	>512 (>0.97)	>512 (>0.97)	>512 (>0.97)
CarboxypyMv-3-glc	>512 (>0.86)	>512 (>0.86)	>512 (>0.86)	>512 (>0.86)	>512 (>0.86)
Red wine carboxypyranoanthocyanin extract (red wine extract)	>512	>512	512 *	>512	>512
VinylpyMv-3-glc-catechin	>512 (>0.59)	>512 (>0.59)	>512 (>0.59)	>512 (>0.59)	>512 (>0.59)

* Only in these cases, the MBC assay could be performed, yet, MBC was >512 μg/mL.

3.1.2. Inhibition of Biofilm Formation

Bacteria tend to naturally form biofilms, in which bacterial aggregates live encased in a matrix that consists of extracellular polymeric substances (EPS) produced by the bacteria [31]. The biofilm alternative lifestyle presents a self-organization, gene expression and growth rate that is entirely distinct from the planktonic (free-living) state. One of the main concerns about bacterial biofilms is their increased resistance to antimicrobial agents and difficulty of eradication. *P. aeruginosa* and *S. aureus* are some of the primary pathogens responsible for biofilm formation in chronic wounds. So, despite the lack of antibacterial activity exhibited by compounds and extracts, their ability to inhibit the biofilm formation of *P. aeruginosa* ATCC 27853 and *S. aureus* ATCC 29213 was evaluated through the crystal violet assay, and the results obtained are shown in Figures 2 and 3, respectively.

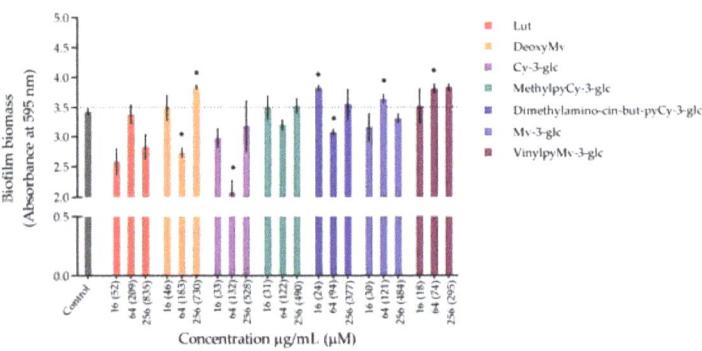

Figure 2. *Cont.*

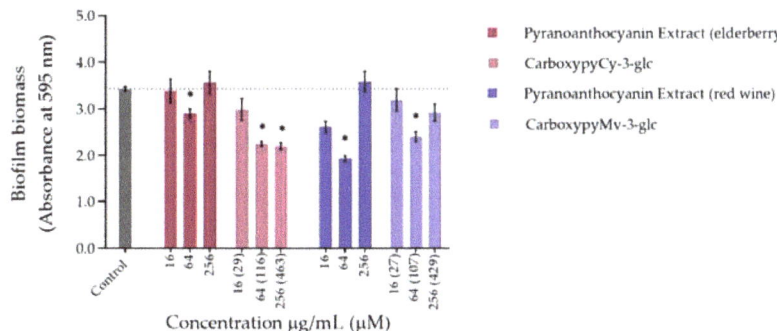

Figure 2. Biomass quantification of biofilms of *P. aeruginosa* ATCC 27853 formed in the absence (control) and in the presence of different concentrations of extracts or compounds: 256 µg/mL, 64 µg/mL and 16 µg/mL. Statistically significant differences between biofilms formed in presence of the extract/compound and control biofilm ($p < 0.05$) are marked with an asterisk.

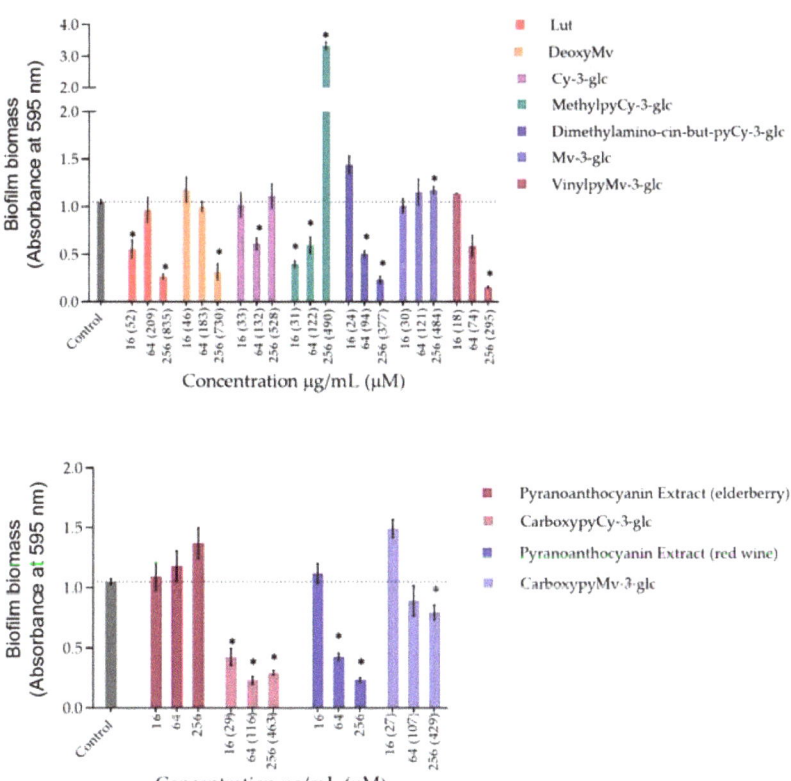

Figure 3. Biomass quantification of biofilms of *S. aureus* ATCC 29213 formed in the absence (control) and in the presence of different concentrations of extracts and compounds: 256 µg/mL, 64 µg/mL and 16 µg/mL. Statistically significant differences between biofilms formed in presence of extract/compound and control biofilm ($p < 0.05$) are marked with an asterisk.

Regarding *P. aeruginosa* biofilm biomass quantification in the presence of the compounds/extracts, it was possible to observe that at both concentrations of 64 and 256 µg/mL, only CarboxypyCy-3-glc significantly affected biofilm formation by *P. aeruginosa*, while at 64 µg/mL more compounds hampered biofilm formation in a significant manner, including deoxyMv, cy-3-glc, dimethylamino-cin-but-pyCy-3-glc and carboxypyMv-3-glc, as well as elderberry and red wine extracts. In some cases, however, an increase in the biofilm biomass was observed.

Concerning *S. aureus* biofilm formation, treatment with red wine extract B significantly affected biofilm formation at both 256 and 64 µg/mL, whereas elderberry extract did not present inhibitory activity at any of the concentrations tested. As can be observed, for most of the other compounds that interfered with biofilm formation, a reduction in biofilm biomass was only observed at one of those two concentrations. In the case of pyrano-derivatives of Cy-3-glc, carboxypyCy-3-glc was particularly efficient, significantly hampering biofilm formation at all three tested concentrations, while MethylpyCy-3-glc, despite clearly hampering biofilm formation at 16 and 64 µg/mL, led to the formation of a precipitate when tested at the highest concentration of 256 µg/mL that could not be removed during the biofilm staining protocol, resulting in a marked absorbance increase at 595 nm.

Furthermore, considering that CarboxypyCy-3-glc is the main component of elderberry extract and CarboxypyMv-3-glc is the major component of red wine extract, and confronting the results obtained for each extract with their main compound in both in *P. aeruginosa* and *S. aureus*, it was possible to draw some conclusions. In the case of CarboxypyCy-3-glc and elderberry extract, the isolated compound exhibited a much higher anti-biofilm activity. In fact, apart from the biomass reduction observed in *P. aeruginosa* when tested at a concentration of 64 µg/mL, elderberry extract did not show evidence of any inhibitory effects. This is possibly caused by antagonistic interactions between the different components of the extract, so that even with CarboxypyCy-3-glc being the major component of the extract (68% of the pyranoanthocyanins content) (Figure S1), its concentration is not enough to hamper biofilm formation and ends up being masked by the other elements: 12% are lipids (palmitic, oleic and stearic acids), 4% are formed by proteins and around 3% correspond to simple sugars (Table S1), which reinforces the importance of studying the compounds in their isolated form [32]. Comparing CarboxypyCy-3-glc with its anthocyanin analogue, Cy-3-glc, the extra pyran ring and carboxylic group appears to be a structural feature beneficial to its anti-biofilm activity. On the other hand, the inhibitory effect of red wine extract was more pronounced than its main component tested in an isolated form, CarboxypyMv-3-glc (considering the total pyranoanthocyanin content was only 30% CarboxypyMv-3-glc), which could indicate the occurrence of additive or synergistic interactions between different constituents: 10% proteins, 5% lipids (palmitic, oleic and stearic acids) and around 2% simple sugars (Table S1), contributing to the extract's having the best performance (Figure S1). It is also worth mentioning that, besides the reduced phenolic content, the huge amount of polymeric phenolic structures likely present in this extract may account for the observed inhibitory effect on biofilm formation. After analysis of proanthocyanin content, no monomeric, dimeric or trimeric structures were identified, although anthocyanin derived polymeric structures may be present (not detected in any of the chromatographic or colorimetric assays). Besides, myricetin-*O*-(*O*-galloyl)arabinoside, myricetin-3-*O*-arabinoside, quercetin 3-methoxyhexoside and quercetin 3-*O*-glucuronide were tentatively identified by mass spectrometry and account for the flavonol content (Table S1), so they may have contributed to the observed effect too.

Most of these molecules impaired biofilm formation only at one or two of the concentrations tested; higher concentration did not mirror a higher inhibition; thus, it can be hypothesized that some of these agents impair biofilm formation at optimum concentrations, not in a dose-response manner [33]. Further, these results reinforce that the mechanism by which these compounds affect biofilm formation is not dependent on their ability to inhibit the bacterial growth but might be related with some interference with the quorum sensing system. In fact, the antibiofilm activities of numerous plant polyphenols, including flavonoids, phenolic acids and tannins, have been reported in previous studies (mostly conducted in *S. aureus*, *E. coli* and *P. aeruginosa*), where biofilm suppression was attributed to the capacity of these compounds to interfere with different bacterial regulatory mechanisms, including quorum sensing [34]. Therefore, it can be of interest to explore these compounds in a future work for their ability to interfere with the quorum sensing of *P. aeruginosa* as well as of *S. aureus*.

Considering that the vast majority of microbial and chronic infections are reported to be related to biofilm formation [35], these results provide a good indicator of the suitability of these compounds for managing biofilm-related diseases and their potential topical application could be an efficient way to hinder biofilm formation and the further development and persistence of infection.

3.2. Solar Protection Factor (SPF)

The use of sunscreens is one of the most widely used and efficient ways to protect the skin against UV-induced damage, by limiting the amount of radiation reaching the epidermal and dermal layers, either by reflecting and scattering (physical filters) or absorbing ultraviolet radiation (chemical filters). The presence of aromatic rings in their flavonoid core structure confers anthocyanins appreciable UV absorptive capacities, so it is no surprise that the application of these pigments has been reframed and proposed as natural UV-filters for photoprotective formulations [36,37].

As an initial screening test, each compound was prepared at a concentration of 0.2 mg/mL in ethanol and its corresponding SPF was determined according to the Mansur equation (Table 3). Overall, the obtained in vitro SPF values of anthocyanins and their structural derivatives support their UV filter activity and further application as additives in UV-protective formulations. Except for vinylpyranomalvidin-3-glucoside-catechin, which exhibited the lowest SPF (8.35), the general values ranged between approximately 14 to 30, with Lut exhibiting the highest SPF (29.82). Although not very marked differences were observed between the compounds, those belonging to the cyanidin group showed slightly higher SPFs compared to their structural analogues of the malvidin group, except for the methylpyranoanthocyanins which had similar values.

Table 3. In vitro solar protection factors (SPF) of anthocyanins and derivatives estimated in the absence and presence of oxybenzone.

Compound (0.2 mg/mL)	SPF	
	-	+ 0.1 mg Oxybenzone/mL
Lut	29.82 ± 0.02	71.89 ± 0.040
DeoxyMv	17.28 ± 0.03	55.25 ± 0.03
Cy-3-glc	22.38 ± 0.01	63.01 ± 0.02
Blackberry anthocyanin extract	20.10 ± 0.06	66.98 ± 0.03
CarboxypyCy-3-glc	20.71 ± 0.18	n.d.
Elderberry carboxypyranoanthocyanin extract	16.03 ± 0.01	64.36 ± 0.03
MethylpyCy-3-glc	18.53 ± 0.15	68.21 ± 0.08
Dimethylamino-cin-but-pyCy-3-glc	14.78 ± 0.02	59.69 ± 0.01
Mv-3 glc	20.96 ± 0.01	n.d.
CarboxypyMv-3-glc	13.92 ± 0.04	67.85 ± 0.04
Red wine carboxypyranoanthocyanin extract	21.60 ± 0.02	67.10 ± 0.02
MethylpyMv-3-glc	19.24 ± 0.01	56.85 ± 0.06
VinylpyMv-3-glc-catechin	8.35 ± 0.06	n.d.
-		41.01 ± 0.38
Oxybenzone	69.03 ± 0.17	

n.d.—not determined.

Oxybenzone, a commercially used chemical UV filter in numerous sunscreen formulations, exhibited a clearly superior UV-absorption capacity, exhibiting SPF values of 41.01 and 69.03, when tested at 0.1 and 0.2 mg/mL, respectively. Nevertheless, when the ethanolic solutions of anthocyanins and derivatives were supplemented with 0.1 mg/mL of oxybenzone, the estimated SPFs were close to that of oxybenzone alone (at 0.2 mg/mL). Overall, the SPF values obtained from the mixture between both agents (pigment + oxybenzone) suggest the occurrence of a cumulative effect. In the cases of MethylpyCy-3-glc and CarboxypyMv-3-glc, however, the resulting SPFs might be indicative of a potentiation effect arising from their combination with the commercial UV filter.

Oxybenzone, along with other conventionally used chemical UV filters such as octinoxate, continues to be allowed in the market (both in the US and EU), but the use of these ingredients remains a controversial topic of discussion. There seems to be no conclusive evidence about the prejudicial effects of oxybenzone to human health, although some reports have raised some concerns about their possible endocrine disruptor effects and photoallergic properties, along with the negative environmental impact regarding marine ecosystems [38,39]. Even though they might not completely replace the traditionally used physical and chemical UV filters, the use of these pigments could be an interesting option for enriching the formulations and allowing for a reduction of the required amounts of conventional filters to obtain a certain level of photoprotection. Additionally, possible synergism between these compounds and other filters could be an alternative strategy for reducing the formation of photodegradation byproducts and the possible phototoxic and photoallergic reactions caused by those reactive intermediates, as well as for preserving the SPF after UV irradiation [40]. This photostability effect has been described in previous studies [41]. To validate these promising yet preliminary results, incorporation of these ingredients in sunscreen formulations is required to understand if and to what extent they can increase SPF values and explore different combinations that could possibly provide synergistic photoprotective effects.

3.3. Cytotoxicity

For the remaining analysis, the group of compounds under study was narrowed, focusing merely on the native anthocyanins and their corresponding deoxyanthocyanins and pyranoanthocyanins. Before performing any other cellular experiments, their possible cytotoxic effects towards human epidermal keratinocytes and dermal fibroblasts were evaluated by MTT assay. Over a period of 48 h of incubation, none of the compounds had significant effects on the cellular viability of either of the two cell lines, up to 100 µM (Figure 4). Prior results with HaCat cells carried out with different anthocyanins and extracts have already demonstrated that Cy3glc has no significant cytotoxicity towards this cell line at concentrations below 100 µM [42]. In this study, pyrano derivatives and deoxyanthocyanins were also screened to identify potential cytotoxicity effects, but similarly to their anthocyanin counterparts, they appear to be safe and suitable for potential application in topical formulations.

3.4. Antioxidant Affect

As discussed earlier, oxidative stress induced by ROS overproduction is acknowledged as one of the most determinant events involved in the age-related decline of skin's structural integrity and function. The use of antioxidants in skin care is one of the possible strategies to efficiently address and attenuate this process and consequent induced cellular and molecular events. With this in mind, ROS production within HaCat and HFF-1 cells was evaluated in the presence of the compounds at a fixed concentration of 50 µM, ensuring the absence of cytotoxicity (Figure 5). Results showed that Cy-3-glc related structures exhibited a more prominent effect on the reduction of the level of ROS, Cy-3-glc and CarboxypyCy-3-glc in particular, 24 h after incubation when compared to the control.

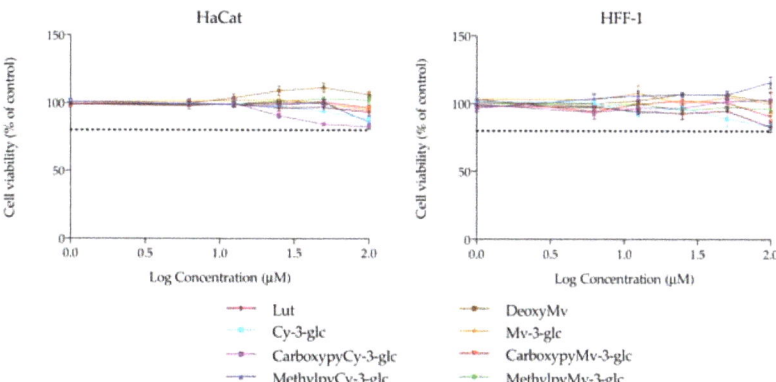

Figure 4. Cell viability of HaCat and HFF-1 cell lines in the presence of increasing concentrations of the compounds, evaluated by MTT assay. Dotted lines represent 80% viability.

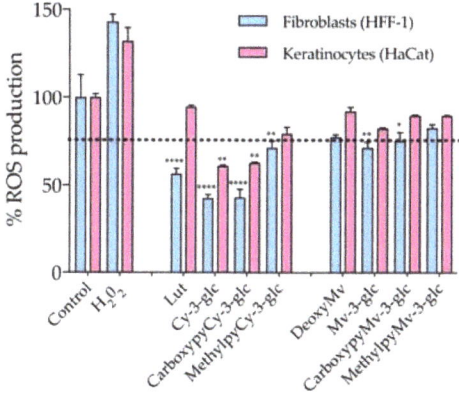

Figure 5. Effect of anthocyanins and related structures on ROS production in HaCat and HFF-1 cell lines, 24 h after incubation with 50 μM of each compound. Hydrogen peroxide (50 μM) was used as a positive control. Statistically significant differences between ROS production in the presence of the different compounds and control group are marked with asterisks: $p < 0.05$ (*), $p < 0.005$ (**) and $p < 0.0001$ (****). Dotted lines represent 80% ROS production.

Apart from that, the antioxidant effect appears to be more pronounced in dermal fibroblasts than in epidermal keratinocytes. In an in vivo context, the proper function of the skin relies on the synergistic interactions established between both cell types, but the primary skin changes occur in the dermal section and aged fibroblasts are the main propagators, by paracrine mechanisms, of epidermal aging [43]. In fact, the oxidative stress environment, arising from both extrinsic and intrinsic sources, contributes to fibroblast collapse, which in turn amplifies the production of ROS, resulting in the simultaneous increased production of ECM degrading enzymes, reduced collagen synthesis and the elevation of multiple pro-inflammatory cytokines, creating an inflammatory microenvironment (commonly referred to as inflammaging) that has a major contribution to skin damage [6]. Therefore, even when considering that it is important to reinforce the antioxidant defense at the epidermal level (which is particularly susceptible to the damaging effects of acute UVR exposure), fibroblasts should be considered as one of the primary targets of antioxidant treatment. Topical application of antioxidants has the advantage of providing them directly to the specific site where their activity is required, supplementing the antioxidant system of the skin and reinforcing protection against oxidative stress. In the case of anthocyanins, besides their recognized ROS-scavenging capacity, several studies have reported their enhancing activity of endogenous antioxidant enzymes, including superoxide dismutase (SOD), catalase (CAT) and glutathione peroxidase (GPx), by stimulating their gene expression, which might have contributed to the observed antioxidant effect [44,45]. Considering the previously discussed UV-filter capacity of these compounds, a formulation containing them would benefit from a dual function of photoprotection. Even though anthocyanins appear to be appropriate ingredients for this type of application, undesirable color changes might occur under pH variations. On the other hand, pyranoanthocyanins exhibit a greater capacity to preserve their color intensity. In that regard, CarboxypyCy-3-glc, which exhibited similar antioxidant effects to Cy-3-glc, might provide an interesting option with regards to ensuring the long-term storage of a cosmetic formulation, given its enhanced structural stability compared to its anthocyanin counterpart.

3.5. Inhibition of Skin Aging Related Enzymes Activity

Hyaluronidase, collagenase and elastase constitute the three main enzymes responsible for the regulation of the structural integrity of the skin layers, being responsible for the degradation of hyaluronic acid, collagen, and elastin, respectively. Their exacerbated activity in the skin aging process and considerable potentiation by UVR exposure contribute to the progressive deterioration of the dermal connective tissue. For that reason, the activity of each of these skin degrading enzymes was monitored in the presence of the different compounds under study and compared to the activity of a control without the compound to determine whether they could reduce their activity. It should be mentioned that these enzymes display some structural differences from their corresponding human analogues. However, they are commonly used as model enzymes in studies, given their commercial availability in great amounts, providing a valuable tool for identifying potential inhibitors, particularly when screening a large number of compounds. The obtained results are summarized in Table 4.

Table 4. Inhibitory activities of anthocyanins and related structures against hyaluronidase, collagenase and elastase. Quercetin at 50 µM, epigallocatechin gallate (EGCG) at 50 µM and N-(Methoxysuccinyl)-Ala-Ala-Pro-Val-chloromethyl ketone (MAAPVCK) at 10 µM were used as positive controls for hyaluronidase, collagenase and elastase, respectively. Results are presented as the mean ± standard error deviation (SEM) of at least 3 independent experiments.

Compound	Hyaluronidase	Collagenase	Elastase
	% Inhibition (50 µM)		
Lut	40.1 ± 2.91	24.2 ± 2.95	27.1 ± 2.71
Cy-3-glc	31.7 ± 4.18	28.5 ± 2.69	13.4 ± 2.57
CarboxypyCy-3-glc	38.1 ± 3.56	40.4 ± 2.59	5.45 ± 1.81
MethylpyCy-3-glc	17.6 ± 1.67	7.33 ± 2.47	23.7 ± 1.87
DeoxyMv	21.8 ± 2.59	n.a.	n.a.
Mv-3-glc	40.8 ± 1.33	n.a.	5.01 ± 3.16
CarboxypyMv-3-glc	28.1 ± 2.67	40.5 ± 4.31	3.54 ± 5.51
MethylpyMv-3-glc	1.92 ± 0.467	8.04 ± 4.48	5.65 ± 5.37
Quercetin	77.6 ± 2.28	n.d.	n.d.
EGCG	n.d.	86.7 ± 5.31	n.d.
MAAPVCK	n.d.	n.d.	94.6 ± 0.759

n.a.—not active; n.d.—not determined.

In the case of elastase, the great majority of the tested compounds exhibited a negligible inhibitory effect, with the exception of Lut and MethylpyCy-3-glc, which presented a moderate rate of inhibition at 50 µM (27.1% and 23.7%, respectively). With respect to collagenase inhibition, both carboxypyranoanthocyanins stood out amongst the remaining compounds, resulting in an inhibition rate of 40%, which is significantly different behavior from that observed in the case of their methylpyrano counterparts, which revealed minor effects on the activity of the enzyme. Concerning hyaluronidase, apart from MethylpyMv-

3-glc, all the compounds tested were able to interfere with the activity of the enzyme, exhibiting moderate inhibition rates ranging from 20 to 40%. Lut, CarboxypyCy-3-glc and Mv-3-glc exhibited higher inhibitory effects, reaching approximately 40%. When tested at higher concentrations (up to 200 µM), the inhibition rate increased to 64.5% in the case of Lut, 81.7% for CarboxypyCy-3-glc and 67.4% in the presence of Mv-3-glc (Figure S2) evidencing a dose dependent enzymatic inhibition.

Although the compounds were mostly tested at a fixed concentration of 50 µM in order to understand their relative inhibition potency within the specific set of conditions defined in this study, higher concentrations could and should be explored in the conception of topical formulations. The apparent absence of cytotoxicity issues at higher concentrations, evidenced by the above-mentioned cell viability results, supports the safety of these compounds as natural anti-aging components. It is also important to point out that in an in vivo context, topically administered compounds must cross the stratum corneum and the epidermal layer in order to reach the deeper skin layers, so higher doses should be considered in order to achieve the desired biological effects.

3.6. Molecular Docking Study with Hyaluronidase

Considering the overall better capacity of the compounds to modulate the activity of hyaluronidase, their interaction in the active site of the enzyme was also assessed by molecular docking. To validate the docking protocol, the X-ray tetrasaccharide was re-docked into the active site of the hyaluronidase, exhibiting a binding energy of −3.55 kcal/mol (Figure S3). Both X-ray and docking poses of the tetrasaccharide are very similar (root-mean-score deviation (RMSd) of 0.60 Å), and the main interactions with the enzyme were maintained. The tetrasaccharide established hydrophilic interactions with the Tyr55, Asp111, Glu113, Tyr184, Tyr227, Gln271, Ser303 and Ser304 residues as well as hydrophobic contacts with the Ile53 and Trp301.

Hyaluronidase catalyzes an acid/base reaction mechanism, in which the Glu113 acts as a proton donor and the acetamido group of hyaluronic acid acts as a nucleophilic base [25]. The relevance and the identification of the Glu113 as a catalytic residue is in line with studies of mutagenesis in the human sperm protein, hyaluronidase PH-20. Its substitution by a glutamine in the PH-20 protein resulted in a protein without activity, indicating that it is essential for the enzymatic reaction [46]. In addition, the aromatic triad (Tyr184, Tyr227 and Trp301) and the Asp111 and Gln271 residues were pointed out as relevant to keep the substrate in the appropriate position for catalysis (see Figure S4) [25]. Given that the alignment of the bee venom and human hyaluronidase sequences proved the conservation of the active site residues, it is possible to infer that they have similar catalytic mechanisms [25].

According to the literature, the hyaluronidase inhibition mechanism by phenolic compounds is competitive [26,47]. Therefore, the polyphenolic compounds used in the in vitro enzymatic inhibition assay were docked into the active site of the enzyme. Table S2 displays their binding energies ($\Delta G_{binding}$) and the nearest ligand group to the catalytic Glu113. Overall, compounds showed a good affinity for the enzyme ($\Delta G_{binding}$ between −4.17 and −8.06 kcal/mol), with their binding beng more favorable than the tetrasaccharide. These affinity values are similar to those previously suggested for several phenolic compounds (including Que-3-glc) from *Ravenala madagascariensis* ($\Delta G_{binding}$ between −4.02 and −7.12 kcal/mol) [26]. However, the order of affinity predicted by molecular docking is not in agreement with the order obtained in experimental kinetic assays, where it was observed that Que exhibited the highest percentage of inhibition among the tested compounds. Previous studies [26] also reported similar differences for related compounds targeting the hyaluronidase. Epicatechin, for example, showed a greater inhibition capacity than rutin (34.4% and 23.7%, respectively), whereas the results obtained from the molecular docking suggested the opposite ($\Delta G_{binding}$ for epicatechin and rutin were determined to be −4.85 and −7.12 kcal/mol, respectively). This fact might be due to the significant differences in molecular sizes, as larger compounds may establish more interactions with the enzyme, favoring their binding energies. However, other properties (e.g., charge polarization) may influence their inhibitory abilities. In this way, the modes of interaction of the various anthocyanins, as well as the main intermolecular interactions, namely with the catalytic Glu113, were analyzed, in order to understand the inhibitory activities obtained from the in vitro enzymatic experiments.

As mentioned, Que and Que-3-glc are considered good hyaluronidase inhibitors [26]. However, their docking binding affinities are slightly lower than those obtained for the other compounds (which can be due to the error range expected for this method) [48]. Figure 6 displays the best docking poses for the two molecules. Que has a $\Delta G_{binding}$ of -5.94 kcal/mol, interacting via its ring B (Figure 6a), in agreement with previous studies that predicted a $\Delta G_{binding}$ of -5.15 kcal/mol and a similar interaction mode [49]. Like the tetrasaccharide, Que interacts with Glu113 at a distance of less than 3 Å. In addition, it establishes hydrogen interactions with Asp111, Tyr184, Ser304 and Asp305 residues and interacts by stacking π-π with the Tyr55 and Trp301 residues. Regarding the Que-3-glc, it can interact with hyaluronidase by different moieties (glucose, ring B or rings A–C). Although binding through the glucose slightly favors the affinity, in this situation the ligand is further away from Glu113 and there is a loss of the π-π stacking with Tyr55 (Figure 6b). The interaction through ring B is very similar to the Que (Figure 6c). The interaction mode by rings A–C is in agreement with those obtained in the literature [26] (Figure 6d). The proximity to the catalytic Glu113 is largely favored when the interaction occurs via the B ring. Based on this, the binding of the Que-3-glc should be similar to the respective aglycone (please see Figure 6c).

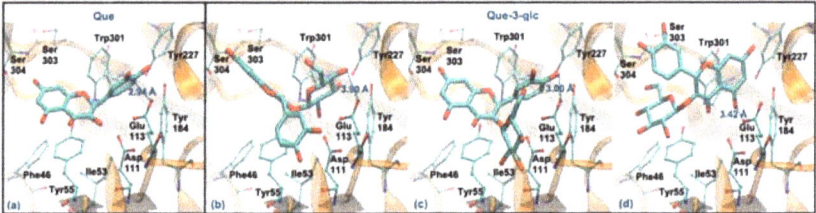

Figure 6. Representation of the structure of hyaluronidase complexed with Que (**a**) and Que-3-glc (interaction by glucose—(**b**), interaction by ring B—(**c**), interaction by rings A and C—(**d**)), showing the interacting residues of the active site. The enzyme is depicted in cartoon and colored in orange, the ligands are represented with sticks and colored by atom type, whilst the interacting residues are depicted in ball-and-sticks and colored by atom type. Hydrogen atoms are not represented to simplify the visualization.

Cy-3-glc (pseudobase carbinol) and Lut (pseudobase carbinol) have the greatest affinities for the enzyme when interacting through the ring B. In fact, the interaction mode of ring B and the main intermolecular interactions of Cy-3-glc are very similar to those of Que (Figure 7a). Curiously, when it interacts through the glucose, the distance to Glu113 and the main interactions are quite similar (Figure 7b). In the form of chalcone, Cy-3-glc has a lower affinity for the enzyme. This structure interacts through ring B, but it is much further away from Glu113 (distance > 4 Å) and loses its π-π stacking with the Tyr55 (Figure 7c). Lut also interacts through the ring B, in a very similar way to Que. However, it slightly deviates from Glu113, and reduces the interaction with Asp111 due to the absence of any substituent on C3 (hydroxyl group or glucose unit) (Figure 7d). The chalcone form of Lut binds much further away from Glu113 (distance > 4 Å) and Tyr55 and does not interact with the Ser303, Ser304 and Asp305 residues (Figure 7e). The breaking of the C ring on the chalcone forms could be responsible for their weaker binding because it allows higher freedom of movement, which may reduce interaction with the aromatic residues of the enzyme. These results agree with those obtained experimentally, assuming that the majority forms in solution are those of the pseudobase carbinol, since a high percentage of inhibition was observed for these compounds.

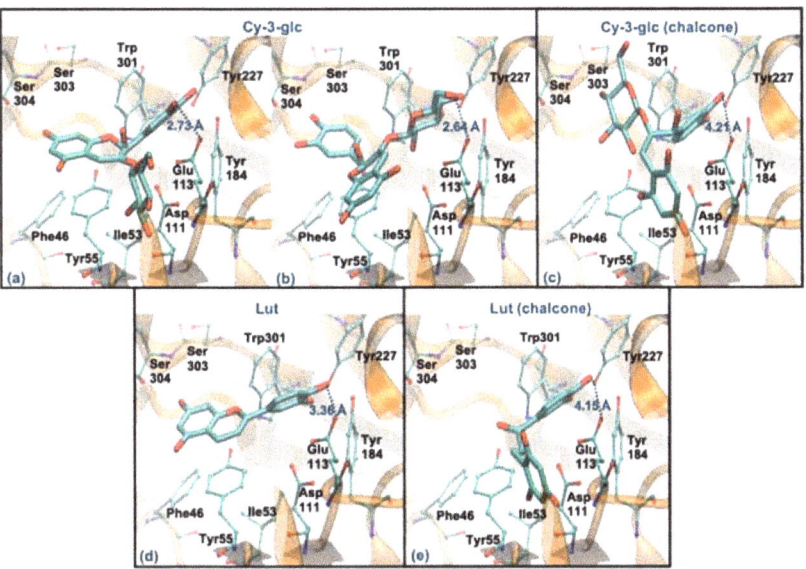

Figure 7. Representation of the structure of hyaluronidase complexed with Cy-3-glc—pseudobase carbinol (interaction by ring B—(**a**), interaction by glucose—(**b**)) and chalcone (interaction by ring B—(**c**))—and Lut–pseudobase carbinol (interaction by ring B—(**d**)) and chalcone (interaction by ring B—(**e**))—showing the interacting residues of the active site. The enzyme is depicted in cartoon and colored in orange, the ligands are represented with sticks and colored by atom type, whilst the interacting residues are depicted in ball-and-sticks and colored by atom type. Hydrogen atoms are not represented to simplify the visualization.

Regarding CarboxypyCy-3-glc, it can interact through the glucose or via its ring B. However, the former binding mode is plainly favored ($\Delta G_{binding}$ of −8.06 kcal/mol vs. −6.06 kcal/mol and distance to Glu113 of 2.61 Å vs. 4.59 Å). Intermolecular interactions with the key active site residues are maintained. Despite the ligand being slightly further away from Tyr55, it made a perpendicular stacking with the pyran group (Figure 8a). Oppositely, when it interacted through the ring B, the parallel stacking with Tyr55 was strongly favored, which can support a competition between the two different interaction modes (see Figure 8b). MethylpyCy-3-glc interacts by its glucose unit ($\Delta G_{binding}$ of −7.15 kcal/mol) and despite its proximity to Glu113 (distance < 3 Å), the remaining groups of the compound bind in a shallow mode, reducing the interactions with the enzyme (Figure 8c).

Mv-3-glc (pseudobase carbinol) can interact with the enzyme by the ring B, glucose or rings A-C. The former binding mode is similar to Que and Cy-3-glc, however, the presence of methoxy groups in ring B hinders the proximity to Glu113 (staying at a distance of 4.55 Å) (Figure 9a). The two latter binding modes clearly favor proximity to Glu113 (distance < 3 Å), the parallel stacking with Tyr55 and/or the perpendicular π-π stacking with Trp301 and Tyr227 as well as dispersive/hydrophobic contacts favored by the presence of methoxy groups (Figure 9b,c). In the form of chalcone, it can interact by the rings A and C or by glucose (in a similar way to those described for Mv-3-glc). These binding modes may be favored, which justify the good inhibitory capacity of this compound (Figure 9d,e). Analyzing the results obtained for DeoxyMv, the mode of interaction by ring B is very similar to that described for Mv-3-glc and for Lut. However, the presence of methoxy groups in ring B hinders proximity to Glu113 (distance of 3.89 Å) (Figure 9f). The same is observed for chalcone (distance of 4.26 Å) (Figure 9g). This higher distance to Glu113 (+0.5 Å) may be responsible for the lower inhibitory activity of this compound.

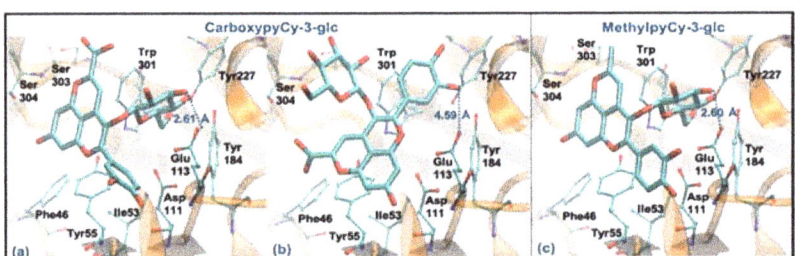

Figure 8. Representation of the structure of hyaluronidase complexed with CarboxypyCy-3-glc (interaction by glucose—(**a**), interaction by ring B—(**b**)) and MethylpyCy-3-glc ((interaction by glucose—(**c**)), showing the interacting residues of the active site. The enzyme is depicted in cartoon and colored in orange, the ligands are represented with sticks and colored by atom type, whilst the interacting residues are depicted in ball-and-sticks and colored by atom type. Hydrogen atoms are not represented to simplify the visualization.

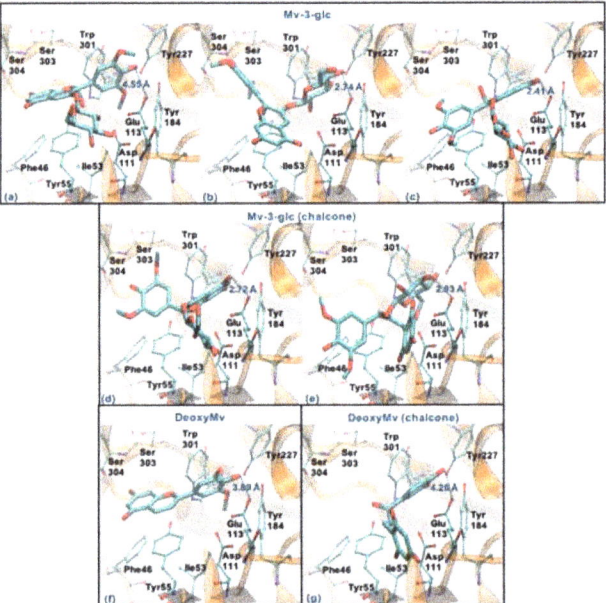

Figure 9. Representation of the structure of hyaluronidase complexed with Mv-3-glc—pseudobase carbinol (interaction by ring B—(**a**), interaction by glucose—(**b**), interaction by rings A and C—(**c**)) and chalcone (interaction by rings A and C—(**d**), interaction by glucose—(**e**))—and DeoxyMv–pseudobase carbinol (interaction by ring B—(**f**)) and chalcone (interaction by ring B—(**g**))—showing the interacting residues of the active site. The enzyme is depicted in cartoon and colored in orange, the ligands are represented with sticks and colored by atom type, whilst the interacting residues are depicted in ball-and-sticks and colored by atom type. Hydrogen atoms are not represented to simplify the visualization.

Regarding the two pyrano derivatives of Mv-3-glc, CarboxypyMv-3-glc and MethylpyMv-3-glc, these compounds interact by ring B, with $\Delta G_{binding}$ values between −6.77 and −6.15 kcal/mol. These molecules are docked far away from Glu113 (distances > 4 Å), probably due to the presence of methoxy groups in the ring B. In addition, as the bulky pyrano group binds in a shallow mode, it is much further away from the Asp111, Tyr227, Tyr265 and Trp301 residues (Figure 10a–c).

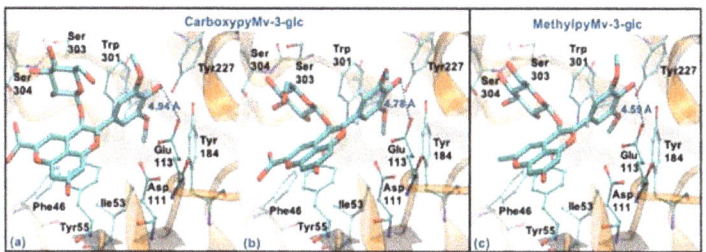

Figure 10. Representation of the structure of hyaluronidase complexed with CarboxypyMv-3-glc (interaction by ring B—(**a**,**b**)) and MethylpyMv-3-glc (interaction by ring B—(**c**)), showing the interacting residues of the active site. The enzyme is depicted in cartoon and colored in orange, the ligands are represented with sticks and colored by atom type, whilst the interacting residues are depicted in ball-and-sticks and colored by atom type. Hydrogen atoms are not represented to simplify the visualization.

Overall, the structural analysis of the docking data suggests that the interactions of anthocyanins with residues Tyr55, Glu113, Tyr184 and Trp301 are determinant of their inhibitory capacity. In addition, contacts with residues Asp111 and Tyr227 are important, but not essential (evidenced, for example, by the interaction mode of the potent inhibitor Lut). The binding of the compounds is plainly favored by a hydrophilic interaction with the catalytic Glu113 (that can occur via ring B, rings A and C or the glucose unit of Cy-3-glc derivatives), as well as by a narrow π-π stacking with Tyr55 and Trp301 residues.

3.7. Transport Efficiency

Despite the beneficial effects that the potential topical application of these compounds might offer, as suggested by the results presented so far, the efficiency of such treatment ultimately depends on the capacity of these bioactives to overcome the stratum corneum barrier for permeation across the skin. However, penetration and permeation studies about these types of compounds are still scarce.

The use of 3D skin models, which faithfully mimic the in vivo epidermis and skin barrier function has emerged as a useful alternative to animal testing. Besides the complex experimental conditions, the large quantities of primary keratinocytes required represent limitations for their application as screening models. The immortalized keratinocyte cell line HaCat could be a solution for overcoming these issues. The HaCaT cell line is widely used in keratinocyte monolayer culture models [50] and responds to differentiation-promoting stimuli, such as contact inhibition and high calcium concentrations in the culture medium [51], but the transcriptional expression pattern of cornified envelope-associated proteins, such as filaggrin, loricrin and involucrin is abnormal compared to normal human primary keratinocytes [52]. Considering this, primary normal human epidermal keratinocytes (Heka) were chosen to develop the optimal conditions of cellular differentiation and create a proper skin barrier model. Given the overall good performance of CarboxyCy-3-glc, it was selected for the transport experiments as a representative compound of the anthocyanin derivatives, along with its corresponding native anthocyanin, Cy-3-glc, in order to investigate how their structural differences might affect the transport profile. Cells were grown in low calcium medium (0.06 mM) until reaching confluence. At the 4th day of culture, medium was switched to high calcium (1.8 mM). Only Heka monolayers with an integrity equivalent to a transepithelial electrical resistance (TEER) higher than 450 $\Omega.cm^{-2}$ were used for the transport studies. These values were reached after a total of 8 days in culture (Figure 11).

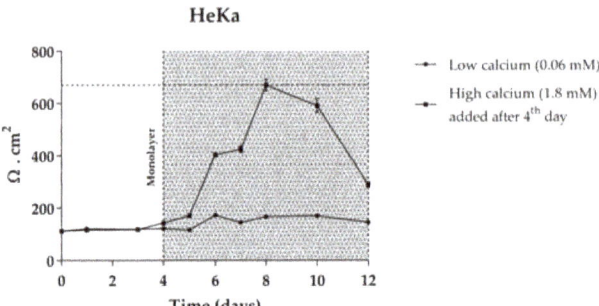

Figure 11. TEER measurements of HeKa cell monolayer during 12 days of culture. Cells were kept for 4 days in low calcium medium (0.06 mM) to allow monolayer formation. For differentiation, in the last 8 days medium was changed to high calcium (1.8 mM).

Comparing the transport profile of both compounds in the first 2 h of culture, transport appears to be slightly slower in the case of CarboxypyCy-3-glc, which could be due to its higher structural complexity compared to Cy-3-glc (Figure 12a). However, throughout the 24 h period, a continuous increase in the amount of the carboxypyrano derivative transported across the barrier could be detected, contrary to what was observed for Cy-3-glc, since the transport rate decreased after 2 h in culture. A reduction in the apical amount of Cy-3-glc available for uptake was observed but does not justify the reduction in the transport efficiency detected in the basolateral side after 3 h (Figure 12). In fact, this apparent reduction in the transport efficiency of Cy-3-glc can be explained by its lower stability in comparison with its corresponding carboxypyrano derivative in pH and temperature conditions (Figure 12b). In this system, the cell culture medium lacks the presence of fetal bovine serum, which eliminates the influence of the enzymatic machinery on the stability of the compounds. In fact, previous research on the stability of anthocyanins in cell culture medium showed that the concentration of Cy-3-glc decreased after 3 h of incubation, from 100 µM to 88.0 µM [53].

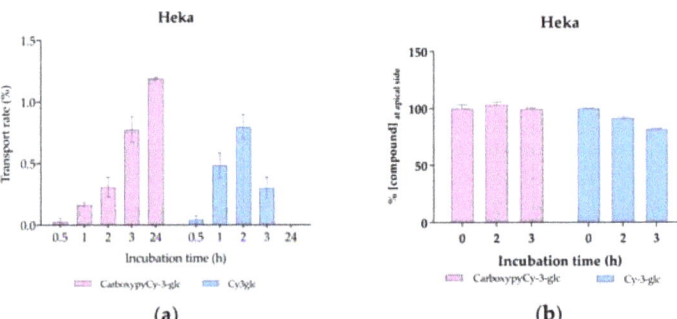

Figure 12. Transport efficiency of 200 µM of Cy3glc and CarboxypyCy-3-glc through HeKa cells (apical → basolateral) monitored for 24 h at the (**a**) basolateral and (**b**) apical side.

The observed uptake of both Cy-3-glc and CarboxypyCy-3-glc may result from the involvement of glucose transporters, namely GLUT1, 2, 3 and 5 expressed in keratinocytes [54], as previously described for other barrier models [55].

The greater molecular weight of CarboxypyCy-3-glc did not pose a constraint on its transport across the cellular barrier. Interestingly, a recent analysis concerning the release of anthocyanins from a lipophilic formulation and their skin penetration capacity through the stratum corneum, carried out in both porcine and human skin samples, revealed that anthocyanins from both elderberry (with molecular weights ranging from 449 to 581 Da) and red radish (933–1019 Da) successfully penetrated into the skin. Pigments were found to reach relevant depths to exert their biological activity, indicating that the higher molecular weight of red radish anthocyanins did not prevent their diffusion across the skin [56].

4. Conclusions

Overall, the results presented herein shed some light on some of the skin-health promoting effects of this group of pigments through distinct levels of action. Topical routes of administration of these compounds have been an increasingly explored topic, providing a targeted and apparently safe therapy. However, to ensure the effectiveness of their biological activities, different parts of the equation must be taken into consideration when conceiving a topical formulation, including the properties of the compounds and of the formulation in which they are incorporated, which will determine their capacity to overcome the stratum corneum. Further tests focused on the skin penetration behavior of these compounds and their quantification within the skin layers are crucial to determine the required doses to achieve the expected benefits in vivo and guide the optimization process of concentrations and compounds ratios.

Furthermore, the use of natural extracts rather than isolated compounds is commonly claimed to be more effective due to the potential beneficial synergistic interactions between their different constituents. However, the opposite effect, antagonism, should also be considered, as the effects of active agents might be masked by other compounds present in the same mixture, as demonstrated in the results regarding the inhibition of biofilm formation. Therefore, the study of highly purified compounds, although representing a time-consuming process, is an important tool for evaluating and comprehending the full potential of each molecule in terms of its biological effects.

Although anthocyanins and anthocyanin-rich sources have long provided solid evidence of their skin-protective properties, their applicability is constantly haunted by stability issues. The inclusion of anthocyanin structural derivatives represents an appealing alternative to overcome this issue. Among all anthocyanin-related structures tested, Carboxypyranocyanidin-3-O-glucoside in particular appeared to be a promising candidate given its overall good performance in the different staged experiments and its higher structural stability.

5. Patents

Provisional patent application N. 117058: Process for extraction and hemi-synthesis of pyranoanthocyanins and skincare cosmetic formulations containing them.

Supplementary Materials: The following are available online at https://www.mdpi.com/article/10.3390/antiox10071038/s1, Figure S1: Chromatographic profile of (a) blackberry anthocyanins, (b) elderberry and (c) red wine pyranoanthocyanins, at 520 nm. Figure S2: Hyaluronidase inhibition rates in the presence of increasing concentrations of Lut, CarboxypyCy-3-glc and Mv-3-glc. Figure S3: Superimposition of the docking and crystallographic geometries of the tetrasaccharide bound into the active site of the hyaluronidase. Enzyme is depicted in cartoon and colored in orange, while the tetrasaccharide is represented with sticks and colored in blue (docking pose) or orange (X-ray pose). Hydrogen atoms are not represented to simplify the visualization, Figure S4: Representation of the structure of hyaluronidase complexed with tetrasaccharide, showing the interacting residues of the active site. The arrow is pointing to the atom where the cleavage occurs. The enzyme is depicted in cartoon and colored in orange, the tetrasaccharide is represented with sticks and colored by atom type, whilst the interacting residues are depicted in ball-and-sticks and colored by atom type. Hydrogen atoms are not represented to simplify the visualization. Table S1: Chemical composition and antioxidant activity of the anthocyanin and pyranoanthocyanin extracts. Table S2: Values of

ΔG$_{binding}$ for the best molecular docking solutions obtained for each compound. The closest group to Glu113 was also identified as well as the respective distance between oxygen atoms. The interacting residues of the active site were identified.

Author Contributions: Conceptualization, J.O. and I.F.; methodology, P.C. (Patrícia Correia), P.A., C.R., H.O., A.R.P., P.C. (Patrícia Coelho), L.J.B., N.F.B., I.F.; validation, P.C. (Patrícia Correia), P.A., C.R., H.O., A.R.P., P.C. (Patrícia Coelho), L.J.B., N.F.B. and I.F.; formal analysis, P.C. (Patrícia Correia), P.A., C.R., H.O., A.R.P., P.C. (Patrícia Coelho), L.J.B., N.F.B. and I.F.; investigation, P.C. (Patrícia Correia), P.A., C.R., H.O., A.R.P., P.C. (Patrícia Coelho), L.J.B., N.F.B., J.O. and I.F.; resources, N.M., V.d.F., P.G., J.O. and I.F.; writing—original draft preparation, P.C. (Patrícia Correia), L.J.B., H.O., N.F.B., C.R. and I.F.; writing—review and editing, N.M., V.d.F., P.G., L.J.B., J.O. and I.F.; visualization, P.C. (Patrícia Correia), C.R., H.O., P.C. (Patrícia Coelho), L.J.B., N.F.B. and I.F.; supervision, J.O. and I.F.; project administration, J.O. and I.F.; funding acquisition, N.M., V.d.F., P.G., J.O. and I.F. All authors have read and agreed to the published version of the manuscript.

Funding: This work was financial supported by the project PTDC/QUI-OUT/29013/2017 funded by FCT and FEDER.

Institutional Review Board Statement: Not applicable.

Informed Consent Statement: Not applicable.

Data Availability Statement: Data is contained within the article and supplementary material.

Acknowledgments: P.A.: A.R.P. and P.C. gratefully acknowledge their doctoral grants from FCT (SFRH/BD/143309/2019, SFRH/BD/146549/2019 and SFRH/BD/150661/2020, respectively). J.O. and N.F.B. would like to thank the FCT for their IF and CEEC contracts (IF/00225/2015 and CEECIND/02017/2018, respectively), H.O. and I.F for their research contracts (PTDC/QUI-OUT/29013/2017 and SFRH/BPD/86173/2012, respectively). This work was supported by the Associated Laboratory for Sustainable Chemistry, Clean Processes and Technologies LAQV through the national funds from UIDB/50006/2020. This research was supported by AgriFood XXI I&D&I project (NORTE-01-0145-FEDER-000041 cofinanced by European Regional Development Fund (ERDF), through the NORTE 2020 (Programa Operacional Regional do Norte 2014/2020).

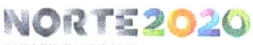 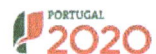 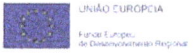

Conflicts of Interest: The authors declare no conflict of interest.

References

1. Rittié, L.; Fisher, G.J. Natural and sun-induced aging of human skin. *Cold Spring Harb. Perspect. Med.* **2015**, *5*, a015370. [CrossRef] [PubMed]
2. Krutmann, J.; Bouloc, A.; Sore, G.; Bernard, B.A.; Passeron, T. The skin aging exposome. *J. Dermatol. Sci.* **2017**, *85*, 152–161. [CrossRef] [PubMed]
3. Orioli, D.; Dellambra, E. Epigenetic Regulation of Skin Cells in Natural Aging and Premature Aging Diseases. *Cells* **2018**, *7*, 268. [CrossRef] [PubMed]
4. Shin, J.W.; Kwon, S.H.; Choi, J.Y.; Na, J.I.; Huh, C.H.; Choi, H.R.; Park, K.C. Molecular Mechanisms of Dermal Aging and Antiaging Approaches. *Int. J. Mol. Sci.* **2019**, *20*, 2126. [CrossRef]
5. Fisher, G.J.; Kang, S.; Varani, J.; Bata-Csorgo, Z.; Wan, Y.; Datta, S.; Voorhees, J.J. Mechanisms of photoaging and chronological skin aging. *Arch. Dermatol.* **2002**, *138*, 1462–1470. [CrossRef]
6. Tu, Y.; Quan, T. Oxidative Stress and Human Skin Connective Tissue Aging. *Cosmetics* **2016**, *3*, 28. [CrossRef]
7. Natarajan, V.T.; Ganju, P.; Ramkumar, A.; Grover, R.; Gokhale, R.S. Multifaceted pathways protect human skin from UV radiation. *Nat. Chem. Biol.* **2014**, *10*, 542–551. [CrossRef]
8. Xu, Y.; Fisher, G.J. Ultraviolet (UV) light irradiation induced signal transduction in skin photoaging. *J. Dermatol. Sci. Suppl.* **2005**, *1*, S1–S8. [CrossRef]
9. Byrd, A.L.; Belkaid, Y.; Segre, J.A. The human skin microbiome. *Nat. Rev. Microbiol.* **2018**, *16*, 143–155. [CrossRef]
10. Hernandez, D.F.; Cervantes, E.L.; Luna-Vital, D.A.; Mojica, L. Food-derived bioactive compounds with anti-aging potential for nutricosmetic and cosmeceutical products. *Crit. Rev. Food Sci. Nutr.* **2020**, 1–16. [CrossRef]
11. Li, D.; Wang, P.; Luo, Y.; Zhao, M.; Chen, F. Health benefits of anthocyanins and molecular mechanisms: Update from recent decade. *Crit. Rev. Food Sci. Nutr.* **2017**, *57*, 1729–1741. [CrossRef]

12. Li, K.; Zhang, M.; Chen, H.; Peng, J.; Jiang, F.; Shi, X.; Bai, Y.; Jian, M.; Jia, Y. Anthocyanins from black peanut skin protect against UV-B induced keratinocyte cell and skin oxidative damage through activating Nrf 2 signaling. *Food Funct.* **2019**, *10*, 6815–6828. [CrossRef]
13. Bucci, P.; Prieto, M.J.; Milla, L.; Calienni, M.N.; Martinez, L.; Rivarola, V.; Alonso, S.; Montanari, J. Skin penetration and UV-damage prevention by nanoberries. *J. Cosmet. Dermatol.* **2018**, *17*, 889–899. [CrossRef]
14. Peng, Z.; Hu, X.; Li, X.; Jiang, X.; Deng, L.; Hu, Y.; Bai, W. Protective effects of cyanidin-3-O-glucoside on UVB-induced chronic skin photodamage in mice via alleviating oxidative damage and anti-inflammation. *Food Front.* **2020**, *1*, 213–223. [CrossRef]
15. Pal, H.C.; Chamcheu, J.C.; Adhami, V.M.; Wood, G.S.; Elmets, C.A.; Mukhtar, H.; Afaq, F. Topical application of delphinidin reduces psoriasiform lesions in the flaky skin mouse model by inducing epidermal differentiation and inhibiting inflammation. *Br. J. Dermatol.* **2015**, *172*, 354–364. [CrossRef]
16. Oliveira, J.; Mateus, N.; de Freitas, V. Previous and recent advances in pyranoanthocyanins equilibria in aqueous solution. *Dyes Pigment.* **2014**, *100*, 190–200. [CrossRef]
17. Xiong, Y.; Zhang, P.; Warner, R.D.; Fang, Z. 3-Deoxyanthocyanidin Colorant: Nature, Health, Synthesis, and Food Applications. *Compr. Rev. Food Sci. Food Saf.* **2019**, *18*, 1533–1549. [CrossRef]
18. Al Bittar, S.; Mora, N.; Loonis, M.; Dangles, O. A simple synthesis of 3-deoxyanthocyanidins and their O-glucosides. *Tetrahedron* **2016**, *72*, 4294–4302. [CrossRef]
19. Oliveira, J.; Fernandes, V.; Miranda, C.; Santos-Buelga, C.; Silva, A.; de Freitas, V.; Mateus, N. Color Properties of Four Cyanidin–Pyruvic Acid Adducts. *J. Agric. Food Chem.* **2006**, *54*, 6894–6903. [CrossRef]
20. Lu, Y.; Foo, L.Y. Unusual anthocyanin reaction with acetone leading to pyranoanthocyanin formation. *Tetrahedron Lett.* **2001**, *42*, 1371–1373. [CrossRef]
21. Oliveira, J.A.P.; Fernandes, A.; Mateus, N.; de Freitas, V. Synthesis and structural characterization of amino-based pyranoanthocyanins with extended electronic delocalization. *Synlett* **2016**, *27*, 2459–2462. [CrossRef]
22. Mateus, N.; Oliveira, J.; Santos-Buelga, C.; Silva, A.M.S.; de Freitas, V. NMR structure characterization of a new vinylpyranoanthocyanin–catechin pigment (a portisin). *Tetrahedron Lett.* **2004**, *45*, 3455–3457. [CrossRef]
23. CLSI. *Methods for Dilution of Antimicrobial Susceptibility Tests for Bacteria That Grow Aerobically: Approved Standard*, 10th ed.; CLSI: Wayne, PA, USA, 2015; Volume 35, pp. M-07–A-10.
24. Bessa, L.J.; Eaton, P.; Dematei, A.; Placido, A.; Vale, N.; Gomes, P.; Delerue-Matos, C.; Sa Leite, J.R.; Gameiro, P. Synergistic and antibiofilm properties of ocellatin peptides against multidrug-resistant Pseudomonas aeruginosa. *Future Microbiol.* **2018**, *13*, 151–163. [CrossRef]
25. Marković-Housley, Z.; Miglierini, G.; Soldatova, L.; Rizkallah, P.J.; Müller, U.; Schirmer, T. Crystal Structure of Hyaluronidase, a Major Allergen of Bee Venom. *Structure* **2000**, *8*, 1025–1035. [CrossRef]
26. Mohamed, E.M.; Hetta, M.H.; Rateb, M.E.; Selim, M.A.; AboulMagd, A.M.; Badria, F.A.; Abdelmohsen, U.R.; Alhadrami, H.A.; Hassan, H.M. Bioassay-Guided Isolation, Metabolic Profiling, and Docking Studies of Hyaluronidase Inhibitors from Ravenala madagascariensis. *Molecules* **2020**, *25*, 1714. [CrossRef]
27. Hanwell, M.D.; Curtis, D.E.; Lonie, D.C.; Vandermeersch, T.; Zurek, E.; Hutchison, G.R. Avogadro: An Advanced Semantic Chemical Editor, Visualization, and Analysis Platform. *J. Cheminform.* **2012**, *4*, 1–17. [CrossRef]
28. Morris, G.M.; Huey, R.; Lindstrom, W.; Sanner, M.F.; Belew, R.K.; Goodsell, D.S.; Olson, A.J. AutoDock4 and AutoDockTools4: Automated Docking with Selective Receptor Flexibility. *J. Comput. Chem.* **2009**, *30*, 2785–2791. [CrossRef]
29. Dolinsky, T.J.; Nielsen, J.E.; McCammon, J.A.; Baker, N.A. PDB2PQR: An Automated Pipeline for the Setup of Poisson-Boltzmann Electrostatics Calculations. *Nucleic Acids Res.* **2004**, *32*, 665–667. [CrossRef]
30. Humphrey, W.; Dalke, A.; Schulten, K. VMD: Visual Molecular Dynamics. *J. Mol. Graph.* **1996**, *14*, 33–38. [CrossRef]
31. Hall-Stoodley, L.; Costerton, J.W.; Stoodley, P. Bacterial biofilms: From the Natural environment to infectious diseases. *Nat. Rev. Microbiol.* **2004**, *2*, 95–108. [CrossRef]
32. Caesar, L.K.; Cech, N.B. Synergy and antagonism in natural product extracts: When 1 + 1 does not equal 2. *Nat. Prod. Rep.* **2019**, *36*, 869–888. [CrossRef] [PubMed]
33. Cady, N.C.; McKean, K.A.; Behnke, J.; Kubec, R.; Mosier, A.P.; Kasper, S.H.; Burz, D.S.; Musah, R.A. Inhibition of biofilm formation, quorum sensing and infection in Pseudomonas aeruginosa by natural products-inspired organosulfur compounds. *PLoS ONE* **2012**, *7*, e38492. [CrossRef] [PubMed]
34. Slobodníková, L.; Fialová, S.; Rendeková, K.; Kováč, J.; Mučaji, P. Antibiofilm Activity of Plant Polyphenols. *Molecules* **2016**, *21*, 1717. [CrossRef] [PubMed]
35. Sitarek, P.; Merecz-Sadowska, A.; Kowalczyk, T.; Wieczfinska, J.; Zajdel, R.; Śliwiński, T. Potential Synergistic Action of Bioactive Compounds from Plant Extracts against Skin Infecting Microorganisms. *Int. J. Mol. Sci.* **2020**, *21*, 5105. [CrossRef]
36. Cefali, L.C.; Franco, J.G.; Nicolini, G.F.; Ataide, J.A.; Mazzola, P.G. In vitro antioxidant activity and solar protection factor of blackberry and raspberry extracts in topical formulation. *J. Cosmet. Dermatol.* **2019**, *18*, 539–544. [CrossRef]
37. Chan, C.F.; Lien, C.Y.; Lai, Y.C.; Huang, C.L.; Liao, W.C. Influence of purple sweet potato extracts on the UV absorption properties of a cosmetic cream. *J. Cosmet. Sci.* **2010**, *61*, 333–341.
38. Suh, S.; Pham, C.; Smith, J.; Mesinkovska, N.A. The banned sunscreen ingredients and their impact on human health: A systematic review. *Int. J. Dermatol.* **2020**, *59*, 1033–1042. [CrossRef]

39. Sabzevari, N.; Qiblawi, S.; Norton, S.A.; Fivenson, D. Sunscreens: UV filters to protect us: Part 1: Changing regulations and choices for optimal sun protection. *Int. J. Women's Dermatol.* **2021**, *7*, 28–44. [CrossRef]
40. de Oliveira, C.A.; Dario, M.F. Bioactive Cosmetics. In *Handbook of Ecomaterials*; Martínez, L.M.T., Kharissova, O.V., Kharisov, B.I., Eds.; Springer International Publishing: Cham, Switzerland, 2017; pp. 1–23. [CrossRef]
41. Hubner, A.; Sobreira, F.; Vetore Neto, A.; Pinto, C.; Dario, M.F.; Díaz, I.E.C.; Lourenço, F.R.; Rosado, C.; Baby, A.R.; Bacchi, E.M. The Synergistic Behavior of Antioxidant Phenolic Compounds Obtained from Winemaking Waste's Valorization, Increased the Efficacy of a Sunscreen System. *Antioxidants* **2019**, *8*, 530. [CrossRef]
42. Évora, A.; de Freitas, V.; Mateus, N.; Fernandes, I. Effect of anthocyanins from red wine and blackberry on the integrity of a keratinocyte model using ECIS. *Food Funct.* **2017**. submitted. [CrossRef]
43. Lewis, D.A.; Krbanjevic, A.; Travers, J.B.; Spandau, D.F. Aging-Associated Nonmelanoma Skin Cancer: A Role for the Dermis. In *Textbook of Aging Skin*; Farage, M.A., Miller, K.W., Maibach, H.I., Eds.; Springer: Berlin/Heidelberg, Germany, 2017; pp. 913–930. [CrossRef]
44. Fallah, A.A.; Sarmast, E.; Jafari, T. Effect of dietary anthocyanins on biomarkers of oxidative stress and antioxidative capacity: A systematic review and meta-analysis of randomized controlled trials. *J. Funct. Foods* **2020**, *68*, 103912. [CrossRef]
45. Xiang, Y.; Lai, F.; He, G.; Li, Y.; Yang, L.; Shen, W.; Huo, H.; Zhu, J.; Dai, H.; Zhang, Y. Alleviation of Rosup-induced oxidative stress in porcine granulosa cells by anthocyanins from red-fleshed apples. *PLoS ONE* **2017**, *12*, e0184033. [CrossRef]
46. Arming, S.; Strobl, B.; Wechselberger, C.; Kreil, G. In vitro Mutagenesis of PH-20 Hyaluronidase from Human Sperm. *Eur. J. Biochem.* **1997**, *247*, 810–814. [CrossRef]
47. Kuppusamy, U.R.; Khoo, H.E.; Das, N.P. Structure-Activity Studies of Flavonoids as Inhibitors of Hyaluronidase. *Biochem. Pharmacol.* **1990**, *40*, 397–401. [CrossRef]
48. Fukunishi, Y.; Yamashita, Y.; Mashimo, T.; Nakamura, H. Prediction of Protein−compound Binding Energies from Known Activity Data: Docking-score-based Method and its Applications. *Mol. Inform.* **2018**, *37*, 1–11. [CrossRef]
49. Ahmed, M.; Aldesouki, H.; Badria, F. Effect of Phenolic Compounds from the Rind of Punica granatum on the Activity of Three Metabolism-related Enzymes. *Biotechnol. Appl. Biochem.* **2019**, *1*, 1–13. [CrossRef]
50. Oliveira, H.; Correia, P.; Bessa, L.J.; Guimarães, M.; Gameiro, P.; Freitas, V.D.; Mateus, N.; Cruz, L.; Fernandes, I. Cyanidin-3-Glucoside Lipophilic Conjugates for Topical Application: Tuning the Antimicrobial Activities with Fatty Acid Chain Length. *Processes* **2021**, *9*, 340. [CrossRef]
51. Three-Dimensional In Vitro Skin and Skin Cancer Models Based on Human Fibroblast-Derived Matrix. *Tissue Eng. Part C Methods* **2015**, *21*, 958–970. [CrossRef]
52. Wan, H.; Yuan, M.; Simpson, C.; Allen, K.; Gavins, F.N.E.; Ikram, M.S.; Basu, S.; Baksh, N.; O'Toole, E.A.; Hart, I.R. Stem/Progenitor Cell-Like Properties of Desmoglein 3dim Cells in Primary and Immortalized Keratinocyte Lines. *Stem Cells* **2007**, *25*, 1286–1297. [CrossRef]
53. Zhang, J.; Giampieri, F.; Afrin, S.; Battino, M.; Zheng, X.; Reboredo-Rodriguez, P. Structure-stability relationship of anthocyanins under cell culture condition. *Int. J. Food Sci. Nutr.* **2019**, *70*, 285–293. [CrossRef]
54. Shen, S.; Sampson, S.R.; Tennenbaum, T.; Wertheimer, E. Characterization of Glucose Transport System in Keratinocytes: Insulin and IGF-1 Differentially Affect Specific Transporters. *J. Investig. Dermatol.* **2000**, *115*, 949–954. [CrossRef]
55. Oliveira, H.; Roma-Rodrigues, C.; Santos, A.; Veigas, B.; Brás, N.; Faria, A.; Calhau, C.; de Freitas, V.; Baptista, P.V.; Mateus, N.; et al. GLUT1 and GLUT3 involvement in anthocyanin gastric transport- Nanobased targeted approach. *Sci. Rep.* **2019**, *9*, 789. [CrossRef]
56. Westfall, A.; Sigurdson, G.T.; Rodriguez-Saona, L.E.; Giusti, M.M. Ex Vivo and In Vivo Assessment of the Penetration of Topically Applied Anthocyanins Utilizing ATR-FTIR/PLS Regression Models and HPLC-PDA-MS. *Antioxidants* **2020**, *9*, 486. [CrossRef]

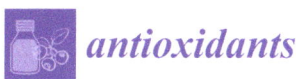

Article

MEK1/2-ERK Pathway Alterations as a Therapeutic Target in Sporadic Alzheimer's Disease: A Study in Senescence-Accelerated OXYS Rats

Natalia A. Muraleva *, Nataliya G. Kolosova and Natalia A. Stefanova

Institute of Cytology and Genetics (ICG), Siberian Branch of Russian Academy of Sciences (SB RAS), 10 Lavrentieva Avenue, 630090 Novosibirsk, Russia; kolosova@bionet.nsc.ru (N.G.K.); stefanovan@mail.ru (N.A.S.)
* Correspondence: myraleva@bionet.nsc.ru

Citation: Muraleva, N.A.; Kolosova, N.G.; Stefanova, N.A. MEK1/2-ERK Pathway Alterations as a Therapeutic Target in Sporadic Alzheimer's Disease: A Study in Senescence-Accelerated OXYS Rats. *Antioxidants* **2021**, *10*, 1058. https://doi.org/10.3390/antiox10071058

Academic Editors: Daniela-Saveta Popa, Laurian Vlase, Marius Emil Rusu and Ionel Fizesan

Received: 2 June 2021
Accepted: 27 June 2021
Published: 30 June 2021

Publisher's Note: MDPI stays neutral with regard to jurisdictional claims in published maps and institutional affiliations.

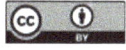

Copyright: © 2021 by the authors. Licensee MDPI, Basel, Switzerland. This article is an open access article distributed under the terms and conditions of the Creative Commons Attribution (CC BY) license (https://creativecommons.org/licenses/by/4.0/).

Abstract: Alzheimer's disease (AD) is a progressive neurodegenerative disorder and the most common cause of dementia worldwide, with no cure. There is growing interest in mitogen-activated protein kinases (MAPKs) as possible pathogenesis-related therapeutic targets in AD. Previously, using senescence-accelerated OXYS rats, which simulate key characteristics of the sporadic AD type, we have shown that prolonged treatment with mitochondria-targeted antioxidant plastoquinonyl-decyltriphenylphosphonium (SkQ1) during active progression of AD-like pathology improves the activity of many signaling pathways (SPs) including the p38 MAPK SP. In this study, we continued to investigate the mechanisms behind anti-AD effects of SkQ1 in OXYS rats and focused on hippocampal extracellular regulated kinases' (ERK1 and -2) activity alterations. According to high-throughput RNA sequencing results, SkQ1 eliminated differences in the expression of eight out of nine genes involved in the ERK1/2 SP, compared to untreated control (Wistar) rats. Western blotting and immunofluorescent staining revealed that SkQ1 suppressed ERK1/2 activity via reductions in the phosphorylation of kinases ERK1/2, MEK1, and MEK2. SkQ1 decreased hyperphosphorylation of tau protein, which is present in pathological aggregates in AD. Thus, SkQ1 alleviates AD pathology by suppressing MEK1/2-ERK1/2 SP activity in the OXYS rat hippocampus and may be a promising candidate drug for human AD.

Keywords: Alzheimer's disease; extracellular regulated kinase (ERK1/2); mitogen-activated protein kinases (MAPK); mitochondria-targeted antioxidant; SkQ1; OXYS rats

1. Introduction

Alzheimer's disease (AD) is a progressive neurodegenerative disorder and the most common cause of dementia worldwide, with no cure. The prevalence of AD is increasing dramatically due to the aging of the world population. At present, there is no effective drug for this complex disease [1], even though the investigation into the mechanisms of AD is very active. There is growing interest in mitogen-activated protein kinases (MAPKs) as potential targets for pathogenesis-directed therapy of AD. Numerous reports have revealed a relationship between the activation of MAPKs and accumulation of pathological aggregates of beta-amyloid (Aβ) and hyperphosphorylated tau protein in neurofibrillary plaques [2,3] as well as neuroinflammation [4], oxidative stress, and other hallmarks of AD. Zhu and coauthors have demonstrated that there are differences in the activation of various MAPKs during AD development in comparison with healthy people [5]. p38 MAPK activity is associated with mild and severe stages of AD, whereas extracellular regulated kinases' (ERK1/2) activities are altered at all the stages of this disease, including stages with limited pathological signs [5].

MAPK pathways are the key mechanism that transmits extracellular signals, including inflammatory cytokines and reactive oxygen species, from the plasma membrane to the nucleus. Among them, the ERK1/2 pathway is important for the central nervous system [6]. It participates in the regulation of differentiation, maturation, and migration of cells, thereby contributing to the establishment of their phenotype [7]. It is noteworthy that the ERK pathway is involved in the regulation of neurogenesis both during brain formation and in adulthood [8]. The ERK pathway actively participates in mechanisms of synaptogenesis, in the transmission of cellular signals, and in the changes related to neural plasticity, including those linked with learning and memory processes, and configures specific networks for the correct processing of emotional signals [6]. Disturbances of ERK pathway activity are associated with neurological syndromes such as autism [9]. Some of the proteins that give rise to pathological deposits in the brain during AD, including tau protein and Aβ, are cytosolic targets of ERK, which take part in the establishment of pathological hallmarks and in neurodegeneration [10,11]. Faucher and colleagues have shown that Aβ aggregates trigger the ERK1/2 signaling pathway (SP) in the brain at early stages of AD [12]. Other authors have found that ERK1/2 activity is implicated in tau phosphorylation during AD [2,3,13]. Greater amounts of phospho-ERK (p-ERK) have been found in brain extracts from AD patients [14]. Thus, the ERK1/2 SP is strongly implicated in AD development and can become a promising therapeutic target. Currently, there are no effective therapeutic agents targeting the ERK1/2 SP for AD treatment. Researchers are focusing their efforts on the determination of selectivity profiles when designing kinase inhibitors that can cross the blood–brain barrier and on the optimization of their therapeutic index [4]. In the present study, we hypothesized that mitochondria-targeted antioxidant plastoquinonyl-decyltriphenylphosphonium (SkQ1) globally affects the activities of MAPK-related SPs; the ability of SkQ1 to delay the development and suppress the progression of AD-like pathology in a rat model of a sporadic type of the disease has previously been reported by us [15–18].

This work is continuation of a series of studies on the identification of AD mechanisms and effective targets for devising therapeutic and preventive strategies against AD as a complicated multifactorial disorder. Using nontransgenic senescence-accelerated OXYS rats, which develop neurodegenerative changes that are similar to the signs of the sporadic type (>90% of cases) of AD in humans [19], we have previously reported that treatment with SkQ1 between ages 12 and 18 months—that is, during active progression of AD-like pathology in these animals—alleviates structural neurodegenerative alterations, improves the structural and functional state of mitochondria, prevents the neuronal loss and synaptic damage, enhances a neurotrophic supply, and decreases $A\beta_{1-42}$ peptide levels and tau hyperphosphorylation in the hippocampus, thus resulting in improvements in learning ability and memory [15–17]. Via transcriptomic approaches, we then found that the anti-AD properties of SkQ1 are related to improvements in the activities of many intracellular processes and SPs in the prefrontal cortex and hippocampus, including the p38 MAPK SP [20,21], which is launched during the development of AD-like pathology in OXYS rats [22]. In this study, we continued to investigate the mechanisms of the anti-AD effects of SkQ1 in OXYS rats at an advanced stage of AD-like pathology and focused on MEK1/2-ERK pathway alterations in the hippocampus.

2. Materials and Methods

2.1. Ethics Statement

All experiments were approved by (and conducted in accordance with the guidelines of) the Ethics Committee on animal testing of the Institute of Cytology and Genetics, Novosibirsk, Russia (the decree of the Presidium of the Russian Academy of Sciences No. 12000-496 of 2 April 1980).

2.2. Animals and Diet

The effect of SkQ1 dietary supplementation was investigated with senescence-accelerated OXYS rats (with Wistar rats as the control) obtained from the Center for Genetic Resources of Laboratory Animals at the ICG SB RAS (Novosibirsk, Russia), which were kept under standard laboratory conditions. One group ($n = 8$) consumed a diet supplemented with

SkQ1 (250 nmol/[kg body weight]) on dried bread slices between ages 12 and 18 months every day. Twelve-month-old OXYS and Wistar rats ($n = 8$) that ingested dried bread without the drug served as controls. SkQ1 was kindly provided by Skulachev Vladimir, from Institute of Mitoengineering of Moscow State University, Moscow, Russia.

2.3. Tissue Preparation

Untreated 18-month-old OXYS and Wistar rats and OXYS rats after the dietary supplementation with SkQ1 ($n = 3$) were euthanized by CO_2 asphyxiation and used for RNA-seq analysis. The right brain hemisphere of the remaining animals in each group ($n = 5$) was excised on ice and fixed under standard conditions (buffered 4% paraformaldehyde for 48 h). Then, the fixed brain was transferred to 30% sucrose for 48 h incubation. The hippocampus from the left hemisphere of the rat brains ($n = 5$ per group) was isolated on ice and put in clean tubes for Western blot analysis. The samples of brain tissue were stored at $-70\,^\circ$C until analysis.

2.4. Gene Expression Analysis

RNA isolation, Illumina sequencing, and sequencing data processing were performed as described elsewhere [20]. The genes with an adjusted p value of <0.05 were defined as differentially expressed. The list of genes related to ERK1/2 SP was compiled by comparing the gene lists in the Rat Genome Database (RGD; 123 rat genes, https://rgd.mcw.edu/ (accessed on 12 January 2021) and Kyoto Encyclopedia of Genes and Genomes (KEGG; https://www.genome.jp/kegg (accessed on 12 January 2021).

2.5. Western Blotting

The hippocampus from OXYS and Wistar rats ($n = 5$ per group) at the age of 18 months after the supplementation with SkQ1 was subjected to Western blotting. Frozen tissue samples of the hippocampus were homogenized in protein radioimmune precipitation buffer (50 mM Tris-HCl pH 7.4, 150 mM NaCl, 1% Triton X-100, 1% sodium deoxycholate, 0.1% sodium dodecyl sulfate, and 1 mM ethylenediaminetetraacetic acid) supplemented with a protease inhibitor cocktail (P8340; Sigma-Aldrich, St. Louis, MO, USA). After incubation for 20 min on ice, the samples were centrifuged at $12,000\times g$ for 30 min at $4\,^\circ$C. The resultant supernatants were collected as a detergent-soluble fraction. The pellets were resuspended in an equal volume of SDS sample buffer, rehomogenized, sonicated, and centrifuged at $14,000\times g$ for 10 min at $4\,^\circ$C. The supernatants were transferred into new tubes as a detergent-insoluble fraction. Total protein was quantified by means of the Bio-Rad Bradford Kit (Bio-Rad Laboratories, Hercules, CA, USA). The protein fractions were transferred onto a nitrocellulose membrane. After blockage with 5% bovine serum albumin (BSA; cat. #SLBJ8588V; Sigma-Aldrich, St. Louis, MO, USA) in phosphate buffered saline with 0.1% Tween 20 for 1 h, the membranes were incubated at $4\,^\circ$C overnight with one of the following primary antibodies: anti alpha B crystallin antibody, anti-phospho-S45 CryaB antibody, anti-ERK1/2 antibody, anti-ERK1/2 (phospho T202, T185) antibody, anti-MEK1/2 antibody, anti-MEK1/2 (phospho S218, S222) antibody, anti-tau, anti-phospho-tau (T181), and anti-β-actin and anti-GAPDH antibodies (cat. # ab76467, ab5598, ab184699, ab201015, ab178876, ab194754, ab1801, and ab8245, respectively; Abcam, Waltham, MA, USA; 1:1000 dilution). We incubated the membrane with secondary antibodies (cat. # ab97046 and ab6721; Abcam, Waltham, MA, USA; 1:5000) for 1 h. The intensity of chemiluminescent signals of the bands was quantified using ImageJ software (NIH, Bethesda, MD, USA).

2.6. Immunofluorescent Staining

The brain tissue slices (16 μm thick) of OXYS and Wistar rats were placed onto Polysine glass slides (Menzel-Glaser; Thermo Scientific, Braunschweig, Germany) and incubated for 1 h in a blocking solution consisting of 1% BSA (Sigma-Aldrich, St. Louis, MO, USA) in PBS with 0.1% Triton X-100 (PBS-T). The slices were incubated overnight at $4\,^\circ$C with the same primary antibody (as in Western blotting) diluted 1:250 with the blocking solution.

After serial washes in PBS, the slices were probed for 1 h in the dark at room temperature with a secondary antibody (cat. # ab150170, ab175472, and ab150075; Abcam, Waltham, MA, USA; 1:5000) diluted 1:300 in a 1% BSA solution in PBS. Next, the slices were washed with PBS and coverslipped with Fluoro-shield mounting medium containing 4′,6-diamidino-2-phenylindole (DAPI; cat. # ab104139; Abcam, Waltham, MA, USA). Negative controls were processed in an identical manner except that the primary antibody was omitted. The experiment included a negative control. The immunofluorescent signals were visualized by means of an Axioplan 2 fluorescence microscope (Carl Zeiss, Jena, Germany).

2.7. Statistical Analysis

The Newman-Keuls post hoc test in Statistica 8.0 software (StatSoft, Tulsa, OK, USA) was applied to significant main effects and interactions in order to evaluate the differences between some sets of means. One-way ANOVA was performed for pairwise group comparisons. The data are presented as mean ± SEM. Differences were regarded as statistically significant at $p < 0.05$.

3. Results

3.1. Dietary Supplementation with SkQ1 Reverses Up- and Downregulation of the Genes Associated with the ERK1/2 SP in the Hippocampus of OXYS Rats

Recently, we showed that the hippocampus of 18-month-old OXYS rats features 1159 differentially expressed genes relative to Wistar rats, and that treatment with SkQ1 from age 12 to 18 months decreases their number by twofold [20]. In untreated (control) OXYS rats, the most significant specific feature was the number of differentially expressed genes associated with mitochondrial function, whereas SkQ1 eliminated differences in the expression of 76% of them (93 of 122 genes). Out of ~300 differentially expressed genes whose products participate in SPs, 26 genes encode proteins taking part in MAPK signaling cascades, of which 13 are involved in the p38 MAPK SP (out of 57 known genes of the p38 MAPK SP) [22]. In the present study, the analysis of the ERK1/2 SP identified nine genes (out of 54 known genes of the ERK1/2 SP) whose expression differed in the hippocampus between 18-month-old OXYS and Wistar rats (Figure 1a). The expression of genes *Atp6v0c*, *Ddt*, *Rgs14*, and *Rps6ka2* was higher, while the expression of genes *Ankrd26*, *Map3k1*, *Ranbp9*, *Nras*, and *Spp1* was lower in untreated OXYS rats (Figure 1). Treatment with SkQ1 eliminated the differences in the expression of these genes except for *Spp1*. In addition, SkQ1 decreased the mRNA level of *Mturn* (Figure 1a,b).

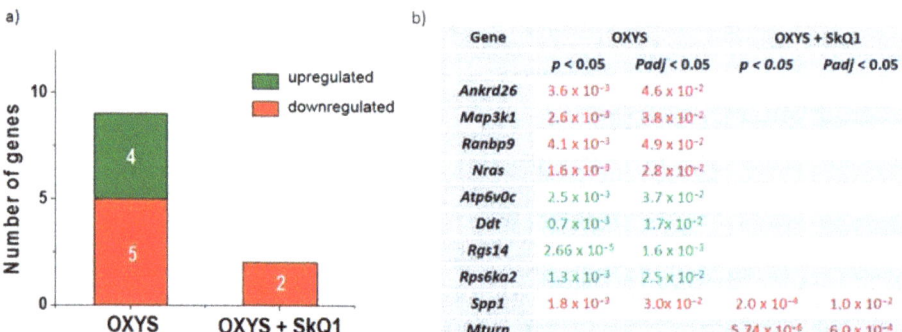

Figure 1. The effects of the dietary supplementation with SkQ1 in OXYS rats on the expression of the genes whose products play a role in the ERK1/2 SP (**a**). Differentially expressed genes of the ERK1/2 SP in untreated (control) OXYS rats and the influence of prolonged treatment with SkQ1 (**b**). Differential expression means a comparison with the parental control strain (Wistar). The data are marked in green if upregulated and red if downregulated of genes. p: probability values; p_{adj}: adjusted p values.

3.2. SkQ1 Reduces the Amounts of Proteins ERK1 and ERK2 and Their Phosphorylation in the OXYS Hippocampus

Western blotting revealed that the combined level of proteins ERK1 and ERK2 in the hippocampus was higher in OXYS rats than in Wistar rats ($p < 0.05$; Figure 2a). The combined amount of proteins p-ERK1 and p-ERK2 was significantly higher in OXYS rats than Wistar rats ($p < 0.05$). Figure 2a,b presents the ratio of p-ERK1/2 to total ERK1/2 proteins. These results suggested that the ERK pathway was activated in OXYS rats with age, and the expression of key proteins of the pathway significantly increased.

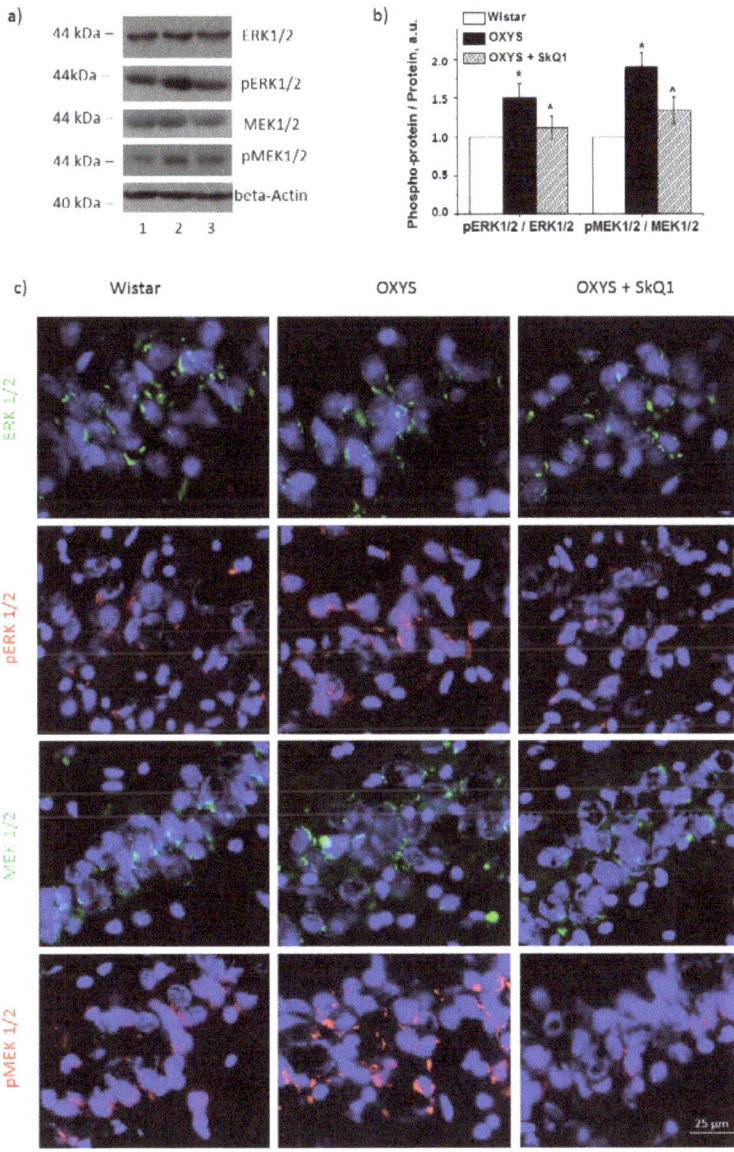

Figure 2. The impact of SkQ1 supplementation in OXYS rats between ages 12 and 18 months on protein levels of ERK1/2 SP components in the hippocampus. (**a**) Representative Western blot images of proteins

ERK1/2, p-ERK1/2, MEK1/2, and p-MEK1/2: Wistar rats (1), OXYS rats (2), and OXYS rats after the supplementation with SkQ1 (3). Graphical presentation of the ratios of proteins p-ERK1/2 to ERK1/2 and p-MEK1/2 to MEK1/2 in the hippocampi of untreated Wistar and OXYS rats and in OXYS rats after the supplementation with SkQ1 (**b**). The protein amounts were normalized to beta-actin or GAPDH and then were normalized to the data from Wistar rats. The results are presented as mean ± SEM of five independent experiments. * Statistically significant differences between the strains of the same age; ˆ the effect of the supplementation with SkQ1 ($p < 0.05$). Immunostaining of ERK1/2, p-ERK1/2, MEK1/2, and p-MEK1/2 in the hippocampus of untreated Wistar and OXYS rats and OXYS rats taking SkQ1 (**c**). Nuclei were stained with 4′,6-diamidino-2-phenylindole dihydrochloride(DAPI) (blue). Scale bars: 25 μm.

After the supplementation with SkQ1, ERK1 and ERK2 became less active. SkQ1 had no effect on the combined ERK1 and ERK2 protein level in OXYS rats but reduced their phosphorylation ($p < 0.05$, Figure 2b). One-way ANOVA revealed a decrease in p-ERK1/2 content ($p < 0.05$) in OXYS rats after the supplementation with SkQ1, but it remained higher than that in the control Wistar rats. The ratio of p-ERK1/2 to total ERK1/2 indicated that the supplementation with SkQ1 reduced ERK1/2 phosphorylation (Figure 2b). Similar data were obtained by immunostaining of the brain from untreated Wistar and OXYS rats and OXYS rats treated with SkQ1 (Figure 2c). These findings indicated that the ERK pathway in the hippocampus of OXYS rats was inactivated by the SkQ1 administration.

3.3. SkQ1 Reduces MER1/2 and p-MEK1/2 Protein Amounts in the Hippocampus of OXYS Rats

Proteins MEK1 and MEK2 are located upstream of the ERK1/2 SP and regulate the activity of ERK1 and ERK2 by means of their phosphorylation. As expected, we registered increased levels of combined MEK1/2 phosphorylation in 18-month-old OXYS rats compared with Wistar rats (Figure 2a,b). The level of p-MEK1/2 proteins was significantly higher in OXYS rats ($p < 0.05$). Nevertheless, total MEK1/2 content was not different between the two strains.

As displayed in Figure 2a,b, the supplementation with SkQ1 decreased the phosphorylation of MEK1/2 in OXYS rats. Statistical analysis indicated that the decrease in the ratio of p-MEK1/2 to total MEK1/2 was due to a significant decrease in the level of MEK1/2 ($p < 0.05$, Figure 2a). Similar results were obtained after the immunostaining of rat brains (Figure 2c).

3.4. SkQ1 Decreases CryaB and p-Ser45-CryaB Protein Amounts in the Hippocampus of OXYS Rats

To confirm the inhibitory influence of SkQ1 on the ERK1/2 SP, we estimated the extent of phosphorylation of one of its target proteins—molecular chaperone CryaB—at the Ser45 position. Phosphorylation of CryaB promotes the formation of strong crosslinks with its target proteins and its transfer into a detergent-insoluble fraction. Accordingly, we quantified p-Ser45-CryaB in the detergent-soluble fraction and detergent-insoluble fraction of the protein homogenates. At first, we noted CryaB hyperphosphorylation in the detergent-insoluble fraction of the OXYS rat hippocampus at the age of 18 months ($p < 0.05$; Figure 3a,b). In the detergent-soluble fraction, the CryaB and p-Ser45-CryaB protein amounts did not differ between the strains. The SkQ1 supplementation did not have an impact on CryaB content of the detergent-soluble fraction. The CryaB amount in the detergent-insoluble fraction was lower in SkQ1-treated OXYS rats than in control OXYS rats ($p < 0.05$; Figure 3b). Statistical analysis indicated that SkQ1 significantly reduced the level of p-Ser45-CryaB in the detergent-insoluble protein fractions of the hippocampus from OXYS rats ($p < 0.05$; Figure 3b), but this parameter remained significantly higher than that in untreated Wistar rats ($p < 0.05$). The Western blotting data were confirmed by immunostaining results (Figure 3c).

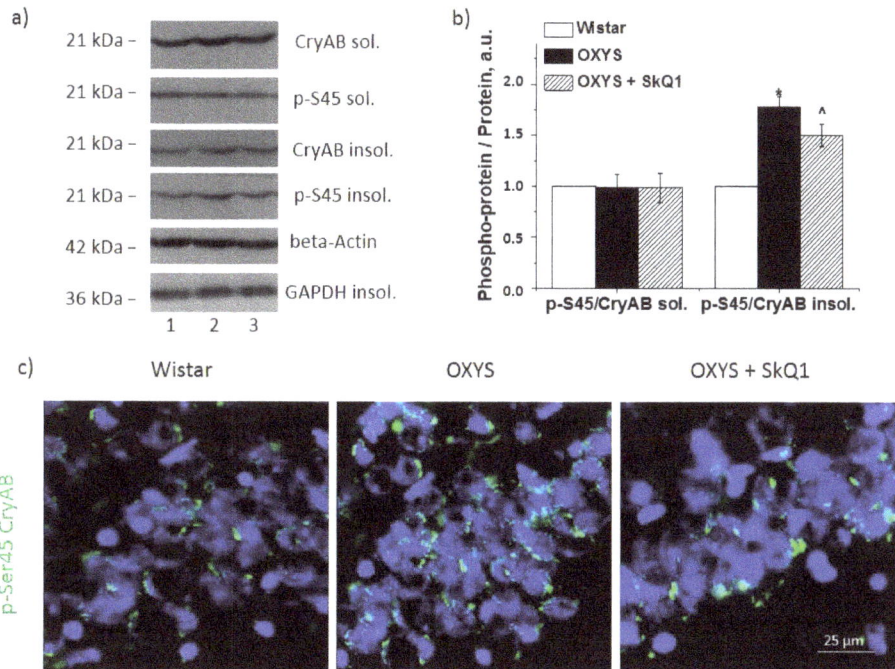

Figure 3. The effect of SkQ1 supplementation in OXYS rats from age 12 to 18 months on the protein levels of CryaB and p-Ser45-CryaB in the hippocampus. Representative Western blots of total and phosphorylated CryaB and p-Ser45-CryaB in the detergent-soluble and detergent-insoluble fractions from the hippocampus of untreated Wistar (1) and OXYS rats (2) and OXYS rats treated with SkQ1 (3) (**a**). Graphical presentation of the ratios of proteins p-Ser45-CryaB to CryaB in the hippocampus of untreated Wistar and OXYS rats and OXYS rats taking SkQ1 after normalization to beta-actin for the detergent-soluble protein fraction and to GAPDH for the detergent-insoluble fraction (**b**). Data are presented as mean ± SEM of five independent experiments. Immunostaining for p-Ser45-CryaB (**c**) in the hippocampus of untreated Wistar and OXYS rats and OXYS rats taking SkQ1. The nuclei were stained with DAPI (blue). Scale bars: 25 μm. ^ Statistically significant differences between the strains of the same age; * the effect of supplementation with SkQ1 ($p < 0.05$). sol.: detergent-soluble protein fraction of hippocampus; insol.: detergent-insoluble protein fraction.

3.5. SkQ1 Prevents Tau Protein Hyperphosphorylation in the Hippocampus of OXYS Rats

According to Western blot findings, OXYS rats after the supplementation with SkQ1 showed significantly lower expression of total tau and p-Thr181-tau ($p < 0.05$ and <0.01, respectively; Figure 4a,b). The Western blotting data were confirmed by immunostaining results (Figure 4c).

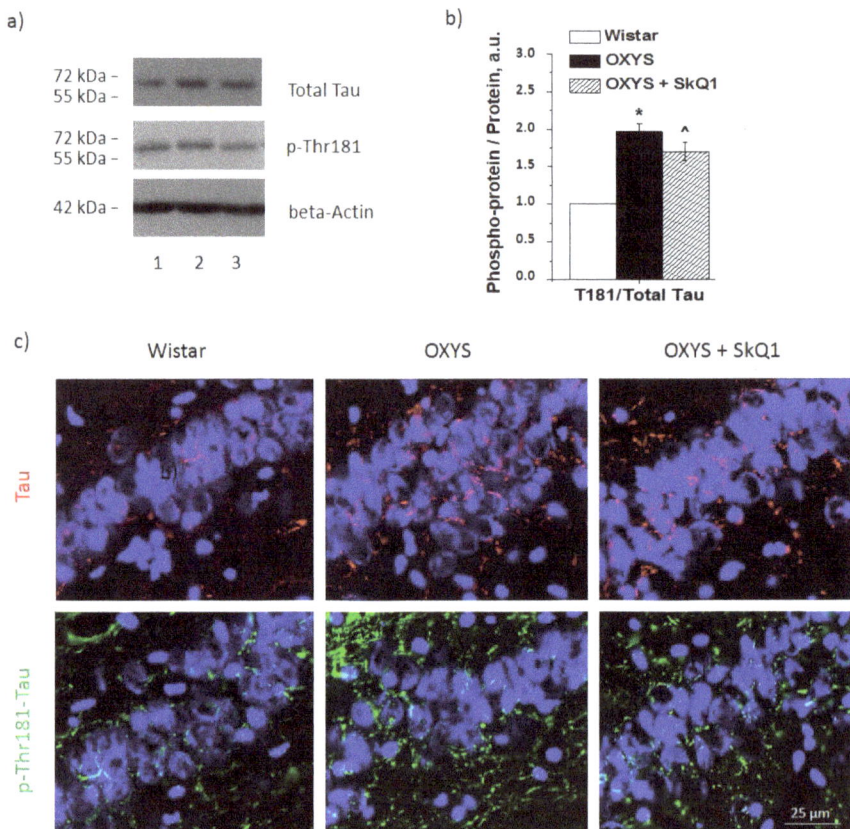

Figure 4. The effects of SkQ1 supplementation in OXYS rats from age 12 to 18 months on protein levels of tau and p-Thr181-tau in the hippocampus. Representative Western blots of total and phosphorylated tau and p-Thr181-tau in the hippocampus of untreated Wistar (1) and OXYS rats (2) and of OXYS rats treated with SkQ1 (3) (**a**). Graphical presentation of the ratios of proteins p-Thr181-tau to tau in the hippocampus of untreated Wistar and OXYS rats and OXYS rats taking SkQ1 after normalization to beta-actin (**b**). Data are presented as mean ± SEM of five independent experiments. Immunostaining for tau and p-Thr181-tau (**c**) in the hippocampus of untreated Wistar and OXYS rats and OXYS rats taking SkQ1. Nuclei were visualized with DAPI (blue). Scale bars: 25 μm. ^ Statistically significant differences between the strains of the same age; * the effect of supplementation with SkQ1 ($p < 0.05$).

4. Discussion

As members of the MAPK family, ERK1 and ERK2 perform functions at every stage of the growth and formation of cells, including proliferation, differentiation, migration, senescence, and apoptosis. They are also important components of the response to stress during AD development. Here, we showed for the first time that the progression of AD-like pathology in OXYS rats takes place simultaneously with alterations in the expression of nine genes encoding proteins participating in the ERK1/2 SP, whereas dietary supplementation with SkQ1 normalizes the expression of eight of these genes. In our previous studies, we have demonstrated that after supplementation with SkQ1 in OXYS rats, the expression of 14 genes involved in MAPK signaling cascades changes [20], of which 12 are affiliated with the p38 MAPK SP [21]. In the present study, we found that products of the remaining two genes take part in the ERK1/2 SP. Although we did not notice any changes in mRNA levels of the key genes of this SP, the increased expression of *Rgs14* (regulator of G protein signaling 14) in the hippocampus of untreated OXYS rats is interesting. The product of this gene is a suppressor of synaptic plasticity in CA2 neurons and hippocampus-based learning and memory [23]. There are reports that RGS14 inhibition holds promise for normalizing a cognitive impairment [24].

The activation of the ERK1/2 SP in OXYS rats can be confirmed by overexpression of D-dopachrome tautomerase (*Ddt*). The DDT protein participates in the activation of kinases ERK1 and ERK2 [25], ultimately launching the expression of proinflammatory genes and neuroinflammation. In addition, the observed increased expression of ATPase H^+-transporting V0 subunit C (*Atp6v0c*) suggests a high demand for autophagy [26]. This is an enzyme transporter that acidifies intracellular compartments, and this alteration is necessary for such processes as receptor-mediated endocytosis and establishment of the proton gradient of synaptic vesicles. The disturbance of *Atp6v0c* expression implies a contribution to the onset and progression of an age-related neurodegenerative disease [27]. Among the analyzed differentially expressed genes with downregulation here, secreted phosphoprotein 1 (*Spp1*, also known as osteopontin) is noteworthy. Recently, it was shown to have a potential role in macrophage-mediated Aβ clearance [28]. Therefore, the reduced expression of *Spp1* can promote and/or exacerbate the accumulation of pathological Aβ aggregates and the progression of neurodegeneration in OXYS rats. It can be assumed that all these alterations contribute to the progression of the AD-like pathology in OXYS rats.

Pathological Aβ accumulation may be a prerequisite for ERK1/2 pathway activation in OXYS rats; this accumulation in OXYS rats starts at age 7 months, i.e., at the stage of AD-like pathology manifestation [19]. Similar activation of ERK in hippocampi of a transgenic animal model of AD has been documented during Aβ accumulation [29]. Moreover, ERK1/2 pathway activation with high levels of kinases p-ERK1 and p-ERK2 has been detected in patients with dementia at various stages of behavioral disturbances [5,14].

Additionally, we quantified kinases upstream of the ERK1/2 SP. As expected, kinases MEK1 and MEK2, which act upstream of this SP, turned out to be activated. Elevated amounts of p-MEK1/2 were found in the hippocampus of 18-month-old OXYS rats in comparison with disease-free age-matched Wistar rats. Kinases MEK1 and -2 are activators of ERK1 and -2 and have very narrow substrate specificity. These observations are consistent with the overactivity of the ERK1/2 SP observed here in OXYS rats at the stage of progression of AD-like pathology signs and are similar to findings about other disease models [29]. It should be noted that MEK-ERK pathway activation may be associated with mutations in BRAF or RAS as its upstream activator [30]. On the other hand, in another study on OXYS rats, we did not find mutations in the genes involved in the ERK1/2 pathway [31].

Cytoplasmic targets of p-ERK ensure proteostasis in the cell. There are 200 substrates of ERK1 and ERK2 that have been identified to date [32,33], including tau protein, whose hyperphosphorylation is regarded as one of the main AD characteristics. Here, we confirmed that the progression of AD-like pathology in OXYS rats is concurrent with increases in both the total level of tau protein and its phosphorylation [16]. These data are consistent with the increased ERK1/2 signaling activity in OXYS rats. Furthermore, as a criterion for assessing ERK1/2 signaling activity, we evaluated changes in ERK1/2-dependent phosphorylation of a small protein chaperone, CryaB. As expected, the increased ERK1/2 signaling upregulated p-Ser45-CryaB in the detergent-insoluble fraction of the 18-month-old OXYS rat hippocampus. The phosphorylation of CryaB enhances its ability to form strong bonds with neurotoxic proteins, including Aβ, and makes CryaB insoluble. Elevated CryaB phosphorylation has also been uncovered by other authors in an AD study, where this phenomenon was associated with pathologically aggregated proteins [34].

Here, we hypothesized that one of the mechanisms behind the beneficial effect of SkQ1 is mediated by ERK1/2 pathway inhibition. Indeed, the OXYS rats on the diet supplemented with SkQ1 manifested a decrease in the p-ERK1/2 level, but not total ERK1/2, in the hippocampus. In addition, we registered decreased phosphorylation of kinases MER1 and -2, which are kinase activators functioning upstream of the ERK1/2 SP. In addition, we noticed decreased phosphorylation of cytosolic targets of this pathway:

tau protein and CryaB. A decrease in tau hyperphosphorylation is thought to be a positive prognostic sign during the treatment of AD. Together with a decrease in Aβ accumulation, this change alleviates the toxic load on neurons. Accordingly, the obtained data mean that SkQ1 inhibits the ERK1/2 SP by blocking kinases MER1 and -2.

Activation of ERK1/2 signal transduction is involved in aberrations of the mitochondrial fission/fusion ratio and defects in mitochondrial function. Ganand and coauthors have demonstrated that ERK inactivation normalizes anomalous mitochondrial dynamics in AD [35]. This observation can explain the previously reported strong connection between the neuroprotective property of SkQ1 and an improvement in the structure and functions of mitochondria [17,18] and in the expression of genes related to mitochondrial function [20]. Furthermore, the suppression of ERK1/2 phosphorylation protects neuronal cell lines and primary cultured neurons from direct oxidative stress [31].

ERK1/2 signaling plays an important role in the regulation of synaptic plasticity in AD. Upregulation of total ERK is associated with deficient memory task performance in a transgenic mouse model of AD [23]. Alterations in ERK1/2 signaling induce Aβ-associated behavioral deficits in an animal model of AD [36]. Conversely, ERK1/2 pathway inhibition eliminates memory deficits in a transgenic model of AD [29], in agreement with our finding that SkQ1 has a beneficial impact on the behavior of OXYS rats [15].

Thus, in our study, we demonstrated that active progression of AD-like pathology in OXYS rats is associated with alterations of the ERK1/2 SP. The mitochondria-targeted antioxidant SkQ1, which alleviated AD pathology through MEK1/2-ERK1/2 pathway suppression in the OXYS rat hippocampus, can be regarded as a promising therapeutic agent against human AD.

Author Contributions: Conceptualization, all the authors; Investigation, N.A.M. and N.A.S.; Supervision, N.G.K.; Writing—Original Draft, N.A.M. and N.G.K.; and Writing—Review and Editing: all the authors. All authors have read and agreed to the published version of the manuscript.

Funding: This work was supported by the Russian Foundation for Basic Research (grant number 19-15-00044). The sponsors had no role in study design; in the collection, analysis, and interpretation of the data; in the writing of the report; or in the decision to submit the manuscript for publication.

Institutional Review Board Statement: All experiments were approved by (and conducted in accordance with the guide-lines of) the Ethics Committee on animal testing of the Institute of Cytology and Genetics, Novosibirsk, Russia (the decree of the Presidium of the Russian Academy of Sciences No. 12000-496 of 2 April 1980).

Informed Consent Statement: Not applicable.

Data Availability Statement: Data is contained within the article.

Acknowledgments: Microscopy was performed at the Microscopy Center of the ICG SB RAS, Russia.

Conflicts of Interest: The authors declare that they have no competing interest.

References

1. Rao, C.V.; Asch, A.S.; Carr, D.; Yamada, H.Y. "Amyloid-beta accumulation cycle" as a prevention and/or therapy target for Alzheimer's disease. *Aging Cell* **2020**, *19*, e13109. [CrossRef]
2. Kirouac, L.; Rajic, A.J.; Cribbs, D.H.; Padmanabhan, J. Activation of Ras-ERK Signaling and GSK-3 by Amyloid Precursor Protein and Amyloid Beta Facilitates Neurodegeneration in Alzheimer's Disease. *eNeuro* **2017**, *4*, ENEURO.0149-16.2017. [CrossRef]
3. Sun, J.; Nan, G. The extracellular signal-regulated kinase 1/2 pathway in neurological diseases: A potential therapeutic target (Review). *Int. J. Mol. Med.* **2017**, *39*, 1338–1346. [CrossRef]
4. Ahmed, T.; Zulfiqar, A.; Arguelles, S.; Rasekhian, M.; Nabavi, S.F.; Silva, A.S.; Nabavi, S.M. Map kinase signaling as therapeutic target for neurodegeneration. *Pharmacol. Res.* **2020**, *160*, 105090. [CrossRef]
5. Zhu, X.; Castellani, R.J.; Takeda, A.; Nunomura, A.; Atwood, C.S.; Perry, G.; Smith, M.A. Differential activation of neuronal ERK, JNK/SAPK and p38 in Alzheimer disease: The 'two hit' hypothesis. *Mech. Ageing Dev.* **2001**, *123*, 39–46. [CrossRef]
6. Albert-Gascó, H.; Ros-Bernal, F.; Castillo-Gómez, E.; Olucha-Bordonau, F.E. MAP/ERK Signaling in Developing Cognitive and Emotional Function and Its Effect on Pathological and Neurodegenerative Processes. *Int. J. Mol. Sci.* **2020**, *21*, 4471. [CrossRef]

7. Hausott, B.; Schlick, B.; Vallant, N.; Dorn, R.; Klimaschewski, L. Promotion of neurite outgrowth by fibroblast growth factor receptor 1 overexpression and lysosomal inhibition of receptor degradation in pheochromocytoma cells and adult sensory neurons. *Neuroscience* **2008**, *153*, 461–473. [CrossRef]
8. Fournier, N.M.; Lee, B.; Banasr, M.; Elsayed, M.; Duman, R.S. Vascular endothelial growth factor regulates adult hippocampal cell proliferation through MEK/ERK- and PI3K/Akt-dependent signaling. *Neuropharmacology* **2012**, *63*, 642–652. [CrossRef]
9. Wen, Y.; Alshikho, M.J.; Herbert, M.R. Pathway network analyses for autism reveal multisystem involvement, major overlaps with other diseases and convergence upon MAPK and calcium signaling. *PLoS ONE* **2016**, *11*, e0153329. [CrossRef] [PubMed]
10. Gerfen, C.R.; Miyachi, S.; Paletzki, R.; Brown, P. D1 dopamine receptor supersensitivity in the dopamine-depleted striatum results from a switch in the regulation of ERK1/2/MAP kinase. *J. Neurosci.* **2002**, *22*, 5042–5054. [CrossRef]
11. Grazia Spillantini, M.; Crowther, R.A.; Jakes, R.; Hasegawa, M.; Goedert, M. α-Synuclein in filamentous inclusions of Lewy bodies from Parkinson's disease and dementia with Lewy bodies. *Proc. Natl. Acad. Sci. USA* **1998**, *95*, 6469–6473. [CrossRef] [PubMed]
12. Faucher, P.; Mons, N.; Micheau, J.; Louis, C.; Beracochea, D.J. Hippocampal Injections of Oligomeric Amyloid β-peptide (1-42) Induce Selective Working Memory Deficits and Long-lasting Alterations of ERK Signaling Pathway. *Front. Aging Neurosci.* **2016**, *7*, 245. [CrossRef] [PubMed]
13. Ferrer, I.; Blanco, R.; Carmona, M.; Ribera, R.; Goutan, E.; Puig, B.; Rey, M.J.; Cardozo, A.; Viñals, F.; Ribalta, T. Phosphorylated map kinase (ERK1, ERK2) expression is associated with early tau deposition in neurones and glial cells, but not with increased nuclear DNA vulnerability and cell death, in Alzheimer disease, Pick's disease, progressive supranuclear palsy and corticobasal degeneration. *Brain Pathol.* **2001**, *11*, 144–158.
14. Russo, C.; Dolcini, V.; Salis, S.; Venezia, V.; Zambrano, N.; Russo, T.; Schettini, G. Signal transduction through tyrosine-phosphorylated C-terminal fragments of amyloid precursor protein via an enhanced interaction with Shc/Grb2 adaptor proteins in reactive astrocytes of Alzheimer's disease brain. *J. Biol. Chem.* **2002**, *277*, 35282–35288. [CrossRef]
15. Stefanova, N.A.; Fursova, A.Z.; Kolosova, N.G. Behavioral effects induced by mitochondria-targeted antioxidant SkQ1 in Wistar and senescence-accelerated OXYS rats. *JAD* **2010**, *21*, 479–491. [CrossRef] [PubMed]
16. Stefanova, N.A.; Muraleva, N.A.; Skulachev, V.P.; Kolosova, N.G. Alzheimer's disease-like pathology in senescence-accelerated OXYS rats can be partially retarded with mitochondria-targeted antioxidant SkQ1. *JAD* **2014**, *38*, 681–694. [CrossRef] [PubMed]
17. Stefanova, N.A.; Muraleva, N.A.; Maksimova, K.Y.; Rudnitskaya, E.A.; Kiseleva, E.; Telegina, D.V.; Kolosova, N.G. An antioxidant specifically targeting mitochondria delays progression of Alzheimer's disease-like pathology. *Aging* **2016**, *8*, 2713–2733. [CrossRef]
18. Kolosova, N.G.; Tyumentsev, M.A.; Muraleva, N.A.; Kiseleva, E.; Vitovtov, A.O.; Stefanova, N.A. Antioxidant SkQ1 alleviates signs of Alzheimer's disease-like pathology in old OXYS rats by reversing mitochondrial deterioration. *Curr. Alzheimer Res.* **2017**, *14*, 1283–1292. [CrossRef]
19. Stefanova, N.A.; Kozhevnikova, O.S.; Vitovtov, A.O.; Maksimova, K.Y.; Logvinov, S.V.; Rudnitskaya, E.A.; Korbolina, E.E.; Muraleva, N.A.; Kolosova, N.G. Senescence-accelerated OXYS rats: A model of age-related cognitive decline with relevance to abnormalities in Alzheimer disease. *Cell Cycle* **2014**, *13*, 898–909. [CrossRef]
20. Stefanova, N.A.; Ershov, N.I.; Kolosova, N.G. Suppression of Alzheimer's Disease-Like Pathology Progression by Mitochondria-Targeted Antioxidant SkQ1: A Transcriptome Profiling Study. *Oxid. Med. Cell Longev.* **2019**, *2019*, 3984906. [CrossRef]
21. Muraleva, N.A.; Stefanova, N.A.; Kolosova, N.G. SkQ1 Suppresses the p38 MAPK Signaling Pathway Involved in Alzheimer's Disease-Like Pathology in OXYS Rats. *Antioxidants* **2020**, *9*, 676. [CrossRef]
22. Muraleva, N.A.; Kolosova, N.G.; Stefanova, N.A. p38 MAPK-dependent alphaB-crystallin phosphorylation in Alzheimer's disease-like pathology in OXYS rats. *Exp. Gerontol.* **2019**, *119*, 45–52. [CrossRef]
23. Evans, C.E.; Thomas, R.S.; Freeman, T.J.; Hvoslef-Eide, M.; Good, M.A.; Kidd, E.J. Selective reduction of APP-BACE1 activity improves memory via NMDA-NR2B receptor-mediated mechanisms in aged PDAPP mice. *Neurobiol. Aging* **2019**, *75*, 136–149. [CrossRef]
24. Lee, S.E.; Simons, S.B.; Heldt, S.A.; Zhao, M.; Schroeder, J.P.; Vellano, C.P.; Cowan, D.P.; Ramineni, S.; Yates, C.K.; Feng, Y.; et al. RGS14 is a natural suppressor of both synaptic plasticity in CA2 neurons and hippocampal-based learning and memory. *Proc. Natl. Acad. Sci. USA* **2010**, *107*, 16994–16998. [CrossRef]
25. Merk, M.; Zierow, S.; Leng, L.; Das, R.; Du, X.; Schulte, W.; Fan, J.; Lue, H.; Chen, Y.; Xiong, H.; et al. The D-dopachrome tautomerase (DDT) gene product is a cytokine and functional homolog of macrophage migration inhibitory factor (MIF). *Proc. Natl. Acad. Sci. USA* **2011**, *108*, E577–E585. [CrossRef]
26. Higashida, H.; Yokoyama, S.; Tsuji, C.; Muramatsu, S.I. Neurotransmitter release: Vacuolar ATPase V0 sector c-subunits in possible gene or cell therapies for Parkinson's, Alzheimer's, and psychiatric diseases. *JPS* **2017**, *67*, 11–17. [CrossRef]
27. Mangieri, L.R.; Mader, B.J.; Thomas, C.E.; Taylor, C.A.; Luker, A.M.; Tse, T.E.; Huisingh, C.; Shacka, J.J. ATP6V0C knock-down in neuroblastoma cells alters autophagy-lysosome pathway function and metabolism of proteins that accumulate in neurodegenerative disease. *PLoS ONE* **2014**, *9*, e93257. [CrossRef]
28. Rentsendorj, A.; Sheyn, J.; Fuchs, D.T.; Daley, D.; Salumbides, B.C.; Schubloom, H.E.; Hart, N.J.; Li, S.; Hayden, E.Y.; Teplow, D.B.; et al. A novel role for osteopontin in macrophage-mediated amyloid-β clearance in Alzheimer's models. *Brain Behav. Immun.* **2018**, *67*, 163–180. [CrossRef]

29. Feld, M.; Krawczyk, M.C.; Sol Fustiñana, M.; Blake, M.G.; Baratti, C.M.; Romano, A.; Boccia, M.M. Decrease of ERK/MAPK overactivation in prefrontal cortex reverses early memory deficit in a mouse model of Alzheimer's disease. *JAD* **2014**, *40*, 69–82. [CrossRef] [PubMed]
30. Xu, J.; Pfarr, N.; Endris, V.; Mai, E.K.; Md Hanafiah, N.H.; Lehners, N.; Penzel, R.; Weichert, W.; Ho, A.D.; Schirmacher, P.; et al. Molecular signaling in multiple myeloma: Association of RAS/RAF mutations and MEK/ERK pathway activation. *Oncogenesis* **2017**, *6*, e337. [CrossRef]
31. Devyatkin, V.A.; Redina, O.E.; Kolosova, N.G.; Muraleva, N.A. Single-Nucleotide Polymorphisms Associated with the Senescence-Accelerated Phenotype of OXYS Rats: A Focus on Alzheimer's Disease-Like and Age-Related-Macular-Degeneration-Like Pathologies. *JAD* **2020**, *73*, 1167–1183. [CrossRef]
32. von Kriegsheim, A.; Baiocchi, D.; Birtwistle, M.; Sumpton, D.; Bienvenut, W.; Morrice, N.; Yamada, K.; Lamond, A.; Kalna, G.; Orton, R.; et al. Cell fate decisions are specified by the dynamic ERK interactome. *Nat. Cell Biol.* **2009**, *11*, 1458–1464. [CrossRef]
33. Yoon, S.; Seger, R. The extracellular signal-regulated kinase: Multiple substrates regulate diverse cellular functions. *Growth Factors* **2006**, *24*, 21–44. [CrossRef]
34. Kato, K.; Inaguma, Y.; Ito, H.; Iida, K.; Iwamoto, I.; Kamei, K.; Ochi, N.; Ohta, H.; Kishikawa, M. Ser-59 is the major phosphorylation site in alphaB-crystallin accumulated in the brains of patients with Alexander's disease. *J. Neurochem.* **2001**, *76*, 730–736. [CrossRef]
35. Gan, X.; Huang, S.; Wu, L.; Wang, Y.; Hu, G.; Li, G.; Zhang, H.; Yu, H.; Swerdlow, R.H.; Chen, J.X.; et al. Inhibition of ERK-DLP1 signaling and mitochondrial division alleviates mitochondrial dysfunction in Alzheimer's disease cybrid cell. *Biochim. Biophys. Acta* **2014**, *1842*, 220–231. [CrossRef]
36. Caccamo, A.; Majumder, S.; Richardson, A.; Strong, R.; Oddo, S. Molecular interplay between mammalian target of rapamycin (mTOR), amyloid-β and Tau: Effects on cognitive impairments. *J. Biol. Chem.* **2010**, *285*, 13107–13120. [CrossRef]

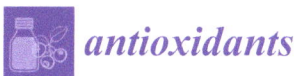

Review

Naturally Occurring Antioxidant Therapy in Alzheimer's Disease

Andrila E. Collins, Tarek M. Saleh and Bettina E. Kalisch *

Department of Biomedical Sciences and Collaborative Specialization in Neuroscience Program, University of Guelph, Guelph, ON N1G 2W1, Canada; andrila@uoguelph.ca (A.E.C.); tsaleh@uoguelph.ca (T.M.S.)
* Correspondence: bkalisch@uoguelph.ca

Abstract: It is estimated that the prevalence rate of Alzheimer's disease (AD) will double by the year 2040. Although currently available treatments help with symptom management, they do not prevent, delay the progression of, or cure the disease. Interestingly, a shared characteristic of AD and other neurodegenerative diseases and disorders is oxidative stress. Despite profound evidence supporting the role of oxidative stress in the pathogenesis and progression of AD, none of the currently available treatment options address oxidative stress. Recently, attention has been placed on the use of antioxidants to mitigate the effects of oxidative stress in the central nervous system. In preclinical studies utilizing cellular and animal models, natural antioxidants showed therapeutic promise when administered alone or in combination with other compounds. More recently, the concept of combination antioxidant therapy has been explored as a novel approach to preventing and treating neurodegenerative conditions that present with oxidative stress as a contributing factor. In this review, the relationship between oxidative stress and AD pathology and the neuroprotective role of natural antioxidants from natural sources are discussed. Additionally, the therapeutic potential of natural antioxidants as preventatives and/or treatment for AD is examined, with special attention paid to natural antioxidant combinations and conjugates that are currently being investigated in human clinical trials.

Keywords: antioxidants; oxidative stress; amyloid-beta; Alzheimer's disease; clinical trials

Citation: Collins, A.E.; Saleh, T.M.; Kalisch, B.E. Naturally Occurring Antioxidant Therapy in Alzheimer's Disease. *Antioxidants* **2022**, *11*, 213. https://doi.org/10.3390/antiox11020213

Academic Editors: Daniela-Saveta Popa, Laurian Vlase, Marius Emil Rusu and Ionel Fizesan

Received: 30 December 2021
Accepted: 19 January 2022
Published: 23 January 2022

Publisher's Note: MDPI stays neutral with regard to jurisdictional claims in published maps and institutional affiliations.

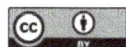

Copyright: © 2022 by the authors. Licensee MDPI, Basel, Switzerland. This article is an open access article distributed under the terms and conditions of the Creative Commons Attribution (CC BY) license (https://creativecommons.org/licenses/by/4.0/).

1. Introduction

Mild declines in cognitive and motor abilities are common aspects of human aging. However, the development of neurodegenerative diseases and neurological conditions is not. Interestingly, although the brain is arguably the most essential organ in the human body, it remains susceptible to its own degradation. As a highly metabolically active organ, the brain's oxygen demand is high [1]. As a result, free radicals are produced as the brain's requirement for oxygen increases [2]. The brain contains high amounts of polyunsaturated fatty acids, which are quickly oxidized by reactive oxygen species (ROS) but lacks essential enzymes that metabolize several toxic oxygen-containing reactants into harmless compounds [3]. This susceptibility to oxidative damage is observed in several neurodegenerative diseases. Alzheimer's disease (AD), Huntington's disease (HD), Parkinson's disease (PD), amyotrophic lateral sclerosis (ALS) and stroke, among many others (see Table 1), possess this shared pathology of oxidative stress. Recently, considerable attention has been placed on the use of naturally occurring (non-synthetic) antioxidants to mitigate the effects of oxidative stress in the central nervous system (CNS). More recently, the concept of combination antioxidant therapy has been explored as a novel approach to preventing and treating neurodegenerative conditions that present oxidative stress as a contributing factor to the pathogenesis and/or progression of the disease. This review explores the relationship between AD pathology and oxidative stress and the therapeutic potential of natural antioxidants as preventatives and/or treatments for AD, with an emphasis on natural antioxidant combinations and conjugates that are currently being investigated in human clinical trials.

Table 1. Some neurodegenerative diseases and conditions associated with oxidative stress.

Disease or Condition
Alzheimer's disease [4,5]
Amyotrophic lateral sclerosis [6,7]
Corticobasal degeneration [8]
Creutzfeldt-Jakob disease (Prion disease) [9]
Down syndrome [10]
Diabetic neuropathy [11,12]
Friedreich's ataxia [13]
Huntington's disease [14–16]
Lewy body disease [17]
Multiple sclerosis [18,19]
Neiman-Pick C disease [20,21]
Neuromyelitis optica [22]
Parkinson's disease [23–25]
Progressive supranuclear palsy [26]
Spinocerebellar ataxia [27–29]
Stroke [30–32]
Traumatic brain injury [33–35]

2. Antioxidants and Oxidative Stress

Antioxidants are compounds that protect the body from damage due to oxidative stress. Oxidative stress occurs when there is an imbalance between antioxidants and the production and accumulation of ROS [reviewed in 4]. ROS can be defined as oxygen-containing reactive molecules that are endogenously generated through mitochondrial oxygen metabolism [36]. ROS can also be produced through interplay with exogenous substances such as xenobiotic compounds [36]. This collective term includes compounds such as hydrogen peroxide (H_2O_2), superoxide ($O_2^{\bullet-}$), hydroxyl radical ($^{\bullet}OH$), nitric oxide ($^{\bullet}NO$) and singlet oxygen ($^1O_2$) [37]. During oxidative stress, an insufficient or dysfunctional antioxidant defence system permits damage to important cellular structures such as proteins, lipids, and nucleic acids [37,38], and is implicated in several pathologies of neurodegeneration [38] and aging [39]. Although ROS are damaging in excess, ROS maintain several endogenous functions at low levels. Under normal circumstances, low levels of ROS are produced through ordinary aerobic metabolism and any damage to cells is rapidly repaired through deployment of the antioxidant defence system [40]. ROS perform a critical role in cellular signalling processes, also known as redox signalling [41]. Therefore, to maintain adequate cellular homeostasis, a balance must be established between the production and depletion of ROS. This occurs through the protective mechanisms of antioxidants, which limit the damage induced by ROS and the eventual development of diseases and accelerated aging [39].

2.1. Antioxidant Classification and Mechanisms of Action

Antioxidants can be classified into two main categories: natural antioxidants and synthetic antioxidants. Synthetic antioxidants are artificially generated using a variety of chemical synthesis techniques [40,41]. Natural antioxidants are found in plants and animals and perform various biological roles, including but not limited to anti-inflammatory, anticancer and antiaging effects [42–45]. Natural antioxidants can be further divided into enzymatic and non-enzymatic antioxidants.

2.1.1. Enzymatic Antioxidants

Enzymatic antioxidants are enzymes produced within the body that possess free radical scavenging abilities and perform antioxidant functions. This group includes primary enzymes such as superoxide dismutase (SOD), catalase (CAT), and glutathione peroxidase (GPx), and secondary enzymes including glutathione reductase (GR) and glucose-6-phosphate dehydrogenase (G6PDH) [46]. SOD eliminates $O_2^{\bullet-}$ radicals by catalyzing the reduction of $O_2^{\bullet-}$ anions to H_2O_2 [15]. SOD is present in its many forms in several cellular locations, including the cytosol (Cu-Zn SOD1 or SOD1), mitochondria (Mn SOD or SOD2) and the extracellular space (SOD3) [47]. In turn, CAT is responsible for the decomposition of H_2O_2 into water and oxygen molecules [48]. In the absence of CAT, H_2O_2 can react with metal ions to form toxic $^{\bullet}OH$ radicals that further perpetuate the effects of oxidative stress [49]. GPx refers to a family of selenocysteine-containing enzymes, including GPx-1, which is predominantly found in the cytoplasm, that utilize glutathione (GSH) as a co-substrate to catalyze the reduction of H_2O_2 to water and oxidized glutathione (GSSG), and reduce other hydroperoxide substrates to alcohols [50,51]. It was suggested that a cooperative activity between CAT and GPx is required to achieve cellular protection against harmful peroxides [52]. However, differences in the antioxidant capacity of these compounds regarding the rate of removal and the capacity to ravage H_2O_2 were also identified [53]. GSSG is then reduced to GSH by nicotinamide adenine dinucleotide phosphate (NADPH). G6PDH, which produces NADPH, and GR, which recycles GSSG using NADPH, are considered secondary enzymatic antioxidants (Figure 1). The processes involved in the breakdown and elimination of elevated/toxic oxidative compounds may also include the presence of essential cofactors such as zinc (Zn), copper (Cu), iron (Fe), selenium (Se) and manganese (Mn) [54].

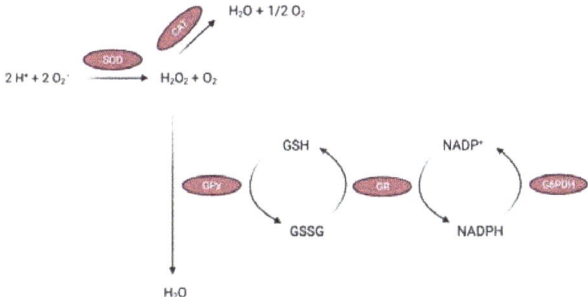

Figure 1. Schematic representation of enzymatic antioxidant mechanisms of action. Created with BioRender.com. SOD, superoxide dismutase; CAT, catalase; GPx, glutathione peroxidase; GR, glutathione reductase; G6PDH, glucose-6-phosphate dehydrogenase.

2.1.2. Non-Enzymatic Antioxidants

Non-enzymatic antioxidants can further be divided into groups of vitamins, carotenoids, polyphenols, and minerals [55]. Vitamins are a group of micronutrients that cannot be produced within the body; hence, they require supplementation through the diet [56]. Vitamins perform various functions within the body that are vital for human health and metabolism and are categorized into two groups based on solubility: fat-soluble vitamins and water-soluble vitamins [56]. Fat-soluble vitamins include vitamins A, D, E and K, which are dissolved in fat prior to their absorption into the bloodstream [56]. Water-soluble vitamins include the group of B-complex vitamins and vitamin C, which are dissolved in water [56].

Vitamin A

Sources of vitamin A include dietary supplements, animal products such as fish, meat, poultry, and dairy products, as well as plant products including fruits and vegetables that contain the provitamin A carotenoids (described below) such as beta-carotene, which is endogenously converted to vitamin A [57]. Vitamin A maintains essential roles in vision and synaptic function [58], bone growth and development [59], gene expression [60], cell division [61], reproduction [62], the maintenance of epithelial cells in respiratory, intestinal and urinary tracts, and a healthy immune system [63,64].

Vitamin D

Vitamin D, also known as vitamin D_3 (cholecalciferol) and vitamin D_2 (ergocalciferol), is predominantly produced endogenously within the skin from the provitamins 7-dehydrocholesterol (7-DHC) and ergosterol [65]. Skin exposure to ultraviolet-B stimulates the synthesis of pre-vitamin D_3, followed by thermal isomerization, producing vitamin D_3 [65]. Vitamins D_3 and D_2 can be obtained from the diet in supplements and fortified foods. Dietary vitamin D is predominantly absorbed in the small intestine by chylomicrons, before entering the lymphatic system and then the bloodstream [66]. Once in the bloodstream, from skin or intestinal absorption, vitamin D is converted into 25-hydroxyvitamin D in the liver, which undergoes further conversion to its active form 1,25-dihydrovitamin D in the kidneys [67–69]. Both compounds circulate in the blood bound to the vitamin D-binding protein. Once released from vitamin D-binding protein at tissues sites, 1,25-dihydrovitamin D binds to intracellular vitamin D receptors to elicit various metabolic functions throughout the body such as cell differentiation and proliferation, and calcium and phosphorus homeostasis [70,71].

Vitamin E

Vitamin E (α-tocopherol) acts as an antioxidant by protecting membrane components such as polyunsaturated fatty acids from lipid peroxidation by free radicals. Notably, vitamin E has been found to protect low-density lipoproteins from oxidation [72] and is present in high levels within the membranes of red blood cells, mitochondria, and endoplasmic reticulum [73–76]. Since vitamin E is predominantly synthesized in plants, it can be found in plant products such as nuts, seeds, vegetable oils and leafy green vegetables [77]. Vitamin E maintains various other biological functions, in addition to its role as an antioxidant, including its impact on signal transduction and gene expression [78], and its capacity to regulate enzymatic activity such as protein kinase C, which is important for regulating processes such as cell proliferation and inflammatory responses [79–82]. The effects of vitamin E may also differ between the four isoforms (α, β, γ and δ), with some studies reporting contradictory effects between these isoforms [82,83]. The ability of vitamin E to donate protons, and thereby saturate and detoxify unpaired electrons on highly reactive radicals such as •OH, support its recognition as a potent antioxidant [84]. The importance of vitamin E in brain health is observed in its ability to inhibit the production and progression of chain reactions that lead to lipid peroxidation by hindering the oxidation of unsaturated side chains present within lipid membranes [85]. This role highlights vitamin E as a potential therapeutic agent for neurological conditions, particularly those characterized by oxidative damage. For example, cerebral ischemia and subsequent infarction are consequences of oxidative stress in which vitamin E provides protection [86]. In addition to scavenging free radicals, studies report that vitamin E reduces the toxic effects of •NO by converting it to a less toxic nitrite ester in vitro and decreases the production of •NO and $O_2^{•-}$ within the brain [87,88].

Vitamin K

Vitamin K is bio-actively found in two forms, vitamins K_1 and K_2. Vitamin K_1 (phylloquinone) is predominately found in green leafy plants and can also be found in animals and further converted to vitamin K_2 (menaquinone) by anaerobic gut bacteria in animals [89,90]. Vitamin K_2 is primarily known for its role in blood-clotting by synthesizing coagulation proteins. It exerts its primary function by creating gamma-carboxyglutamate residues during the production of clotting factors by combining glutamate residues with carboxylic acids [91]. The addition of two carboxylic acid groups to an individual carbon present within a gamma-carboxyglutamate residue permits it to chelate calcium ions. Calcium ion binding is essential for vitamin K-dependent clotting factors, resulting in continued clotting cascades [92]. In a process called the vitamin K cycle, vitamin K is reduced to its metabolic form, vitamin K hydroquinone, by vitamin K epoxide reductase (VKOR), within the cell [93]. In turn, vitamin K hydroquinone is oxidized by vitamin K-dependent carboxylase. This enzyme then carboxylates glutamate residues to gamma-carboxyglutamate residues, ultimately producing vitamin K epoxide [94]. Both carboxylation and epoxidation reactions occur simultaneously. Vitamin K epoxide is then converted to vitamin K by VKOR [95–97]. Since vitamin K is continuously recycled within cells, vitamin K deficiency is uncommon in humans. The health benefits of vitamin K extend beyond coagulation to include hepatic functions [95]. More recently, vitamin K's role in preventing and treating cancer [96] has been explored, as well as its implication in age-related diseases such as osteoporosis and osteoarthrosis, cardiovascular diseases, and neurodegenerative diseases [97–99].

B Vitamins

B vitamins constitute a cluster of seven essential water-soluble vitamins; B_1 (thiamine), B_2 (riboflavin), B_3 (niacin), B_5 (pantothenic acid), B_6 (pyridoxine), B_9 (folate) and B_{12} (cobalamin). B vitamins are primarily produced within the mitochondria, chloroplasts, and the cytosol of plants, and play essential roles in energy production, and the composition and alteration of bioactive compounds through catabolic and anabolic processes, respectively [100]. In a significant portion of enzymatic processes, B vitamins carry out physiological functions by acting as coenzymes. As coenzymes, the biologically active forms of B vitamins tightly bind to the apoenzyme of a protein, producing a holoenzyme that is complete and catalytically active [101]. Through this binding activity, B vitamins play various ubiquitous roles in cellular functioning. The ubiquitous role of B vitamins is demonstrated by vitamin B_6. Vitamin B_6 functions primarily through its bioactive form, pyridoxal 5′-phosphate. Pyridoxal 5′-phosphate is an important cofactor that influences the functionality of several enzymes that are necessary for the production, degeneration, and conversion of amino acids in all organisms [101]. The essential requirement of B vitamins is also observed with coenzyme A (CoA), the bioactive coenzyme of vitamin B_5. CoA is a compulsory co-factor for approximately 4% of mammalian enzymes functioning as a carbonyl-activating group and acyl carrier in numerous biochemical transformation reactions [102]. B vitamins may also act as precursors of metabolic substances, although this is less frequent. CoA also provides a good example of this. CoA can be further acetylated by acetyltransferase enzymes to produce acetyl-CoA, which participates in the biochemical metabolism of proteins, carbohydrates, and lipids, as well as energy production [103]. Notably, B vitamins possess various brain-specific functions. Vitamin B_1 plays a critical role in the synthesis of amino acid precursors for neurotransmitters such as acetylcholine (Ach) and was reported to have neuromodulatory functions, including alterations to cholinergic transmission [104]. Vitamin B_1 plays structural and functional roles within cell membranes, including in neurons and neuroglia [105] and vitamin B_1 deficiency resulted in AD-like abnormalities, such as dysregulation of the cholinergic system, reduced neurotransmitter levels and memory deficits, in preclinical mouse models [106–108].

Vitamin C

Vitamin C (ascorbic acid) is predominately found within cells in its redox state, ascorbate [109]. Since humans are unable to endogenously produce vitamin C, the nutrient is obtained from fruit and vegetable sources such as citrus fruits (orange, berries, tomatoes) and leafy green vegetables (broccoli, brussels sprouts). Vitamin C primarily functions as a cofactor for many enzymes, such as hydroxylases, that are implicated in collagen synthesis [110]. More importantly, vitamin C acts as a potent antioxidant through attenuating lipid peroxidation. Lipid peroxidation is a form of radical chain reaction that is initiated by ROS-mediated dissociation of hydrogen atoms from C-H bonds producing lipid radicals [111]. ROS are often entrenched within lipid bilayers [111]. This renders lipids susceptible to the harmful effects of free radicals. Vitamin C can prevent lipid peroxidation by scavenging ROS and working synergistically with other antioxidant compounds, such as vitamin E, to reduce radical formation through the vitamin E redox cycle [112]. Vitamin C is also an exceptional source of electrons. Vitamin C can donate electrons to free radicals that seek out electrons from cellular components such as lipids, proteins, and DNA [111]. By donating an electron to free radicals, vitamin C stabilizes these volatile compounds, reducing their reactivity and the subsequent cellular damage. Vitamin C is constantly recycled within the cell, which increases its antioxidant activity [113]. As a donor of high-energy electrons, vitamin C is oxidized to dehydroascorbic acid. Dehydroascorbic acid can be converted back to vitamin C by dehydroascorbate reductase to be reused or further metabolized, which releases more electrons for ROS stabilization [110,111]. However, the ability of vitamin C to act as a reducing agent for metals such as Cu and Fe heightens the pro-oxidant composition and activity of these metals [114]. Therefore, vitamin C can behave as an antioxidant and a pro-oxidant, and this may depend on its concentration. The pro-oxidant role of vitamin C was initially reported to occur at low concentrations and the antioxidant activities at high concentrations [114]. However, more recent reports contradict these findings and suggest a switch-like behaviour of vitamin C, where it possesses bimodal activity as an antioxidant under normal conditions and switches over to a pro-oxidant at high concentrations and/or under pathophysiological conditions [115,116]. This raises questions regarding the therapeutic use of vitamin C when there is uncertainty of its antioxidant status within the literature [113,114]. Nonetheless, the potential health benefits of vitamin C continue to be explored for their therapeutic effectiveness in several diseases such as cancer, cardiovascular disease, diabetes, immunity, and neurodegenerative disorders [116–119].

Vitamin C assists in maintaining the function and integrity of various processes within the CNS including antioxidant protection, neuronal development and differentiation, myelination, catecholamine synthesis and regulation of neurotransmission [120]. Studies using animal models have reported detrimental impacts on the brain when vitamin C is decreased, such as enhanced oxidative stress, increased mortality, and the acceleration of amyloid plaque development and aggregation [121–123]. Vitamin C deficiency also reduced blood glucose levels and caused oxidative damage to proteins and lipids in the cortex of mice [122,124]. Dopamine and serotonin metabolites in the cortex and striatum of mice and physical strength and locomotor activity were decreased, and treatment with vitamin C was able to restore these deficits [125]. Since the highest concentrations of vitamin C are found in the brain [126] and several neurodegenerative diseases are characterized by oxidative stress, the protective role that vitamin C may play in altering the development and progression of neurological disease such as AD is being investigated.

Carotenoids

Carotenoids are a group of natural pigments that exist ubiquitously across all organisms [127]. Carotenoids perform active roles in photosynthesis in plants and function primarily through photoprotection in non-photosynthetic organisms [127]. In humans, carotenoids, which are found in blood and tissues, are essential precursors of vitamin A. Carotenoids maintain their status as antioxidants through their efficiency in chemically and physically quenching singlet oxygen and scavenging other ROS [127,128]. The structure of carotenoids is the most significant characteristic, contributing to their protective effects. Carotenoids are comprised of several conjugated double bonds, which are essential for photoprotection in all living organisms and light absorption in photosynthetic organisms [128]. Additionally, carotenoids are lipophilic compounds; therefore, they primarily reside within cell membranes.

The most commonly described carotenoids include β-carotene, α-carotene, lutein, lycopene, and zeaxanthin. β-carotene and lycopene are examples of rigid hydrocarbons that are entirely organized within the inner portion of the lipid bilayer [129]. Lutein and zeaxanthin are polar compounds that contain oxygen atoms and exist horizontally to the membrane surface, exposing their hydrophilic segments to the aqueous surroundings [129,130]. It is suggested that the inclusion of carotenoids may impact membrane properties such as permeability, thickness, fluidity, and rigidity, all of which are essential for maintaining membrane integrity [131]. Membrane modifications by carotenoids may enhance resistance to ROS, thereby reducing susceptibility to ROS. Several reports have described the participation of carotenoids in various biological systems and general physiology. These include modulating gap junction communication via intracellular signaling pathways [131] and regulating cell cycle, differentiation, and growth factors [132]. Carotenoids and their metabolites have been implicated as having functions in human health and providing protection in various ROS-induced disorders. These roles include but are not limited to cognitive functions [133–135], cancer prevention [131,136], immune stimulation/modulation [137], fertility [138,139] and genomic impacts on transcription and translation [140].

Polyphenols

Polyphenols are naturally occurring compounds found in food sources such as beverages, cereals, fruits, and vegetables and are classified based on chemical structure and resulting activity. The primary classes of polyphenols are phenolic acids, flavonoids, lignans and stilbenes [141]. Phenolic acids are further divided into two classes: hydroxybenzoic acids and hydroxycinnamic acids. Hydroxybenzoic acids are less common than hydroxycinnamic acids and consist of compounds such as gallic and vanillic acid [142]. Hydroxycinnamic acids include caffeic, ferulic, ρ-coumaric and sinapic acids [142]. Flavonoids are the most highly studied cluster of polyphenols. Compounds within this group share a primary structure consisting of two aromatic rings, held by three carbon atoms creating an oxygenated heterocycle [143]. Flavonoids are separated into six subdivisions: anthocyanins, flavan-3-ols, flavonols, flavones, flavanones and isoflavones (Figure 2). Variations within these clusters are derived from differences in the composition and number of hydroxyl groups and their degree of glycosylation and/or alkylation [143]. The most widely studied flavonoids Are catechins, commonly found in green tea, quercetin, found in red wine and foods, and myricetin, which is also commonly found in medicinal plants [144–146]. Lignans are referred to as diphenolic compounds, formed by two cinnamic acid residues dimerizing to create a 2,3-dibenxylbutane structure. Many lignans, such as secoisolariciresinol, are regarded as phytoestrogens, possessing antioxidation and antitumor bioactivities [144]. Stilbenes are primarily found in grape skins and berries, and the most prevalent of this subdivision are resveratrol and its derivative pterostilbene [145]. Stilbenes, although low in the human diet, have been implicated for their potential for treating human disease due to their antioxidant and anti-inflammatory activities [145,146]. Other polyphenols include curcumin and gingerol, which have both been reported to provide health benefits and restoration to normal physiology in diseased states [146–148]. Overall, there is evidence to support the protective role of polyphenols in multiple disease conditions, such as cancer [149–151], cardiovascular disease [152], type 2 diabetes and obesity [149,153], inflammation [154] and neurodegenerative diseases [155–157]. Notable polyphenolic compounds studied for their neuroprotective effects include resveratrol, curcumin, quercetin, and epigallocatechin-3-gallate (EGCG) [158]. Recent studies examining cognitive deficits in transgenic AD mice report improvements in AD-like cognitive deficits through anti-amyloidogenic, anti-inflammatory and anti-apoptotic effects of polyphenolic compounds [159–162].

Minerals

Recently, minerals have been studied for their participation in the antioxidant defence system [163–171]. Cu is one of many trace elements that are essential to the biochemistry of active organisms due to its activity as a cofactor and a constituent of metalloenzymes [163]. Cu participates in electron transfer catalysis due to its ability to maintain two oxidation states [164]. Modest amounts of Cu are necessary and beneficial in maintaining metal homeostatic levels; however, the accumulation of redox transition metals such as excess Cu within tissues is cytotoxic [164]. Disturbances in metal homeostasis stimulate the development of oxidative stress and free radical formation, targeting membranes and essential molecules. At high levels, Cu has been implicated in the pathology of neurodegenerative conditions [163]. A study examining the effects of excess Cu showed significantly lower SOD and GSH activity in the brain tissue of Cu-intoxicated rats [163]. Similarly, Fe can result in comparable toxicity due to its ability to donate and accept electrons. Redox-active Fe is a significant contributor to oxidative damage in cellular compartments through the generation of free radicals from ROS by reducing H_2O_2 to produce •OH radicals [165]. This eventually results in damage to several cellular structures, as the •OH radical formed by Fe and even Cu can react with H_2O_2 to stimulate lipid peroxidation [166]. For this reason, Fe is predominantly bound to other molecules for transport and storage, leaving minuscule amounts of redox-active Fe in the labile pool. Even then, Fe does not remain unbound, as it forms complexes with carboxylates, phosphates, and peptides within the labile pool [166].

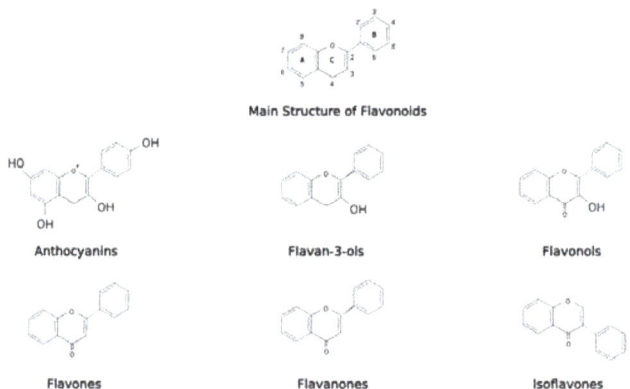

Figure 2. Chemical structure of flavonoid polyphenols. Created with BioRender.com. The flavonoid subclass of polyphenols is further classified into six main groups: anthocyanins, flavan-3-ols, flavonols, flavone, flavanones and isoflavones. Differences in chemical structure arise based on variations in the placement and number of hydroxyl groups and unsaturated bonds.

Mn is an essential element in the synthesis and activation of several enzymes. Its main antioxidant activity occurs through its role as a metalloenzyme via SOD2 to reduce mitochondrial oxidative stress [167]. SOD2 is the principal antioxidant that probes for $O_2^{•−}$, produced within the mitochondria to protect against oxidative stress [167]. SOD2 has also been suggested to provide protection for several disease states such as atherosclerosis, metabolic syndrome, and obesity [167]. Se is another natural trace element. Se is necessary for the composition of selenoproteins, which have been reported to play a critical role in the antioxidant defence system. The activity of GPx, one of the most efficient enzymatic antioxidants, is relatively dependent on Se [168]. Se is inorganically present as selenates, selenides, and selenite, which are more toxic than the organic states selenomethionine and selenocysteine [168]. Se present with GPx has been implicated in the repair of damaged DNA, and the ability to increase GPx activity contributes to the potential benefits of increased Se intake [169].

Zn has been considered an essential metal since its deficiency in humans was first recognized over 50 years ago [170,171]. Zn acts as an antioxidant through multiple mechanisms. Zn can compete with Cu and Fe for binding to proteins and cell membranes, which displaces redox-active Cu and Fe, resulting in the generation of •OH from H_2O_2. Zn can also protect biomolecules such as sulfhydryl groups by binding to them, preventing oxidation [172]. Zn is also capable of enhancing the activation of antioxidant enzymes CAT, SOD and GSH, and diminishing the activity of pro-oxidant enzymes such as inducible

•NO synthase and NADPH oxide, while blocking the production of lipid peroxidation products [172]. Interestingly, Zn has been reported to upregulate nuclear erythroid 2-related factor 2 (Nrf2) activity, resulting in reduced oxidative stress [173,174]. Nrf2 is a member of the "cap'n'collar" subfamily of basic region leucine zipper transcription factors [175]. Nrf2 regulates the gene expression of many antioxidant and detoxifying enzymes such as SOD and GSH, and glutathione-S-transferase-1 and heme oxygenase-1, respectively. The binding activity of Nrf2 to the antioxidant response element found in the promoter of these target genes leads to the production of enzymes that function as part of the antioxidant defence system [176].

Estrogens

Neuroprotective antioxidants also include compounds such as hormones that are capable of exerting antioxidant effects within the body. Estrogens have been of particular interest as they are well-documented for their neuroprotective roles as steroid hormone antioxidants [177]. The neuroprotective effects of estrogen are proposed to occur through several mechanisms, including estrogen receptor (ER)-dependent and ER-independent actions, and several studies have explored the effects of estrogens in the aging brain and cognition. Estrogens are reportedly involved in learning and memory [178,179] and protect against neurodegenerative conditions such as AD [180,181]. Studies have explored the potential of estrogen replacement therapy (ERT) on improvements in cognitive function. These reports support the postulation of estrogen-mediated enhancements of cognitive function in women across age ranges and defer the onset of AD [182–184]. While estrogens have been reported to provide benefits against disease onset and progression, several findings contradict the role of estrogens in neurodegenerative diseases such as AD, reporting minimal differences in cognitive function between placebo and estrogen-treated groups [185–187]. These discrepancies leave room for further clarification and investigations into the therapeutic impacts of estrogens by means of ERT. Therefore, although it appears that estrogens may provide protective effects against the onset of AD, further clarification is required to determine whether estrogens are effective once neurodegenerative conditions have already developed.

In summary, antioxidants function through three main mechanisms of action: they (1) act as scavengers to terminate or prevent the production of free radicals; (2) inhibit chain initiation and proliferation reactions; and (3) repair damaged DNA, proteins, and lipid biomolecules. A schematic representation of the classification of natural antioxidants is depicted in Figure 3.

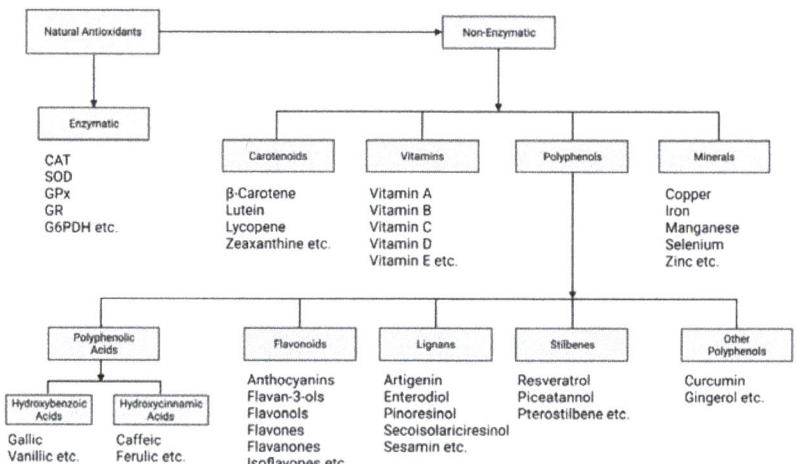

Figure 3. Schematic diagram of classification of natural antioxidants. Created with BioRender.com. CAT, catalase; SOD, superoxide dismutase; GPx, glutathione peroxidase; GR, glutathione reductase; G6PDH, glucose-6-phosphate dehydrogenase.

3. Oxidative Stress in Alzheimer's Disease

The role of oxidative stress in the pathogenesis of AD is well-established in the literature [188–202]. To this effect, the oxidative stress hypothesis of AD development postulates potential mechanisms by which oxidative damage causes and/or contributes to the development and progression of AD [203]. This hypothesis is supported by findings from molecular, genetic, and biochemical studies and highlights the detrimental role of ROS in AD onset and progression. Heightened levels of biomarkers of oxidative stress, impairments in the antioxidant defence system, gene mutations and mitochondrial dysfunction have all been implicated [194,196]. As previously mentioned, highly reactive molecules such as ROS target biomolecules such as DNA, proteins, and lipids and, in the instance of AD, mitochondrial dysfunction is proposed to underlie the increase in ROS [191–203]. Neuronal mitochondria consume high amounts of intracellular oxygen to perform essential functions including energy metabolism, the metabolism of amino acids, fatty acids and lipids, intracellular calcium homeostasis, ROS generation and regulation and more [204]. During mitochondrial respiration, $O_2^{\bullet-}$, a by-product of adenosine triphosphate production, is created. In large amounts, $O_2^{\bullet-}$ contributes to oxidative stress by oxidizing cellular targets directly or indirectly by reacting with other molecules and oxidants to form additional ROS and reactive nitrogen species [204]. Mitochondria also produce H_2O_2, which can further exacerbate oxidative stress by the endogenous conversion reaction of H_2O_2 to $^{\bullet}OH$ by Fe^{2+} via the Fenton reaction [190,204]. Although the primary generation sites of $O_2^{\bullet-}$ are mitochondrial respiratory transport chains I and III, additional cellular sources that could contribute to neuronal oxidative stress include xanthine oxidase, NADPH oxidase and cytochrome P450 enzymes. To prevent a cascade of ROS production, $O_2^{\bullet-}$ is neutralized by SOD (Figure 1). Oxidative stress does not exist alone as a potential cause or contributing factor to AD [205–209]. Oxidative stress is reported to contribute to other hypotheses of AD, which implicate the aggregation of intracellular tau, elastin degradation, N-methyl-D-aspartate receptor (NMDAR)-mediated cell stress and abnormal extracellular amyloid accumulation as the primary cause [210–221].

The tau hypothesis of AD is widely described in the literature and explains the role of tau-induced neurotoxicity via abnormal hyperphosphorylation of the microtubule-associated protein, tau [222–231]. Under normal physiological conditions, tau proteins stabilize microtubules within healthy neurons, which maintains neuron morphology and facilitates the transport of enzymes and organelles along the cytoskeleton [224–226]. This action is regulated by the level of tau phosphorylation, which primarily depends on the balance between phosphorylation and dephosphorylation, resulting in the activity of various tau kinases and phosphatases, respectively [223–225]. Tau hyperphosphorylation reduces the tau microtubule-binding affinity, resulting in the destabilization of microtubules and oligomerization of hyperphosphorylated tau monomers [226–228]. In turn, tau oligomers aggregate to form neurofibrillary tangles that induce neurotoxicity and eventual cell death [229–231]. The link between oxidative stress and tauopathies is also well-described and attributes tauopathy to oxidative stress-induced aggregate formation that results in the degradation of the microtubule network [232–236].

A recent review by Atlante et al. [237] explains the active and reciprocal relationship between oxidative stress and tau pathology in AD. The researchers report both oxidative stress-induced tau phosphorylation and tau-induced oxidative stress as contributors to the development of AD due to factors, including reductions in cytoplasmic SOD1 and mitochondrial SOD2, which increases the profile of tau phosphorylation and the induction of mitochondrial dysfunction, resulting in H_2O_2 production by hippocampal tau phosphorylation, respectively [237–240]. In vitro, the inhibition of glutathione, which triggered mild oxidative stress, increased the levels of phosphorylated tau [234] and the oxidation of fatty acids stimulated tau polymerization [241]. Several reports demonstrate that oxidative stress-induced increases in metal ion redox potential also stimulate the upregulation of tau kinases [242–250]. Amyloid-beta (Aβ) is also implicated as a contributor to the cascade of molecular events that result in tau hyperphosphorylation and the inhibition of tau binding to microtubules by promoting glycogen synthase kinase 3 (GSK3) activation [251–257].

Recently, researchers have identified elastin degradation as a potential contributor to aging, oxidative stress and AD pathology [258–267]. Elastin is an essential protein that maintains the structural matrix of organs and tissues, including the skin, lungs, cartilage, and blood vessels [258–260]. Although elastin is structurally stable, it readily undergoes proteolytic degradation, producing elastin-derived peptides (EDPs) [261–263]. Utilizing in vivo and in vitro models, researchers have found that EDPs enhance Aβ formation, which could contribute to subsequent AD development [257,264]. Additionally, EDPs released from elastin due to proteolytic degradation gradually develop into amyloid-like structures [265,266]. Interestingly, like tau, described above, a recent review by Szychowski and Skóra examined the reciprocal relationship between the production of ROS and EDPs [268]. An essential factor in the mechanism of action of EDPs is the peroxisome proliferator-activated receptor gamma (PPARγ) pathway, which is reported to increase the production of ROS by increasing calcium (Ca^{2+}) influx and disrupting the activity and expression of antioxidant enzymes [268–270]. PPARγ is reported to enhance SOD, CAT and GPx activity and increase lipid peroxidation [271,272]. Resveratrol, a PPAR agonist, is an example of an antioxidant compound that exerts these neuroprotective properties and was examined for its therapeutic potential in AD [273,274]. Interestingly, in other forms of neurodegeneration, such as ischemia, EDPs are formed in the brain post-injury, which is also when Aβ formation is induced [275]. Some reports have demonstrated EDP-induced increases in ROS in the brain in neuronal stem cells as well as astrocytes [270,272,276]. In turn, EDPs are reported to induce Aβ formation by inducing the overexpression of γ-secretase, which results in excess cleavage activities and the overproduction of Aβ [265]. A few studies suggest that proteoglycans, which are present in the extracellular matrix, may contribute to AD pathogenesis by promoting the fibrilization of Aβ and tau and protecting Aβ from proteolytic degradation [277,278]. The presence and accumulation of EDPs in the brain are also associated with age and correspond with the incidence of AD [275,279]. Increased levels of EDPs have also been detected in CSF patients following a stroke [275,280]. Taken together, these findings suggest the presence of EDPs as potential biomarkers of neurodegenerative disease and that therapies directed at elastin degradation may be useful in the treatment of AD.

The NMDAR hypothesis suggests that excess NMDAR activation leads to the neurodegeneration that occurs in AD [281,282]. Under normal conditions, excitatory neurotransmission by glutamate through the NMDAR is essential for synaptic plasticity and the survival of neurons [281,282]. However, the superfluous activity of the NMDAR induces excitotoxicity causing neuron death, which is a foundational mechanism of the neurodegeneration observed in AD [281,282]. Since the NMDAR mediates Ca^{2+} regulation and influx [283–286], dysregulation and overactivity are reported to induce oxidative stress by enhancing the production of ROS within the brain through mechanisms involving EDPs [287,288]. Ca^{2+} channel blockers such as nifedipine and verapamil are also reported to attenuate ROS production induced by EDP fragments, influence EDP levels in the brain and possibly delay the progression of AD [276,289,290].

Several reports support the involvement of oxidative stress in Aβ toxicity involving metal ions [291–305]. Extracellular senile plaques/fibrils comprised of aggregated Aβ peptides exist with metal ions such as Fe, Cu and Zn [293–295]. These redox-active metal ions can catalyze the production of ROS when bound to Aβ [296–305]. Subsequently, newly generated ROS can oxidize both Aβ peptides as well as surrounding biomolecules such as lipids, nucleic acids, and proteins [306–315]. The oxidation of lipids such as cholesterol within neuronal membranes obstructs membrane integrity [313,314]. In addition, the oxidation of Aβ by ROS and redox-active metal ions impairs its clearance by low-density lipoprotein receptor-related proteins, which could contribute to the accumulation of Aβ in AD [315,316].

Oxidative stress, caused by the production of ROS, creates a favourable environment for Aβ synthesis and accumulation through transcriptional, translational, and epigenetic mechanisms [317–328]. Researchers have found that the activation of stress-related signalling pathways stimulates the transcription of amyloid precursor protein (APP) and beta-secretase 1 (BACE1), an essential enzyme for Aβ production [318–320]. Additionally, an enhanced protein expression of BACE1 due to ROS such as H_2O_2 has been reported and is proposed to be regulated by eukaryotic translational initiation factor-2alpha (eIF2α), which was implicated in AD when activated via phosphorylation [321,322]. Several studies have established the role of epigenetic modifications, such as DNA methylation, histone acetylation and chromatin remodelling, in changes to Aβ and AD progression [323–327]. More recently, researchers have demonstrated a link between oxidative stress and epigenetic changes in Aβ production. Gu et al. showed that when neuroblastoma cells were treated with H_2O_2, a significant decrease in DNA methylation and an increase in histone acetylation occurred [328]. This resulted in increased APP and BACE1 transcription, which was followed by enhanced Aβ production and plaque accumulation [328].

In turn, Aβ exerts its toxic effects through several mechanisms, including oxidative stress. Aβ has been reported to alter mitochondrial function by localizing within the mitochondrial membrane, where it blocks the transport of nuclear-encoded mitochondrial proteins [236–329]. Additionally, Aβ prevents normal neuronal functions by interacting with mitochondrial proteins, dysregulating the electron transport chain, and stimulating the production of ROS [237–339]. Additional actions include Aβ-mediated dysregulation of Ca^{2+} homeostasis, ion leakage through pore formation and depletion of membrane potential [340–342]. As a result, this disrupts the cytoskeleton, causes synaptic dysfunction, and stimulates neuronal apoptosis [343]. The examination of human brains from patients diagnosed with AD showed a high degree of membrane damage due to oxidation within the cerebral cortex [344]. Evidence supports the validation of the oxidation of proteins as biomarkers of AD, as enhanced levels of carboxylate proteins have been reported in the hippocampus and parietal cortex [345–347].

Considering that ROS production can be a product of tissue injury [348–350], it is currently unclear whether oxidative stress is a primary or secondary cause of AD. Even as a secondary cause, oxidative stress perpetuates a detrimental cascade of toxic events that ultimately result in neuron loss. Despite profound evidence supporting the role of oxidative stress in the pathogenesis and progression of AD, none of the currently available treatment options are designed to address oxidative stress. The development of innovative therapies that target the pathological contributors of the disease, such as ROS, could substantially improve the care of patients with AD.

4. Current Treatments for Alzheimer's Disease

Currently, the only United States Food and Drug Administration (FDA)- and Health Canada-approved medications for AD fall under the classifications of acetylcholinesterase (AChE) inhibitors and NMDAR antagonists [351–353]. Donepezil, galantamine and rivastigmine fall under the category of cholinesterase inhibitors. AChE is found predominantly in neuromuscular junctions and synapses of cholinergic neurons in the periphery and CNS, where it rapidly degrades ACh. This neurotransmitter is reported to be involved in learning and memory [354], and the loss of cholinergic neurons projecting from the basal forebrain to the hippocampus and cortex increases as AD progresses [355]. Donepezil and galantamine act by reversibly binding to AChE, which inhibits the hydrolysis (breakdown) of ACh, increasing its levels at synapses throughout the CNS [356]. Rivastigmine also acts to enhance cholinergic communication by binding to and inhibiting AChE, as well as butyrylcholinesterase [357]. These drugs are indicated as long-term symptomatic treatments of AD; however, these drugs lose their efficacy as fewer cholinergic neurons remain in the brain as AD progresses [355]. Donepezil is approved for all stages of AD, while rivastigmine and galantamine are recommended for patients exhibiting mild to moderate symptoms [358]. Memantine, an NMDAR antagonist, acts by blocking the flow of ions through the NMDAR ion channel [359]. Memantine is indicated for moderate to severe AD [360]. Manufactured conjugate (combination) drugs, comprised of donepezil and memantine as extended-release capsules, also exist to alleviate the pill burden of taking multiple medications and increase patient compliance, while mitigating challenges with swallowing that are often associated with AD [361].

Non-pharmacological treatment options include identifying any potential harmful supplements and medications and removing them from the patient's regimen [362]. First-line treatments for the neuropsychiatric symptoms and behavioural issues associated with the disease include repetitive evaluations, identifying triggers, providing psychoeducation, and modifying both behavioural and environmental interventions [362,363].

The currently available treatments for AD are ineffective in preventing, delaying progression, or curing disease [351]. This necessitates the development of novel disease-modifying therapies that target the pathological hallmarks of the disease, such as tau protein hyperphosphorylation, the development and accumulation of Aβ, inflammation, and oxidative stress [351]. Recently, aducanumab, the only potential disease-modifying therapy, was approved by the FDA through the FDA's accelerated approval program. Aducanumab is a human monoclonal antibody that significantly reduced the formation and increased the clearance of existing Aβ plaques in mouse models of AD [364–366]. However, there is controversy regarding whether the drug slows disease progression in humans, as findings from currently available clinical trial data indicate strategies that reduce amyloid levels do not significantly improve cognition [367]. Biogen, the drug company that created aducanumab, is conducting additional studies to assess the clinical benefit of aducanumab post-approval. If the additional studies fail to show evidence of a clinical benefit, the FDA can withdraw drug approval. Phase 4 clinical trial results for aducanumab are expected to be accessible as early as 2030.

Despite tremendous efforts to find a cure or an effective treatment, AD remains progressive and incurable. Studies utilizing animal models to depict AD show improvements in AD-like phenotypes when utilizing novel therapies such as antioxidants [368–370]. Some epidemiological studies also show a reduced risk of AD due to the dietary intake of antioxidants [371–373]. Recently, researchers have begun exploring the use of antioxidants in combination with other antioxidant compounds, as well as drugs that are currently being used to treat neurogenerative diseases. This is referred to as combination or conjugate therapy.

5. Conjugate Therapies and the Blood Brain Barrier

The concept of conjugate drug therapy was initially developed as a novel avenue for cancer treatment and has now produced treatment strategies such as antibody–drug conjugates (ADCs). ADCs are designed to target and destroy cancer cells while preserving healthy cells by chemically linking two or more distinct substances [374]. ADCs utilize monoclonal antibodies to deliver cytotoxic agents to antigen-expressing target cells. This approach to treatment has been applied to various types of cancer, such as breast cancer, non-small-cell lung cancer and ovarian cancer, to name a few [375–377]. The impact of oxidative stress as a contributing factor to the development of various cancers is well-studied [378–384], which makes it a primary target in the development of anti-cancer drugs. Interestingly, researchers also utilize the harmful effects of ROS as a tool to target cancer cells [385–390]. This includes activating ROS-specific cell death mechanisms such as apoptosis, autophagy, ferroptosis (Fe-dependent) and necrotic cell death in tumour targeted therapy [385–390]. An example of the application of ROS in cancer therapy is through targeted tyrosine therapies, which include monoclonal antibodies and small-molecule inhibitors that have been shown to elicit anticancer ROS-mediated effects [391–396]. More recently, ADCs have been applied to neurological cancers and neurodegenerative diseases. One example is glioblastoma, an aggressive form of brain cancer that can develop within the brain and spinal cord [397]. However, the efficacy and applications of ADCs within the CNS have been reported to be limited due to the inability of these large drug conjugates to cross the blood–brain barrier (BBB) [398].

When developing novel therapies for neurodegenerative disorders, several factors must be considered for effective drug delivery. One of the most significant is BBB permeability. Unfortunately, the effectiveness of various antioxidants, alone or in conjugated form, are limited by their inability to cross the BBB [399]. The BBB functions as the brain's endogenous defence system, by excluding non-lipophilic and high-molecular-weight compounds. For a drug or compound to elicit its desired effects, it must first permeate the BBB to reach its drug targets. BBB permeation can occur through several mechanisms, including transmembrane diffusion, saturable transporters, absorption via endocytosis and other extracellular pathways [399]. Several drugs cross the BBB through transmembrane diffusion. This mechanism largely depends on the drug or compound's ability to cross the cell membrane, which depends on the exogenous compound's molecular weight, charge, and degree of lipid solubility [400]. Once a drug or compound has diffused through the lipid membranes of the BBB, it will enter the brain's aqueous environment before reaching its therapeutic target. Therefore, the substance must possess a desirable level of lipid solubility but not be "too lipid soluble", so that it does not get trapped within the BBB [399]. Saturable transport systems are also an advantageous mechanism of drug delivery and transport across the BBB. Transporters increase the rate of uptake across the BBB compared to what a drug would achieve through transmembrane diffusion alone [401]. However, uptake is limited, as transport occurs via saturable transport systems [401]. The BBB also contains transporters that remove compounds from the brain. These transporters assist with removing toxins from the brain but can also reduce the effectiveness of some therapeutics by increasing their efflux [402]. Under normal conditions, BBB uptake and efflux transporters adapt to meet the needs of the CNS; however, during diseased states, dysregulation can occur. This is observed in AD, for example. Deposition of Aβ damages the BBB and, inversely, reduces Aβ efflux, which contributes to the disease cyclically, as disturbances in BBB function further provoke Aβ deposition [403,404]. BBB dysregulation can be further exacerbated by oxidative stress, either directly or by stimulating the damaging effects of the Aβ peptide (discussed above).

Several antioxidants, including non-traditional antioxidants such as ebselen, have been explored for their ability to cross the BBB and exert neuroprotective roles within the brain when administered alone, in combination, or conjugated with other compounds. Ebselen, a Se-containing compound, has also been assessed for its GPx-like effects [405,406]. As previously mentioned, Se is an essential trace element that maintains antioxidant activity within the brain through oxidative stress resistance [407]. Ebselen has been shown to mitigate the impacts of AD pathology in cell line and primary culture models, as well as triple transgenic AD mouse models. A study conducted by Xie et al. demonstrated the ability of ebselen to inhibit oxidative stress in both cellular and mouse models of AD through enhancing GPx and SOD activity while reducing the activity of p38 mitogen-activated protein kinases [408]. Additionally, ebselen was able to reduce oligomeric Aβ levels within the brains of AD mice by diminishing the expression of APP and BACE-1, both of which are involved in the amyloidogenic pathway of Aβ synthesis [408]. Similar mechanisms have also been reported for other antioxidant compounds that have shown promise in studies utilizing animal subjects to model the onset and course of progression of AD, and the impacts of novel drugs and/or compounds as therapeutic options. Antioxidants that have been explored in combination with other compounds in both cellular and animal models of AD including but not limited to ebselen and donepezil [409], lipoic acid and donepezil [410], ferulic acid and tacrine (the first AChE inhibitor approved for AD, but now discontinued) [411], and polyphenolic hybrids [412,413].

Researchers are currently exploring the neuroprotective roles of antioxidants in humans when these drugs are administered alone, in combination with other antioxidants or drugs but not chemically linked, or in conjugated form with other antioxidants or drugs. To be effective, potential antioxidant drug compounds must be lipid-soluble, small molecule, and/or be chauffeured by other mobilizing non-toxic substances from the bloodstream, through the BBB and into the brain. Instead of utilizing only one antioxidant compound, a combination of antioxidant compounds would increase the overall antioxidant capacity of the drug therapy, heighten the bioavailability to various cellular locations and increase the functionality of antioxidant molecules, such as through facilitating redox cycling [414].

6. Clinical Trials

Various studies have explored the role of compounds with antioxidant activity for the prevention and treatment of cognitive decline and dementia caused by AD. Table 2 summarizes the data from human clinical trials investigating antioxidants in AD. This summary includes results published within the last two decades and those available from on-going clinical trials. Data from clinical trials were collected from the NIH U.S National Library of Medicine site: ClinicalTrials.gov. The inclusion criteria for the clinical trials for this review required that the study (1) includes participants diagnosed with a neurodegenerative disease with evidence of oxidative stress such as AD, (2) utilized at least one natural antioxidant as a form of treatment or preventative therapy, (3) utilized more than one natural antioxidant as combination treatment, and/or (4) utilized a natural antioxidant in combination with a drug currently used to treat AD.

Table 2. Summary of clinical trials utilizing combination/conjugate antioxidants as preventative therapy or treatment in AD. ADCS-ADL: Alzheimer's Disease Cooperative Study—Activity of Daily Living; ADAS-Cog: Alzheimer's Disease Assessment Scale (Cog: Cognitive score).

Classification	Compound(s)	Participants	Intervention	Primary Outcome Measures	Main Results	In-Text Reference
Vitamins	Vitamin E + Selegiline	341 patients with moderate AD	2000 IU vitamin E, 10 mg selegiline, both or placebo daily for 2 years	Time until occurrence of death, institutionalization, loss of ability to perform activities of daily living, or severe dementia	Treatment with vitamin E or selegiline slowed the progression of disease in patients with moderately severe impairment from AD	[415]
	Vitamin E + Donepezil	790 patients with mild cognitive impairment (MCI)	2000 IU vitamin E, 10 mg donepezil or placebo, daily for 3 years	Clinically possible or probable AD	Vitamin E had no benefit. Donepezil was associated with a lower rate of progression in first 12 months	[416]
	Vitamin E + Memantine	613 patients with mild to moderate AD	2000 IU vita-min E, 20 mg memantine, both or placebo daily for 5 years	ADCS-ADL	2000 IU/day of vitamin E compared to placebo slowed functional decline. No difference between groups receiving memantine alone or memantine + vitamin E	[417]
	Vitamin E + Vitamin C + Alpha-Lipoic Acid	75 patients with mild to moderate AD	800 IU vitamin E + 500 mg vitamin C + 900 mg alpha-lipoic acid, 400 mg coenzyme Q10 3 times/day or placebo daily for 16 weeks	Changes in cerebral spinal fluid (CSF) biomarkers related to AD and oxidative stress, cognition and function	Antioxidants did not influence CSF biomarkers related to amyloid or tau pathology	[418]
	B Vitamins	340 patients with mild to moderate AD	5 mg folate + 25 mg vitamin B_6 + 1 mg vitamin B_{12} or placebo daily for 18 months	Changes in the cognitive subscale of the ADAS-Cog	Regimen of high-dose B vitamin supplements does not slow cognitive decline in individuals with mild to moderate AD	[419]
	Vitamin D + Memantine	90 patients with moderate AD	100,000 IU vitamin D_3 (every 4 weeks) + 20 mg memantine or placebo daily for 24 weeks	Change of cognitive performance	Ongoing	[420]

Table 2. Cont.

Classification	Compound(s)	Participants	Intervention	Primary Outcome Measures	Main Results	In-Text Reference
	Multivitamin	135 patients with AD or MCI	Nutraceutical formulation (NF) of: 400 ug folic acid, 6 ug vitamin B_{12}, 30 IU vitamin E, 400 mg S-adenosylmethionine, 600 mg N-acetyl cysteine, 500 mg acetyl-L-carnitine daily for 1 year	Cognitive improvement or maintenance of cognitive performance	NF maintained or improved cognitive performance and mood/behaviour	[421]
Polyphenols	Resveratrol	39 patients with mild to moderate AD	5 mg resveratrol + 5 mg dextrose + 5 mg malate or placebo twice daily for 1 year	Evaluate the safety, tolerability and efficacy of resveratrol, glucose and malate in slowing the progression of AD	Low-dose resveratrol is safe and well-tolerated	[422]
	Resveratrol	119 patients with mild to moderate AD	Up to 1 mg resveratrol twice daily or placebo for 52 weeks	Safety and tolerability of treatment with resveratrol and change in ADL	Resveratrol decreases CSF biomarkers, modulates neuro-inflammation and induces adaptive immunity	[423]
	Curcumin	36 patients with mild to moderate AD	2 g or 4 g curcumin or placebo daily for 24 weeks	Examine safety and tolerability of curcumin and determine its side effects on patients	Curcumin well-tolerated. Unable to demonstrate clinical or biochemical evidence of efficacy of curcumin C3 complex. Data suggest limited bioavailability	[424]
	Curcumin	36 patients with dementia, presumed AD	1 g curcumin + 120 mg ginkgo leaf extract, 4 g curcumin + ginkgo leaf extract or placebo daily for 6 months	Change in isoprostane levels in plasma and change in beta-amyloid levels in serum	Serum beta-amyloid rose on curcumin. Fewer adverse events reported	[425]
	Quercetin	48 patients with MCI or early AD	1000 mg quercetin or 100 mg dasatinib or placebo daily for 2 days	Serious adverse events and adverse events, and change in cellular senescence blood markers	Ongoing	[426]
	Quercetin	Recruiting patients with early AD	Quercetin + dasatinib for 2 days on, 14 days off for 12 weeks (6 cycles)	Brain penetrance of dasatinib and quercetin	Ongoing	[427]
	EGCG	21 patients with early AD	200 mg, 400 mg, 600 mg and 800 mg EGCG tri-monthly or placebo for 18 months	ADAS-Cog	Ongoing	[428]
	EGCG	200 patients with AD carrying ApoE4 allele	260–520 mg EGCG + personalized intervention or placebo + non personalized intervention or 260–520 mg EGCG + non personalized intervention or placebo to personalized intervention, daily for 15 months	Evaluate the efficacy of multimodal intervention (dietary, physical and cognition) combined with EGCG in slowing down cognitive decline	Ongoing	[429]

Table 2. Cont.

Classification	Compound(s)	Participants	Intervention	Primary Outcome Measures	Main Results	In-Text Reference
	Genistein	27 patients with mild AD	60 mg genistein or placebo daily for 360 days	Changes in amyloid beta concentration of CSF	Ongoing	[430]
	Genistein + Daidzein	72 patients with AD	100 mg of soy isoflavones or placebo daily for 6 months	Cognitive outcomes: language execution function, verbal memory and recall, attention, visual memory and planning	Six months of 100 mg/day isoflavones did not benefit cognition in older men and women with AD	[431]
	Alpha-Lipoic Acid + Omega-3 Fatty Acids	39 patients with mild AD	600 mg alpha-lipoic acid + 3 g fish oil, 3 g fish oil alone or placebo daily for 12 months	Peripheral F2-isoprostane levels (oxidative stress measure)	Combination of alpha lipoic acid with omega-3 fatty acids slowed cognitive and functional decline	[432]
Minerals	Copper	68 patients with mild to moderate AD	8 mg copper or placebo daily for 1 year	Change in cognitive function, measured by ADAS-Cog	Results not yet published	[433]
	Selenium + Vitamin E	7540 participants with dementia	200 µg Selenium + 400 IU Vitamin E, 200 µg selenium + placebo or 400 IU vitamin E + placebo or placebo + placebo daily for 7–12 years	Incidence of dementia (including AD)	Neither supplement prevented dementia	[434]

6.1. Vitamins

Studies have reported that vitamins may delay the progression of AD in patients with moderate to severe AD [435–437]. Notably, due to the findings from preclinical data supporting the potent effects of vitamin E [438–442], it has been explored as a suitable antioxidant treatment in humans. In addition, vitamin E has been tested in combination with other vitamins and drugs that are currently being used to treat AD for its neuroprotective effects. A randomized, controlled, double-blind study compared the effects of daily administration of 2000 IU vitamin E or 10 mg selegiline, administered alone or in combination, compared to a placebo over 2 years in 341 patients with moderate AD [415]. Selegiline is a selective irreversible monoamine oxidase B (MAO-B) inhibitor that increases the level of dopamine within the synapse by inhibiting dopamine metabolism and is primarily indicated for the treatment of PD [443]. However, earlier trials showed promise for its role in treating AD [444,445], which led researchers to explore the potential benefit of selegiline when combined with other promising compounds such as vitamin E. Based on the primary outcome measures from this study, including the time until death, institutionalization, loss of ability to perform activities of daily living, or severe dementia, this study reported that treatment with both vitamin E and selegiline slowed the progression of disease in patients with moderately severe impairment from AD [444]. The effects of vitamin E have also been examined compared to the AD drug donepezil [416]. However, this study, which included 790 patients with mild cognitive impairment (MCI) and probable AD, showed findings that conflict with other clinical trials involving vitamin E. Patients received 2000 IU vitamin E, 10 mg donepezil or placebo, daily for 3 years. The main findings from this double-blind study showed that vitamin E had no benefit, while donepezil was associated with a lower rate of progression in the first 12 months [416]. In contrast, patients with mild to moderate AD receiving 2000 IU vitamin E, 20 mg memantine or both daily for 5 years showed improvements compared to placebo in another randomized clinical trial [417]. Although a daily dose of 2000 IU vitamin E alone slowed functional decline, there was no difference between the groups receiving memantine alone or with vitamin E [417]. Vitamin E was also tested in combination with other vitamins and minerals [434]. A randomized control trial assessed the changes in cerebrospinal fluid (CSF) biomarkers related to AD and oxidative stress, cognition, and function after antioxidant administration in 75 patients with mild to moderate AD who received 800 IU vitamin E in combination with 500 mg vitamin C, 900 mg ALA and 400 mg coenzyme Q10 3 times/day or placebo daily for 16 weeks. The researchers found that these antioxidants did not influence CSF biomarkers related to amyloid or tau pathology. Although markers of oxidative stress in the brain were reduced, the researchers raised concerns that this antioxidant combination may promote cognitive decline, which would have to be assessed on a long-term basis [418].

B vitamins have also been investigated for their potential protective role in AD in human clinical trials. Although several studies are still ongoing, B vitamins are being explored for their impacts on factors such as changes in phosphorylated tau, brain energy metabolism, oxidative stress, and cognitive function [446,447]. One randomized clinical trial assessed the role of high-dose vitamin B supplementation on homocysteine levels among 340 patients with mild to moderate AD [419]. Elevated homocysteine levels are reported to be a risk factor for dementias such as AD and are attenuated by B vitamin supplementation [448–452]. In this study, patients received a combination of 5 mg folate, 25 mg vitamin B6 and 1 mg vitamin B12 or a placebo, daily for 18 months with the objective of assessing changes in the cognitive subscale of the Alzheimer's Disease Assessment Scale (ADAS-Cog) [419]. The results indicated that although high-dose B vitamin supplementation reduced homocysteine levels, it did not slow cognitive decline in individuals with mild to moderate AD. The researchers note that several factors could have influenced this negative result. One of them is a difference in the reduction of homocysteine levels observed in participants with milder AD symptoms compared to those with moderate AD, which may indicate a need for further studies that separate the cohorts based on stage, as supplementation may be more beneficial in older individuals with higher homocysteine levels [419]. Additionally, factors such as mental health, diet, supplements, and the activity of the patients should be considered when monitoring or assessing cognitive decline in patients with AD as they may contribute to the worsening of symptoms over time.

Vitamin D has also been explored, notably in combination with memantine [420]. Although this study is ongoing, researchers have set the criteria to assess the effects of vitamin D and memantine in 90 patients with moderate AD. Patients will receive 100,000 IU vitamin D_3 (every 4 weeks), in combination with 20 mg memantine or placebo, daily for 24 weeks. The primary objective is to measure changes in cognitive performance measured with the ADAS-Cog and Mini-Mental State Examination (MMSE). Additional measures include changes in functional performance, posture and gait, and comparisons of compliance and tolerance to treatment.

A multivitamin approach was also explored as a treatment for AD [421,453]. In one study including 135 patients with AD or MCI, patients received a multivitamin in the form of a nutraceutical formulation (NF) of 400 ug folic acid, 6 ug vitamin B12, 30 UI vitamin E, 400 mg S-adenosyl methionine, 600 mg N-acetyl cysteine, 500 mg, and acetyl-L-carnitine, daily for 1 year [421]. The primary outcome measures were cognitive improvement or maintenance of cognitive performance, rated by caregivers using the Dementia Rating Scale (DMS), CLOX-1 clock drawing test and the Neuropsychiatric Inventory Questionnaire (NPI-Q). The phase II study reported that patients who received the NF showed improvements compared to the placebo cohort, demonstrating a maintained or improved cognitive performance and mood/behaviour based on the DMS and CLOX-1 measurements. However, no significant improvements were reported in NPI-Q scores. These findings support the conclusions of the phase I study that reported maintenance and/or improvements in cognitive performance and mood/behaviour [453].

6.2. Polyphenols

Polyphenolic compounds are also being explored for their potential as antioxidant treatments for AD. Resveratrol, a potent stilbene antioxidant, has been assessed for its safety, tolerability and efficacy and its role in impacting biomarkers associated with AD. A pilot study involving 39 patients with mild to moderate AD showed that low-dose resveratrol was as safe and well-tolerated as a placebo when administered at 5 mg resveratrol in combination with 5 mg dextrose and 5 mg malate twice daily for 1 year [422]. However, a larger study was necessary to evaluate its beneficial effects. Another study that included 119 patients with mild to moderate AD receiving up to 1 mg resveratrol twice daily or placebo for 52 weeks demonstrated that resveratrol decreased CSF biomarkers, modulated neuro-inflammation, and induced adaptive immunity, which are linked to the progression of AD [423].

Curcumin is another polyphenol that showed promise in preclinical studies. However, these data lack translation in human clinical trials. Although human clinical trials are ongoing, some studies report that curcumin may not be as beneficial for the treatment of AD as some researchers had hoped. One study that included 36 patients with mild to moderate AD who were given 2 g or 4 g curcumin or placebo, daily for 24 weeks showed that although curcumin was well-tolerated, there was no clinical or biochemical evidence of efficacy [424]. In addition, the data suggested the limited bioavailability of curcumin [424]. This is supported by other reports describing fewer adverse events but a concern of elevated serum Aβ in patients receiving either 1 g curcumin or 4 g curcumin in combination with 120 mg ginkgo leaf extract daily for 6 months when compared to a placebo [425]. However, it is possible that this finding was the result of the other compounds consumed in combination with curcumin.

Quercetin and EGCG are also popular antioxidants that are currently under investigation in ongoing trials recruiting patients with early AD and/or patients that are carriers of the ApoE4 allele [426–429,454]. Carriers of the ApoE4 allele present an increased susceptibility and risk of developing AD [449]. One ongoing study is exploring the role of quercetin on changes in cellular senescence blood markers in patients with early AD [426]. Patients will receive a combination of 1000 mg quercetin and 100 mg dasatinib, a tyrosine receptor inhibitor, or placebo for 2 consecutive days followed by a 13-day +/− no drug period for 12 weeks. Another ongoing study is examining the cognitive impacts of EGCG treatment in patients with early AD [428]. Patients will receive daily treatments of tri-monthly increasing doses of 200 mg, 400 mg, 600 mg, and 800 mg EGCG or placebo for 18 months. Cognitive improvements will be assessed using the ADAS-Cog scale.

Genistein, an isoflavone, has also been investigated both alone and in combination with other compounds for its potential neuroprotective effects in AD [430,431]. Ongoing trials are evaluating genistein-induced changes in Aβ concentrations in the CSF of patients with mild AD [430]. Genistein has also been tested for its effects on cognition in combination with other soy isoflavones such as daidzein [431]. A study of 72 patients with mild AD who received 100 mg of soy isoflavones or placebo daily for 6 months was tested for cognitive outcomes [431]. The 100 mg soy isoflavones combination consisted of genistein and daidzein in equal 50 mg capsules. Cognitive outcomes included language execution function, verbal memory and recall, attention, visual memory, and planning. However, the main findings from this study demonstrated that, after 6 months, the combination treatment of isoflavones genistein and daidzein did not benefit cognition in older men and women with AD [431]. This study was one of the first to examine the function of soy isoflavones in older adults with cognitive decline and AD. The researchers propose that these findings are likely influenced by individual differences in isoflavone metabolism.

ALA has been explored in combination with omega fatty acids [432]. In a pilot trial, 39 patients with mild AD received 600 mg ALA and 3 g fish oil, 3 g fish oil only or placebo daily for 12 months. The results showed that the combination of ALA with omega-3 fatty acids slowed cognitive and functional decline compared to placebo. However, since the size of study participants is relatively small, future studies that include larger sample sizes are essential to determine the neuroprotective benefits of this antioxidant combination as a treatment for AD.

6.3. Minerals

Minerals such as Cu and Se have also been explored for their role in AD and potential to act as a form of therapy. An ongoing trial is evaluating the role of Cu on cognitive function in patients with mild to moderate AD [433]. Patients will receive 8 mg of Cu or placebo daily for 1 year. Changes in cognitive function will be measured using the ADAS-Cog scale. Se has also been studied for its potential role in AD when administered in combination with vitamin E [434]. The Prevention of Alzheimer's Disease by Vitamin E and Selenium (PREADVISE) trial recruited 7540 men, of which 3786 participated and received 200 μg Se in combination with 400 IU Vitamin E, 200 μg Se + placebo, or 400 IU vitamin E + placebo or placebo + placebo, daily for 7–12 years [434]. The primary outcome was to assess the incidence of dementia (including AD); however, findings showed that neither supplement prevented the development of dementia or the progression from mild cognitive impairment to AD.

Conflicting clinical trial data perpetuate the ongoing disposition on the benefits of antioxidants in AD treatment. Researchers have postulated that these disparities may be due to a variety of factors. Firstly, the equilibrium status between the production of oxidants and the presence of antioxidants is relatively unknown, and this creates a greater challenge when testing human subjects that may present remarkably different profiles of adequacy in endogenous antioxidant defence [455]. Secondly, factors such as the insufficiency of utilizing only one antioxidant compound in a treatment plan should be considered in addition to correcting for the dosages that would provide the most desirable effects specific to the patient [456,457]. Another factor, and arguably the most significant, is BBB permeability. There may be individual differences in BBB permeability; however, results from animal studies indicate that several antioxidants, alone and in combination, can permeate the BBB to some degree [458–463]. More recently, novel avenues for drug delivery have emerged to tackle this challenge. These include the utilization of nanoparticles as a strategy to deliver drugs into the CNS [464], as well as synthesizing antioxidant compounds that are chemically linked and developed to meet the criteria for BBB permeation [464–466]. Therefore, it is reasonable to conclude that the use of conjugated antioxidants, establishing a reliable profile of biomarkers for each patient and addressing BBB permeation may result in more conclusive findings regarding the effects of antioxidant therapy in AD.

7. Conclusions

AD is currently the leading cause of dementia worldwide, with a prevalence of more than 20 million, which is expected to double by 2040 [286]. Although research has progressed in investigating the etiology and pathogenesis of the disease, much remains unknown about AD. This review describes the well-documented role of oxidative stress in AD; however, the ability of antioxidants to prevent and/or mitigate the impacts of oxidative stress in AD remains uncertain. Compounds such as vitamins, carotenoids, polyphenols, and minerals have shown promise in cellular and animal-based models of AD, prompting their investigation in human clinical trials for their neuroprotective effects, both alone and in combination with other antioxidants or drugs that are currently approved for the treatment of AD. In general, results from previous and ongoing clinical trials remain inconclusive.

Although antioxidants show promise as potential therapies for AD, limitations exist regarding their capacity to treat AD. These limitations include challenges with dosing and determining appropriate timepoints and intervals for intervention, the probability that factors other than oxidative stress may be the predominant cause or propagator of neurodegeneration or that one antioxidant compound may not sufficiently combat oxidative stress to have an impact on disease development or progression. The latter consideration supports the need to explore the use of combination and/or conjugate antioxidant therapy where more than one antioxidant is utilized as a novel approach to treating AD and other neurogenerative conditions that include oxidative stress as a contributing factor. Other considerations for the development of therapies that target ROS-mediated harm in AD, include employing strategies that enhance the activity of molecular targets such as Nrf2 to increase the production of antioxidant enzymes and strengthen the endogenous antioxidant defence system. These approaches will enhance the understanding and application of antioxidant therapies in ROS-mediated neurodegenerative disease.

Author Contributions: Conceptualization, A.E.C.; data curation, A.E.C.; writing—original draft preparation, A.E.C.; writing—review and editing, B.E.K. and T.M.S. All authors have read and agreed to the published version of the manuscript.

Funding: This research received no external funding.

Acknowledgments: The authors would like to thank the Ontario Veterinary College and the Department of Biomedical Sciences at the University of Guelph for supporting this work. A.E.C. is the recipient of an Ontario Veterinary College Graduate Scholarship.

Conflicts of Interest: The authors declare no conflict of interest.

References

1. Halliwell, B. Reactive Oxygen Species and the Central Nervous System. *J. Neurochem.* **1992**, *59*, 1609–1623. [CrossRef] [PubMed]
2. Shukla, V.; Mishra, S.K.; Pant, H.C. Oxidative Stress in Neurodegeneration. *Adv. Pharmacol. Sci.* **2011**, *2011*, 572634. [CrossRef] [PubMed]
3. Perry, G.; Nunomura, A.; Hirai, K.; Zhu, X.; Pérez, M.; Avila, J.; Castellani, R.J.; Atwood, C.S.; Aliev, G.; Sayre, L.M.; et al. Is Oxidative Damage the Fundamental Pathogenic Mechanism of Alzheimer's and Other Neurodegenerative Diseases? *Free Radic. Biol. Med.* **2002**, *33*, 1475–1479. [CrossRef]
4. Huang, W.-J.; Zhang, X.; Chen, W.-W. Role of Oxidative Stress in Alzheimer's Disease. *Biomed. Rep.* **2016**, *4*, 519–522. [CrossRef] [PubMed]
5. Frontiers | Mitochondrial Dysfunction and Oxidative Stress in Alzheimer's Disease | Aging Neuroscience. Available online: https://www.frontiersin.org/articles/10.3389/fnagi.2021.617588/full (accessed on 28 December 2021).
6. Barber, S.C.; Shaw, P.J. Oxidative Stress in ALS: Key Role in Motor Neuron Injury and Therapeutic Target. *Free Radic. Biol. Med.* **2010**, *48*, 629–641. [CrossRef]
7. Oxidative Stress in ALS: A Mechanism of Neurodegeneration and a Therapeutic Target—ScienceDirect. Available online: https://www.sciencedirect.com/science/article/pii/S0925443906000524 (accessed on 28 December 2021).
8. Castellani, R.; Smith, M.A.; Richey, P.L.; Kalaria, R.; Gambetti, P.; Perry, G. Evidence for Oxidative Stress in Pick Disease and Corticobasal Degeneration. *Brain Res.* **1995**, *696*, 268–271. [CrossRef]
9. Prasad, K.N.; Bondy, S.C. Oxidative and Inflammatory Events in Prion Diseases: Can They Be Therapeutic Targets? *Curr. Aging Sci.* **2018**, *11*, 216–225. [CrossRef]
10. Muchová, J.; Žitňanová, I.; Ďuračková, Z. Oxidative Stress and Down Syndrome. Do Antioxidants Play a Role in Therapy? *Physiol. Res.* **2014**, *63*, 535–542. [CrossRef]
11. Pop-Busui, R.; Sima, A.; Stevens, M. Diabetic Neuropathy and Oxidative Stress. *Diabetes Metab. Res. Rev.* **2006**, *22*, 257–273. [CrossRef]
12. Hosseini, A.; Abdollahi, M. Diabetic Neuropathy and Oxidative Stress: Therapeutic Perspectives. *Oxid. Med. Cell. Longev.* **2013**, *2013*, 168039. [CrossRef]
13. Lupoli, F.; Vannocci, T.; Longo, G.; Niccolai, N.; Pastore, A. The Role of Oxidative Stress in Friedreich's Ataxia. *FEBS Lett.* **2018**, *592*, 718–727. [CrossRef]
14. Frontiers | Impaired Redox Signaling in Huntington's Disease: Therapeutic Implications | Molecular Neuroscience. Available online: https://www.frontiersin.org/articles/10.3389/fnmol.2019.00068/full (accessed on 28 December 2021).
15. Velusamy, T.; Panneerselvam, A.S.; Purushottam, M.; Anusuyadevi, M.; Pal, P.K.; Jain, S.; Essa, M.M.; Guillemin, G.J.; Kandasamy, M. Protective Effect of Antioxidants on Neuronal Dysfunction and Plasticity in Huntington's Disease. *Oxidative Med. Cell. Longev.* **2017**, *2017*, e3279061. [CrossRef]
16. Túnez, I.; Sánchez-López, F.; Agüera, E.; Fernández-Bolaños, R.; Sánchez, F.M.; Tasset-Cuevas, I. Important Role of Oxidative Stress Biomarkers in Huntington's Disease. *J. Med. Chem.* **2011**, *54*, 5602–5606. [CrossRef] [PubMed]
17. Dalfó, E.; Portero-Otín, M.; Ayala, V.; Martínez, A.; Pamplona, R.; Ferrer, I. Evidence of Oxidative Stress in the Neocortex in Incidental Lewy Body Disease. *J. Neuropathol. Exp. Neurol.* **2005**, *64*, 816–830. [CrossRef] [PubMed]
18. Ohl, K.; Tenbrock, K.; Kipp, M. Oxidative Stress in Multiple Sclerosis: Central and Peripheral Mode of Action. *Exp. Neurol.* **2016**, *277*, 58–67. [CrossRef] [PubMed]
19. Adamczyk, B.; Adamczyk-Sowa, M. New Insights into the Role of Oxidative Stress Mechanisms in the Pathophysiology and Treatment of Multiple Sclerosis. *Oxid. Med. Cell. Longev.* **2016**, *2016*, 1973834. [CrossRef] [PubMed]
20. Fu, R.; Yanjanin, N.M.; Bianconi, S.; Pavan, W.J.; Porter, F.D. Oxidative Stress in Niemann-Pick Disease, Type C. *Mol. Genet. Metab.* **2010**, *101*, 214–218. [CrossRef]
21. Vázquez, M.C.; Balboa, E.; Alvarez, A.R.; Zanlungo, S. Oxidative Stress: A Pathogenic Mechanism for Niemann-Pick Type C Disease. *Oxidative Med. Cell. Longev.* **2012**, *2012*, e205713. [CrossRef]

22. Pentón-Rol, G.; Cervantes-Llanos, M.; Martínez-Sánchez, G.; Cabrera-Gómez, J.A.; Valenzuela-Silva, C.M.; Ramírez-Nuñez, O.; Casanova-Orta, M.; Robinson-Agramonte, M.A.; Lopategui-Cabezas, I.; López-Saura, P.A. TNF-α and IL-10 Downregulation and Marked Oxidative Stress in Neuromyelitis Optica. *J. Inflamm.* **2009**, *6*, 18. [CrossRef]
23. Blesa, J.; Trigo-Damas, I.; Quiroga-Varela, A.; Jackson-Lewis, V.R. Oxidative Stress and Parkinson's Disease. *Front. Neuroanat.* **2015**, *9*, 91. [CrossRef]
24. Wei, Z.; Li, X.; Li, X.; Liu, Q.; Cheng, Y. Oxidative Stress in Parkinson's Disease: A Systematic Review and Meta-Analysis. *Front. Mol. Neurosci.* **2018**, *11*, 236. [CrossRef] [PubMed]
25. Puspita, L.; Chung, S.Y.; Shim, J. Oxidative Stress and Cellular Pathologies in Parkinson's Disease. *Mol. Brain* **2017**, *10*, 53. [CrossRef] [PubMed]
26. Aoyama, K.; Matsubara, K.; Kobayashi, S. Aging and Oxidative Stress in Progressive Supranuclear Palsy. *Eur. J. Neurol.* **2006**, *13*, 89–92. [CrossRef] [PubMed]
27. Dennis, A.-G.; Almaguer-Mederos, L.E.; Raúl, R.-A.; Roberto, R.-L.; Luis, V.-P.; Dany, C.-A.; Yanetza, G.-Z.; Yaimeé, V.-M.; Annelié, E.-D.; Arnoy, P.-A.; et al. Redox Imbalance Associates with Clinical Worsening in Spinocerebellar Ataxia Type 2. *Oxidative Med. Cell. Longev.* **2021**, *2021*, e9875639. [CrossRef] [PubMed]
28. Wang, Y.-C.; Lee, C.-M.; Lee, L.-C.; Tung, L.-C.; Hsieh-Li, H.-M.; Lee-Chen, G.-J.; Su, M.-T. Mitochondrial Dysfunction and Oxidative Stress Contribute to the Pathogenesis of Spinocerebellar Ataxia Type 12 (SCA12). *J. Biol. Chem.* **2011**, *286*, 21742–21754. [CrossRef]
29. Torres-Ramos, Y.; Montoya-Estrada, A.; Cisneros, B.; Tercero-Pérez, K.; León-Reyes, G.; Leyva-García, N.; Hernández-Hernández, O.; Magaña, J.J. Oxidative Stress in Spinocerebellar Ataxia Type 7 Is Associated with Disease Severity. *Cerebellum* **2018**, *17*, 601–609. [CrossRef]
30. Allen, C.L.; Bayraktutan, U. Oxidative Stress and Its Role in the Pathogenesis of Ischaemic Stroke. *Int. J. Stroke* **2009**, *4*, 461–470. [CrossRef]
31. Žitňanová, I.; Šiarnik, P.; Kollár, B.; Chomová, M.; Pazderová, P.; Andrezálová, L.; Ježovičová, M.; Koňariková, K.; Laubertová, L.; Krivošíková, Z.; et al. Oxidative Stress Markers and Their Dynamic Changes in Patients after Acute Ischemic Stroke. *Oxidative Med. Cell. Longev.* **2016**, *2016*, e9761697. [CrossRef]
32. Komsiiska, D. Oxidative Stress and Stroke: A Review of Upstream and Downstream Antioxidant Therapeutic Options. *Comp. Clin. Pathol.* **2019**, *28*, 915–926. [CrossRef]
33. Cornelius, C.; Crupi, R.; Calabrese, V.; Graziano, A.; Milone, P.; Pennisi, G.; Radak, Z.; Calabrese, E.J.; Cuzzocrea, S. Traumatic Brain Injury: Oxidative Stress and Neuroprotection. *Antioxid. Redox Signal.* **2013**, *19*, 836–853. [CrossRef]
34. Ismail, H.; Shakkour, Z.; Tabet, M.; Abdelhady, S.; Kobaisi, A.; Abedi, R.; Nasrallah, L.; Pintus, G.; Al-Dhaheri, Y.; Mondello, S.; et al. Traumatic Brain Injury: Oxidative Stress and Novel Anti-Oxidants Such as Mitoquinone and Edaravone. *Antioxidants* **2020**, *9*, 943. [CrossRef] [PubMed]
35. Mendes Arent, A.; de Souza, L.F.; Walz, R.; Dafre, A.L. Perspectives on Molecular Biomarkers of Oxidative Stress and Antioxidant Strategies in Traumatic Brain Injury. *Biomed. Res. Int.* **2014**, *2014*, e723060. [CrossRef] [PubMed]
36. Ray, P.D.; Huang, B.-W.; Tsuji, Y. Reactive Oxygen Species (ROS) Homeostasis and Redox Regulation in Cellular Signaling. *Cell. Signal.* **2012**, *24*, 981–990. [CrossRef] [PubMed]
37. Li, R.; Jia, Z.; Trush, M.A. Defining ROS in Biology and Medicine. *React. Oxyg. Species* **2016**, *1*, 9–21. [CrossRef] [PubMed]
38. Haigis, M.C.; Yankner, B.A. The Aging Stress Response. *Mol. Cell* **2010**, *40*, 333–344. [CrossRef]
39. Yu, B.P. Cellular Defenses against Damage from Reactive Oxygen Species. *Physiol. Rev.* **1994**, *74*, 139–162. [CrossRef]
40. Khajeh Dangolani, S.; Panahi, F.; Tavaf, Z.; Nourisefat, M.; Yousefi, R.; Khalafi-Nezhad, A. Synthesis and Antioxidant Activity Evaluation of Some Novel Aminocarbonitrile Derivatives Incorporating Carbohydrate Moieties. *ACS Omega* **2018**, *3*, 10341–10350. [CrossRef]
41. Mohana, K.N.; Kumar, C.B.P. Synthesis and Antioxidant Activity of 2-Amino-5-Methylthiazol Derivatives Containing 1,3,4-Oxadiazole-2-Thiol Moiety. *ISRN Org. Chem.* **2013**, *2013*, e620718. [CrossRef]
42. Li, A.-N.; Li, S.; Zhang, Y.-J.; Xu, X.-R.; Chen, Y.-M.; Li, H.-B. Resources and Biological Activities of Natural Polyphenols. *Nutrients* **2014**, *6*, 6020–6047. [CrossRef]
43. Zhou, Y.; Li, Y.; Zhou, T.; Zheng, J.; Li, S.; Li, H.-B. Dietary Natural Products for Prevention and Treatment of Liver Cancer. *Nutrients* **2016**, *8*, 156. [CrossRef]
44. Peng, C.; Wang, X.; Chen, J.; Jiao, R.; Wang, L.; Li, Y.M.; Zuo, Y.; Liu, Y.; Lei, L.; Ma, K.Y.; et al. Biology of Ageing and Role of Dietary Antioxidants. *Biomed. Res. Int.* **2014**, *2014*, 831841. [CrossRef] [PubMed]
45. Arulselvan, P.; Fard, M.T.; Tan, W.S.; Gothai, S.; Fakurazi, S.; Norhaizan, M.E.; Kumar, S.S. Role of Antioxidants and Natural Products in Inflammation. *Oxid. Med. Cell. Longev.* **2016**, *2016*, 5276130. [CrossRef] [PubMed]
46. Biotransformation of Waste Biomass into High Value Biochemicals. Available online: https://www.springerprofessional.de/en/biotransformation-of-waste-biomass-into-high-value-biochemicals/1889608 (accessed on 28 December 2021).
47. Fukai, T.; Ushio-Fukai, M. Superoxide Dismutases: Role in Redox Signaling, Vascular Function, and Diseases. *Antioxid. Redox Signal.* **2011**, *15*, 1583–1606. [CrossRef] [PubMed]
48. Marín-García, J. Chapter 14—Oxidative Stress and Cell Death in Cardiovascular Disease: A Post-Genomic Appraisal. In *Post-Genomic Cardiology*, 2nd ed.; Marín-García, J., Ed.; Academic Press: Boston, MA, USA, 2014; pp. 471–498. [CrossRef]

49. van Lith, R.; Ameer, G.A. Chapter Ten—Antioxidant Polymers as Biomaterial. In *Oxidative Stress and Biomaterials*; Dziubla, T., Butterfield, D.A., Eds.; Academic Press: Cambridge, MA, USA, 2016; pp. 251–296. [CrossRef]
50. Lubos, E.; Loscalzo, J.; Handy, D.E. Glutathione Peroxidase-1 in Health and Disease: From Molecular Mechanisms to Therapeutic Opportunities. *Antioxid. Redox Signal.* **2011**, *15*, 1957–1997. [CrossRef]
51. Dalvi, S.M.; Patil, V.W.; Ramraje, N.N. The Roles of Glutathione, Glutathione Peroxidase, Glutathione Reductase and the Carbonyl Protein in Pulmonary and Extra Pulmonary Tuberculosis. *J. Clin. Diagn. Res.* **2012**, *6*, 1462–1465. [CrossRef]
52. Baud, O.; Greene, A.E.; Li, J.; Wang, H.; Volpe, J.J.; Rosenberg, P.A. Glutathione Peroxidase-Catalase Cooperativity Is Required for Resistance to Hydrogen Peroxide by Mature Rat Oligodendrocytes. *J. Neurosci.* **2004**, *24*, 1531–1540. [CrossRef]
53. Mulholland, C.W.; Elwood, P.C.; Davis, A.; Thurnham, D.I.; Kennedy, O.; Coulter, J.; Fehily, A.; Strain, J.J. Antioxidant Enzymes, Inflammatory Indices and Lifestyle Factors in Older Men: A Cohort Analysis. *QJM Int. J. Med.* **1999**, *92*, 579–585. [CrossRef]
54. Nimse, S.B.; Pal, D. Free Radicals, Natural Antioxidants, and Their Reaction Mechanisms. *RSC Adv.* **2015**, *5*, 27986–28006. [CrossRef]
55. Shahidi, F.; Zhong, Y. Novel Antioxidants in Food Quality Preservation and Health Promotion. *Eur. J. Lipid Sci. Technol.* **2010**, *112*, 930–940. [CrossRef]
56. Reddy, P.; Jialal, I. Biochemistry, Fat Soluble Vitamins. In *StatPearls*; StatPearls Publishing: Treasure Island, FL, USA, 2021.
57. Micronutrients, I. *Vitamin A*; National Academies Press: Cambridge, MA, USA, 2001.
58. Dowling, J.E. Vitamin A: Its Many Roles-from Vision and Synaptic Plasticity to Infant Mortality. *J. Comp. Physiol. A Neuroethol. Sens. Neural. Behav. Physiol.* **2020**, *206*, 389–399. [CrossRef]
59. Tanumihardjo, S.A. Vitamin A and Bone Health: The Balancing Act. *J. Clin. Densitom.* **2013**, *16*, 414–419. [CrossRef] [PubMed]
60. McGrane, M.M. Vitamin A Regulation of Gene Expression: Molecular Mechanism of a Prototype Gene. *J. Nutr. Biochem.* **2007**, *18*, 497–508. [CrossRef] [PubMed]
61. Pozniakov, S.P. Mechanism of action of vitamin A on cell differentiation and function. *Ontogenez* **1986**, *17*, 578–586. [PubMed]
62. Clagett-Dame, M.; Knutson, D. Vitamin A in Reproduction and Development. *Nutrients* **2011**, *3*, 385–428. [CrossRef]
63. Bar-El Dadon, S.; Reifen, R. Vitamin A and the Epigenome. *Crit. Rev. Food Sci. Nutr.* **2017**, *57*, 2404–2411. [CrossRef]
64. Cantorna, M.T.; Snyder, L.; Arora, J. Vitamin A and Vitamin D Regulate the Microbial Complexity, Barrier Function, and the Mucosal Immune Responses to Ensure Intestinal Homeostasis. *Crit. Rev. Biochem. Mol. Biol.* **2019**, *54*, 184–192. [CrossRef]
65. Holick, M.F. Chapter 4—Photobiology of Vitamin D. In *Vitamin D*, 4th ed.; Feldman, D., Ed.; Academic Press: Cambridge, MA, USA, 2018; pp. 45–55. [CrossRef]
66. Jones, G. Metabolism and Biomarkers of Vitamin D. *Scand. J. Clin. Lab. Investig. Suppl.* **2012**, *243*, 7–13. [CrossRef]
67. Jones, G.; Prosser, D.E.; Kaufmann, M. Cytochrome P450-Mediated Metabolism of Vitamin D. *J. Lipid. Res.* **2014**, *55*, 13–31. [CrossRef]
68. Jones, G.; Prosser, D.E.; Kaufmann, M. 25-Hydroxyvitamin D-24-Hydroxylase (CYP24A1): Its Important Role in the Degradation of Vitamin D. *Arch. Biochem. Biophys.* **2012**, *523*, 9–18. [CrossRef]
69. Norman, A.W. From Vitamin D to Hormone D: Fundamentals of the Vitamin D Endocrine System Essential for Good Health. *Am. J. Clin. Nutr.* **2008**, *88*, 491S–499S. [CrossRef]
70. Samuel, S.; Sitrin, M.D. Vitamin D's role in cell proliferation and differentiation. *Nutr. Rev.* **2008**, *66*, S116–S124. [CrossRef]
71. Shaker, J.L.; Deftos, L. Calcium and Phosphate Homeostasis. In *Endotext*; Feingold, K.R., Anawalt, B., Boyce, A., Chrousos, G., de Herder, W.W., Dhatariya, K., Dungan, K., Hershman, J.M., Hofland, J., Kalra, S., et al., Eds.; MDText.com, Inc.: South Dartmouth, MA, USA, 2000.
72. Bowry, V.W.; Ingold, K.U.; Stocker, R. Vitamin E in Human Low-Density Lipoprotein. When and How This Antioxidant Becomes a pro-Oxidant. *Biochem. J.* **1992**, *288 Pt 2*, 341–344. [CrossRef] [PubMed]
73. Jilani, T.; Iqbal, M.P. Does Vitamin E Have a Role in Treatment and Prevention of Anemia? *Pak. J. Pharm. Sci.* **2011**, *24*, 237–242. [PubMed]
74. Napolitano, G.; Fasciolo, G.; Di Meo, S.; Venditti, P. Vitamin E Supplementation and Mitochondria in Experimental and Functional Hyperthyroidism: A Mini-Review. *Nutrients* **2019**, *11*, 2900. [CrossRef] [PubMed]
75. Chow, C.K. Vitamin E Regulation of Mitochondrial Superoxide Generation. *Biol. Signals Recept.* **2001**, *10*, 112–124. [CrossRef]
76. Bozaykut, P.; Ekren, R.; Sezerman, O.U.; Gladyshev, V.N.; Ozer, N.K. High-Throughput Profiling Reveals Perturbation of Endoplasmic Reticulum Stress-Related Genes in Atherosclerosis Induced by High-Cholesterol Diet and the Protective Role of Vitamin E. *Biofactors* **2020**, *46*, 653–664. [CrossRef]
77. Office of Dietary Supplements—Vitamin E. Available online: https://ods.od.nih.gov/factsheets/VitaminE-HealthProfessional/ (accessed on 28 December 2021).
78. Zingg, J.-M. Vitamin E: A Role in Signal Transduction. *Annu. Rev. Nutr.* **2015**, *35*, 135–173. [CrossRef]
79. Boscoboinik, D.; Szewczyk, A.; Azzi, A. Alpha-Tocopherol (Vitamin E) Regulates Vascular Smooth Muscle Cell Proliferation and Protein Kinase C Activity. *Arch. Biochem. Biophys.* **1991**, *286*, 264–269. [CrossRef]
80. Boscoboinik, D.; Szewczyk, A.; Hensey, C.; Azzi, A. Inhibition of Cell Proliferation by Alpha-Tocopherol. Role of Protein Kinase C. *J. Biol. Chem.* **1991**, *266*, 6188–6194. [CrossRef]
81. Lloret, A.; Esteve, D.; Monllor, P.; Cervera-Ferri, A.; Lloret, A. The Effectiveness of Vitamin E Treatment in Alzheimer's Disease. *Int. J. Mol. Sci.* **2019**, *20*, 879. [CrossRef]

82. Berdnikovs, S.; Abdala-Valencia, H.; McCary, C.; Somand, M.; Cole, R.; Garcia, A.; Bryce, P.; Cook-Mills, J.M. Isoforms of Vitamin E Have Opposing Immunoregulatory Functions during Inflammation by Regulating Leukocyte Recruitment. *J. Immunol.* **2009**, *182*, 4395–4405. [CrossRef]
83. Cook-Mills, J.M. Isoforms of Vitamin E Differentially Regulate PKC α and Inflammation: A Review. *J. Clin. Cell. Immunol.* **2013**, *4*, 1000137. [CrossRef]
84. Njus, D.; Kelley, P.M. Vitamins C and E donate single hydrogen atoms in vivo. *FEBS Lett.* **1991**, *284*, 147–151. [CrossRef]
85. Sultana, R.; Perluigi, M.; Butterfield, D.A. Lipid Peroxidation Triggers Neurodegeneration: A Redox Proteomics View into the Alzheimer Disease Brain. *Free Radic. Biol. Med.* **2013**, *62*, 157–169. [CrossRef]
86. Neelamegam, M.; Looi, I.; Ng, K.S.; Malavade, S.S. Vitamin E Supplementation for Preventing Recurrent Stroke and Other Vascular Events in Patients with Stroke or Transient Ischaemic Attack. *Cochrane Database Syst. Rev.* **2017**, *2017*, CD010797. [CrossRef]
87. Chow, C.K.; Hong, C.B. Dietary Vitamin E and Selenium and Toxicity of Nitrite and Nitrate. *Toxicology* **2002**, *180*, 195–207. [CrossRef]
88. d'Ischia, M.; Novellino, L. Nitric Oxide-Induced Oxidation of Alpha-Tocopherol. *Bioorg. Med. Chem.* **1996**, *4*, 1747–1753. [CrossRef]
89. Booth, S.L. Vitamin K: Food Composition and Dietary Intakes. *Food Nutr. Res.* **2012**, *56*, 5505. [CrossRef]
90. Imbrescia, K.; Moszczynski, Z. Vitamin K. In *StatPearls*; StatPearls Publishing: Treasure Island, FL, USA, 2021.
91. Tie, J.-K.; Stafford, D.W. Chapter Fourteen—Functional Study of the Vitamin K Cycle Enzymes in Live Cells. In *Methods in Enzymology*; Gelb, M.H., Ed.; Enzymology at the Membrane Interface: Intramembrane Proteases; Academic Press: Cambridge, MA, USA, 2017; Volume 584, pp. 349–394. [CrossRef]
92. Tie, J.-K.; Stafford, D.W. Structural and Functional Insights into Enzymes of the Vitamin K Cycle. *J. Thromb. Haemost.* **2016**, *14*, 236–247. [CrossRef]
93. Oldenburg, J.; Bevans, C.G.; Müller, C.R.; Watzka, M. Vitamin K Epoxide Reductase Complex Subunit 1 (VKORC1): The Key Protein of the Vitamin K Cycle. *Antioxid. Redox Signal.* **2006**, *8*, 347–353. [CrossRef] [PubMed]
94. Suttie, J.W. Vitamin K-Dependent Carboxylase. *Annu. Rev. Biochem.* **1985**, *54*, 459–477. [CrossRef] [PubMed]
95. The Vitamin K Cycle—STAFFORD—2005—Journal of Thrombosis and Haemostasis—Wiley Online Library. Available online: https://onlinelibrary.wiley.com/doi/full/10.1111/j.1538-7836.2005.01419.x (accessed on 28 December 2021).
96. Lanzkowsky, P. Chapter 7—Megaloblastic Anemia. In *Lanzkowsky's Manual of Pediatric Hematology and Oncology*, 6th ed.; Lanzkowsky, P., Lipton, J.M., Fish, J.D., Eds.; Academic Press: San Diego, CA, USA, 2016; pp. 84–101. [CrossRef]
97. Xv, F.; Chen, J.; Duan, L.; Li, S. Research Progress on the Anticancer Effects of Vitamin K2 (Review). *Oncol. Lett.* **2018**, *15*, 8926–8934. [CrossRef] [PubMed]
98. Harshman, S.G.; Shea, M.K. The Role of Vitamin K in Chronic Aging Diseases: Inflammation, Cardiovascular Disease, and Osteoarthritis. *Curr. Nutr. Rep.* **2016**, *5*, 90–98. [CrossRef] [PubMed]
99. Ferland, G. Vitamin K and the Nervous System: An Overview of Its Actions. *Adv. Nutr.* **2012**, *3*, 204–212. [CrossRef]
100. Kennedy, D.O. B Vitamins and the Brain: Mechanisms, Dose and Efficacy—A Review. *Nutrients* **2016**, *8*, 68. [CrossRef]
101. Wilson, D.; Branda, N.R. Turning "On" and "Off" a Pyridoxal 5′-Phosphate Mimic Using Light. *Angew. Chem. Int. Ed.* **2012**, *51*, 5431–5434. [CrossRef]
102. Daugherty, M.; Polanuyer, B.; Farrell, M.; Scholle, M.; Lykidis, A.; de Crécy-Lagard, V.; Osterman, A. Complete Reconstitution of the Human Coenzyme A Biosynthetic Pathway via Comparative Genomics. *J. Biol. Chem.* **2002**, *277*, 21431–21439. [CrossRef]
103. Shi, L.; Tu, B.P. Acetyl-CoA and the Regulation of Metabolism: Mechanisms and Consequences. *Curr. Opin. Cell. Biol.* **2015**, *33*, 125–131. [CrossRef]
104. New Considerations on the Neuromodulatory Role of Thiamine—Abstract—Pharmacology 2012. Volume 89, No. 1–2—Karger Publishers. Available online: https://www.karger.com/Article/Abstract/336339 (accessed on 28 December 2021).
105. Dias, C.; Nylandsted, J. Plasma Membrane Integrity in Health and Disease: Significance and Therapeutic Potential. *Cell Discov.* **2021**, *7*, 4. [CrossRef]
106. Sharma, A.; Bist, R. Alteration in Cholinesterases, γ-Aminobutyric Acid and Serotonin Level with Respect to Thiamine Deficiency in Swiss Mice. *Turk. J. Biochem.* **2019**, *44*, 218–223. [CrossRef]
107. Zhao, N.; Zhong, C.; Wang, Y.; Zhao, Y.; Gong, N.; Zhou, G.; Xu, T.; Hong, Z. Impaired Hippocampal Neurogenesis Is Involved in Cognitive Dysfunction Induced by Thiamine Deficiency at Early Pre-Pathological Lesion Stage. *Neurobiol. Dis.* **2008**, *29*, 176–185. [CrossRef] [PubMed]
108. Barclay, L.L.; Gibson, G.E.; Blass, J.P. Impairment of Behavior and Acetylcholine Metabolism in Thiamine Deficiency. *J. Pharm. Exp.* **1981**, *217*, 537–543.
109. Pinnell, S.R. Regulation of Collagen Biosynthesis by Ascorbic Acid: A Review. *Yale J. Biol. Med.* **1985**, *58*, 553–559. [PubMed]
110. Buettner, G.R. The Pecking Order of Free Radicals and Antioxidants: Lipid Peroxidation, Alpha-Tocopherol, and Ascorbate. *Arch. Biochem. Biophys.* **1993**, *300*, 535–543. [CrossRef] [PubMed]
111. Traber, M.G.; Stevens, J.F. Vitamins C and E: Beneficial Effects from a Mechanistic Perspective. *Free Radic. Biol. Med.* **2011**, *51*, 1000–1013. [CrossRef]
112. Wilson, J.X. Regulation of Vitamin C Transport. *Annu. Rev. Nutr.* **2005**, *25*, 105–125. [CrossRef]

113. Buettner, G.R.; Jurkiewicz, B.A. Catalytic Metals, Ascorbate and Free Radicals: Combinations to Avoid. *Radiat. Res.* **1996**, *145*, 532–541. [CrossRef]
114. Kaźmierczak-Barańska, J.; Boguszewska, K.; Adamus-Grabicka, A.; Karwowski, B.T. Two Faces of Vitamin C—Antioxidative and Pro-Oxidative Agent. *Nutrients* **2020**, *12*, 1501. [CrossRef]
115. Chakraborthy, A.; Ramani, P.; Sherlin, H.J.; Premkumar, P.; Natesan, A. Antioxidant and Pro-Oxidant Activity of Vitamin C in Oral Environment. *Indian J. Dent. Res.* **2014**, *25*, 499–504. [CrossRef]
116. Cameron, E.; Pauling, L. Supplemental Ascorbate in the Supportive Treatment of Cancer: Prolongation of Survival Times in Terminal Human Cancer. *Proc. Natl. Acad. Sci. USA* **1976**, *73*, 3685–3689. [CrossRef]
117. Pfister, R.; Sharp, S.J.; Luben, R.; Wareham, N.J.; Khaw, K.-T. Plasma Vitamin C Predicts Incident Heart Failure in Men and Women in European Prospective Investigation into Cancer and Nutrition-Norfolk Prospective Study. *Am. Heart. J.* **2011**, *162*, 246–253. [CrossRef] [PubMed]
118. Osganian, S.K.; Stampfer, M.J.; Rimm, E.; Spiegelman, D.; Hu, F.B.; Manson, J.E.; Willett, W.C. Vitamin C and Risk of Coronary Heart Disease in Women. *J. Am. Coll. Cardiol.* **2003**, *42*, 246–252. [CrossRef]
119. Moretti, M.; Fraga, D.B.; Rodrigues, A.L.S. Preventive and Therapeutic Potential of Ascorbic Acid in Neurodegenerative Diseases. *CNS Neurosci.* **2017**, *23*, 921–929. [CrossRef]
120. Hansen, S.N.; Tveden-Nyborg, P.; Lykkesfeldt, J. Does Vitamin C Deficiency Affect Cognitive Development and Function? *Nutrients* **2014**, *6*, 3818–3846. [CrossRef] [PubMed]
121. Dixit, S.; Bernardo, A.; Walker, M.J.; Kennard, J.A.; Kim, G.Y.; Kessler, E.S.; Harrison, F.E. Vitamin C Deficiency in the Brain Impairs Cognition, Increases Amyloid Accumulation and Deposition, and Oxidative Stress in APP/PSEN1 and Normally-Aging Mice. *ACS Chem. Neurosci.* **2015**, *6*, 570–581. [CrossRef]
122. Harrison, F.E.; Green, R.J.; Dawes, S.M.; May, J.M. Vitamin C Distribution and Retention in the Mouse Brain. *Brain Res.* **2010**, *1348*, 181–186. [CrossRef]
123. Harrison, F.E.; May, J.M.; McDonald, M.P. Vitamin C Deficiency Increases Basal Exploratory Activity but Decreases Scopolamine-Induced Activity in APP/PSEN1 Transgenic Mice. *Pharm. Biochem. Behav.* **2010**, *94*, 543–552. [CrossRef]
124. Ghosh, M.K.; Chattopadhyay, D.J.; Chatterjee, I.B. Vitamin C Prevents Oxidative Damage. *Free Radic. Res.* **1996**, *25*, 173–179. [CrossRef]
125. Ward, M.S.; Lamb, J.; May, J.M.; Harrison, F.E. Behavioral and Monoamine Changes Following Severe Vitamin C Deficiency. *J. Neurochem.* **2013**, *124*, 363–375. [CrossRef]
126. Harrison, F.E.; May, J.M. Vitamin C Function in the Brain: Vital Role of the Ascorbate Transporter (SVCT2). *Free Radic. Biol. Med.* **2009**, *46*, 719–730. [CrossRef]
127. Landrum, J.T. (Ed.) *Carotenoids: Physical, Chemical, and Biological Functions and Properties*; CRC Press: Boca Raton, FL, USA, 2009. [CrossRef]
128. Fiedor, J.; Fiedor, L.; Haessner, R.; Scheer, H. Cyclic Endoperoxides of Beta-Carotene, Potential pro-Oxidants, as Products of Chemical Quenching of Singlet Oxygen. *Biochim. Biophys. Acta* **2005**, *1709*, 1–4. [CrossRef] [PubMed]
129. Wisniewska, A.; Subczynski, W.K. Effects of Polar Carotenoids on the Shape of the Hydrophobic Barrier of Phospholipid Bilayers. *Biochim. Biophys. Acta* **1998**, *1368*, 235–246. [CrossRef]
130. Accumulation of Macular Xanthophylls in Unsaturated Membrane Domains—Abstract—Europe PMC. Available online: https://europepmc.org/article/med/16678020 (accessed on 28 December 2021).
131. Bertram, J.S. Cancer Prevention by Carotenoids. Mechanistic Studies in Cultured Cells. *Ann. N. Y. Acad. Sci.* **1993**, *691*, 177–191. [CrossRef]
132. Krinsky, N.I. Micronutrients and Their Influence on Mutagenicity and Malignant Transformation. *Ann. N. Y. Acad. Sci.* **1993**, *686*, 229–242. [CrossRef]
133. Walk, A.M.; Khan, N.A.; Barnett, S.M.; Raine, L.B.; Kramer, A.F.; Cohen, N.J.; Moulton, C.J.; Renzi-Hammond, L.M.; Hammond, B.R.; Hillman, C.H. From Neuro-Pigments to Neural Efficiency: The Relationship between Retinal Carotenoids and Behavioral and Neuroelectric Indices of Cognitive Control in Childhood. *Int. J. Psychophysiol.* **2017**, *118*, 1–8. [CrossRef]
134. Grodstein, F.; Kang, J.H.; Glynn, R.J.; Cook, N.R.; Gaziano, J.M. A Randomized Trial of Beta Carotene Supplementation and Cognitive Function in Men: The Physicians' Health Study II. *Arch. Intern. Med.* **2007**, *167*, 2184–2190. [CrossRef]
135. Johnson, E.J.; McDonald, K.; Caldarella, S.M.; Chung, H.-Y.; Troen, A.M.; Snodderly, D.M. Cognitive Findings of an Exploratory Trial of Docosahexaenoic Acid and Lutein Supplementation in Older Women. *Nutr. Neurosci.* **2008**, *11*, 75–83. [CrossRef]
136. Rowles, J.L.; Erdman, J.W. Carotenoids and Their Role in Cancer Prevention. *Biochim. Biophys. Acta BBA Mol. Cell Biol. Lipids* **2020**, *1865*, 158613. [CrossRef]
137. Jonasson, L.; Wikby, A.; Olsson, A.G. Low Serum Beta-Carotene Reflects Immune Activation in Patients with Coronary Artery Disease. *Nutr. Metab. Cardiovasc. Dis.* **2003**, *13*, 120–125. [CrossRef]
138. Adewoyin, M.; Ibrahim, M.; Roszaman, R.; Md Isa, M.L.; Mat Alewi, N.A.; Abdul Rafa, A.A.; Anuar, M.N.N. Male Infertility: The Effect of Natural Antioxidants and Phytocompounds on Seminal Oxidative Stress. *Diseases* **2017**, *5*, 9. [CrossRef]
139. Pike, T.W.; Blount, J.D.; Lindström, J.; Metcalfe, N.B. Dietary Carotenoid Availability, Sexual Signalling and Functional Fertility in Sticklebacks. *Biol. Lett.* **2010**, *6*, 191–193. [CrossRef] [PubMed]

140. Sharoni, Y.; Linnewiel-Hermoni, K.; Zango, G.; Khanin, M.; Salman, H.; Veprik, A.; Danilenko, M.; Levy, J. The Role of Lycopene and Its Derivatives in the Regulation of Transcription Systems: Implications for Cancer Prevention. *Am. J. Clin. Nutr.* **2012**, *96*, 1173S–1178S. [CrossRef] [PubMed]
141. Kumar, N.; Goel, N. Phenolic Acids: Natural Versatile Molecules with Promising Therapeutic Applications. *Biotechnol. Rep. Amst.* **2019**, *24*, e00370. [CrossRef] [PubMed]
142. Fernandes, I.; Pérez-Gregorio, R.; Soares, S.; Mateus, N.; de Freitas, V. Wine Flavonoids in Health and Disease Prevention. *Molecules* **2017**, *22*, 292. [CrossRef] [PubMed]
143. Musial, C.; Kuban-Jankowska, A.; Gorska-Ponikowska, M. Beneficial Properties of Green Tea Catechins. *Int. J. Mol. Sci.* **2020**, *21*, 1744. [CrossRef]
144. Sultana, B.; Anwar, F. Flavonols (Kaempeferol, Quercetin, Myricetin) Contents of Selected Fruits, Vegetables and Medicinal Plants. *Food Chem.* **2008**, *108*, 879–884. [CrossRef]
145. Reinisalo, M.; Kårlund, A.; Koskela, A.; Kaarniranta, K.; Karjalainen, R.O. Polyphenol Stilbenes: Molecular Mechanisms of Defence against Oxidative Stress and Aging-Related Diseases. *Oxidative Med. Cell. Longev.* **2015**, *2015*, 340520. [CrossRef]
146. Al-Suhaimi, E.A.; Al-Riziza, N.A.; Al-Essa, R.A. Physiological and Therapeutical Roles of Ginger and Turmeric on Endocrine Functions. *Am. J. Chin. Med.* **2011**, *39*, 215–231. [CrossRef]
147. Eren, D.; Betul, Y.M. Revealing the Effect of 6-Gingerol, 6-Shogaol and Curcumin on MPGES-1, GSK-3β and β-Catenin Pathway in A549 Cell Line. *Chem. Biol. Interact.* **2016**, *258*, 257–265. [CrossRef] [PubMed]
148. Zhou, Y.; Zheng, J.; Li, Y.; Xu, D.-P.; Li, S.; Chen, Y.-M.; Li, H.-B. Natural Polyphenols for Prevention and Treatment of Cancer. *Nutrients* **2016**, *8*, E515. [CrossRef]
149. Fujiki, H.; Sueoka, E.; Watanabe, T.; Suganuma, M. Primary Cancer Prevention by Green Tea, and Tertiary Cancer Prevention by the Combination of Green Tea Catechins and Anticancer Compounds. *J. Cancer Prev.* **2015**, *20*, 1–4. [CrossRef] [PubMed]
150. Sirerol, J.A.; Rodríguez, M.L.; Mena, S.; Asensi, M.A.; Estrela, J.M.; Ortega, A.L. Role of Natural Stilbenes in the Prevention of Cancer. *Oxidative Med. Cell. Longev.* **2015**, *2016*, e3128951. [CrossRef] [PubMed]
151. Guo, R.; Li, W.; Liu, B.; Li, S.; Zhang, B.; Xu, Y. Resveratrol Protects Vascular Smooth Muscle Cells against High Glucose-Induced Oxidative Stress and Cell Proliferation in Vitro. *Med. Sci. Monit. Basic Res.* **2014**, *20*, 82–92. [CrossRef] [PubMed]
152. Yamagata, K.; Tagami, M.; Yamori, Y. Dietary Polyphenols Regulate Endothelial Function and Prevent Cardiovascular Disease. *Nutrition* **2015**, *31*, 28–37. [CrossRef]
153. Xiao, J.B.; Högger, P. Dietary Polyphenols and Type 2 Diabetes: Current Insights and Future Perspectives. *Curr. Med. Chem.* **2015**, *22*, 23–38. [CrossRef]
154. Zhang, H.; Tsao, R. Dietary Polyphenols, Oxidative Stress and Antioxidant and Anti-Inflammatory Effects. *Curr. Opin. Food Sci.* **2016**, *8*, 33–42. [CrossRef]
155. Rossi, L.; Mazzitelli, S.; Arciello, M.; Capo, C.R.; Rotilio, G. Benefits from Dietary Polyphenols for Brain Aging and Alzheimer's Disease. *Neurochem. Res.* **2008**, *33*, 2390–2400. [CrossRef]
156. Noguchi-Shinohara, M.; Yuki, S.; Dohmoto, C.; Ikeda, Y.; Samuraki, M.; Iwasa, K.; Yokogawa, M.; Asai, K.; Komai, K.; Nakamura, H.; et al. Consumption of Green Tea, but Not Black Tea or Coffee, Is Associated with Reduced Risk of Cognitive Decline. *PLoS ONE* **2014**, *9*, e96013. [CrossRef] [PubMed]
157. Aquilano, K.; Baldelli, S.; Rotilio, G.; Ciriolo, M.R. Role of Nitric Oxide Synthases in Parkinson's Disease: A Review on the Antioxidant and Anti-Inflammatory Activity of Polyphenols. *Neurochem. Res.* **2008**, *33*, 2416–2426. [CrossRef]
158. Bao, J.; Liu, W.; Zhou, H.-Y.; Gui, Y.-R.; Yang, Y.-H.; Wu, M.-J.; Xiao, Y.-F.; Shang, J.-T.; Long, G.-F.; Shu, X.-J. Epigallocatechin-3-Gallate Alleviates Cognitive Deficits in APP/PS1 Mice. *Curr. Med. Sci.* **2020**, *40*, 18–27. [CrossRef]
159. Broderick, T.L.; Rasool, S.; Li, R.; Zhang, Y.; Anderson, M.; Al-Nakkash, L.; Plochocki, J.H.; Geetha, T.; Babu, J.R. Neuroprotective Effects of Chronic Resveratrol Treatment and Exercise Training in the 3xTg-AD Mouse Model of Alzheimer's Disease. *Int. J. Mol. Sci.* **2020**, *21*, 7337. [CrossRef]
160. Lim, G.P.; Chu, T.; Yang, F.; Beech, W.; Frautschy, S.A.; Cole, G.M. The Curry Spice Curcumin Reduces Oxidative Damage and Amyloid Pathology in an Alzheimer Transgenic Mouse. *J. Neurosci.* **2001**, *21*, 8370–8377. [CrossRef] [PubMed]
161. Moreno, L.C.G.E.I.; Puerta, E.; Suárez-Santiago, J.E.; Santos-Magalhães, N.S.; Ramirez, M.J.; Irache, J.M. Effect of the oral administration of nanoencapsulated quercetin on a mouse model of Alzheimer's disease. *Int. J. Pharm.* **2017**, *517*, 50–57. [CrossRef] [PubMed]
162. Spagnuolo, C.; Napolitano, M.; Tedesco, I.; Moccia, S.; Milito, A.; Russo, G.L. Neuroprotective Role of Natural Polyphenols. *Curr. Top. Med. Chem.* **2016**, *16*, 1943–1950. [CrossRef]
163. Waggoner, D.J.; Bartnikas, T.B.; Gitlin, J.D. The Role of Copper in Neurodegenerative Disease. *Neurobiol. Dis.* **1999**, *6*, 221–230. [CrossRef] [PubMed]
164. Ozcelik, D.; Uzun, H. Copper Intoxication; Antioxidant Defenses and Oxidative Damage in Rat Brain. *Biol. Trace Elem. Res.* **2009**, *127*, 45–52. [CrossRef] [PubMed]
165. Hirayama, K.; Yasutake, A.; Inoue, M. Free Radicals and Trace Elements. *Prog. Clin. Biol. Res.* **1993**, *380*, 257–268. [CrossRef]
166. Hentze, M.W.; Muckenthaler, M.U.; Galy, B.; Camaschella, C. Two to Tango: Regulation of Mammalian Iron Metabolism. *Cell* **2010**, *142*, 24–38. [CrossRef] [PubMed]
167. Li, L.; Yang, X. The Essential Element Manganese, Oxidative Stress, and Metabolic Diseases: Links and Interactions. *Oxidative Med. Cell. Longev.* **2018**, *2018*, e7580707. [CrossRef]

168. Coskun, M.; Kayis, T.; Gulsu, E.; Alp, E. Effects of Selenium and Vitamin E on Enzymatic, Biochemical, and Immunological Biomarkers in *Galleria mellonella* L. *Sci. Rep.* **2020**, *10*, 9953. [CrossRef]
169. Jerome-Morais, A.; Bera, S.; Rachidi, W.; Gann, P.H.; Diamond, A.M. The Effects of Selenium and the GPx-1 Selenoprotein on the Phosphorylation of H2AX. *Biochim. Biophys. Acta* **2013**, *1830*, 3399–3406. [CrossRef] [PubMed]
170. Prasad, A.S.; Miale, A.; Farid, Z.; Sandstead, H.H.; Schulert, A.R. Zinc Metabolism in Patients with the Syndrome of Iron Deficiency Anemia, Hepatosplenomegaly, Dwarfism, and Hypognadism. *J. Lab. Clin. Med.* **1963**, *61*, 537–549. [PubMed]
171. Bao, B.; Ahmad, A.; Azmi, A.; Li, Y.; Prasad, A.; Sarkar, F.H. Chapter 2—The Biological Significance of Zinc in Inflammation and Aging. In *Inflammation, Advancing Age and Nutrition*; Rahman, I., Bagchi, D., Eds.; Academic Press: San Diego, FL, USA, 2014; pp. 15–27. [CrossRef]
172. Ha, K.-N.; Chen, Y.; Cai, J.; Sternberg, P., Jr. Increased Glutathione Synthesis through an ARE-Nrf2–Dependent Pathway by Zinc in the RPE: Implication for Protection against Oxidative Stress. *Investig. Ophthalmol. Vis. Sci.* **2006**, *47*, 2709–2715. [CrossRef]
173. Kaufman, Z.; Salvador, G.A.; Liu, X.; Oteiza, P.I. Zinc and the Modulation of Nrf2 in Human Neuroblastoma Cells. *Free Radic. Biol. Med.* **2020**, *155*, 1–9. [CrossRef]
174. Li, B.; Cui, W.; Tan, Y.; Luo, P.; Chen, Q.; Zhang, C.; Qu, W.; Miao, L.; Cai, L. Zinc Is Essential for the Transcription Function of Nrf2 in Human Renal Tubule Cells in Vitro and Mouse Kidney in Vivo under the Diabetic Condition. *J. Cell. Mol. Med.* **2014**, *18*, 895–906. [CrossRef]
175. Kocot, J.; Luchowska-Kocot, D.; Kiełczykowska, M.; Musik, I.; Kurzepa, J. Does Vitamin C Influence Neurodegenerative Diseases and Psychiatric Disorders? *Nutrients* **2017**, *9*, 659. [CrossRef]
176. Ma, Q. Role of Nrf2 in Oxidative Stress and Toxicity. *Annu. Rev. Pharm. Toxicol.* **2013**, *53*, 401–426. [CrossRef]
177. Norbury, R.; Cutter, W.; Compton, J.; Robertson, D.; Craig, M.; Whitehead, M.; Murphy, D. The Neuroprotective Effects of Estrogen on the Aging Brain. *Exp. Gerontol.* **2003**, *38*, 109–117. [CrossRef]
178. Sherwin, B.B. Estrogen Effects on Cognition in Menopausal Women. *Neurology* **1997**, *48*, S21–S26. [CrossRef]
179. Sherwin, B.B. Estrogenic Effects on Memory in Women. *Ann. N. Y. Acad. Sci.* **1994**, *743*, 213–230; discussion 230–231. [CrossRef]
180. Henderson, V.W.; Watt, L.; Buckwalter, J.G. Cognitive Skills Associated with Estrogen Replacement in Women with Alzheimer's Disease. *Psychoneuroendocrinology* **1996**, *21*, 421–430. [CrossRef]
181. Birge, S.J. The Role of Estrogen in the Treatment of Alzheimer's Disease. *Neurology* **1997**, *48*, S36–S41. [CrossRef] [PubMed]
182. Fillit, H. Estrogens in the Pathogenesis and Treatment of Alzheimer's Disease in Postmenopausal Women. *Ann. N. Y. Acad. Sci.* **1994**, *743*, 233–238; discussion 238–239. [CrossRef] [PubMed]
183. Paganini-Hill, A.; Henderson, V.W. Estrogen Deficiency and Risk of Alzheimer's Disease in Women. *Am. J. Epidemiol.* **1994**, *140*, 256–261. [CrossRef] [PubMed]
184. Fillit, H.; Weinreb, H.; Cholst, I.; Luine, V.; McEwen, B.; Amador, R.; Zabriskie, J. Observations in a Preliminary Open Trial of Estradiol Therapy for Senile Dementia-Alzheimer's Type. *Psychoneuroendocrinology* **1986**, *11*, 337–345. [CrossRef]
185. Barrett-Connor, E.; Kritz-Silverstein, D. Estrogen Replacement Therapy and Cognitive Function in Older Women. *JAMA* **1993**, *269*, 2637–2641. [CrossRef]
186. Mulnard, R.A.; Cotman, C.W.; Kawas, C.; van Dyck, C.H.; Sano, M.; Doody, R.; Koss, E.; Pfeiffer, E.; Jin, S.; Gamst, A.; et al. Estrogen Replacement Therapy for Treatment of Mild to Moderate Alzheimer Disease: A Randomized Controlled Trial. Alzheimer's Disease Cooperative Study. *JAMA* **2000**, *283*, 1007–1015. [CrossRef]
187. Brenner, D.E.; Kukull, W.A.; Stergachis, A.; van Belle, G.; Bowen, J.D.; McCormick, W.C.; Teri, L.; Larson, E.B. Postmenopausal Estrogen Replacement Therapy and the Risk of Alzheimer's Disease: A Population-Based Case-Control Study. *Am. J. Epidemiol.* **1994**, *140*, 262–267. [CrossRef]
188. Sultana, R.; Butterfield, D.A. Role of Oxidative Stress in the Progression of Alzheimer's Disease. *J. Alzheimer's Dis.* **2010**, *19*, 341–353. [CrossRef]
189. Chen, Z.; Zhong, C. Oxidative Stress in Alzheimer's Disease. *Neurosci. Bull.* **2014**, *30*, 271–281. [CrossRef]
190. Wang, X.; Wang, W.; Li, L.; Perry, G.; Lee, H.; Zhu, X. Oxidative Stress and Mitochondrial Dysfunction in Alzheimer's Disease. *Biochim. Biophys. Acta BBA Mol. Basis Dis.* **2014**, *1842*, 1240–1247. [CrossRef] [PubMed]
191. Padurariu, M.; Ciobica, A.; Hritcu, L.; Stoica, B.; Bild, W.; Stefanescu, C. Changes of Some Oxidative Stress Markers in the Serum of Patients with Mild Cognitive Impairment and Alzheimer's Disease. *Neurosci. Lett.* **2010**, *469*, 6–10. [CrossRef] [PubMed]
192. Guglielmotto, M.; Giliberto, L.; Tamagno, E.; Tabaton, M. Oxidative Stress Mediates the Pathogenic Effect of Different Alzheimer's Disease Risk Factors. *Front. Aging Neurosci.* **2010**, *2*, 3. [CrossRef] [PubMed]
193. Darvesh, A.S.; Carroll, R.T.; Bishayee, A.; Geldenhuys, W.J.; Van der Schyf, C.J. Oxidative Stress and Alzheimer's Disease: Dietary Polyphenols as Potential Therapeutic Agents. *Exp. Rev. Neurother.* **2010**, *10*, 729–745. [CrossRef] [PubMed]
194. Torres, L.L.; Quaglio, N.B.; de Souza, G.T.; Garcia, R.T.; Dati, L.M.M.; Moreira, W.L.; de Melo Loureiro, A.P.; de souza-Talarico, J.N.; Smid, J.; Porto, C.S.; et al. Peripheral Oxidative Stress Biomarkers in Mild Cognitive Impairment and Alzheimer's Disease. *J. Alzheimer's Dis.* **2011**, *26*, 59–68. [CrossRef] [PubMed]
195. Sutherland, G.T.; Chami, B.; Youssef, P.; Witting, P.K. Oxidative Stress in Alzheimer's Disease: Primary Villain or Physiological by-Product? *Redox Rep.* **2013**, *18*, 134–141. [CrossRef] [PubMed]
196. Chang, Y.-T.; Chang, W.-N.; Tsai, N.-W.; Huang, C.-C.; Kung, C.-T.; Su, Y.-J.; Lin, W.-C.; Cheng, B.-C.; Su, C.-M.; Chiang, Y.-F.; et al. The Roles of Biomarkers of Oxidative Stress and Antioxidant in Alzheimer's Disease: A Systematic Review. *BioMed. Res. Int.* **2014**, *2014*, e182303. [CrossRef]

197. Meraz-Ríos, M.A.; Franco-Bocanegra, D.; Toral Rios, D.; Campos-Peña, V. Early Onset Alzheimer's Disease and Oxidative Stress. *Oxidative Med. Cell. Longev.* **2014**, *2014*, e375968. [CrossRef]
198. Bonda, D.J.; Lee, H.; Blair, J.A.; Zhu, X.; Perry, G.; Smith, M.A. Role of Metal Dyshomeostasis in Alzheimer's Disease. *Metallomics* **2011**, *3*, 267–270. [CrossRef]
199. Pohanka, M. Alzheimer´s Disease and Oxidative Stress: A Review. *Curr. Med. Chem.* **2014**, *21*, 356–364. [CrossRef]
200. Du, X.; Wang, X.; Geng, M. Alzheimer's Disease Hypothesis and Related Therapies. *Transl. Neurodegener.* **2018**, *7*, 2. [CrossRef] [PubMed]
201. Luca, M.; Luca, A.; Calandra, C. The Role of Oxidative Damage in the Pathogenesis and Progression of Alzheimer's Disease and Vascular Dementia. *Oxidative Med. Cell. Longev.* **2015**, *2015*, e504678. [CrossRef] [PubMed]
202. Wojtunik-Kulesza, K.A.; Oniszczuk, A.; Oniszczuk, T.; Waksmundzka-Hajnos, M. The Influence of Common Free Radicals and Antioxidants on Development of Alzheimer's Disease. *Biomed. Pharmacother.* **2016**, *78*, 39–49. [CrossRef] [PubMed]
203. Padurariu, M.; Ciobica, A.; Lefter, R.; Serban, I.L.; Stefanescu, C.; Chirita, R. The Oxidative Stress Hypothesis in Alzheimer's Disease. *Psychiatr. Danub.* **2013**, *25*, 401–409.
204. Hung, C.H.-L.; Cheng, S.S.-Y.; Cheung, Y.-T.; Wuwongse, S.; Zhang, N.Q.; Ho, Y.-S.; Lee, S.M.-Y.; Chang, R.C.-C. A Reciprocal Relationship between Reactive Oxygen Species and Mitochondrial Dynamics in Neurodegeneration. *Redox Biol.* **2018**, *14*, 7–19. [CrossRef] [PubMed]
205. Agostinho, P.; Cunha, R.A.; Oliveira, C. Neuroinflammation, Oxidative Stress and the Pathogenesis of Alzheimer's Disease. *Curr. Pharm. Des.* **2010**, *16*, 2766–2778. [CrossRef]
206. Ganguly, G.; Chakrabarti, S.; Chatterjee, U.; Saso, L. Proteinopathy, Oxidative Stress and Mitochondrial Dysfunction: Cross Talk in Alzheimer's Disease and Parkinson's Disease. *Drug. Des. Devel.* **2017**, *11*, 797–810. [CrossRef]
207. González-Reyes, R.E.; Nava-Mesa, M.O.; Vargas-Sánchez, K.; Ariza-Salamanca, D.; Mora-Muñoz, L. Involvement of Astrocytes in Alzheimer's Disease from a Neuroinflammatory and Oxidative Stress Perspective. *Front. Mol. Neurosci.* **2017**, *10*, 427. [CrossRef] [PubMed]
208. Verri, M.; Pastoris, O.; Dossena, M.; Aquilani, R.; Guerriero, F.; Cuzzoni, G.; Venturini, L.; Ricevuti, G.; Bongiorno, A.I. Mitochondrial Alterations, Oxidative Stress and Neuroinflammation in Alzheimer's Disease. *Int. J. Immunopathol. Pharm.* **2012**, *25*, 345–353. [CrossRef]
209. Butterfield, D.A.; Boyd-Kimball, D. Oxidative Stress, Amyloid-β Peptide, and Altered Key Molecular Pathways in the Pathogenesis and Progression of Alzheimer's Disease. *J. Alzheimer's Dis.* **2018**, *62*, 1345–1367. [CrossRef] [PubMed]
210. Takahashi, R.H.; Nagao, T.; Gouras, G.K. Plaque Formation and the Intraneuronal Accumulation of β-Amyloid in Alzheimer's Disease. *Pathol. Int.* **2017**, *67*, 185–193. [CrossRef] [PubMed]
211. Tillement, L.; Lecanu, L.; Papadopoulos, V. Alzheimer's Disease: Effects of β-Amyloid on Mitochondria. *Mitochondrion* **2011**, *11*, 13–21. [CrossRef] [PubMed]
212. Viola, K.L.; Klein, W.L. Amyloid β Oligomers in Alzheimer's Disease Pathogenesis, Treatment, and Diagnosis. *Acta Neuropathol.* **2015**, *129*, 183–206. [CrossRef] [PubMed]
213. Cheng, Y.; Bai, F. The Association of Tau With Mitochondrial Dysfunction in Alzheimer's Disease. *Front. Neurosci.* **2018**, *12*, 163. [CrossRef] [PubMed]
214. Pooler, A.M.; Polydoro, M.; Maury, E.A.; Nicholls, S.B.; Reddy, S.M.; Wegmann, S.; William, C.; Saqran, L.; Cagsal-Getkin, O.; Pitstick, R.; et al. Amyloid Accelerates Tau Propagation and Toxicity in a Model of Early Alzheimer's Disease. *Acta Neuropathol. Commun.* **2015**, *3*, 14. [CrossRef] [PubMed]
215. Medina, M.; Avila, J. New Perspectives on the Role of Tau in Alzheimer's Disease. Implications for Therapy. *Biochem. Pharmacol.* **2014**, *88*, 540–547. [CrossRef] [PubMed]
216. Malinow, R. New Developments on the Role of NMDA Receptors in Alzheimer's Disease. *Curr. Opin. Neurobiol.* **2012**, *22*, 559–563. [CrossRef]
217. Zhang, Y.; Li, P.; Feng, J.; Wu, M. Dysfunction of NMDA Receptors in Alzheimer's Disease. *Neurol. Sci.* **2016**, *37*, 1039–1047. [CrossRef]
218. Bordji, K.; Becerril-Ortega, J.; Buisson, A. Synapses, NMDA Receptor Activity and Neuronal Aβ Production in Alzheimer's Disease. *Gruyter* **2011**, *22*, 285–294. [CrossRef]
219. Mota, S.I.; Ferreira, I.L.; Rego, A.C. Dysfunctional Synapse in Alzheimer's Disease—A Focus on NMDA Receptors. *Neuropharmacology* **2014**, *76*, 16–26. [CrossRef]
220. Foster, T.C.; Kyritsopoulos, C.; Kumar, A. Central Role for NMDA Receptors in Redox Mediated Impairment of Synaptic Function during Aging and Alzheimer's Disease. *Behav. Brain Res.* **2017**, *322*, 223–232. [CrossRef] [PubMed]
221. Kamat, P.K.; Kalani, A.; Rai, S.; Swarnkar, S.; Tota, S.; Nath, C.; Tyagi, N. Mechanism of Oxidative Stress and Synapse Dysfunction in the Pathogenesis of Alzheimer's Disease: Understanding the Therapeutics Strategies. *Mol. Neurobiol.* **2016**, *53*, 648–661. [CrossRef] [PubMed]
222. Beyrent, E.; Gomez, G. Oxidative Stress Differentially Induces Tau Dissociation from Neuronal Microtubules in Neurites of Neurons Cultured from Different Regions of the Embryonic Gallus Domesticus Brain. *J. Neurosci. Res.* **2020**, *98*, 734–747. [CrossRef] [PubMed]
223. Cassidy, L.; Fernandez, F.; Johnson, J.B.; Naiker, M.; Owoola, A.G.; Broszczak, D.A. Oxidative Stress in Alzheimer's Disease: A Review on Emergent Natural Polyphenolic Therapeutics. *Complement. Ther. Med.* **2020**, *49*, 102294. [CrossRef] [PubMed]

224. Šerý, O.; Povová, J.; Míšek, I.; Pešák, L.; Janout, V. Molecular Mechanisms of Neuropathological Changes in Alzheimer's Disease: A Review. *Folia Neuropathol.* **2013**, *51*, 1–9. [CrossRef]
225. Lasagna-Reeves, C.A.; Castillo-Carranza, D.L.; Sengupta, U.; Sarmiento, J.; Troncoso, J.; Jackson, G.R.; Kayed, R. Identification of Oligomers at Early Stages of Tau Aggregation in Alzheimer's Disease. *FASEB J.* **2012**, *26*, 1946–1959. [CrossRef]
226. Evans, D.B.; Rank, K.B.; Bhattacharya, K.; Thomsen, D.R.; Gurney, M.E.; Sharma, S.K. Tau Phosphorylation at Serine 396 and Serine 404 by Human Recombinant Tau Protein Kinase II Inhibits Tau's Ability to Promote Microtubule Assembly. *J. Biol. Chem.* **2000**, *275*, 24977–24983. [CrossRef]
227. Andorfer, C. Cell-Cycle Reentry and Cell Death in Transgenic Mice Expressing Nonmutant Human Tau Isoforms. *J. Neurosci.* **2005**, *25*, 5446–5454. [CrossRef]
228. Steinhilb, M.L.; Dias-Santagata, D.; Fulga, T.A.; Felch, D.L.; Feany, M.B. Tau Phosphorylation Sites Work in Concert to Promote Neurotoxicity In Vivo. *MBoC* **2007**, *18*, 5060–5068. [CrossRef]
229. Alonso, A.; Grundke-Iqbal, I.; Iqbal, K. Alzheimer's Disease Hyperphosphorylated Tau Sequesters Normal Tau into Tangles of Filaments and Disassembles Microtubules. *Nat. Med.* **1996**, *2*, 783–787. [CrossRef]
230. Chung, C.-W.; Song, Y.-H.; Kim, I.-K.; Yoon, W.-J.; Ryu, B.-R.; Jo, D.-G.; Woo, H.-N.; Kwon, Y.-K.; Kim, H.-H.; Gwag, B.-J.; et al. Proapoptotic Effects of Tau Cleavage Product Generated by Caspase-3. *Neurobiol. Dis.* **2001**, *8*, 162–172. [CrossRef] [PubMed]
231. Braak, H.; Braak, E. Neuropathological Stageing of Alzheimer-Related Changes. *Acta Neuropathol.* **1991**, *82*, 239–259. [CrossRef] [PubMed]
232. Melov, S.; Adlard, P.A.; Morten, K.; Johnson, F.; Golden, T.R.; Hinerfeld, D.; Schilling, B.; Mavros, C.; Masters, C.L.; Volitakis, I.; et al. Mitochondrial Oxidative Stress Causes Hyperphosphorylation of Tau. *PLoS ONE* **2007**, *2*, e536. [CrossRef] [PubMed]
233. Yu, L.; Wang, W.; Pang, W.; Xiao, Z.; Jiang, Y.; Hong, Y. Dietary Lycopene Supplementation Improves Cognitive Performances in Tau Transgenic Mice Expressing P301L Mutation via Inhibiting Oxidative Stress and Tau Hyperphosphorylation. *J. Alzheimer's Dis.* **2017**, *57*, 475–482. [CrossRef] [PubMed]
234. Su, B.; Wang, X.; Lee, H.; Tabaton, M.; Perry, G.; Smith, M.A.; Zhu, X. Chronic Oxidative Stress Causes Increased Tau Phosphorylation in M17 Neuroblastoma Cells. *Neurosci. Lett.* **2010**, *468*, 267–271. [CrossRef]
235. Egaña, J.T.; Zambrano, C.; Nuñez, M.T.; Gonzalez-Billault, C.; Maccioni, R.B. Iron-Induced Oxidative Stress Modify Tau Phosphorylation Patterns in Hippocampal Cell Cultures. *Biometals* **2003**, *16*, 215–223. [CrossRef]
236. Wang, D.-L.; Ling, Z.-Q.; Cao, F.-Y.; Zhu, L.-Q.; Wang, J.-Z. Melatonin Attenuates Isoproterenol-Induced Protein Kinase A Overactivation and Tau Hyperphosphorylation in Rat Brain. *J. Pineal Res.* **2004**, *37*, 11–16. [CrossRef]
237. Atlante, A.; Valenti, D.; Latina, V.; Amadoro, G. Role of Oxygen Radicals in Alzheimer's Disease: Focus on Tau Protein. *Oxygen* **2021**, *1*, 96–120. [CrossRef]
238. Kandimalla, R.; Manczak, M.; Yin, X.; Wang, R.; Reddy, P.H. Hippocampal Phosphorylated Tau Induced Cognitive Decline, Dendritic Spine Loss and Mitochondrial Abnormalities in a Mouse Model of Alzheimer's Disease. *Hum. Mol. Genet.* **2018**, *27*, 30–40. [CrossRef]
239. Horiguchi, T.; Uryu, K.; Giasson, B.I.; Ischiropoulos, H.; LightFoot, R.; Bellmann, C.; Richter-Landsberg, C.; Lee, V.M.-Y.; Trojanowski, J.Q. Nitration of Tau Protein Is Linked to Neurodegeneration in Tauopathies. *Am. J. Pathol.* **2003**, *163*, 1021–1031. [CrossRef]
240. Torres, A.K.; Jara, C.; Olesen, M.A.; Tapia-Rojas, C. Pathologically Phosphorylated Tau at S396/404 (PHF-1) Is Accumulated inside of Hippocampal Synaptic Mitochondria of Aged Wild-Type Mice. *Sci. Rep.* **2021**, *11*, 4448. [CrossRef] [PubMed]
241. Gamblin, T.C.; King, M.E.; Kuret, J.; Berry, R.W.; Binder, L.I. Oxidative Regulation of Fatty Acid-Induced Tau Polymerization. *Biochemistry* **2000**, *39*, 14203–14210. [CrossRef] [PubMed]
242. Zhou, F.; Chen, S.; Xiong, J.; Li, Y.; Qu, L. Luteolin Reduces Zinc-Induced Tau Phosphorylation at Ser262/356 in an ROS-Dependent Manner in SH-SY5Y Cells. *Biol. Trace Elem. Res.* **2012**, *149*, 273–279. [CrossRef]
243. Yamamoto, A.; Shin, R.-W.; Hasegawa, K.; Naiki, H.; Sato, H.; Yoshimasu, F.; Kitamoto, T. Iron (III) Induces Aggregation of Hyperphosphorylated τ and Its Reduction to Iron (II) Reverses the Aggregation: Implications in the Formation of Neurofibrillary Tangles of Alzheimer's Disease. *J. Neurochem.* **2002**, *82*, 1137–1147. [CrossRef]
244. Yang, L.; Ksiezak-Reding, H. Ca^{2+} and Mg^{2+} Selectively Induce Aggregates of PHF-Tau but Not Normal Human Tau. *J. Neurosci. Res.* **1999**, *55*, 36–43. [CrossRef]
245. Bihaqi, S.W.; Bahmani, A.; Adem, A.; Zawia, N.H. Infantile Postnatal Exposure to Lead (Pb) Enhances Tau Expression in the Cerebral Cortex of Aged Mice: Relevance to AD. *Neurotoxicology* **2014**, *44*, 114–120. [CrossRef]
246. Jiang, L.-F.; Yao, T.-M.; Zhu, Z.-L.; Wang, C.; Ji, L.-N. Impacts of Cd(II) on the Conformation and Self-Aggregation of Alzheimer's Tau Fragment Corresponding to the Third Repeat of Microtubule-Binding Domain. *Biochim. Biophys. Acta BBA Proteins Proteom.* **2007**, *1774*, 1414–1421. [CrossRef]
247. Olivieri, G.; Brack, C.; Müller-Spahn, F.; Stähelin, H.B.; Herrmann, M.; Renard, P.; Brockhaus, M.; Hock, C. Mercury Induces Cell Cytotoxicity and Oxidative Stress and Increases β-Amyloid Secretion and Tau Phosphorylation in SHSY5Y Neuroblastoma Cells. *J. Neurochem.* **2000**, *74*, 231–236. [CrossRef]
248. Walton, J.R. An Aluminum-Based Rat Model for Alzheimer's Disease Exhibits Oxidative Damage, Inhibition of PP2A Activity, Hyperphosphorylated Tau, and Granulovacuolar Degeneration. *J. Inorg. Biochem.* **2007**, *101*, 1275–1284. [CrossRef]

249. Prema, A.; Justin Thenmozhi, A.; Manivasagam, T.; Mohamed Essa, M.; Guillemin, G.J. Fenugreek Seed Powder Attenuated Aluminum Chloride-Induced Tau Pathology, Oxidative Stress, and Inflammation in a Rat Model of Alzheimer's Disease. *J. Alzheimer's Dis.* **2017**, *60*, S209–S220. [CrossRef]
250. Kim, A.C.; Lim, S.; Kim, Y.K. Metal Ion Effects on Aβ and Tau Aggregation. *Int. J. Mol. Sci.* **2018**, *19*, 128. [CrossRef]
251. Yao, K.; Zhao, Y.-F.; Zu, H.-B. Melatonin Receptor Stimulation by Agomelatine Prevents Aβ-Induced Tau Phosphorylation and Oxidative Damage in PC12 Cells. *Drug Des. Dev.* **2019**, *13*, 387–396. [CrossRef]
252. Busciglio, J.; Lorenzo, A.; Yeh, J. β-Amyloid fibrils induce tau phosphorylation and loss of microtubule binding. *Neuron* **1995**, *14*, 879–888. [CrossRef]
253. Hernández, F.; Gómez de Barreda, E.; Fuster-Matanzo, A.; Lucas, J.J.; Avila, J. GSK3: A Possible Link between Beta Amyloid Peptide and Tau Protein. *Exp. Neurol.* **2010**, *223*, 322–325. [CrossRef]
254. Hanger, D.P.; Anderton, B.H.; Noble, W. Tau Phosphorylation: The Therapeutic Challenge for Neurodegenerative Disease. *Trends Mol. Med.* **2009**, *15*, 112–119. [CrossRef]
255. Noble, W.; Planel, E.; Zehr, C.; Olm, V.; Meyerson, J.; Suleman, F.; Gaynor, K.; Wang, L.; LaFrancois, J.; Feinstein, B.; et al. Inhibition of Glycogen Synthase Kinase-3 by Lithium Correlates with Reduced Tauopathy and Degeneration in Vivo. *Proc. Natl. Acad. Sci. USA* **2005**, *102*, 6990–6995. [CrossRef] [PubMed]
256. Takashima, A.; Honda, T.; Yasutake, K.; Michel, G.; Murayama, O.; Murayama, M.; Ishiguro, K.; Yamaguchi, H. Activation of Tau Protein Kinase I/Glycogen Synthase Kinase-3β by Amyloid β Peptide (25–35) Enhances Phosphorylation of Tau in Hippocampal Neurons. *Neurosci. Res.* **1998**, *31*, 317–323. [CrossRef]
257. Terwel, D.; Muyllaert, D.; Dewachter, I.; Borghgraef, P.; Croes, S.; Devijver, H.; Van Leuven, F. Amyloid Activates GSK-3β to Aggravate Neuronal Tauopathy in Bigenic Mice. *Am. J. Pathol.* **2008**, *172*, 786–798. [CrossRef]
258. Ma, J.; Ma, C.; Li, J.; Sun, Y.; Ye, F.; Liu, K.; Zhang, H. Extracellular Matrix Proteins Involved in Alzheimer's Disease. *Chem. A Eur. J.* **2020**, *26*, 12101–12110. [CrossRef]
259. Debelle, L.; Tamburro, A.M. Elastin: Molecular Description and Function. *Int. J. Biochem. Cell Biol.* **1999**, *31*, 261–272. [CrossRef]
260. Sandberg, L.B.; Soskel, N.T.; Leslie, J.G. Elastin Structure, Biosynthesis, and Relation to Disease States. Available online: https://www.nejm.org/doi/pdf/10.1056/NEJM198103053041004 (accessed on 29 December 2021). [CrossRef]
261. Powell, J.T.; Vine, N.; Crossman, M. On the Accumulation of D-Aspartate in Elastin and Other Proteins of the Ageing Aorta. *Atherosclerosis* **1992**, *97*, 201–208. [CrossRef]
262. Robert, L.; Molinari, J.; Ravelojaona, V.; Andrès, E.; Robert, A.M. Age- and Passage-Dependent Upregulation of Fibroblast Elastase-Type Endopeptidase Activity. Role of Advanced Glycation Endproducts, Inhibition by Fucose- and Rhamnose-Rich Oligosaccharides. *Arch. Gerontol. Geriatr.* **2010**, *50*, 327–331. [CrossRef]
263. Fulop, T.; Khalil, A.; Larbi, A. The Role of Elastin Peptides in Modulating the Immune Response in Aging and Age-Related Diseases. *Pathol. Biol.* **2012**, *60*, 28–33. [CrossRef]
264. Edgar, S.; Hopley, B.; Genovese, L.; Sibilla, S.; Laight, D.; Shute, J. Effects of Collagen-Derived Bioactive Peptides and Natural Antioxidant Compounds on Proliferation and Matrix Protein Synthesis by Cultured Normal Human Dermal Fibroblasts. *Sci. Rep.* **2018**, *8*, 10474. [CrossRef]
265. Ma, C.; Su, J.; Sun, Y.; Feng, Y.; Shen, N.; Li, B.; Liang, Y.; Yang, X.; Wu, H.; Zhang, H.; et al. Significant Upregulation of Alzheimer's β-Amyloid Levels in a Living System Induced by Extracellular Elastin Polypeptides. *Angew. Chem. Int. Ed.* **2019**, *58*, 18703–18709. [CrossRef]
266. Bochicchio, B.; Lorusso, M.; Pepe, A.; Tamburro, A.M. On Enhancers and Inhibitors of Elastin-Derived Amyloidogenesis. Available online: https://www.futuremedicine.com/doi/abs/10.2217/17435889.4.1.31 (accessed on 29 December 2021).
267. Bochicchio, B.; Pepe, A.; Delaunay, F.; Lorusso, M.; Baud, S.; Dauchez, M. Amyloidogenesis of Proteolytic Fragments of Human Elastin. *RSC Adv.* **2013**, *3*, 13273–13285. [CrossRef]
268. Szychowski, K.A.; Skóra, B. Review of the Relationship between Reactive Oxygen Species (ROS) and Elastin-Derived Peptides (EDPs). *Appl. Sci.* **2021**, *11*, 8732. [CrossRef]
269. Lehrke, M.; Lazar, M.A. The Many Faces of PPARγ. *Cell* **2005**, *123*, 993–999. [CrossRef]
270. Szychowski, K.A.; Gmiński, J. Impact of Elastin-Derived VGVAPG Peptide on Bidirectional Interaction between Peroxisome Proliferator-Activated Receptor Gamma (Pparγ) and Beta-Galactosidase (β-Gal) Expression in Mouse Cortical Astrocytes in Vitro. *Naunyn-Schmiedeberg's Arch Pharm.* **2019**, *392*, 405–413. [CrossRef]
271. Gmiński, J.; Węglarz, L.; Dróżdż, M.; Goss, M. Pharmacological Modulation of the Antioxidant Enzymes Activities and the Concentration of Peroxidation Products in Fibroblasts Stimulated with Elastin Peptides. *Gen. Pharmacol. Vasc. Syst.* **1991**, *22*, 495–497. [CrossRef]
272. Szychowski, K.A.; Skóra, B.; Wójtowicz, A.K. Elastin-Derived Peptides in the Central Nervous System: Friend or Foe. *Cell Mol. Neurobiol.* **2021**, 1–15. [CrossRef]
273. Calleri, E.; Pochetti, G.; Dossou, K.S.S.; Laghezza, A.; Montanari, R.; Capelli, D.; Prada, E.; Loiodice, F.; Massolini, G.; Bernier, M.; et al. Resveratrol and Its Metabolites Bind to PPARs. *Chembiochem* **2014**, *15*, 1154–1160. [CrossRef]
274. Ma, T.; Tan, M.-S.; Yu, J.-T.; Tan, L. Resveratrol as a Therapeutic Agent for Alzheimer's Disease. *BioMed. Res. Int.* **2014**, *2014*, e350516. [CrossRef]
275. Nicoloff, G.; Tzvetanov, P.; Christova, P.; Baydanoff, S. Detection of Elastin Derived Peptides in Cerebrospinal Fluid of Patients with First Ever Ischaemic Stroke. *Neuropeptides* **2008**, *42*, 277–282. [CrossRef]

276. Szychowski, K.A.; Gmiński, J. The VGVAPG Peptide Regulates the Production of Nitric Oxide Synthases and Reactive Oxygen Species in Mouse Astrocyte Cells In Vitro. *Neurochem. Res.* **2019**, *44*, 1127–1137. [CrossRef]
277. van Horssen, J.; Wesseling, P.; van den Heuvel, L.P.; de Waal, R.M.; Verbeek, M.M. Heparan Sulphate Proteoglycans in Alzheimer's Disease and Amyloid-related Disorders. *Lancet Neurol.* **2003**, *2*, 482–492. [CrossRef]
278. Karamanos, N.K.; Piperigkou, Z.; Theocharis, A.D.; Watanabe, H.; Franchi, M.; Baud, S.; Brézillon, S.; Götte, M.; Passi, A.; Vigetti, D.; et al. Proteoglycan Chemical Diversity Drives Multifunctional Cell Regulation and Therapeutics. *Chem. Rev.* **2018**, *118*, 9152–9232. [CrossRef]
279. Kawecki, C.; Hézard, N.; Bocquet, O.; Poitevin, G.; Rabenoelina, F.; Kauskot, A.; Duca, L.; Blaise, S.; Romier, B.; Martiny, L.; et al. Elastin-Derived Peptides Are New Regulators of Thrombosis. *Arter. Thromb. Vasc. Biol.* **2014**, *34*, 2570–2578. [CrossRef]
280. Tzvetanov, P.; Nicoloff, G.; Rousseff, R.; Christova, P. Increased Levels of Elastin-Derived Peptides in Cerebrospinal Fluid of Patients with Lacunar Stroke. *Clin. Neurol. Neurosurg.* **2008**, *110*, 239–244. [CrossRef]
281. Wang, R.; Reddy, P.H. Role of Glutamate and NMDA Receptors in Alzheimer's Disease. *J. Alzheimers Dis.* **2017**, *57*, 1041–1048. [CrossRef]
282. Liu, J.; Chang, L.; Song, Y.; Li, H.; Wu, Y. The Role of NMDA Receptors in Alzheimer's Disease. *Front. Neurosci.* **2019**, *13*, 43. [CrossRef]
283. Xia, Z.; Dudek, H.; Miranti, C.K.; Greenberg, M.E. Calcium Influx via the NMDA Receptor Induces Immediate Early Gene Transcription by a MAP Kinase/ERK-Dependent Mechanism. *J. Neurosci.* **1996**, *16*, 5425–5436. [CrossRef]
284. Evans, R.C.; Morera-Herreras, T.; Cui, Y.; Du, K.; Sheehan, T.; Kotaleski, J.H.; Venance, L.; Blackwell, K.T. The Effects of NMDA Subunit Composition on Calcium Influx and Spike Timing-Dependent Plasticity in Striatal Medium Spiny Neurons. *PLoS Comput. Biol.* **2012**, *8*, e1002493. [CrossRef]
285. Paoletti, P.; Neyton, J. NMDA Receptor Subunits: Function and Pharmacology. *Curr. Opin. Pharmacol.* **2007**, *7*, 39–47. [CrossRef]
286. Paoletti, P.; Bellone, C.; Zhou, Q. NMDA Receptor Subunit Diversity: Impact on Receptor Properties, Synaptic Plasticity and Disease. *Nat. Rev. Neurosci.* **2013**, *14*, 383–400. [CrossRef]
287. Kamat, P.K.; Rai, S.; Swarnkar, S.; Shukla, R.; Ali, S.; Najmi, A.K.; Nath, C. Okadaic Acid-Induced Tau Phosphorylation in Rat Brain: Role of NMDA Receptor. *Neuroscience* **2013**, *238*, 97–113. [CrossRef]
288. Bezprozvanny, I.; Mattson, M.P. Neuronal Calcium Mishandling and the Pathogenesis of Alzheimer's Disease. *Trends Neurosci.* **2008**, *31*, 454–463. [CrossRef]
289. Ahmed, H.A.; Ismael, S.; Mirzahosseini, G.; Ishrat, T. Verapamil Prevents Development of Cognitive Impairment in an Aged Mouse Model of Sporadic Alzheimer's Disease. *Mol. Neurobiol.* **2021**, *58*, 3374–3387. [CrossRef]
290. Jomsky, M.; Kerna, N. Nifedipine: Can This Calcium Channel Blocker Be Used "Off Label" to Inhibit the Development and Symptoms of Alzheimer's Disease and Related Beta-Amyloid-Producing Syndromes? *EC Pharmacol. Toxicol.* **2019**. [CrossRef]
291. Pithadia, A.S.; Lim, M.H. Metal-Associated Amyloid-β Species in Alzheimer's Disease. *Curr. Opin. Chem. Biol.* **2012**, *16*, 67–73. [CrossRef]
292. Greenough, M.A.; Camakaris, J.; Bush, A.I. Metal Dyshomeostasis and Oxidative Stress in Alzheimer's Disease. *Neurochem. Int.* **2013**, *62*, 540–555. [CrossRef] [PubMed]
293. Das, N.; Raymick, J.; Sarkar, S. Role of Metals in Alzheimer's Disease. *Metab. Brain Dis.* **2021**, *36*, 1627–1639. [CrossRef]
294. Tiiman, A.; Palumaa, P.; Tõugu, V. The Missing Link in the Amyloid Cascade of Alzheimer's Disease—Metal Ions. *Neurochem. Int.* **2013**, *62*, 367–378. [CrossRef]
295. Wang, L.; Yin, Y.-L.; Liu, X.-Z.; Shen, P.; Zheng, Y.-G.; Lan, X.-R.; Lu, C.-B.; Wang, J.-Z. Current Understanding of Metal Ions in the Pathogenesis of Alzheimer's Disease. *Transl. Neurodegener.* **2020**, *9*, 10. [CrossRef] [PubMed]
296. Strodel, B.; Coskuner-Weber, O. Transition Metal Ion Interactions with Disordered Amyloid-β Peptides in the Pathogenesis of Alzheimer's Disease: Insights from Computational Chemistry Studies. *J. Chem. Inf. Model.* **2019**, *59*, 1782–1805. [CrossRef]
297. Bagheri, S.; Squitti, R.; Haertlé, T.; Siotto, M.; Saboury, A.A. Role of Copper in the Onset of Alzheimer's Disease Compared to Other Metals. *Front. Aging Neurosci.* **2018**, *9*, 446. [CrossRef]
298. Kepp, K.P. Alzheimer's Disease: How Metal Ions Define β-Amyloid Function. *Coord. Chem. Rev.* **2017**, *351*, 127–159. [CrossRef]
299. Watt, A.D.; Villemagne, V.L.; Barnham, K.J. Metals, Membranes, and Amyloid-β Oligomers: Key Pieces in the Alzheimer's Disease Puzzle? *J. Alzheimer's Dis.* **2013**, *33*, S283–S293. [CrossRef]
300. Roberts, B.R.; Ryan, T.M.; Bush, A.I.; Masters, C.L.; Duce, J.A. The Role of Metallobiology and Amyloid-β Peptides in Alzheimer's Disease. *J. Neurochem.* **2012**, *120*, 149–166. [CrossRef]
301. Tõugu, V.; Tiiman, A.; Palumaa, P. Interactions of Zn(II) and Cu(II) Ions with Alzheimer's Amyloid-Beta Peptide. Metal Ion Binding, Contribution to Fibrillization and Toxicity. *Metallomics* **2011**, *3*, 250–261. [CrossRef]
302. Dahms, S.O.; Könnig, I.; Roeser, D.; Gührs, K.-H.; Mayer, M.C.; Kaden, D.; Multhaup, G.; Than, M.E. Metal Binding Dictates Conformation and Function of the Amyloid Precursor Protein (APP) E2 Domain. *J. Mol. Biol.* **2012**, *416*, 438–452. [CrossRef]
303. Kozin, S.A.; Mezentsev, Y.V.; Kulikova, A.A.; Indeykina, M.I.; Golovin, A.V.; Ivanov, A.S.; Tsvetkov, P.O.; Makarov, A.A. Zinc-Induced Dimerization of the Amyloid-β Metal-Binding Domain 1–16 Is Mediated by Residues 11–14. *Mol. Biosyst.* **2011**, *7*, 1053–1055. [CrossRef]
304. Cheignon, C.; Tomas, M.; Bonnefont-Rousselot, D.; Faller, P.; Hureau, C.; Collin, F. Oxidative Stress and the Amyloid Beta Peptide in Alzheimer's Disease. *Redox Biol.* **2018**, *14*, 450–464. [CrossRef]

305. Girvan, P.; Teng, X.; Brooks, N.J.; Baldwin, G.S.; Ying, L. Redox Kinetics of the Amyloid-β-Cu Complex and Its Biological Implications. *Biochemistry* **2018**, *57*, 6228–6233. [CrossRef]
306. Ayala, A.; Muñoz, M.F.; Argüelles, S. Lipid Peroxidation: Production, Metabolism, and Signaling Mechanisms of Malondialdehyde and 4-Hydroxy-2-Nonenal. *Oxid. Med. Cell Longev.* **2014**, *2014*, 360438. [CrossRef]
307. Lipinski, M.M.; Zheng, B.; Lu, T.; Yan, Z.; Py, B.F.; Ng, A.; Xavier, R.J.; Li, C.; Yankner, B.A.; Scherzer, C.R.; et al. Genome-Wide Analysis Reveals Mechanisms Modulating Autophagy in Normal Brain Aging and in Alzheimer's Disease. *Proc. Natl. Acad. Sci. USA* **2010**, *107*, 14164–14169. [CrossRef]
308. Kaur, U.; Banerjee, P.; Bir, A.; Sinha, M.; Biswas, A.; Chakrabarti, S. Reactive Oxygen Species, Redox Signaling and Neuroinflammation in Alzheimer's Disease: The NF-KB Connection. *Curr. Top. Med. Chem.* **2015**, *15*, 446–457. [CrossRef]
309. Mota, S.I.; Costa, R.O.; Ferreira, I.L.; Santana, I.; Caldeira, G.L.; Padovano, C.; Fonseca, A.C.; Baldeiras, I.; Cunha, C.; Letra, L.; et al. Oxidative Stress Involving Changes in Nrf2 and ER Stress in Early Stages of Alzheimer's Disease. *Biochim. Biophys. Acta BBA Mol. Basis Dis.* **2015**, *1852*, 1428–1441. [CrossRef]
310. Patten, D.A.; Germain, M.; Kelly, M.A.; Slack, R.S. Reactive Oxygen Species: Stuck in the Middle of Neurodegeneration. *J. Alzheimer's Dis.* **2010**, *20*, S357–S367. [CrossRef]
311. Caldeira, G.L.; Ferreira, I.L.; Rego, A.C. Impaired Transcription in Alzheimer's Disease: Key Role in Mitochondrial Dysfunction and Oxidative Stress. *J. Alzheimer's Dis.* **2013**, *34*, 115–131. [CrossRef]
312. Nesi, G.; Sestito, S.; Digiacomo, M.; Rapposelli, S. Oxidative Stress, Mitochondrial Abnormalities and Proteins Deposition: Multitarget Approaches in Alzheimer's Disease. *Curr. Top. Med. Chem.* **2017**, *17*, 3062–3079. [CrossRef] [PubMed]
313. Buccellato, F.R.; D'Anca, M.; Fenoglio, C.; Scarpini, E.; Galimberti, D. Role of Oxidative Damage in Alzheimer's Disease and Neurodegeneration: From Pathogenic Mechanisms to Biomarker Discovery. *Antioxidants* **2021**, *10*, 1353. [CrossRef] [PubMed]
314. Uddin, M.S.; Tewari, D.; Sharma, G.; Kabir, M.T.; Barreto, G.E.; Bin-Jumah, M.N.; Perveen, A.; Abdel-Daim, M.M.; Ashraf, G.M. Molecular Mechanisms of ER Stress and UPR in the Pathogenesis of Alzheimer's Disease. *Mol. Neurobiol.* **2020**, *57*, 2902–2919. [CrossRef] [PubMed]
315. Lane, D.J.R.; Ayton, S.; Bush, A.I. Iron and Alzheimer's Disease: An Update on Emerging Mechanisms. *J. Alzheimer's Dis.* **2018**, *64*, S379–S395. [CrossRef] [PubMed]
316. Sharma, C.; Kim, S.R. Linking Oxidative Stress and Proteinopathy in Alzheimer's Disease. *Antioxidants* **2021**, *10*, 1231. [CrossRef] [PubMed]
317. Zuo, L.; Hemmelgarn, B.T.; Chuang, C.-C.; Best, T.M. The Role of Oxidative Stress-Induced Epigenetic Alterations in Amyloid-β Production in Alzheimer's Disease. *Oxid. Med. Cell Longev.* **2015**, *2015*, 604658. [CrossRef]
318. Lin, H.-C.; Hsieh, H.-M.; Chen, Y.-H.; Hu, M.-L. S-Adenosylhomocysteine Increases Beta-Amyloid Formation in BV-2 Microglial Cells by Increased Expressions of Beta-Amyloid Precursor Protein and Presenilin 1 and by Hypomethylation of These Gene Promoters. *Neurotoxicology* **2009**, *30*, 622–627. [CrossRef]
319. Sung, H.Y.; Choi, E.N.; Ahn Jo, S.; Oh, S.; Ahn, J.-H. Amyloid Protein-Mediated Differential DNA Methylation Status Regulates Gene Expression in Alzheimer's Disease Model Cell Line. *Biochem. Biophys. Res. Commun.* **2011**, *414*, 700–705. [CrossRef]
320. Mouton-Liger, F.; Paquet, C.; Dumurgier, J.; Bouras, C.; Pradier, L.; Gray, F.; Hugon, J. Oxidative Stress Increases BACE1 Protein Levels through Activation of the PKR-EIF2α Pathway. *Biochim. Biophys. Acta* **2012**, *1822*, 885–896. [CrossRef]
321. Ma, T.; Trinh, M.A.; Wexler, A.J.; Bourbon, C.; Gatti, E.; Pierre, P.; Cavener, D.R.; Klann, E. Suppression of EIF2α Kinases Alleviates AD-Related Synaptic Plasticity and Spatial Memory Deficits. *Nat. Neurosci.* **2013**, *16*, 1299–1305. [CrossRef]
322. Oliveira, M.M.; Klann, E. EIF2-Dependent Translation Initiation: Memory Consolidation and Disruption in Alzheimer's Disease. *Semin. Cell Dev. Biol.* **2021**. [CrossRef] [PubMed]
323. Wang, S.-C.; Oelze, B.; Schumacher, A. Age-Specific Epigenetic Drift in Late-Onset Alzheimer's Disease. *PLoS ONE* **2008**, *3*, e2698. [CrossRef] [PubMed]
324. Scarpa, S.; Cavallaro, R.A.; D'Anselmi, F.; Fuso, A. Gene Silencing through Methylation: An Epigenetic Intervention on Alzheimer Disease. *J. Alzheimers Dis.* **2006**, *9*, 407–414. [CrossRef] [PubMed]
325. Lithner, C.U.; Hernandez, C.; Sweatt, J.D.; Nordberg, A. O3-05-05: Epigenetic Effects of Aβ and the Implication on the Pathophysiology in Alzheimer's Disease. *Alzheimer's Dement.* **2011**, *7*, S508. [CrossRef]
326. Marques, S.C.F.; Lemos, R.; Ferreiro, E.; Martins, M.; de Mendonça, A.; Santana, I.; Outeiro, T.F.; Pereira, C.M.F. Epigenetic Regulation of BACE1 in Alzheimer's Disease Patients and in Transgenic Mice. *Neuroscience* **2012**, *220*, 256–266. [CrossRef]
327. Chouliaras, L.; Mastroeni, D.; Delvaux, E.; Grover, A.; Kenis, G.; Hof, P.R.; Steinbusch, H.W.M.; Coleman, P.D.; Rutten, B.P.F.; van den Hove, D.L.A. Consistent Decrease in Global DNA Methylation and Hydroxymethylation in the Hippocampus of Alzheimer's Disease Patients. *Neurobiol. Aging* **2013**, *34*, 2091–2099. [CrossRef]
328. Gu, X.; Sun, J.; Li, S.; Wu, X.; Li, L. Oxidative Stress Induces DNA Demethylation and Histone Acetylation in SH-SY5Y Cells: Potential Epigenetic Mechanisms in Gene Transcription in Aβ Production. *Neurobiol. Aging* **2013**, *34*, 1069–1079. [CrossRef]
329. Luque-Contreras, D.; Carvajal, K.; Toral-Rios, D.; Franco-Bocanegra, D.; Campos-Peña, V. Oxidative Stress and Metabolic Syndrome: Cause or Consequence of Alzheimer's Disease? *Oxidative Med. Cell. Longev.* **2014**, *2014*, e497802. [CrossRef]
330. Massaad, C.A. Neuronal and Vascular Oxidative Stress in Alzheimer's Disease. *Curr. Neuropharmacol.* **2011**, *9*, 662–673. [CrossRef]
331. Hamilton, A.; Holscher, C. The Effect of Ageing on Neurogenesis and Oxidative Stress in the APPswe/PS1deltaE9 Mouse Model of Alzheimer's Disease. *Brain Res.* **2012**, *1449*, 83–93. [CrossRef]

332. Sultana, R.; Mecocci, P.; Mangialasche, F.; Cecchetti, R.; Baglioni, M.; Butterfield, D.A. Increased Protein and Lipid Oxidative Damage in Mitochondria Isolated from Lymphocytes from Patients with Alzheimer's Disease: Insights into the Role of Oxidative Stress in Alzheimer's Disease and Initial Investigations into a Potential Biomarker for This Dementing Disorder. *J. Alzheimer's Dis.* **2011**, *24*, 77–84. [CrossRef]
333. Readnower, R.D.; Sauerbeck, A.D.; Sullivan, P.G. Mitochondria, Amyloid β, and Alzheimer's Disease. *Int. J. Alzheimer's Dis.* **2011**, *2011*, e104545. [CrossRef] [PubMed]
334. Sun, X.; Chen, W.-D.; Wang, Y.-D. β-Amyloid: The Key Peptide in the Pathogenesis of Alzheimer's Disease. *Front. Pharmacol.* **2015**, *6*, 221. [CrossRef] [PubMed]
335. Reddy, P.H.; Tripathi, R.; Troung, Q.; Tirumala, K.; Reddy, T.P.; Anekonda, V.; Shirendeb, U.P.; Calkins, M.J.; Reddy, A.P.; Mao, P.; et al. Abnormal Mitochondrial Dynamics and Synaptic Degeneration as Early Events in Alzheimer's Disease: Implications to Mitochondria-Targeted Antioxidant Therapeutics. *Biochim. Biophys. Acta BBA Mol. Basis Dis.* **2012**, *1822*, 639–649. [CrossRef] [PubMed]
336. Sirk, D.; Zhu, Z.; Wadia, J.S.; Shulyakova, N.; Phan, N.; Fong, J.; Mills, L.R. Chronic Exposure to Sub-Lethal Beta-Amyloid (Abeta) Inhibits the Import of Nuclear-Encoded Proteins to Mitochondria in Differentiated PC12 Cells. *J. Neurochem.* **2007**, *103*, 1989–2003. [CrossRef]
337. Crouch, P.J.; Blake, R.; Duce, J.A.; Ciccotosto, G.D.; Li, Q.X.; Barnham, K.J.; Curtain, C.C.; Cherny, R.A.; Cappai, R.; Dyrks, T.; et al. Copper-Dependent Inhibition of Human Cytochrome c Oxidase by a Dimeric Conformer of Amyloid-Beta(1-42). *J. Neurosci.* **2005**, *25*, 672–679. [CrossRef]
338. Chen, J.X.; Yan, S.D. Amyloid-β-Induced Mitochondrial Dysfunction. *J. Alzheimers Dis.* **2007**, *12*, 177–184. [CrossRef]
339. Reddy, P.H.; Beal, M.F. Amyloid Beta, Mitochondrial Dysfunction and Synaptic Damage: Implications for Cognitive Decline in Aging and Alzheimer's Disease. *Trends Mol. Med.* **2008**, *14*, 45–53. [CrossRef]
340. Ferreira, I.L.; Bajouco, L.M.; Mota, S.I.; Auberson, Y.P.; Oliveira, C.R.; Rego, A.C. Amyloid Beta Peptide 1-42 Disturbs Intracellular Calcium Homeostasis through Activation of GluN2B-Containing N-Methyl-d-Aspartate Receptors in Cortical Cultures. *Cell Calcium.* **2012**, *51*, 95–106. [CrossRef]
341. Shirwany, N.A.; Payette, D.; Xie, J.; Guo, Q. The Amyloid Beta Ion Channel Hypothesis of Alzheimer's Disease. *Neuropsychiatr. Dis. Treat.* **2007**, *3*, 597–612.
342. Magi, S.; Castaldo, P.; Macrì, M.L.; Maiolino, M.; Matteucci, A.; Bastioli, G.; Gratteri, S.; Amoroso, S.; Lariccia, V. Intracellular Calcium Dysregulation: Implications for Alzheimer's Disease. *Biomed. Res. Int.* **2016**, *2016*, 6701324. [CrossRef] [PubMed]
343. Parihar, M.S.; Brewer, G.J. Amyloid Beta as a Modulator of Synaptic Plasticity. *J. Alzheimers Dis.* **2010**, *22*, 741–763. [CrossRef] [PubMed]
344. Granold, M.; Moosmann, B.; Staib-Lasarzik, I.; Arendt, T.; Del Rey, A.; Engelhard, K.; Behl, C.; Hajieva, P. High Membrane Protein Oxidation in the Human Cerebral Cortex. *Redox Biol.* **2015**, *4*, 200–207. [CrossRef] [PubMed]
345. Butterfield, D.A.; Reed, T.; Newman, S.F.; Sultana, R. Roles of Amyloid β-Peptide-Associated Oxidative Stress and Brain Protein Modifications in the Pathogenesis of Alzheimer's Disease and Mild Cognitive Impairment. *Free Radic. Biol. Med.* **2007**, *43*, 658–677. [CrossRef] [PubMed]
346. Rothman, S.M.; Mattson, M.P. Adverse Stress, Hippocampal Networks, and Alzheimer's Disease. *Neuromol. Med.* **2010**, *12*, 56–70. [CrossRef]
347. Venkateshappa, C.; Harish, G.; Mahadevan, A.; Srinivas Bharath, M.M.; Shankar, S.K. Elevated Oxidative Stress and Decreased Antioxidant Function in the Human Hippocampus and Frontal Cortex with Increasing Age: Implications for Neurodegeneration in Alzheimer's Disease. *Neurochem. Res.* **2012**, *37*, 1601–1614. [CrossRef] [PubMed]
348. Müller, W.E.; Eckert, A.; Kurz, C.; Eckert, G.P.; Leuner, K. Mitochondrial Dysfunction: Common Final Pathway in Brain Aging and Alzheimer's Disease—Therapeutic Aspects. *Mol. Neurobiol.* **2010**, *41*, 159–171. [CrossRef]
349. Sivanandam, T.M.; Thakur, M.K. Traumatic Brain Injury: A Risk Factor for Alzheimer's Disease. *Neurosci. Biobehav. Rev.* **2012**, *36*, 1376–1381. [CrossRef]
350. Johnson, V.E.; Stewart, W.; Smith, D.H. Traumatic Brain Injury and Amyloid-β Pathology: A Link to Alzheimer's Disease? *Nat. Rev. Neurosci.* **2010**, *11*, 361–370. [CrossRef]
351. Yiannopoulou, K.G.; Papageorgiou, S.G. Current and Future Treatments in Alzheimer Disease: An Update. *J. Cent. Nerv. Syst. Dis.* **2020**, *12*, 1179573520907397. [CrossRef]
352. Government of Canada, H.C. Drug Product Database Online Query. Available online: https://health-products.canada.ca/dpd-bdpp/info.do?lang=en&code=93258 (accessed on 28 December 2021).
353. Government of Canada, H.C. Drug Product Database Online Query. Available online: https://health-products.canada.ca/dpd-bdpp/info.do?lang=en&code=80954 (accessed on 28 December 2021).
354. Hasselmo, M.E. The Role of Acetylcholine in Learning and Memory. *Curr. Opin. Neurobiol.* **2006**, *16*, 710–715. [CrossRef] [PubMed]
355. Ferreira-Vieira, T.H.; Guimaraes, I.M.; Silva, F.R.; Ribeiro, F.M. Alzheimer's Disease: Targeting the Cholinergic System. *Curr. Neuropharmacol.* **2016**, *14*, 101–115. [CrossRef] [PubMed]
356. Kumar, A.; Gupta, V.; Sharma, S. Donepezil. In *StatPearls*; StatPearls Publishing: Treasure Island, FL, USA, 2021.
357. Müller, T. Rivastigmine in the Treatment of Patients with Alzheimer's Disease. *Neuropsychiatr. Dis. Treat.* **2007**, *3*, 211–218. [CrossRef] [PubMed]

358. Razay, G.; Wilcock, G.K. Galantamine in Alzheimer's Disease. *Exp. Rev. Neurother.* **2008**, *8*, 9–17. [CrossRef]
359. Johnson, J.W.; Kotermanski, S.E. Mechanism of Action of Memantine. *Curr. Opin. Pharm.* **2006**, *6*, 61–67. [CrossRef]
360. Reisberg, B.; Doody, R.; Stöffler, A.; Schmitt, F.; Ferris, S.; Möbius, H.J.; Memantine Study Group. Memantine in Moderate-to-Severe Alzheimer's Disease. *N. Engl. J. Med.* **2003**, *348*, 1333–1341. [CrossRef]
361. Deardorff, W.J.; Grossberg, G.T. A Fixed-Dose Combination of Memantine Extended-Release and Donepezil in the Treatment of Moderate-to-Severe Alzheimer's Disease. *Drug Des. Dev.* **2016**, *10*, 3267–3279. [CrossRef]
362. InformedHealth.org. *Non-Drug Interventions for Alzheimer's Disease*; Institute for Quality and Efficiency in Health Care (IQWiG): Cologne, Germany, 2017.
363. Non-pharmacological Treatment of Alzheimer's | IntechOpen. Available online: https://www.intechopen.com/chapters/65852 (accessed on 28 December 2021).
364. Bastrup, J.; Hansen, K.H.; Poulsen, T.B.G.; Kastaniegaard, K.; Asuni, A.A.; Christensen, S.; Belling, D.; Helboe, L.; Stensballe, A.; Volbracht, C. Anti-Aβ Antibody Aducanumab Regulates the Proteome of Senile Plaques and Closely Surrounding Tissue in a Transgenic Mouse Model of Alzheimer's Disease. *J. Alzheimer's Dis.* **2021**, *79*, 249–265. [CrossRef]
365. Sevigny, J.; Chiao, P.; Bussière, T.; Weinreb, P.H.; Williams, L.; Maier, M.; Dunstan, R.; Salloway, S.; Chen, T.; Ling, Y.; et al. The Antibody Aducanumab Reduces Aβ Plaques in Alzheimer's Disease. *Nature* **2016**, *537*, 50–56. [CrossRef]
366. Leinenga, G.; Koh, W.K.; Götz, J. A Comparative Study of the Effects of Aducanumab and Scanning Ultrasound on Amyloid Plaques and Behavior in the APP23 Mouse Model of Alzheimer Disease. *Alzheimers Res.* **2021**, *13*, 76. [CrossRef]
367. Knopman, D.S.; Jones, D.T.; Greicius, M.D. Failure to Demonstrate Efficacy of Aducanumab: An Analysis of the EMERGE and ENGAGE Trials as Reported by Biogen, December 2019. *Alzheimers Dement.* **2021**, *17*, 696–701. [CrossRef] [PubMed]
368. Boonruamkaew, P.; Chonpathompikunlert, P.; Vong, L.B.; Sakaue, S.; Tomidokoro, Y.; Ishii, K.; Tamaoka, A.; Nagasaki, Y. Chronic Treatment with a Smart Antioxidative Nanoparticle for Inhibition of Amyloid Plaque Propagation in Tg2576 Mouse Model of Alzheimer's Disease. *Sci. Rep.* **2017**, *7*, 3785. [CrossRef] [PubMed]
369. El Sayed, N.S.; Ghoneum, M.H. Antia, a Natural Antioxidant Product, Attenuates Cognitive Dysfunction in Streptozotocin-Induced Mouse Model of Sporadic Alzheimer's Disease by Targeting the Amyloidogenic, Inflammatory, Autophagy, and Oxidative Stress Pathways. *Oxid. Med. Cell Longev.* **2020**, *2020*, 4386562. [CrossRef] [PubMed]
370. Nicolakakis, N.; Aboulkassim, T.; Ongali, B.; Lecrux, C.; Fernandes, P.; Rosa-Neto, P.; Tong, X.-K.; Hamel, E. Complete Rescue of Cerebrovascular Function in Aged Alzheimer's Disease Transgenic Mice by Antioxidants and Pioglitazone, a Peroxisome Proliferator-Activated Receptor Gamma Agonist. *J. Neurosci.* **2008**, *28*, 9287–9296. [CrossRef] [PubMed]
371. Veurink, G.; Perry, G.; Singh, S.K. Role of Antioxidants and a Nutrient Rich Diet in Alzheimer's Disease. *Open Biol.* **2020**, *10*, 200084. [CrossRef] [PubMed]
372. Mielech, A.; Puścion-Jakubik, A.; Markiewicz-Żukowska, R.; Socha, K. Vitamins in Alzheimer's Disease—Review of the Latest Reports. *Nutrients* **2020**, *12*, 3458. [CrossRef]
373. Fenech, M. Vitamins Associated with Brain Aging, Mild Cognitive Impairment, and Alzheimer Disease: Biomarkers, Epidemiological and Experimental Evidence, Plausible Mechanisms, and Knowledge Gaps. *Adv. Nutr.* **2017**, *8*, 958–970. [CrossRef]
374. Antibody–Drug Conjugates: A Comprehensive Review | Molecular Cancer Research. Available online: https://mcr.aacrjournals.org/content/18/1/3 (accessed on 28 December 2021).
375. Barroso-Sousa, R.; Tolaney, S.M. Clinical Development of New Antibody–Drug Conjugates in Breast Cancer: To Infinity and Beyond. *BioDrugs* **2021**, *35*, 159–174. [CrossRef]
376. Li, B.T.; Smit, E.F.; Goto, Y.; Nakagawa, K.; Udagawa, H.; Mazières, J.; Nagasaka, M.; Bazhenova, L.; Saltos, A.N.; Felip, E.; et al. DESTINY-Lung01 Trial Investigators. Trastuzumab Deruxtecan in HER2-Mutant Non-Small-Cell Lung Cancer. *N. Engl. J. Med.* **2021**, *386*, 241–251. [CrossRef]
377. Calo, C.A.; O'Malley, D.M. Antibody-Drug Conjugates for the Treatment of Ovarian Cancer. *Exp. Opin. Biol.* **2021**, *21*, 875–887. [CrossRef]
378. Prasad, S.; Gupta, S.C.; Pandey, M.K.; Tyagi, A.K.; Deb, L. Oxidative Stress and Cancer: Advances and Challenges. *Oxidative Med. Cell. Longev.* **2016**, *2016*, e5010423. [CrossRef] [PubMed]
379. Sosa, V.; Moliné, T.; Somoza, R.; Paciucci, R.; Kondoh, H.; LLeonart, M.E. Oxidative Stress and Cancer: An Overview. *Ageing Res. Rev.* **2013**, *12*, 376–390. [CrossRef] [PubMed]
380. Reuter, S.; Gupta, S.C.; Chaturvedi, M.M.; Aggarwal, B.B. Oxidative Stress, Inflammation, and Cancer: How Are They Linked? *Free Radic. Biol. Med.* **2010**, *49*, 1603–1616. [CrossRef] [PubMed]
381. Andrisic, L.; Dudzik, D.; Barbas, C.; Milkovic, L.; Grune, T.; Zarkovic, N. Short Overview on Metabolomics Approach to Study Pathophysiology of Oxidative Stress in Cancer. *Redox Biol.* **2018**, *14*, 47–58. [CrossRef]
382. Barrera, G. Oxidative Stress and Lipid Peroxidation Products in Cancer Progression and Therapy. *ISRN Oncol.* **2012**, *2012*, 1–21. [CrossRef]
383. Thanan, R.; Oikawa, S.; Hiraku, Y.; Ohnishi, S.; Ma, N.; Pinlaor, S.; Yongvanit, P.; Kawanishi, S.; Murata, M. Oxidative Stress and Its Significant Roles in Neurodegenerative Diseases and Cancer. *Int. J. Mol. Sci.* **2015**, *16*, 193–217. [CrossRef]
384. Hayes, J.D.; Dinkova-Kostova, A.T.; Tew, K.D. Oxidative Stress in Cancer. *Cancer Cell* **2020**, *38*, 167–197. [CrossRef]
385. Zou, Z.; Chang, H.; Li, H.; Wang, S. Induction of Reactive Oxygen Species: An Emerging Approach for Cancer Therapy. *Apoptosis* **2017**, *22*, 1321–1335. [CrossRef]

386. Chen, P.; Luo, X.; Nie, P.; Wu, B.; Xu, W.; Shi, X.; Chang, H.; Li, B.; Yu, X.; Zou, Z. CQ Synergistically Sensitizes Human Colorectal Cancer Cells to SN-38/CPT-11 through Lysosomal and Mitochondrial Apoptotic Pathway via P53-ROS Cross-Talk. *Free Radic. Biol. Med.* **2017**, *104*, 280–297. [CrossRef]
387. Dewangan, J.; Tandon, D.; Srivastava, S.; Verma, A.K.; Yapuri, A.; Rath, S.K. Novel Combination of Salinomycin and Resveratrol Synergistically Enhances the Anti-Proliferative and pro-Apoptotic Effects on Human Breast Cancer Cells. *Apoptosis* **2017**, *22*, 1246–1259. [CrossRef]
388. Zhao, Y.; Qu, T.; Wang, P.; Li, X.; Qiang, J.; Xia, Z.; Duan, H.; Huang, J.; Zhu, L. Unravelling the Relationship between Macroautophagy and Mitochondrial ROS in Cancer Therapy. *Apoptosis* **2016**, *21*, 517–531. [CrossRef] [PubMed]
389. Zhang, Y.; Su, S.S.; Zhao, S.; Yang, Z.; Zhong, C.-Q.; Chen, X.; Cai, Q.; Yang, Z.-H.; Huang, D.; Wu, R.; et al. RIP1 Autophosphorylation Is Promoted by Mitochondrial ROS and Is Essential for RIP3 Recruitment into Necrosome. *Nat. Commun.* **2017**, *8*, 14329. [CrossRef] [PubMed]
390. Dixon, S.J.; Lemberg, K.M.; Lamprecht, M.R.; Skouta, R.; Zaitsev, E.M.; Gleason, C.E.; Patel, D.N.; Bauer, A.J.; Cantley, A.M.; Yang, W.S.; et al. Ferroptosis: An Iron-Dependent Form of Nonapoptotic Cell Death. *Cell* **2012**, *149*, 1060–1072. [CrossRef] [PubMed]
391. Yang, Y.; Guo, R.; Tian, X.; Zhang, Z.; Zhang, P.; Li, C.; Feng, Z. Synergistic Anti-Tumor Activity of Nimotuzumab in Combination with Trastuzumab in HER2-Positive Breast Cancer. *Biochem. Biophys. Res. Commun.* **2017**, *489*, 523–527. [CrossRef] [PubMed]
392. Santoro, V.; Jia, R.; Thompson, H.; Nijhuis, A.; Jeffery, R.; Kiakos, K.; Silver, A.R.; Hartley, J.A.; Hochhauser, D. Role of Reactive Oxygen Species in the Abrogation of Oxaliplatin Activity by Cetuximab in Colorectal Cancer. *JNCI J. Natl. Cancer Inst.* **2016**, *108*, djv394. [CrossRef]
393. Combined Oridonin with Cetuximab Treatment Shows Synergistic Anticancer Effects on Laryngeal Squamous Cell Carcinoma: Involvement of Inhibition of EGFR and Activation of Reactive Oxygen Species-Mediated JNK Pathway. Available online: https://www.spandidos-publications.com/10.3892/ijo.2016.3696 (accessed on 29 December 2021).
394. Fack, F.; Espedal, H.; Keunen, O.; Golebiewska, A.; Obad, N.; Harter, P.N.; Mittelbronn, M.; Bähr, O.; Weyerbrock, A.; Stuhr, L.; et al. Bevacizumab Treatment Induces Metabolic Adaptation toward Anaerobic Metabolism in Glioblastomas. *Acta Neuropathol.* **2015**, *129*, 115–131. [CrossRef] [PubMed]
395. Guo, X.; Li, D.; Sun, K.; Wang, J.; Liu, Y.; Song, J.; Zhao, Q.; Zhang, S.; Deng, W.; Zhao, X.; et al. Inhibition of Autophagy Enhances Anticancer Effects of Bevacizumab in Hepatocarcinoma. *J. Mol. Med.* **2013**, *91*, 473–483. [CrossRef]
396. Leone, A.; Roca, M.S.; Ciardiello, C.; Terranova-Barberio, M.; Vitagliano, C.; Ciliberto, G.; Mancini, R.; Di Gennaro, E.; Bruzzese, F.; Budillon, A. Vorinostat Synergizes with EGFR Inhibitors in NSCLC Cells by Increasing ROS via Up-Regulation of the Major Mitochondrial Porin VDAC1 and Modulation of the c-Myc-NRF2-KEAP1 Pathway. *Free Radic. Biol. Med.* **2015**, *89*, 287–299. [CrossRef]
397. Abounader, R.; Schiff, D. The Blood-Brain Barrier Limits the Therapeutic Efficacy of Antibody-Drug Conjugates in Glioblastoma. *Neuro. Oncol.* **2021**, *23*, 1993–1994. [CrossRef]
398. Frontiers | Antibody Drug Conjugates in Glioblastoma—Is There a Future for Them? | Oncology. Available online: https://www.frontiersin.org/articles/10.3389/fonc.2021.718590/full (accessed on 28 December 2021).
399. Banks, W.A. Characteristics of Compounds That Cross the Blood-Brain Barrier. *BMC Neurol.* **2009**, *9*, S3. [CrossRef]
400. Cavaco, M.; Frutos, S.; Oliete, P.; Valle, J.; Andreu, D.; Castanho, M.A.R.B.; Vila-Perelló, M.; Neves, V. Conjugation of a Blood Brain Barrier Peptide Shuttle to an Fc Domain for Brain Delivery of Therapeutic Biomolecules. *ACS Med. Chem. Lett.* **2021**, *12*, 1663–1668. [CrossRef]
401. Oldendorf, W.H. Brain Uptake of Radiolabeled Amino Acids, Amines, and Hexoses after Arterial Injection. *Am. J. Physiol.* **1971**, *221*, 1629–1639. [CrossRef] [PubMed]
402. Taylor, E.M. The Impact of Efflux Transporters in the Brain on the Development of Drugs for CNS Disorders. *Clin. Pharm.* **2002**, *41*, 81–92. [CrossRef] [PubMed]
403. Deane, R.; Sagare, A.; Zlokovic, B. The Role of the Cell Surface LRP and Soluble LRP in Blood-Brain Barrier Abeta Clearance in Alzheimers Disease. *Curr. Pharm. Des.* **2008**, *14*, 1601–1605. [CrossRef]
404. Frontiers | Relationship Between Amyloid-β Deposition and Blood–Brain Barrier Dysfunction in Alzheimer's Disease | Cellular Neuroscience. Available online: https://www.frontiersin.org/articles/10.3389/fncel.2021.695479/full (accessed on 28 December 2021).
405. Sarma, B.K.; Mugesh, G. Glutathione Peroxidase (GPx)-like Antioxidant Activity of the Organoselenium Drug Ebselen: Unexpected Complications with Thiol Exchange Reactions. *J. Am. Chem. Soc.* **2005**, *127*, 11477–11485. [CrossRef] [PubMed]
406. Pearson, J.K.; Boyd, R.J. Effect of Substituents on the GPx-like Activity of Ebselen: Steric versus Electronic. *J. Phys. Chem. A* **2008**, *112*, 1013–1017. [CrossRef]
407. Asbaghi, O.; Zakeri, N.; Rezaei Kelishadi, M.; Naeini, F.; Mirzadeh, E. Selenium Supplementation and Oxidative Stress: A Review. *PharmaNutrition* **2021**, *17*, 100263. [CrossRef]
408. Xie, Y.; Tan, Y.; Zheng, Y.; Du, X.; Liu, Q. Ebselen Ameliorates β-Amyloid Pathology, Tau Pathology, and Cognitive Impairment in Triple-Transgenic Alzheimer's Disease Mice. *J. Biol. Inorg. Chem.* **2017**, *22*, 851–865. [CrossRef]
409. Luo, Z.; Sheng, J.; Sun, Y.; Lu, C.; Yan, J.; Liu, A.; Luo, H.-B.; Huang, L.; Li, X. Synthesis and Evaluation of Multi-Target-Directed Ligands against Alzheimer's Disease Based on the Fusion of Donepezil and Ebselen. *J. Med. Chem.* **2013**, *56*, 9089–9099. [CrossRef]

410. Terra, B.; da Silva, P.; Tramarin, A.; Franco, L.; da Cunha, E.; Macedo Junior, F.; Ramalho, T.; Bartolini, M.; Bolognesi, M.; de Fátima, Â. Two Novel Donepezil-Lipoic Acid Hybrids: Synthesis, Anticholinesterase and Antioxidant Activities and Theoretical Studies. *J. Braz. Chem. Soc.* **2017**, *29*, 738–747. [CrossRef]
411. Pi, R.; Mao, X.; Chao, X.; Cheng, Z.; Liu, M.; Duan, X.; Ye, M.; Chen, X.; Mei, Z.; Liu, P.; et al. Tacrine-6-Ferulic Acid, a Novel Multifunctional Dimer, Inhibits Amyloid-β-Mediated Alzheimer's Disease-Associated Pathogenesis In Vitro and In Vivo. *PLoS ONE* **2012**, *7*, e31921. [CrossRef] [PubMed]
412. Pérez-Cruz, K.; Moncada-Basualto, M.; Morales-Valenzuela, J.; Barriga-González, G.; Navarrete-Encina, P.; Núñez-Vergara, L.; Squella, J.A.; Olea-Azar, C. Synthesis and Antioxidant Study of New Polyphenolic Hybrid-Coumarins. *Arab. J. Chem.* **2018**, *11*, 525–537. [CrossRef]
413. Trang, N.V.; Thuy, P.T.; Thanh, D.T.M.; Son, N.T. Benzofuran–Stilbene Hybrid Compounds: An Antioxidant Assessment—A DFT Study. *RSC Adv.* **2021**, *11*, 12971–12980. [CrossRef]
414. Zhao, Y.; Zhao, B. Oxidative Stress and the Pathogenesis of Alzheimer's Disease. *Oxidative Med. Cell. Longev.* **2013**, *2013*, e316523. [CrossRef] [PubMed]
415. Sano, M.; Ernesto, C.; Thomas, R.G.; Klauber, M.R.; Schafer, K.; Grundman, M.; Woodbury, P.; Growdon, J.; Cotman, C.W.; Pfeiffer, E.; et al. A Controlled Trial of Selegiline, Alpha-Tocopherol, or Both as Treatment for Alzheimer's Disease. The Alzheimer's Disease Cooperative Study. *N. Engl. J. Med.* **1997**, *336*, 1216–1222. [CrossRef] [PubMed]
416. Petersen, R.C.; Thomas, R.G.; Grundman, M.; Bennett, D.; Doody, R.; Ferris, S.; Galasko, D.; Jin, S.; Kaye, J.; Levey, A.; et al. Alzheimer's Disease Cooperative Study Group. Vitamin E and Donepezil for the Treatment of Mild Cognitive Impairment. *N. Engl. J. Med.* **2005**, *352*, 2379–2388. [CrossRef]
417. Dysken, M.W.; Sano, M.; Asthana, S.; Vertrees, J.E.; Pallaki, M.; Llorente, M.; Love, S.; Schellenberg, G.D.; McCarten, J.R.; Malphurs, J.; et al. Effect of Vitamin E and Memantine on Functional Decline in Alzheimer Disease: The TEAM-AD VA Cooperative Randomized Trial. *JAMA* **2014**, *311*, 33–44. [CrossRef]
418. Galasko, D.R.; Peskind, E.; Clark, C.M.; Quinn, J.F.; Ringman, J.M.; Jicha, G.A.; Cotman, C.; Cottrell, B.; Montine, T.J.; Thomas, R.G.; et al. Alzheimer's Disease Cooperative Study. Antioxidants for Alzheimer Disease: A Randomized Clinical Trial with Cerebrospinal Fluid Biomarker Measures. *Arch. Neurol.* **2012**, *69*, 836–841. [CrossRef]
419. Aisen, P.S.; Schneider, L.S.; Sano, M.; Diaz-Arrastia, R.; van Dyck, C.H.; Weiner, M.F.; Bottiglieri, T.; Jin, S.; Stokes, K.T.; Thomas, R.G.; et al. Alzheimer Disease Cooperative Study. High-Dose B Vitamin Supplementation and Cognitive Decline in Alzheimer Disease: A Randomized Controlled Trial. *JAMA* **2008**, *300*, 1774–1783. [CrossRef]
420. Annweiler, C.; Fantino, B.; Parot-Schinkel, E.; Thiery, S.; Gautier, J.; Beauchet, O. Alzheimer's Disease–Input of Vitamin D with MEmantine Assay (AD-IDEA Trial): Study Protocol for a Randomized Controlled Trial. *Trials* **2011**, *12*, 230. [CrossRef]
421. Remington, R.; Bechtel, C.; Larsen, D.; Samar, A.; Doshanjh, L.; Fishman, P.; Luo, Y.; Smyers, K.; Page, R.; Morrell, C.; et al. A Phase II Randomized Clinical Trial of a Nutritional Formulation for Cognition and Mood in Alzheimer's Disease. *J. Alzheimers Dis.* **2015**, *45*, 395–405. [CrossRef] [PubMed]
422. Zhu, C.W.; Grossman, H.; Neugroschl, J.; Parker, S.; Burden, A.; Luo, X.; Sano, M. A Randomized, Double-Blind, Placebo-Controlled Trial of Resveratrol with Glucose and Malate (RGM) to Slow the Progression of Alzheimer's Disease: A Pilot Study. *Alzheimers Dement.* **2018**, *4*, 609–616. [CrossRef] [PubMed]
423. Moussa, C.; Hebron, M.; Huang, X.; Ahn, J.; Rissman, R.A.; Aisen, P.S.; Turner, R.S. Resveratrol Regulates Neuro-Inflammation and Induces Adaptive Immunity in Alzheimer's Disease. *J. Neuroinflamm.* **2017**, *14*, 1. [CrossRef]
424. Ringman, J.M.; Frautschy, S.A.; Teng, E.; Begum, A.N.; Bardens, J.; Beigi, M.; Gylys, K.H.; Badmaev, V.; Heath, D.D.; Apostolova, L.G.; et al. Oral Curcumin for Alzheimer's Disease: Tolerability and Efficacy in a 24-Week Randomized, Double Blind, Placebo-Controlled Study. *Alzheimers Res.* **2012**, *4*, 43. [CrossRef]
425. Baum, L.; Lam, C.W.K.; Cheung, S.K.-K.; Kwok, T.; Lui, V.; Tsoh, J.; Lam, L.; Leung, V.; Hui, E.; Ng, C.; et al. Six-Month Randomized, Placebo-Controlled, Double-Blind, Pilot Clinical Trial of Curcumin in Patients with Alzheimer Disease. *J. Clin. Psychopharmacol.* **2008**, *28*, 110–113. [CrossRef]
426. Pilot Study to Investigate the Safety and Feasibility of Senolytic Therapy to Modulate Progression of Alzheimer's Disease (SToMP-AD). ClinicalTrials.gov Identifier: NCT04063124. Available online: https://www.clinicaltrials.gov/ct2/show/NCT04063124 (accessed on 18 December 2021).
427. Phase II Clinical Trial to Evaluate the Safety and Feasibility of Senolytic Therapy in Alzheimer's Disease. ClinicalTrials.gov Identifier: NCT04685590. Available online: https://www.clinicaltrials.gov/ct2/show/NCT04685590 (accessed on 18 December 2021).
428. Sunphenon EGCg (Epigallocatechin-Gallate) in the Early Stage of Alzheimer´s Disease. ClinicalTrials.gov Identifier: NCT00951834. Available online: https://www.clinicaltrials.gov/ct2/show/NCT00951834 (accessed on 18 December 2021).
429. Prevention of Cognitive Decline in ApoE4 Carriers with Subjective Cognitive Decline After EGCG and a Multimodal Intervention. ClinicalTrials.gov Identifier: NCT03978052. Available online: https://www.clinicaltrials.gov/ct2/show/NCT03978052 (accessed on 18 December 2021).
430. Vina, J. Effect of Activation of the Receptor PPARg/RXR as a Possible Treatment for Alzheimer's Disease. Role of Genistein. Clinical Trial Registration NCT01982578; clinicaltrials.gov, 2021. Available online: https://www.clinicaltrials.gov/ct2/show/NCT01982578 (accessed on 18 December 2021).

431. Gleason, C.E.; Fischer, B.L.; Dowling, N.M.; Setchell, K.D.R.; Atwood, C.S.; Carlsson, C.M.; Asthana, S. Cognitive Effects of Soy Isoflavones in Patients with Alzheimer's Disease. *J. Alzheimers. Dis.* **2015**, *47*, 1009–1019. [CrossRef]
432. Shinto, L.; Quinn, J.; Montine, T.; Dodge, H.H.; Woodward, W.; Baldauf-Wagner, S.; Waichunas, D.; Bumgarner, L.; Bourdette, D.; Silbert, L.; et al. A Randomized Placebo-Controlled Pilot Trial of Omega-3 Fatty Acids and Alpha Lipoic Acid in Alzheimer's Disease. *J. Alzheimers Dis.* **2014**, *38*, 111–120. [CrossRef]
433. Treatment with Copper in Patients with Mild Alzheimer´s Dementia—Full Text View—ClinicalTrials.gov. Available online: https://clinicaltrials.gov/ct2/show/NCT00608946 (accessed on 28 December 2021).
434. Kryscio, R.J.; Abner, E.L.; Caban-Holt, A.; Lovell, M.; Goodman, P.; Darke, A.K.; Yee, M.; Crowley, J.; Schmitt, F.A. Association of Antioxidant Supplement Use and Dementia in the Prevention of Alzheimer's Disease by Vitamin E and Selenium Trial (PREADViSE). *JAMA Neurol.* **2017**, *74*, 567–573. [CrossRef]
435. Morris, M.C.; Evans, D.A.; Bienias, J.L.; Tangney, C.C.; Bennett, D.A.; Aggarwal, N.; Wilson, R.S.; Scherr, P.A. Dietary Intake of Antioxidant Nutrients and the Risk of Incident Alzheimer Disease in a Biracial Community Study. *JAMA* **2002**, *287*, 3230–3237. [CrossRef]
436. Grundman, M.; Grundman, M.; Delaney, P. Antioxidant Strategies for Alzheimer's Disease. *Proc. Nutr. Soc.* **2002**, *61*, 191–202. [CrossRef]
437. Zandi, P.P.; Anthony, J.C.; Khachaturian, A.S.; Stone, S.V.; Gustafson, D.; Tschanz, J.T.; Norton, M.C.; Welsh-Bohmer, K.A.; Breitner, J.C.S.; Cache County Study Group. Reduced Risk of Alzheimer Disease in Users of Antioxidant Vitamin Supplements: The Cache County Study. *Arch. Neurol.* **2004**, *61*, 82–88. [CrossRef]
438. Sung, S.; Yao, Y.; Uryu, K.; Yang, H.; Lee, V.M.-Y.; Trojanowski, J.Q.; Praticò, D. Early Vitamin E Supplementation in Young but Not Aged Mice Reduces Abeta Levels and Amyloid Deposition in a Transgenic Model of Alzheimer's Disease. *FASEB J.* **2004**, *18*, 323–325. [CrossRef]
439. Nakashima, H.; Ishihara, T.; Yokota, O.; Terada, S.; Trojanowski, J.Q.; Lee, V.M.-Y.; Kuroda, S. Effects of Alpha-Tocopherol on an Animal Model of Tauopathies. *Free Radic. Biol. Med.* **2004**, *37*, 176–186. [CrossRef]
440. Giraldo, E.; Lloret, A.; Fuchsberger, T.; Viña, J. Aβ and Tau Toxicities in Alzheimer's Are Linked via Oxidative Stress-Induced P38 Activation: Protective Role of Vitamin E. *Redox Biol.* **2014**, *2*, 873–877. [CrossRef]
441. Veinbergs, I.; Mallory, M.; Sagara, Y.; Masliah, E. Vitamin E Supplementation Prevents Spatial Learning Deficits and Dendritic Alterations in Aged Apolipoprotein E-Deficient Mice. *Eur. J. Neurosci.* **2000**, *12*, 4541–4546.
442. Ishihara, Y.; Itoh, K.; Mitsuda, Y.; Shimada, T.; Kubota, T.; Kato, C.; Song, S.Y.; Kobayashi, Y.; Mori-Yasumoto, K.; Sekita, S.; et al. Involvement of Brain Oxidation in the Cognitive Impairment in a Triple Transgenic Mouse Model of Alzheimer's Disease: Noninvasive Measurement of the Brain Redox State by Magnetic Resonance Imaging. *Free Radic. Res.* **2013**, *47*, 731–739. [CrossRef]
443. Moore, J.J.; Saadabadi, A. Selegiline. In *StatPearls*; StatPearls Publishing: Treasure Island, FL, USA, 2021.
444. Filip, V.; Kolibás, E. Selegiline in the Treatment of Alzheimer's Disease: A Long-Term Randomized Placebo-Controlled Trial. Czech and Slovak Senile Dementia of Alzheimer Type Study Group. *J. Psychiatry Neurosci.* **1999**, *24*, 234–243.
445. Birks, J.; Flicker, L. Selegiline for Alzheimer's Disease. *Cochrane Database Syst. Rev.* **2003**, CD000442. [CrossRef]
446. Calderón-Ospina, C.A.; Nava-Mesa, M.O. B Vitamins in the Nervous System: Current Knowledge of the Biochemical Modes of Action and Synergies of Thiamine, Pyridoxine, and Cobalamin. *CNS Neurosci.* **2019**, *26*, 5–13. [CrossRef]
447. Kim, H.; Kim, G.; Jang, W.; Kim, S.Y.; Chang, N. Association between Intake of B Vitamins and Cognitive Function in Elderly Koreans with Cognitive Impairment. *Nutr. J.* **2014**, *13*, 118. [CrossRef]
448. Morris, M.S. Homocysteine and Alzheimer's Disease. *Lancet Neurol.* **2003**, *2*, 425–428. [CrossRef]
449. Yazdi, D.S.; Bar-Yosef, D.L.; Adsi, H.; Kreiser, T.; Sigal, S.; Bera, S.; Zaguri, D.; Shaham-Niv, S.; Oluwatoba, D.S.; Levy, D.; et al. Homocysteine Fibrillar Assemblies Display Cross-Talk with Alzheimer's Disease β-Amyloid Polypeptide. *Proc. Natl. Acad. Sci. USA* **2021**, *118*, e2017575118C. [CrossRef]
450. Smith, A.D.; Refsum, H.; Bottiglieri, T.; Fenech, M.; Hooshmand, B.; McCaddon, A.; Miller, J.W.; Rosenberg, I.H.; Obeid, R. Homocysteine and Dementia: An International Consensus Statement1. *J. Alzheimers Dis.* **2018**, *62*, 561–570. [CrossRef]
451. Seshadri, S.; Beiser, A.; Selhub, J.; Jacques, P.F.; Rosenberg, I.H.; D'Agostino, R.B.; Wilson, P.W.F.; Wolf, P.A. Plasma Homocysteine as a Risk Factor for Dementia and Alzheimer's Disease. *N. Engl. J. Med.* **2002**, *346*, 476–483. [CrossRef]
452. Strain, J.J.; Dowey, L.; Ward, M.; Pentieva, K.; McNulty, H. B-Vitamins, Homocysteine Metabolism and CVD. *Proc. Nutr. Soc.* **2004**, *63*, 597–603. [CrossRef]
453. Remington, R.; Chan, A.; Paskavitz, J.; Shea, T.B. Efficacy of a Vitamin/Nutriceutical Formulation for Moderate-Stage to Later-Stage Alzheimer's Disease: A Placebo-Controlled Pilot Study. *Am. J. Alzheimers Dis. Other Demen.* **2009**, *24*, 27–33. [CrossRef]
454. Liu, C.-C.; Kanekiyo, T.; Xu, H.; Bu, G. Apolipoprotein E and Alzheimer Disease: Risk, Mechanisms, and Therapy. *Nat. Rev. Neurol.* **2013**, *9*, 106–118. [CrossRef]
455. Lobo, V.; Patil, A.; Phatak, A.; Chandra, N. Free Radicals, Antioxidants and Functional Foods: Impact on Human Health. *Pharm. Rev.* **2010**, *4*, 118–126. [CrossRef]
456. Prasad, K.N.; Hovland, A.R.; Cole, W.C.; Prasad, K.C.; Nahreini, P.; Edwards-Prasad, J.; Andreatta, C.P. Multiple Antioxidants in the Prevention and Treatment of Alzheimer Disease: Analysis of Biologic Rationale. *Clin. Neuropharmacol.* **2000**, *23*, 2–13. [CrossRef]

457. Salehi, B.; Martorell, M.; Arbiser, J.L.; Sureda, A.; Martins, N.; Maurya, P.K.; Sharifi-Rad, M.; Kumar, P.; Sharifi-Rad, J. Antioxidants: Positive or Negative Actors? *Biomolecules* **2018**, *8*, 124. [CrossRef]
458. Figueira, I.; Garcia, G.; Pimpão, R.C.; Terrasso, A.P.; Costa, I.; Almeida, A.F.; Tavares, L.; Pais, T.F.; Pinto, P.; Ventura, M.R.; et al. Polyphenols Journey through Blood-Brain Barrier towards Neuronal Protection. *Sci. Rep.* **2017**, *7*, 11456. [CrossRef] [PubMed]
459. Hall, E.D.; Andrus, P.K.; Smith, S.L.; Fleck, T.J.; Scherch, H.M.; Lutzke, B.S.; Sawada, G.A.; Althaus, J.S.; Vonvoigtlander, P.F.; Padbury, G.E.; et al. Pyrrolopyrimidines: Novel Brain-Penetrating Antioxidants with Neuroprotective Activity in Brain Injury and Ischemia Models. *J. Pharm. Exp.* **1997**, *281*, 895–904.
460. Agus, D.B.; Gambhir, S.S.; Pardridge, W.M.; Spielholz, C.; Baselga, J.; Vera, J.C.; Golde, D.W. Vitamin C Crosses the Blood-Brain Barrier in the Oxidized Form through the Glucose Transporters. *J. Clin. Investig.* **1997**, *100*, 2842–2848. [CrossRef] [PubMed]
461. Spector, R.; Johanson, C.E. Vitamin Transport and Homeostasis in Mammalian Brain: Focus on Vitamins B and E. *J. Neurochem.* **2007**, *103*, 425–438. [CrossRef]
462. Figueira, I.; Tavares, L.; Jardim, C.; Costa, I.; Terrasso, A.P.; Almeida, A.F.; Govers, C.; Mes, J.J.; Gardner, R.; Becker, J.D.; et al. Blood–Brain Barrier Transport and Neuroprotective Potential of Blackberry-Digested Polyphenols: An in Vitro Study. *Eur. J. Nutr.* **2019**, *58*, 113–130. [CrossRef] [PubMed]
463. Milbury, P.E.; Kalt, W. Xenobiotic Metabolism and Berry Flavonoid Transport across the Blood-Brain Barrier. *J. Agric. Food Chem.* **2010**, *58*, 3950–3956. [CrossRef]
464. Teleanu, D.M.; Negut, I.; Grumezescu, V.; Grumezescu, A.M.; Teleanu, R.I. Nanomaterials for Drug Delivery to the Central Nervous System. *Nanomaterials* **2019**, *9*, 371. [CrossRef] [PubMed]
465. Klyachko, N.L.; Manickam, D.S.; Brynskikh, A.M.; Uglanova, S.V.; Li, S.; Higginbotham, S.M.; Bronich, T.K.; Batrakova, E.V.; Kabanov, A.V. Cross-Linked Antioxidant Nanozymes for Improved Delivery to CNS. *Nanomedicine* **2012**, *8*, 119–129. [CrossRef]
466. Khalil, I.; Yehye, W.A.; Etxeberria, A.E.; Alhadi, A.A.; Dezfooli, S.M.; Julkapli, N.B.M.; Basirun, W.J.; Seyfoddin, A. Nanoantioxidants: Recent Trends in Antioxidant Delivery Applications. *Antioxidants* **2019**, *9*, 24. [CrossRef]

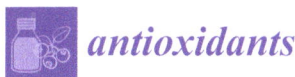

Review

Mechanistic Basis and Clinical Evidence for the Applications of Nicotinamide (Niacinamide) to Control Skin Aging and Pigmentation

Yong Chool Boo

Department of Molecular Medicine, School of Medicine, BK21 Plus KNU Biomedical Convergence Program, Cell and Matrix Research Institute, Kyungpook National University, Daegu 41944, Korea; ycboo@knu.ac.kr; Tel.: +82-53-420-4946

Abstract: Vitamin B3 (nicotinic acid, niacin) deficiency causes the systemic disease pellagra, which leads to dermatitis, diarrhea, dementia, and possibly death depending on its severity and duration. Vitamin B3 is used in the synthesis of the NAD^+ family of coenzymes, contributing to cellular energy metabolism and defense systems. Although nicotinamide (niacinamide) is primarily used as a nutritional supplement for vitamin B3, its pharmaceutical and cosmeceutical uses have been extensively explored. In this review, we discuss the biological activities and cosmeceutical properties of nicotinamide in consideration of its metabolic pathways. Supplementation of nicotinamide restores cellular NAD^+ pool and mitochondrial energetics, attenuates oxidative stress and inflammatory response, enhances extracellular matrix and skin barrier, and inhibits the pigmentation process in the skin. Topical treatment of nicotinamide, alone or in combination with other active ingredients, reduces the progression of skin aging and hyperpigmentation in clinical trials. Topically applied nicotinamide is well tolerated by the skin. Currently, there is no convincing evidence that nicotinamide has specific molecular targets for controlling skin aging and pigmentation. This substance is presumed to contribute to maintaining skin homeostasis by regulating the redox status of cells along with various metabolites produced from it. Thus, it is suggested that nicotinamide will be useful as a cosmeceutical ingredient to attenuate skin aging and hyperpigmentation, especially in the elderly or patients with reduced NAD^+ pool in the skin due to internal or external stressors.

Keywords: nicotinamide; niacinamide; vitamin B3; skin aging; pigmentation; cosmetic; cosmeceutical; metabolism; antioxidant; senescence; inflammation

Citation: Boo, Y.C. Mechanistic Basis and Clinical Evidence for the Applications of Nicotinamide (Niacinamide) to Control Skin Aging and Pigmentation. *Antioxidants* **2021**, *10*, 1315. https://doi.org/10.3390/antiox10081315

Academic Editors: Laurian Vlase, Marius Emil Rusu, Ionel Fizesan and Daniela-Saveta Popa

Received: 28 July 2021
Accepted: 20 August 2021
Published: 21 August 2021

Publisher's Note: MDPI stays neutral with regard to jurisdictional claims in published maps and institutional affiliations.

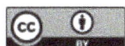

Copyright: © 2021 by the author. Licensee MDPI, Basel, Switzerland. This article is an open access article distributed under the terms and conditions of the Creative Commons Attribution (CC BY) license (https://creativecommons.org/licenses/by/4.0/).

1. Introduction

The primary characteristic of the skin is that it surrounds our body and is directly exposed to the external environment. Skin serves the barrier function to protect the body from external harmful factors and to prevent water loss from the body, as well as the thermoregulation function to keep body temperature constant despite changes in external temperature [1]. However, when the skin is subjected to pathological conditions due to internal and external factors, such as malnutrition, infection, wounds, and exposure to pollutants, abnormalities in the immune system and excessive inflammatory response throughout the body can be induced. Even if the symptoms are limited to the skin, various skin diseases, aging, and cancer can occur, and these are the main research subjects in dermatology.

Another characteristic of the skin is that it is an externally visible organ, and therefore, its health is important from an aesthetic point of view, as well as a medical point of view. The aging of the skin involves both the decline of various biological functions and changes in morphological beauty. In the cosmetic field, skin aging is being studied by dividing it into natural aging, which is a chronological skin change caused by internal factors of the body, and photoaging, which is a skin change caused by exposure to ultraviolet (UV) rays from the sun [2]. Natural aging and photoaging are not mutually exclusive but partly overlap. Clinical observations show that naturally aged skin is thin, dry, and has many fine wrinkles, whereas photoaged skin usually has a leathery and saggy appearance with reduced elasticity, uneven pigmentation, coarse and deep wrinkles, and telangiectasia (appearance of blood vessels) [3]. Changes due to natural aging or photoaging occur in both epidermal and dermal compartments. A decrease in the extracellular matrix (ECM) of the dermis, such as collagen and elastin, is consistently observed in either natural aging or photoaging [4].

Reactive oxygen species (ROS) and free radicals generated over the antioxidant capacity of cells due to external factors, such as UV radiation and pollution, or internal metabolic dysfunction can cause oxidative damage to cells [5]. ROS also induces senescence of cells and degradation of ECM involved in premature skin aging [6,7]. Indeed, ROS plays a pathological role in the development of various skin diseases and cancer [8–10]. Therefore, ingredients that directly remove ROS or enhance the antioxidant capacity of cells are expected to help maintain skin homeostasis [11,12].

Nicotinamide (niacinamide) is the amide form of water-soluble vitamin B3 (nicotinic acid, niacin). Vitamin B3 deficiency causes pellagra [13,14]. Nicotinamide is a component of coenzymes, such as nicotinamide adenine dinucleotide (NAD^+), reduced nicotinamide adenine dinucleotide (NADH), nicotinamide adenine dinucleotide phosphate ($NADP^+$), and reduced nicotinamide adenine dinucleotide phosphate (NADPH) [14,15]. Nicotinamide has the same vitamin activity as nicotinic acid, but other pharmacological actions and side effects are different [16]. Unlike nicotinic acid, nicotinamide does not reduce cholesterol or cause flushing [17]. Supplementation of nicotinamide as an essential nutrient will be beneficial to the health of the whole body and the skin.

In the field of dermatology, many studies on nicotinamide and its analogs have been reported concerning the prevention and treatment of cancer, blistering disorders, acne vulgaris, psoriasis, wound healing, and pigmentation disorders [18–21]. Nicotinamide has also been used in the cosmetic field for decades to prevent skin aging and brighten skin tone [22–25]. However, its mechanism of action in alleviating skin diseases or controlling skin aging and pigmentation is not well understood. In addition, it is unclear whether the efficacy of nicotinamide is its direct effect or its indirect effect acting as a precursor of other active metabolites.

The purpose of this review is to understand the mechanistic basis for the cosmeceutical application of nicotinamide. The pharmaceutical application of nicotinamide is excluded from the scope of this review. First, we briefly review the metabolic process of nicotinamide. Secondly, we examine the antioxidant and anti-inflammatory effects of nicotinamide and its effects on cell senescence and epidermal differentiation. Next, we discuss the effects of nicotinamide on the ECM and skin barrier, which is closely related to skin aging, and on the synthesis and distribution of melanin related to skin pigmentation. Finally, we review the results of clinical trials on the efficacy of cosmetic formulations containing nicotinamide alone or in combination with other active ingredients to control skin aging and pigmentation. It is hoped that this study will help us understand the mechanism of action of nicotinamide and correctly evaluate the potential of nicotinamide as a cosmeceutical.

2. Metabolism of Nicotinamide

2.1. Synthesis and Function of NAD(H) and NADP(H)

The roles of NAD^+ coenzyme in the life system are significant and broad [15,26]. In this section, we briefly review the metabolic pathways of NAD^+ with special attention to nicotinamide (Figure 1).

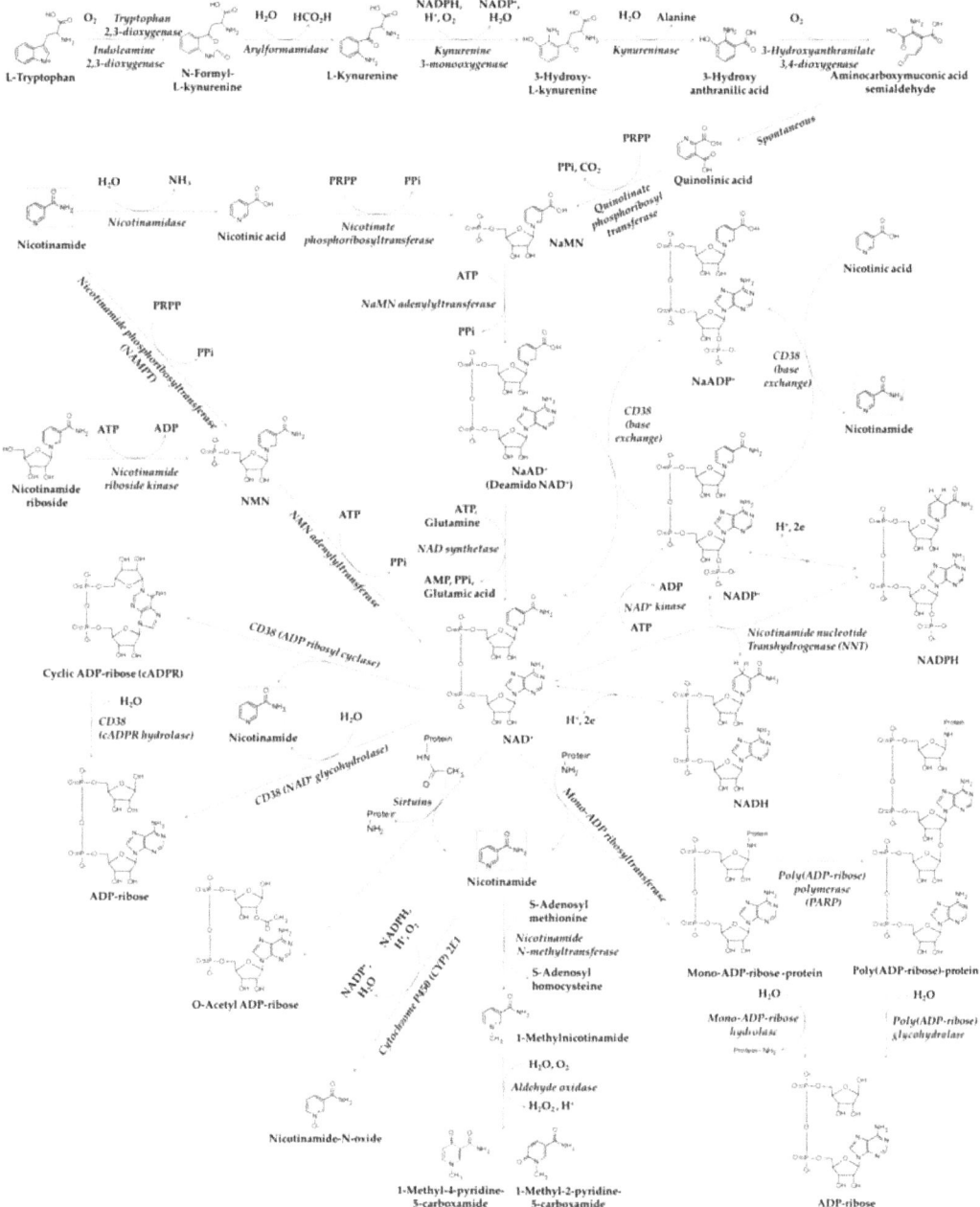

Figure 1. Metabolic pathways related to nicotinamide: ADP, adenosine diphosphate; AMP, adenosine monophosphate; ATP, adenosine triphosphate; cADPR, cyclic ADP-ribose; CYP, cytochrome P450; NaAD$^+$, nicotinic acid adenine dinucleotide; NaADP$^+$, nicotinic acid adenine dinucleotide phosphate; NAD$^+$, nicotinamide adenine dinucleotide; NADH, reduced nicotinamide adenine dinucleotide; NADP$^+$, nicotinamide adenine dinucleotide phosphate; NADPH, reduced nicotinamide adenine dinucleotide phosphate; NaMN, nicotinic acid mononucleotide; NAMPT, nicotinamide phosphoribosyltransferase; NMN, nicotinamide mononucleotide; NNT, nicotinamide nucleotide transhydrogenase; PARP, poly(ADP-ribose) polymerase; PPi, inorganic pyrophosphate; PRPP, phosphoribosyl pyrophosphate.

De novo synthesis of NAD$^+$ starts with oxidation of L-tryptophan to N-formyl-L-kynurenine by tryptophan 2,3-dioxygenase or indoleamine 2,3-dioxygenase [27,28]. N-formyl-L-kynurenine is converted to quinolinic acid via multiple enzymatic and non-enzymatic reactions. Nicotinic acid mononucleotide (NaMN) is synthesized from quinolinic acid and phosphoribosyl pyrophosphate (PRPP) by quinolinate phosphoribosyltransferase, and inorganic pyrophosphate (PPi) and carbon dioxide are released as by-products.

As tryptophan is one of the essential amino acids that cannot be synthesized well by humans, the salvage pathway using nicotinamide or nicotinic acid from dietary sources is important for the synthesis of NAD$^+$ [29]. NaMN is synthesized from nicotinic acid and PRPP by nicotinate phosphoribosyltransferase, and PPi is released as a by-product. Nicotinic acid adenine dinucleotide (NaAD$^+$) is synthesized from NaMN and adenosine triphosphate (ATP) by NaMN adenylyltransferase, releasing PPi as a by-product and is then used in the synthesis of NAD$^+$ by NAD synthetase, which uses glutamine as an amine group donor and energy from ATP hydrolysis to adenosine monophosphate (AMP) and PPi. NAD$^+$ is also synthesized by NMN adenylyltransferase using nicotinamide mononucleotide (NMN) and ATP. Nicotinamide and PRPP are used in the synthesis of NMN by nicotinamide phosphoribosyltransferase (NAMPT), which releases PPi as a by-product. NMN is also synthesized from nicotinamide riboside and ATP by nicotinamide riboside kinase, which releases adenosine diphosphate (ADP) as a by-product.

Conversion of NAD$^+$ to NADP$^+$ is catalyzed by NAD$^+$ kinase consuming ATP molecules for needed free energy [30]. Nicotinamide nucleotide transhydrogenase (NNT) catalyzes a reversible reaction, NADH + NADP$^+$ $\rightleftharpoons$ NAD$^+$ + NADPH [31]. NAD(H) and NADP(H) play as cofactors or coenzymes in a myriad of oxidation-reduction reactions in biological systems [32]. NAD$^+$ serves as an electron acceptor in many enzyme reactions in glycolysis, the citric acid cycle, and β-oxidation of fatty acids, producing NADH. NADH serves as an electron donor in many enzyme reactions, such as NADH dehydrogenase in complex I of mitochondrial electron transport and lactate dehydrogenase in the cytosol. NADP$^+$ serves as an electron acceptor in many enzyme reactions, such as glucose 6-phosphate dehydrogenase in the pentose phosphate pathway and isocitrate dehydrogenase outside the context of the citric acid cycle. NADPH serves as an electron donor in many enzyme reactions, such as NADPH oxidase, cytochrome P450 (CYP), nitric oxide synthase, and glutathione reductase. Glutathione reductase catalyzes a reaction, glutathione disulfide (GSSG) + NADPH → 2 × glutathione (GSH) + NADP$^+$.

2.2. Metabolisms of NAD$^+$ and Nicotinamide

Poly(ADP-ribose) polymerase (PARP) family consists of 18 genes, which encode 17 enzymes with either mono-ADP ribosyltransferase or PARP activity [33]. NAD$^+$ is used as a substrate for mono-ADP-ribosylation of target proteins catalyzed by mono-ADP ribosyltransferase activity, and for poly(ADP-ribose) polymerization catalyzed by PARP activity [34,35]. Nicotinamide is released as a by-product. Hydrolysis of mono- and poly-ADP-ribosylated proteins by mono-ADP-ribose hydrolase and poly(ADP-ribose) hydrolase results in the production of ADP-ribose. These reversible processes are involved in DNA repair, apoptosis, and many other biological processes to maintain cellular homeostasis [36].

Sirtuins are a family of signaling proteins that have a mono-ADP-ribosyltransferase activity or a protein deacylase activity (deacetylase, desuccinylase, demalonylase, demyristoylase, or depalmitoylase activity) and have been hypothesized to play a role in the aging process [37]. Histone deacetylation by sirtuins yields the deacetylated protein, O-acetyl ADP-ribose, and nicotinamide [38]. Sirtuins epigenetically regulate target gene expression involved in stress resistance and energy alertness and directly link cell physiology to the energy status of the cell [39].

CD38 functions as a receptor and a multifunctional enzyme, catalyzing the cleavage of NAD$^+$ into cyclic ADP ribose (cADPR) and nicotinamide, the hydrolysis of cADPR to ADP-ribose, and the direct hydrolysis of NAD$^+$ to ADP-ribose and nicotinamide [40]. CD38 also catalyzes a base exchange reaction that couples the conversion of NADP$^+$ to

NaADP with the conversion of nicotinic acid to nicotinamide [41], or that of NaAD$^+$ to NAD$^+$ [42]. Both cADPR and NaADP$^+$ play essential roles for the regulation of intracellular Ca^{2+} [43,44]. CD38 is considered to play a critical role in keeping a harmonized balance between various NAD$^+$ metabolites.

Nicotinamide is metabolized to 1-methylnicotinamide by nicotinamide N-methyltransferase, which uses S-adenosyl methionine as a methyl group donor [45]. 1-Methylnicotinamide is further oxidized to 1-methyl-2-pyridone-5-carboxamide or 1-methyl-4-pyridone-3-carboxamide by aldehyde oxidase [46]. Nicotinamide is also directly oxidized to nicotinamide N-oxide by CYP 2E1 in human liver microsomes [47]. These enzyme reactions mainly occur in the liver and are considered a clearance mechanism involved in the urinary excretion of nicotinamide.

3. Antioxidant and Anti-Inflammatory Effects of Nicotinamide

3.1. Antioxidant Properties of Nicotinamide

Ingestion of nicotinamide, prevents lipid peroxidation and normalizes the reduced antioxidants and antioxidant enzymes in experimental animal models [48–50].

Kamat et al. showed that nicotinamide scavenged singlet oxygen at the rate constant of 1.8×10^8 M^{-1} s^{-1} and inhibited lipid peroxidation of rat liver microsomes induced by the photosensitized reaction of methylene blue irradiated with visible light in the presence of oxygen [51]. They also showed that nicotinamide inhibited lipid peroxidation induced by NADPH/ADP-Fe^{3+} in rat liver microsomes [51]. Nicotinamide inhibited lipid peroxidation and protein oxidation (carbonylation) induced by the ascorbate–Fe^{2+} system in the rat brain mitochondria, whereas such action was not observed for nicotinic acid [52].

3.2. Protective Effect of Nicotinamide in Cells Exposed to Environmental Stressors

Nicotinamide rescued the viability of a Chinese hamster ovary cell line (CHO AA8) irradiated with UV radiation and prevented apoptosis through mechanisms related to the stabilization of the cytoskeleton proteins, such as F-actin, vimentin, and β-tubulin [53]. Nicotinamide exhibited a protective effect against UVA- and/or UVB-induced DNA damage in normal human epidermal melanocytes, as indicated by decreased levels of cyclobutane pyrimidine dimers and 8-hydroxy-2′-deoxyguanosine [54]. This effect was associated with the enhanced expression of nucleotide excision repair genes, such as sirtuin 1 (SIRT1), tumor suppressor protein P53, damage-specific DNA binding protein (DDB) 1 and 2, 8-oxoguanine glycosylase (OGG) 1, excision repair cross-complementation group (ERCC) 1 and 2, and cyclin-dependent kinase (CDK) 7, and the activation of the nuclear factor erythroid 2-related factor 2 (NRF 2) signaling pathway.

Nicotinamide inhibited the generation of ROS, the oxidation of lipids, proteins, and DNA, cell membrane depolarization, and the apoptosis in human HaCaT keratinocytes cells exposed to particulate matter (PM) 2.5 [55]. Mi et al. examined the protective effect of nicotinamide and 12-hydroxystearic acid in reconstructed human skin equivalents exposed to benzo(a)pyrene as a representative airborne particle-bound organic compound, or to squalene monohydroperoxide as a representative sebum peroxidation product [56]. Individual treatment and co-treatment of the skin equivalents with nicotinamide (5 mM) and 12-hydroxystearic acid (20 μM) ameliorated viability loss, inflammatory response, and pigmentation induced by benzo(a)pyrene or squalene monohydroperoxide.

These studies suggest that the topical application of nicotinamide may alleviate oxidative stress and reduce cytotoxicity, inflammation, and pigmentation in the skin that is exposed to UV or PM.

3.3. Anti-Inflammatory Effects of Nicotinamide

Nicotinamide suppressed interleukin (IL)-8 production at the mRNA and protein levels through modulation of the nuclear factor (NF)-κB and mitogen-activated protein kinase (MAPK) pathways in HaCaT cells and primary keratinocytes stimulated by *Propionibacterium acnes*, the etiological agent causing inflammatory acne vulgaris [57].

Nicotinamide downregulated the expression of IL-6, IL-10, monocyte chemoattractant protein-1 and tumor necrosis factor (TNF)-α in UV-irradiated keratinocytes [58].

Nicotinamide attenuated the synthesis of inflammatory mediators, such as prostaglandin (PG) E_2, IL-6, and IL-8 in human epidermal keratinocytes and in full-thickness three-dimensional skin organotypic models that were stimulated by UV radiation [59]. In a clinical trial, pretreatment with 5% nicotinamide reduced erythema that was induced by UV radiation [59]. Analysis of IL-1α and its receptor antagonist (IL-1αRA) ratios showed that nicotinamide significantly reduced the UV-induced inflammatory response, compared to the control sites.

3.4. Anti-Inflammatory Effects of N-Methylnicotinamide and NMN

Nicotinamide and l-methylnicotinamide exhibit anti-inflammatory effects in several experimental models although the relative activity of these two substances is not consistent. The contact hypersensitivity reaction of CBA/J inbred mice to oxazolone was reduced when the mice were fed with 1-methylnicotinamide or nicotinamide added to the drink, the former being relatively more effective [60]. In an in vitro experiment using CBA/J mouse peritoneal macrophages activated with lipopolysaccharide, nicotinamide inhibited the production of a variety of pro-inflammatory factors, such as TNF-α, IL-6, nitric oxide, and PGE_2, and 1-methylnicotinamide was less effective, although both substances similarly attenuated the generation of ROS [61]. It is considered that the anti-inflammatory activity of these two substances is affected by bioavailability, such as absorption through the digestive tract and cell membrane.

In clinical trials, topical application of a gel containing 0.25% 1-methylnicotinamide twice a day for 4 weeks alleviated rosacea, a chronic facial dermatosis [62]. Intradermal injection of 1-methylnicotinamide or nicotinamide increased skin vascular permeability in rats, the former being more effective [63]. The changes in skin vascular permeability were attenuated by indomethacin and N_ω-nitro-L-arginine methyl ester, indicating the involvement of PGs and nitric oxide (NO). Although the molecular mechanism linking skin vascular permeability and rosacea is unclear, it is considered that 1-methylnicotinamide or nicotinamide directly or indirectly affects vascular endothelial function [64,65].

In a rat model, oral administration of NMN alone or in combination with *Lactobacillus fermentum* TKSN041 reduced UV-induced skin oxidative damage and inflammatory response and restored small molecular antioxidants and antioxidant enzymes in blood and skin tissues [66].

4. Modulation of Cell Senescence and Epidermal Differentiation by Nicotinamide

4.1. Differential Effects of Nicotinamide on Lifespans of Yeast and Mammalian Cells

Nicotinamide is known as an inhibitor of silent information regulator-2 (sir2) deacetylase that mediates lifespan extension by calorie restriction in yeasts (*Saccharomyces cerevisiae*), and nicotinamide depletion or overexpression of nicotinamidase 1 (pyrazinamidase 1) prolongs the lifespan of yeast cells [67].

On the contrary, nicotinamide supplementation to human cells rather prolongs the replicative lifespan and retards the senescence [68,69]. Matuoka et al. observed that nicotinamide reverses the aging phenotypes in human diploid fibroblasts as evaluated by cell morphology, senescence-associated β-galactosidase activity, and cell replication potential, and tentatively attributed this action of nicotinamide to the enhancement of histone acetyltransferase activity and subsequently altered gene expression [68]. Lim et al. demonstrated that that nicotinamide extends the lifespan of primary human diploid somatic fibroblasts (82-6 and IMR-90) via a mechanism largely independent of SIRT1, a close human homolog of yeast sir2 [69].

The discrepancy regarding the effects of nicotinamide on the lifespans of yeast cells vs. mammalian cells could be attributed to differences in intracellular nicotinamide concentrations in situ [70,71]. The 50% inhibitory concentration of nicotinamide on Sir2 is about 50 µM, and this level of nicotinamide concentration can be reached in yeasts [70]. On the other hand, it is difficult to reach this nicotinamide concentration in mammalian cells because the supplied nicotinamide is rapidly metabolized by NAMPT in a mammalian NAD$^+$ salvage pathway [71].

4.2. Antisenescence Effects of Nicotinamide

Cellular NAD$^+$ pool is low in aged skin [72]. Thus, external supplementation of nicotinamide as a primary precursor of NAD$^+$ and related coenzymes may improve the epidermal homeostasis and cellular bioenergetics in aged and stressed cells [73]. Kang et al. proposed that the extension of the lifespan of normal human fibroblasts by nicotinamide might be associated with the reduction in mitochondrial ROS production [74]. The antioxidant activity of nicotinamide reducing ROS production and lipofuscin accumulation correlates with antisenescence activity suppressing the increases in cell size, granule content, and senescence-associated β-galactosidase activity as observed in both rapidly senescing cells (human breast cancer MCF-7 cell line treated with Adriamycin) and already senescent cells (old passage human fibroblasts) [75]. Gene expression of subunits of complexes I to V of mitochondrial electron transport chain was reduced in fibroblasts from older aged donors, and treatment of the cells with nicotinamide restored gene expression and mitochondrial function to younger cell levels [76].

Ectopic expression of NAMPT in human aortic endothelial cells extended replicative lifespan, delayed markers of senescence, and limited ROS accumulation under high glucose conditions [77]. Nicotinamide protected glycolysis and oxidative phosphorylation activities in dermal fibroblasts exposed to oxidative stress through a mechanism partially dependent on NAMPT [78]. NAMPT and NAD$^+$ contents have been shown to decline in primary mouse embryonic fibroblast cells undergoing replicative senescence, whereas constitutive over-expression of NAMPT increases NAD$^+$ content and delays cell senescence, which is associated with increases in the activity of SIRT1 and the expression levels of superoxide dismutase 2 and catalase [79]. FK866, a NAMPT inhibitor, induced premature differentiation and senescence of human primary keratinocytes in multi-dimensional culture, and this effect was competitively attenuated by nicotinamide [80]. Therefore, NAMPT is considered to mediate the antisenescence effects of nicotinamide at least partly.

4.3. Epidermal Stem Cells

Adult stem cells are present in the bulge region of the hair follicles and the basal layer of the interfollicular epidermis and play a critical role in maintaining the structural and functional integrity of the skin through self-renewal and generation of daughter cells that undergo terminal differentiation [81]. Skin aging is more associated with the reduction of healthy stem cells able to respond to proliferative signals rather than the reduction of the total number of stem cells [82]. Liu et al. have proposed a mechanistic model for skin aging based on the competition between epidermal stem cells expressing different levels of hemidesmosome component collagen 17A1 [83]. In this model, the stressed stem cells expressing a low level of collagen 17A1 are delaminated from the basal epidermis, whereas healthy stem cells expressing a high level of collagen 17A1 survive in the aging skin. Regardless of who the final winner is, this competition leads to an eventual loss of collagen 17A1 due to exhaustion of epidermal stem cells and results in skin aging represented by a thin epidermal structure.

Epidermal stem cells can also undergo senescence, accelerating premature aging of the skin [84]. It is hypothesized that the skin aging process may be slowed down by maintaining a young stem cell phenotype [85]. In this regard, sirtuins are viewed as a promising target in slowing down the aging process [86]. Various natural compounds are known to modulate the activity of sirtuins and will be potentially useful for this purpose [87].

4.4. Modulation of Epidermal Differentiation by Nicotinamide

Nicotinamide affects the proliferation and differentiation of various stem cells including human embryonic stem cells [88]. In a study by Tan et al. [80], high concentrations of nicotinamide inhibited the differentiation of the upper epidermal layers and maintained proliferation in the basal layer of a three-dimensional organotypic skin model. Nicotinamide increased the proliferative capacity of human primary keratinocytes and the proportion of human primary keratinocyte stem cells (holoclones), which were reduced by FK866. By contrast, FK866 induced the premature senescence of human primary keratinocyte, which was rescued by nicotinamide. These observations suggest that nicotinamide metabolism through NAMPT can modulate epidermal differentiation and stem cell biology.

5. Enhancement of ECM and Skin Barrier by Nicotinamide

5.1. Changes of ECM by Skin Aging

The main component of ECM is collagen and elastin, and these fibrous components provide the skin's tensile strength, elasticity, and resiliency [89]. In human skin, type I, type III, and type V collagen constitute 80–90%, 8–12%, and less than 5% of total collagen, respectively [90]. Alteration in the amount and structures of collagen and elastin is a common feature of natural aging and photoaging of the skin [4]. The activities of matrix metalloproteinase (MMP) and elastase are increased in aged skin while transforming growth factor (TGF)-β signaling that leads to the synthesis of collagen is reduced [91,92].

ROS increased by internal and external factors stimulates activator protein (AP)-1 and NF-κB through cell signaling systems involving several MAPKs, and increases the expression of MMPs in epidermal keratinocytes and dermal fibroblasts, resulting in collagen degradation [7,89,92,93]. Stratifin, also called 14-3-3σ protein, plays an important role in communication between keratinocytes and fibroblasts, especially for the degradation of dermal collagen associated with premature skin aging [93,94]. Stratifin from the keratinocytes exposed to UV radiation stimulates the fibroblasts in close vicinity to increase MMP 1 expression [95,96].

Other components of the ECM include different types of glycosaminoglycans, such as heparan sulfate/heparin, chondroitin sulfate/dermatan sulfate, keratan sulfate, and hyaluronan and proteoglycans made of glycosaminoglycans (other than hyaluronan) and protein cores [97]. These extremely hydrophilic components reside in the space between the cell and the collagen/elastin fibrils in the dermis and adopt highly extended conformations that enable matrices to hold a high amount of water and to withstand high compressive forces dermis [98]. The levels of different types of glycosaminoglycans and proteoglycans change differently by natural aging and photoaging of the skin [99].

5.2. Effects of Nicotinamide on Collagen and Other ECMs

Nicotinamide and its derivatives have been shown to increase the expression of collagen (type I, III, and V), elastin, and fibrillin (1 and 2), and reduce MMP (1, 3, and 9) and elastase activity in non-irradiated and UVA-irradiated dermal fibroblasts [100,101]. Nicotinamide alone or in combination with other substances, such as L-carnosine, hesperidin, enhanced fibroblast collagen synthesis and cellular proliferation, thereby augmenting wound healing in vitro [102]. Topical nicotinamide improved tissue regeneration by increasing fibroblast proliferation, collagen synthesis, and vascularization in skin wounds of Sprague Dawley rats [103]. These studies provide evidence from various aspects that nicotinamide has the action of promoting the synthesis of dermal collagen and inhibiting its degradation.

5.3. Enhancement of Skin Barrier by Nicotinamide

During aging, the structural and functional integrity of the skin barrier is changed or disturbed [104]. Tanno et al. showed that in cultured human epidermal keratinocytes, nicotinamide could upregulate the synthesis of major components of skin barriers, such as ceramide, other sphingolipid fractions (glucosylceramide and sphingomyelin), free fatty acid, and cholesterol [105]. Supplementation of nicotinamide to cultured normal human epidermal keratinocytes increased the synthesis of involucrin and filaggrin, which are essential proteins for fully integral keratinized corneocytes [106].

A facial moisturizer containing 2% nicotinamide improved skin barriers in patients with rosacea [107]. Myristyl nicotinate enhanced the NAD$^+$ pool, epidermal differentiation, and barrier function in the photoaged skin [108]. Thus, nicotinamide and its metabolism could enhance the structural and functional integrity of the skin barriers.

6. Regulation of Pigmentary Process by Nicotinamide

6.1. Effects of Nicotinamide on Melanogenesis vs. Melanosome Transfer

Nicotinamide has a variable effect on melanin synthesis in melanocyte monoculture. There are reports that nicotinamide increased, decreased, or had no significant effect on tyrosinase activity and melanin synthesis [109,110]. On the other hand, in melanocyte-keratinocyte co-culture, reconstituted skin tissue model, or live skin, nicotinamide consistently decreased melanin content or pigmentation [22,111]. Furthermore, nicotinamide slowed the melanosome transfer from melanocytes to keratinocytes [22,111]. This suggests that the interaction between melanocytes and keratinocytes is important in skin pigmentation and that nicotinamide may affect melanocytes indirectly by primarily affecting keratinocytes.

6.2. Mechanisms for Melanosome Transfer

The transfer of melanosomes from melanocytes to keratinocytes has become a very important and interesting research topic in dermatology [112–115]. Melanosome transfer, the process of transferring a package of organelles from a donor cell to a recipient cell, is a very unique biological process, and various mechanisms, such as cytophagocytosis, membrane fusion, shedding–phagocytosis, and exocytosis–endocytosis, have been proposed to describe this process [115]. The membrane fusion mechanism was supported by Scott et al. [116]. Shedding–phagocytosis mechanisms were supported by Ando et al. [117] and Wu et al. [118]. The exocytosis–endocytosis mechanism was supported by Tarafder et al. [119]. Regardless of the mechanism, the precise nature of the "donate-it" signal that keratinocytes send to melanocytes and the "receive-it" signal that melanocytes send to keratinocytes is not yet clear.

6.3. Modulation of Melanosome Transfer

Protease-activated receptor-2 (PAR-2) is expressed in the skin and plays an important role in the regulation of growth and differentiation of keratinocytes [120,121]. In 2000, Seiberg et al. showed that PAR-2 expressed in keratinocytes could regulate skin pigmentation, although this receptor is not expressed in melanocytes [122]. They further showed that activation of PAR-2 by SLIGRL peptide (a peptide agonist derived from the N-terminus of PAR-2) could enhance melanosome transfer and inhibition of this receptor by RWJ-503530 (a serine protease inhibitor) could reduce melanosome transfer [123].

UV rays increased PAR-2 expression in the upper epidermis of human skin, and the change was more rapid and bigger in dark-skinned people [124]. Optimized concentration of hydrogen peroxide (0.3 mM) increased melanin content and melanosome transfer in melanocyte–keratinocyte co-cultures through upregulating expression levels of PAR-2 and Rab-27A [125]. Activation of keratinocyte PAR-2 stimulated the release of PGE$_2$ and PGF$_{2\alpha}$, the paracrine factors act on EP1, EP3, and FP receptors on melanocytes, increasing the number and length of melanocyte dendrites [126]. PGE$_2$, as well as α-melanocyte-stimulating hormone (MSH), stimulated melanosome transfer in melanocyte–keratinocyte co-cultures [127]. These studies suggest a possible relationship between oxidative stress and PAR-2 activation, and thus, there is a possibility that melanosome transfer may be modulated by certain antioxidants or anti-inflammatory agents. Interestingly, macelignan, a natural product derived from *Myristica fragrans*, attenuated the expression of PAR-2 at the mRNA and protein levels, calcium mobilization, and phagocytic activity of HaCaT keratinocyte cells stimulated with SLIGRL peptide [128]. Macelignan also reduced PGE_2 secretion from HaCaT keratinocytes and dendrite formation of B16F10 melanoma cells in a co-culture model with SLIGRL stimulation [128]. However, it is not known whether nicotinamide affects the expression of PAR-2 and related signaling pathways.

Melanosome transfer is also regulated by other receptors, such as keratinocyte growth factor receptors expressed in keratinocytes [114], N-methyl-D-aspartate receptors [129], transient receptor potential cation channel subfamily M member 1 (TRPM1, melastatin-1) [130], and Toll-like receptors 2/3 [131] expressed in melanocytes. The direct and indirect effects of nicotinamide on cellular signaling related to melanosome transfer involving these receptors remain to be explored [132].

7. Clinical Evidence for Skin Antiaging Efficacy of Nicotinamide

Clinical studies on the skin antiaging efficacy of nicotinamide alone or in combination with other active ingredients are summarized in Table 1. In double-blind, placebo-controlled, split-face, left–right randomized clinical studies, Bissett et al. assessed the effect of nicotinamide on the appearance of aging facial skin [23,24]. Moisturizer product with or without containing 5% nicotinamide was applied on the facial skin for 12 weeks. Nicotinamide at 5% was evaluated to be well tolerated by the skin and to improve a broad array of skin appearance (fine lines/wrinkles, texture, hyperpigmentation spots, red blotchiness, and skin sallowness), and elasticity.

Table 1. Skin antiaging efficacy of cosmeceuticals containing nicotinamide alone or with other active ingredients.

Literature	Study Format	No. of Subjects	Compared Formulations	Treatment	Key Findings
[23]	A double-blind, placebo-controlled, split-face, left–right randomized clinical study	50	An oil-in-water moisturizer (placebo control) / 5% nicotinamide	To each side of the face was applied each product, twice daily for 12 weeks.	Improved fine lines/wrinkles, hyperpigmentation spots, texture, red blotchiness, and skin yellowing (sallowness) compared to the control in endpoints.
[24]	A double-blind, placebo formulation-controlled, split-face study with left–right randomization	50	An oil-in-water moisturizer (placebo control) / 5% nicotinamide	To each side of the face was applied each product, twice daily for 12 weeks.	Reduced fine lines, wrinkles, hyperpigmentation spots, red blotchiness, and skin sallowness (yellowing), and increased elasticity (as measured via cutometry).
[133]	A randomized, double-blind, placebo-controlled, split-face comparative study	27 / 25	An aqueous serum 0.03% kinetin + 4% nicotinamide / An aqueous serum 4% nicotinamide	Test serum was applied evenly to one side of the face and vehicle to the other side twice daily for 12 weeks.	Combination of kinetin and nicotinamide reduced pore, wrinkle, unevenness, erythema, and spot at weeks 8 and 12 and increased corneal moisture at week 12. Nicotinamide alone reduced pore and unevenness at week 8 and wrinkle at week 12.
[134]	A randomized, placebo-controlled, split-face study	30	A vehicle lotion / 4% nicotinamide	The test product was applied on wrinkles of one side and a control product on the other side for 8 weeks.	Test product reduced wrinkle grades and average roughness of skin surface (Ra value) in the tested skin area to lower levels compared to pre-application ($p < 0.001$) and the vehicle control ($p < 0.001$) in endpoints.
[135]	A randomized, parallel-group facial appearance study	99 / 97	A daytime lotion (SPF 30) containing 5% nicotinamide and peptides; a night cream containing nicotinamide and peptides; a wrinkle treatment containing nicotinamide, peptides, and 0.3% retinyl propionate. / 0.02% tretinoin in an emollient base; a sunscreen (SPF 30)	Subjects applied a wrinkle treatment twice daily, a daytime lotion, and the night cream daily.	The cosmetic regimen significantly improved wrinkle appearance after 8 weeks relative to tretinoin in the total population, with comparable benefits in subject cohorts ($n = 25$) who continued treatment for an additional 16 weeks.

Table 1. Cont.

Literature	Study Format	No. of Subjects	Compared Formulations	Treatment	Key Findings
[136]	A randomized, double-blinded, vehicle-controlled, split-face study	40	A simple oil-in-water emulsion 2% gold silk sericin, 5% nicotinamide, 0.1% signaline™ (diacylglycerol and fatty alcohols)	Subjects applied the products twice daily to either the left- or right-hand side of their face at 2 mg cm^{-2}.	Test product improved stratum corneum hydration, barrier function, elasticity, and surface topography compared with the vehicle control in endpoints.
[137]	An open-label, single-center study	25	0.5% retinol, 4.4% nicotinamide, 1% resveratrol, and 1.1% hexylresorcinol	Treatment at night for 10 weeks.	The formulation improved hyperpigmentation, overall skin clarity, evenness of skin tone, and wrinkles compared to baseline at week 4 and through week 10.
[138]	A double-blind, randomized, split-face, vehicle-controlled study	24	2% human adipocyte-derived mesenchymal stem cell-conditioned medium and 2% nicotinamide A vehicle cream	Applied twice daily for 3 weeks after fractional ablative CO$_2$ laser treatment.	The formulation reduced the wrinkle index ($p = 0.036$) and melanin index ($p = 0.043$) compared to the control group.

In a randomized, double-blind, placebo-controlled, split-face comparative study by Chiu et al. [133], 4% nicotinamide alone reduced pores and skin unevenness after 8 weeks and improved wrinkles after 12 weeks. In contrast, the formulation containing 0.03% kinetin + 4% nicotinamide significantly reduced erythema and hyperpigmented spots in addition to pores, roughness, and wrinkles after 8 weeks.

The anti-wrinkle effect of nicotinamide was further examined by Kawada et al. in a randomized, placebo-controlled, split-face study [134]. A cosmetic containing 4% nicotinamide was applied on the wrinkles of one side and a control cosmetic on the other side of the face for 8 weeks. The wrinkle grades in the test area, evaluated by doctors' visual observation, were significantly lower than those before application ($p < 0.001$) or in the control area ($p < 0.001$) at the endpoints. The average surface roughness (Ra value) on the test area, determined using skin replica, was significantly lower, compared to the pre-application values ($p < 0.01$) or those in the control site ($p < 0.05$).

Fu et al. reported significant results in a clinical trial comparing the antiaging effect of the cosmetic regimen using a series of products containing nicotinamide/other active ingredients plus a sunscreen with the sun protection factor (SPF) 30, vs. the use of control products containing 0.02% Tretinoin plus a sunscreen with SPF 30 [135]. However, it is difficult to estimate the relative contribution of nicotinamide to the observed antiaging effects of the cosmetic regimen.

Several other clinical trials have evaluated the efficacy of cosmetics containing nicotinamide and several other active ingredients (silk sericin, diacylglycerol, fatty alcohols, retinol, resveratrol, hexylresorcinol, and/or stem cell culture medium) [136–138]. These products showed a wrinkle improvement effect in common, and certain products were evaluated to have improvement effects on skin moisture, skin barrier, elasticity, surface morphology, skin clarity, and/or pigmentation [136–138]. Again, it is difficult to estimate the contribution of nicotinamide to the clinical trial results obtained using the combination formulation.

8. Clinical Evidence for Skin-Lightening Efficacy of Nicotinamide

8.1. Skin-Lightening Efficacy of Nicotinamide

Clinical studies on the skin-lightening efficacy of nicotinamide as an active ingredient are summarized in Table 2. Hakozaki et al. examined the skin depigmenting efficacy of nicotinamide in humans [22]. In a randomized, split-face, double-blind, paired clinical study involving eighteen Japanese women with multiple types of brown hyperpigmentation, subjects applied a test moisturizer containing 5% nicotinamide and the control moisturizer without nicotinamide to each side of the face twice daily for 8 weeks. The side of the face receiving the test moisturizer showed a significant decrease in the total hyperpigmented area measured by image analysis and a reduction in visually assessed hyperpigmentation degree, compared to the side receiving the control moisturizer after 4 weeks or 8 weeks of treatment.

Table 2. Skin-lightening efficacy of cosmeceuticals containing nicotinamide.

Literature	Study Format	No. of Subjects	Compared Formulations	Treatment	Key Findings
[22]	A randomized, split-face, double-blind, paired clinical study	18	5% nicotinamide	Subjects applied a test or a control moisturizer to each side of the face twice daily for 8 weeks.	The side of the face receiving the test moisturizer showed a significant decrease in the total hyperpigmented area measured by image analysis and a reduction in visually assessed hyperpigmentation degree compared to the side receiving the control moisturizer after 4 weeks or 8 weeks of treatment.
			A control moisturizer		
	A randomized, split-face, double-blind, round-robin design	120	A vehicle moisturizer	Applied two of three different products, each product to each side of their face twice daily for 8 weeks.	After 4 weeks, L* value of the treated sides was highest with a test sunscreen moisturizer, followed by a control sunscreen moisturizer, and a vehicle moisturizer.
			A control sunscreen moisturizer (SPF 15)		
			A test sunscreen moisturizer containing 2% nicotinamide		
[111]	A double-blinded, randomized, vehicle-controlled, split-face design human clinical trial	39	5% nicotinamide	Subjects applied either test or control product to the assigned sides of their faces twice a day for 8 weeks.	5% Nicotinamide-containing moisturizer demonstrated a higher reduction in hyperpigmented spot than the vehicle moisturizer, after 4 and 8 weeks of treatment. 2% Nicotinamide did not show a statistically significant effect compared to the vehicle moisturizer.
			A vehicle moisturizer		
		40	2% nicotinamide		
			A vehicle moisturizer		
[139]	A double-blind, randomized, clinical trial	27	4% nicotinamide	Melasma patients applied a product on the left side of the face and the other on the right side for 8 weeks.	After 8 weeks of treatment, MASI score was decreased, L* value was increased and a* value was unchanged by both treatments compared to the baseline values. Good to excellent improvement was observed in 44% of patients receiving nicotinamide and 55% of patients receiving hydroquinone.
			4% hydroquinone		
[140]	A randomized, double-blind, left–right axilla, placebo-controlled trial	24	4% nicotinamide (n = 16 axillae)	Treatment at night for 9 weeks.	At 9 weeks, L* values in the nicotinamide and desonide groups were increased more compared with the placebo group. Desonide was more effective than nicotinamide ($p = 0.002$).
			0.05% desonide (n = 16 axillae)		
			A placebo cream (n = 16 axillae)		

Nicotinamide has been incorporated into a sunscreen product for added performance. In total, 120 Japanese women with moderate-to-deep facial tan were enrolled in another randomized, split-face, double-blind, round-robin design and were assigned to apply any two of three different products, each product to each side of their face twice daily for eight weeks [22]. Three tested products are a vehicle moisturizer, a control sunscreen moisturizer with SPF 15, and a test sunscreen moisturizer containing 2% nicotinamide. The skin color is expressed with the Commission Internationale de l'Eclairage Lab color space composed of L* value (lightness), a* value (redness), and b* value (blueness) [141]. After 4 weeks of treatment, L* values of the treated sides were the highest for a test sunscreen moisturizer, followed by a control sunscreen moisturizer and a vehicle moisturizer, with statistical significances between test groups. After 4 weeks of treatment, the side of the face receiving a test sunscreen moisturizer showed a significant increase in visually assessed skin lightness, compared to the side receiving a vehicle moisturizer, whereas the side of the face receiving a control sunscreen moisturizer was not lighter than the vehicle moisturizer-treated side.

Dose-dependent efficacy of nicotinamide was examined in a double-blinded, randomized, vehicle-controlled, split-face design human clinical trial that involved 79 Japanese women with multiple types of brown hyperpigmentation on both sides of the face [111]. Group 1 subjects applied a 5% nicotinamide-containing moisturizer and the vehicle moisturizer, and group 2 subjects applied a 2% nicotinamide-containing moisturizer and the vehicle moisturizer to the assigned sides of their faces twice a day for 8 weeks. After

4 or 8 weeks of treatment, the side of the face receiving a 5% nicotinamide-containing moisturizer demonstrated a higher hyperpigmented spot-reduction than the site receiving the vehicle moisturizer, while a 2% nicotinamide-containing moisturizer efficacy did not show a statistically significant effect, compared to the vehicle moisturizer. During the regression period, the spot-reduction efficacy of a 5% nicotinamide-containing moisturizer was gradually reduced to a level not statistically different from the vehicle moisturizer after 42 weeks. Therefore, topical nicotinamide can have dose-dependent and reversible skin depigmenting effects in humans.

Depigmenting efficacy of nicotinamide was compared with other active ingredients. Navarrete-Solís et al. performed a double-blind, randomized clinical trial to compare the efficacy and safety of 4% nicotinamide vs. 4% hydroquinone in the treatment of melisma [139]. For the study, 27 melasma patients applied a product on the left side of the face, and the other on the right side for 8 weeks. After 8 weeks of treatment, melasma area and severity index (MASI) was decreased, L* value was increased and a* value was unchanged by both treatments compared to the baseline values. Good-to-excellent improvement was observed in 44% of patients receiving nicotinamide and 55% of patients receiving hydroquinone. Side effects were noted in 18% of patients receiving nicotinamide and 29% of patients receiving hydroquinone. Therefore, nicotinamide and hydroquinone were considered to have comparable skin depigmenting activity.

Castanedo-Cazares et al. compared the efficacy of nicotinamide and desonide against axillary hyperpigmentation, which is a variant of inflammatory hyperpigmentation [140]. In a clinical trial involving 24 women with hyperpigmented axillae, the emulsions containing 4% nicotinamide or 0.05% desonide (a low potency corticosteroid used against skin inflammation) were applied to the hyperpigmented axillary region for 9 weeks. Both nicotinamide and desonide improved skin lightness, compared with placebo, and the former was slightly less effective than the latter.

8.2. Skin-Lightening Efficacy of Combined Formulations of Nicotinamide and Other Active Ingredients

An improved whitening efficacy can be expected when nicotinamide is used in combination with other active ingredients than when used alone. In addition, it will be possible to enhance the whitening efficacy by increasing the absorption of active ingredients into the skin in a special way rather than simply applying the formulation to the skin. Table 3 introduces several clinical studies that have been conducted based on this reasoning. The composite formulations additionally contain various active ingredients such as arbutin, kojic acid, ascorbic acid, ascorbyl glucoside, tranexamic acid, N-undecylenoyl phenylalanine, N-acetyl glucosamine, *trans*-4-(amino methyl) cyclohexanecarboxylic acid, potassium azeloyl diglycinate, hydroxyethylpiperazineethane sulfonic acid, and/or epidermal growth factor.

Table 3. Skin-lightening efficacy of cosmeceuticals containing nicotinamide in combination with other active ingredients

Literature	Study Format	No. of Subjects	Compared Formulations	Treatment	Key Findings
[142]	A randomized, split-face design	30	No treatment	Subjects used the ultrasound device for 10 min with or without a gel every night for 4 weeks.	Use of ultrasound treatment with a gel reduced hyperpigmentation compared with no treatment or treatment of a gel alone after 4 weeks.
			Ultrasound treatment		
		30	A gel containing 2% ascorbyl glucoside, and 3.5% nicotinamide		
			Ultrasound treatment with a gel		
[143]	Double-blind, left–right, randomized, split-face clinical studies	40	A vehicle emulsion	Treatment in the morning and evening before bedtime for 8 weeks.	Combination formulation and nicotinamide alone reduced the appearance of hyperpigmentation after 8 weeks. The combination was more effective than nicotinamide alone ($p = 0.0003$).
			5% nicotinamide		
		40	5% nicotinamide		
			5% nicotinamide plus 1% n-undecylenoyl phenylalanine		

Table 3. Cont.

Literature	Study Format	No. of Subjects	Compared Formulations	Treatment	Key Findings
[144]	A double-blind, vehicle-controlled, full-face, parallel-group clinical study	101	4% nicotinamide plus 2% N-acetyl glucosamine	Treatment of a sunscreen lotion in the morning and test creams in the evening for 8 weeks.	The formulation reduced the area of facial spots and the appearance of irregular pigmentation at weeks 6 (p = 0.0270 and weeks 8 (p = 0.037).
		101	A vehicle cream		
[145]	A single-center, randomized, double-blind, controlled study	30	trans-4-(amino methyl) cyclohexanecarboxylic acid, potassium azeloyl diglycinate, and nicotinamide	Treatment in the morning and before bedtime for 8 weeks.	The formulation reduced the relative melanin value at week 6 (p = 0.006); Reduced MASI scores at week 4 (p = 0.005).
		30	Emulsion-based control		
[146]	A prospective, randomized, double-blind, vehicle-controlled clinical study	21	2% nicotinamide plus 2% tranexamic acid	Treatment in the morning and evening for 8 weeks.	The formulation reduced melanin index from baseline at weeks 4 (p < 0.001) and 8 (p < 0.001). It reduced the mean pigment intensity score compared with the vehicle control formulation (p = 0.015).
		21	A vehicle cream		
[147]	A clinical study	55	3% tranexamic acid, 1% kojic acid, 5% nicotinamide, and 5% hydroxyethylpiperazineethane sulfonic acid	Treatment in the morning and evening for 12 weeks.	The formulation reduced melanin index and improved the appearance of hyperpigmentation compared to both pre-treatment baselines.
[148]	A prospective, randomized, controlled split-face study	18	SKNB19 formulation containing epidermal growth factor, tranexamic acid, vitamin C, arbutin, nicotinamide, and other ingredients	Treatment in the morning and night for 8 weeks. Hydroquinone application only nightly.	SKNB19 improved the appearance of hyperpigmentation when compared with 4% hydroquinone.
			Standard formulation containing 4% hydroquinone		

In the study of Bissett et al. [143], the whitening efficacies of 5% nicotinamide alone and combined formulation of 5% nicotinamide plus 1% N-undecylenoyl phenylalanine were compared. Significant differences were found after 8 weeks of using these products, the latter being significantly more efficacious. In several other clinical studies, the combined formulation was compared with the vehicle formulation; thus, it is difficult to distinguish the contribution of individual components. In addition, in some studies, the content of active ingredients is not disclosed, and therefore, caution is needed in interpreting the results.

Significantly superior results were observed when the composite formulation (A gel containing 2% ascorbyl glucoside, and 3.5% nicotinamide) was applied with ultrasonic treatment, compared to either conventional application only or ultrasonic treatment only [142]. This study suggests that active ingredients, as well as techniques to increase skin absorption, are important for better clinical benefit.

9. Discussion

9.1. Cosmetic Benefits and Side Effects of Topical Nicotinamide

In cosmetics, nicotinamide is mainly formulated at a concentration of 4 to 5% and is used to control skin aging and pigmentation. Several clinical trials have shown that the formulation containing nicotinamide has the effect of relieving skin aging such as wrinkles, elasticity, and skin color, compared to the control formulation that does not contain nicotine [23,134,135]. When nicotinamide-containing cosmetics are used in a well-planned regimen, you can expect a skin-aging-relieving effect comparable to that of retinol products [135]. To be sure, you can expect a good effect with a combination of nicotinamide and retinol [137]. When products containing nicotinamide are applied to hyperpigmented areas, skin-lightening effects can be expected [22,111]. The facial skin-lightening efficacy of 4% nicotinamide is almost comparable to that of 4% hydroquinone [139]. The underarm skin-lightening efficacy of 4% nicotinamide is slightly weaker than 0.5% desonide [140].

Nicotinamide-containing products can be used together with sunscreen products to attenuate sun-induced skin aging and pigmentation [135,143]. The skin-lightening efficacy of nicotinamide can be expected to increase with the use of a device that helps transdermal absorption of the active ingredient [142]. Nicotinamide can be combined with other active ingredients for added skin-lightening efficacy [143]. If nicotinamide plays a role in inhibiting melanosome transfer in preventing skin pigmentation, combining it with other active ingredients that play a different role would maximize the effect. Potential candidates for combination with nicotinamide for this purpose may include substances that inhibit the expression of enzymes involved in melanin synthesis [149,150], that inhibit the catalytic activity of an enzyme [151–153], and/or that reduce the relative ratio of eumelanin to pheomelanin [154,155].

Although nicotinamide is considered a very safe nutrient, its long-term use at very high doses may cause side effects to the liver or other organs [156]. Serious metabolic and epigenetic changes were observed in rats fed with high doses of nicotinamide over a long period [157]. When 10% nicotinamide was applied to the skin, human subjects did not feel stinging sensation or flushing, and irritation did not appear in a single-use primary irritation test or a cumulative irritation test for 21 days with 5% product [158]. Thus, nicotinamide is well tolerated by the skin at the normally used concentrations (<5%) [159]. Nevertheless, the skin reaction to nicotinamide can vary depending on the skin condition of each individual; thus, it is necessary to consult a doctor if severe side effects exist.

9.2. Mechanisms of Skin Antiaging Action of Nicotinamide

This review highlights the fact that nicotinamide can have a wide range of effects on cellular metabolism; therefore, it is not easy to identify the mechanism of this substance in controlling skin aging. Although nicotinamide, a reaction product of sirtuins or PARPs, can inhibit these enzymes at several tens of micromolar concentrations [160,161], it is unclear whether its intracellular concentrations can reach that high. Nicotinamide is known to be absorbed into cells to some extent, but its transporter has not been identified yet, whereas transporters of nicotinic acid and 1-methylnicotinamide are relatively well known [162]. The different effects of nicotinamide on the lifespans of yeast and mammalian cells [67–69] suggest that in the latter case, the intracellular concentration is lower, and thus, the sirtuins inhibitory concentration cannot be reached. A possible cause is that nicotinamide is rapidly converted to NMN by NAMPT outside the cell. In agreement with this assumption, a secreted form of NAMPT exists outside the cell [163], and a transporter responsible for the intracellular uptake of NMN produced by this enzyme was recently discovered [164]. Accordingly, it is emphasized that the biological effects of nicotinamide can be dependent on the activity of NAMPT, which plays an important role in aging [165].

Natural aging and photoaging commonly accompany cellular senescence, chronic inflammation, and changes in the ECM and skin barrier along with external appearance changes. In senescent cells, NAMPT, NAD^+ pool, and mitochondrial electron transport activity decrease, while ROS production increases [71,73,75]. The supply of nicotinamide helps to normalize these changes, delaying cell senescence and extending its lifespan [72,74,75,77]. Nicotinamide inhibits the production of inflammatory cytokines and PGs in keratinocytes or in three-dimensional skin models that are exposed to UV radiation [58,59]. Nicotinamide decreases ECM-degrading enzymes and increases collagen synthesis in dermal fibroblasts [100–102]. Nicotinamide enhances the structural and functional integrity of the skin barrier by increasing the synthesis of lipid components [105]. Although nicotinamide exhibits various biological activities, the evidence for the existence of a specific molecular target is not clear. For now, it is believed that nicotinamide contributes to skin homeostasis by regulating the redox status of cells along with various metabolites produced from it.

9.3. Mechanisms of Skin Depigmenting Action of Nicotinamide

The effects of nicotinamide on melanin synthesis in mono-cultured melanocytes are diverse [109,110]. It is presumed that nicotinamide can help restore intrinsic melanin synthesis in melanocytes when it is impaired for some reason, whereas it can prevent excessive melanin synthesis stimulated by external signals. In the keratinocyte–melanocyte co-culture system, nicotinamide appears to consistently decrease the amount of melanin delivered to keratinocytes [22,111]. This finding has been confirmed in other independent studies [166,167]. Therefore, the interaction between these two cell types can be modulated by nicotinamide, but the underlying molecular mechanism remains to be explored.

It is worth noting PAR-2 as the main director of melanosome transfer from melanocytes to keratinocytes [122]. The receptor is expressed in keratinocytes, is activated by stimuli, such as UV radiation or hydrogen peroxide, and releases PGE_2, which warns surrounding cells including melanocytes [124,125]. The melanocytes are then activated by this signal to initiate the synthesis of melanin and biogenesis of melanosomes and deliver mature melanosomes to keratinocytes via dendrites [126,127]. In this scenario, if a substance could affect either or both of these two steps, it would exert an inhibitory effect on skin hyperpigmentation. Studying whether nicotinamide affects the PAR-2 mediated signal transduction process will be important in elucidating the mechanism of the pigmentation inhibitory action of this substance.

A recent study showed that NNT could regulate melanin synthesis in the skin [168]. In human melanoma cells, depletion of NNT increased melanin synthesis, which was inhibited by N-acetyl cysteine. Overexpression of NNT decreased eumelanin synthesis, which was attributed to increases in the $NADPH/NADP^+$ ratio and the GSH/GSSG ratio. NNT expression levels were low in post-inflammatory hyperpigmentation or age spots of human skin. It would be interesting to examine the effects of nicotinamide on pigmentation in the skin with altered NNT activity.

9.4. Questions to Be Answered in Future Studies

As discussed above, important and interesting questions about the mechanism of action and biological activity of nicotinamide remain unclear, with the following questions to list a few:

- Is there any specific molecular target of nicotinamide for the control of skin aging or pigmentation?
- Is the antiaging effect of nicotinamide is due to its intrinsic property or its metabolites?
- How does nicotinamide modulate the cell-to-cell interactions in the skin?
- Whether and how does nicotinamide regulate PAR-2 or NNT involved in skin pigmentation?
- Does nicotinamide supplementation affect the $NADPH/NADP^+$ ratio and the GSH/GSSG ratio in the skin?
- Would it be more effective if the dose of nicotinamide is adjusted according to the NAD^+ pool level, which varies depending on the individual skin condition?
- How does nicotinamide affect the self-renewal, proliferation, differentiation, senescence, and eventual exhaustion of epidermal stem cells?

10. Conclusions

The action of nicotinamide in controlling skin aging and pigmentation may be due to the intrinsic properties of nicotinamide, or the properties of other metabolites derived from nicotinamide, or both. Nicotinamide mitigates oxidative stress of cells via a direct ROS/free radical-scavenging action or an indirect action that enhances the antioxidant capacity of cells. Nicotinamide is metabolized by NAMPT to restore the NAD^+ pool and delay the senescence of cells. Both nicotinamide and its metabolites, such as NMN and 1-methylnicotinamide exert anti-inflammatory properties in various experimental models. Therefore, for cosmetic applications of nicotinamide, it is important to consider the biological activities of its metabolites as well as nicotinamide itself.

External stimuli, such as UV light and PM, internal stimuli, and chronological time cause skin aging and hyperpigmentation through direct and indirect paths. When epidermal keratinocytes are activated through ROS-mediated signaling, the expressions of inflammatory cytokines, PGs, and other signaling molecules are induced. Signaling molecules, such as stratifin, secreted from keratinocytes activate dermal fibroblasts to release MMPs for ECM remodeling. PGs secreted from keratinocytes activate epidermal melanocytes to increase melanin synthesis and melanosome biogenesis, and promote intercellular melanosome transfer from melanocytes to keratinocytes. These overall processes can be alleviated by supplementation of nicotinamide, resulting in reduced skin aging and pigmentation.

Therefore, nutritional and pharmacological actions of nicotinamide may be mediated by a complex mechanism including several metabolic pathways and multiple signaling processes. Aside from the identity of the mechanism of action, the results of many clinical trials suggest that nicotinamide is a beneficial cosmetic ingredient that helps skin health and beauty without any severe side effects.

Funding: This research was supported by a grant of the Korea Health Technology R&D Project through the Korea Health Industry Development Institute (KHIDI), funded by the Ministry of Health and Welfare, Republic of Korea (Grant Number: HP20C0004).

Conflicts of Interest: The authors declare no conflict of interest.

Abbreviations

ADP	adenosine diphosphate
AMP	adenosine monophosphate
ATP	adenosine triphosphate
cADPR	cyclic ADP ribose
CYP	cytochrome P450
ECM	extracellular matrix
GSH	glutathione
GSSG	glutathione disulfide
IL	interleukin
MAPK	mitogen-activated protein kinase
MASI	melasma area and severity index
MMP	matrix metalloproteinase
NaAD$^+$	nicotinic acid adenine dinucleotide
NaADP$^+$	nicotinic acid adenine dinucleotide phosphate
NAD$^+$	nicotinamide adenine dinucleotide
NADH	reduced nicotinamide adenine dinucleotide
NADP$^+$	nicotinamide adenine dinucleotide phosphate
NADPH	reduced nicotinamide adenine dinucleotide phosphate
NaMN	nicotinic acid mononucleotide
NAMPT	nicotinamide phosphoribosyltransferase
NF-κB	nuclear factor-κB
NMN	nicotinamide mononucleotide
NNT	nicotinamide nucleotide transhydrogenase
PAR-2	protease-activated receptor-2
PARP	poly(ADP-ribose) polymerase
PG	prostaglandin
PM	particulate matter
PPi	inorganic pyrophosphate
PRPP	phosphoribosyl pyrophosphate
ROS	reactive oxygen species
sir2	silent information regulator-2
SIRT1	sirtruin1
SPF	sun protection factor
TGF-β	transforming growth factor-β
TNF-α	tumor necrosis factor-α
UV	ultraviolet

References

1. Chambers, E.S.; Vukmanovic-Stejic, M. Skin barrier immunity and ageing. *Immunology* **2020**, *160*, 116–125. [CrossRef] [PubMed]
2. Fisher, G.J.; Kang, S.; Varani, J.; Bata-Csorgo, Z.; Wan, Y.; Datta, S.; Voorhees, J.J. Mechanisms of photoaging and chronological skin aging. *Arch. Dermatol.* **2002**, *138*, 1462–1470. [CrossRef] [PubMed]
3. Rittie, L.; Fisher, G.J. Natural and sun-induced aging of human skin. *Cold Spring Harb. Perspect. Med.* **2015**, *5*, a015370. [CrossRef] [PubMed]
4. Tzaphlidou, M. The role of collagen and elastin in aged skin: An image processing approach. *Micron* **2004**, *35*, 173–177. [CrossRef]
5. Pizzino, G.; Irrera, N.; Cucinotta, M.; Pallio, G.; Mannino, F.; Arcoraci, V.; Squadrito, F.; Altavilla, D.; Bitto, A. Oxidative Stress: Harms and Benefits for Human Health. *Oxid. Med. Cell. Longev.* **2017**, *2017*, 8416763. [CrossRef]
6. Gu, Y.; Han, J.; Jiang, C.; Zhang, Y. Biomarkers, oxidative stress and autophagy in skin aging. *Ageing Res. Rev.* **2020**, *59*, 101036. [CrossRef] [PubMed]
7. Kammeyer, A.; Luiten, R.M. Oxidation events and skin aging. *Ageing Res. Rev.* **2015**, *21*, 16–29. [CrossRef]
8. Shah, A.A.; Sinha, A.A. Oxidative stress and autoimmune skin disease. *Eur. J. Dermatol.* **2013**, *23*, 5–13. [CrossRef]
9. Bickers, D.R.; Athar, M. Oxidative stress in the pathogenesis of skin disease. *J. Investig. Dermatol.* **2006**, *126*, 2565–2575. [CrossRef]
10. Awad, F.; Assrawi, E.; Louvrier, C.; Jumeau, C.; Giurgea, I.; Amselem, S.; Karabina, S.A. Photoaging and skin cancer: Is the inflammasome the missing link? *Mech. Ageing Dev.* **2018**, *172*, 131–137. [CrossRef]
11. Boo, Y.C. Natural Nrf2 Modulators for Skin Protection. *Antioxidants* **2020**, *9*, 812. [CrossRef]
12. Baek, J.; Lee, M.G. Oxidative stress and antioxidant strategies in dermatology. *Redox Rep.* **2016**, *21*, 164–169. [CrossRef]
13. Hegyi, J.; Schwartz, R.A.; Hegyi, V. Pellagra: Dermatitis, dementia, and diarrhea. *Int. J. Dermatol.* **2004**, *43*, 1–5. [CrossRef]
14. Kirkland, J.B. Niacin Status, NAD Distribution and ADP-Ribose Metabolism. *Curr. Pharm. Des.* **2009**, *15*, 3–11. [CrossRef] [PubMed]
15. De Figueiredo, L.F.; Gossmann, T.I.; Ziegler, M.; Schuster, S. Pathway analysis of NAD$^+$ metabolism. *Biochem. J.* **2011**, *439*, 341–348. [CrossRef]
16. Mattiussi, A.J.; Blais, D. Niacin Versus Niacinamide. *Can. Med Assoc. J.* **1992**, *147*, 990–991.
17. MacKay, D.; Hathcock, J.; Guarneri, E. Niacin: Chemical forms, bioavailability, and health effects. *Nutr. Rev.* **2012**, *70*, 357–366. [CrossRef]
18. Surjana, D.; Damian, D.L. Nicotinamide in dermatology and photoprotection. *Skinmed* **2011**, *9*, 360–365. [PubMed]
19. Forbat, E.; Al-Niaimi, F.; Ali, F.R. Use of nicotinamide in dermatology. *Clin. Exp. Dermatol.* **2017**, *42*, 137–144. [CrossRef]
20. Ballotti, R.; Healy, E.; Bertolotto, C. Nicotinamide as a chemopreventive therapy of skin cancers. Too much of good thing? *Pigment. Cell Melanoma Res.* **2019**, *32*, 601–602. [CrossRef]
21. Snaidr, V.A.; Damian, D.L.; Halliday, G.M. Nicotinamide for photoprotection and skin cancer chemoprevention: A review of efficacy and safety. *Exp. Dermatol.* **2019**, *28* (Suppl. S1), 15–22. [CrossRef]
22. Hakozaki, T.; Minwalla, L.; Zhuang, J.; Chhoa, M.; Matsubara, A.; Miyamoto, K.; Greatens, A.; Hillebrand, G.G.; Bissett, D.L.; Boissy, R.E. The effect of niacinamide on reducing cutaneous pigmentation and suppression of melanosome transfer. *Br. J. Dermatol.* **2002**, *147*, 20–31. [CrossRef]
23. Bissett, D.L.; Miyamoto, K.; Sun, P.; Li, J.; Berge, C.A. Topical niacinamide reduces yellowing, wrinkling, red blotchiness, and hyperpigmented spots in aging facial skin. *Int. J. Cosmet. Sci.* **2004**, *26*, 231–238. [CrossRef]
24. Bissett, D.L.; Oblong, J.E.; Berge, C.A. Niacinamide: A B vitamin that improves aging facial skin appearance. *Dermatol. Surg.* **2005**, *31*, 860–865; discussion 865. [CrossRef]
25. Otte, N.; Borelli, C.; Korting, H.C. Nicotinamide—Biologic actions of an emerging cosmetic ingredient. *Int. J. Cosmet. Sci.* **2005**, *27*, 255–261. [CrossRef]
26. Braidy, N.; Berg, J.; Clement, J.; Khorshidi, F.; Poljak, A.; Jayasena, T.; Grant, R.; Sachdev, P. Role of Nicotinamide Adenine Dinucleotide and Related Precursors as Therapeutic Targets for Age-Related Degenerative Diseases: Rationale, Biochemistry, Pharmacokinetics, and Outcomes. *Antioxid. Redox Signal.* **2019**, *30*, 251–294. [CrossRef]
27. Fukuwatari, T.; Shibata, K. Nutritional aspect of tryptophan metabolism. *Int. J. Tryptophan Res.* **2013**, *6*, 3–8. [CrossRef]
28. Shibata, K. Organ Co-Relationship in Tryptophan Metabolism and Factors That Govern the Biosynthesis of Nicotinamide from Tryptophan. *J. Nutr. Sci. Vitaminol.* **2018**, *64*, 90–98. [CrossRef]
29. Kennedy, B.E.; Sharif, T.; Martell, E.; Dai, C.; Kim, Y.; Lee, P.W.K.; Gujar, S.A. NAD$^+$ salvage pathway in cancer metabolism and therapy. *Pharmacol. Res.* **2016**, *114*, 274–283. [CrossRef] [PubMed]
30. Tedeschi, P.M.; Bansal, N.; Kerrigan, J.E.; Abali, E.E.; Scotto, K.W.; Bertino, J.R. NAD$^+$ Kinase as a Therapeutic Target in Cancer. *Clin. Cancer Res.* **2016**, *22*, 5189–5195. [CrossRef] [PubMed]
31. Zhang, Q.; Padayatti, P.S.; Leung, J.H. Proton-Translocating Nicotinamide Nucleotide Transhydrogenase: A Structural Perspective. *Front. Physiol.* **2017**, *8*, 1089. [CrossRef]
32. Chini, C.C.S.; Zeidler, J.D.; Kashyap, S.; Warner, G.; Chini, E.N. Evolving concepts in NAD$^+$ metabolism. *Cell Metab.* **2021**, *33*, 1076–1087. [CrossRef]
33. Schweiker, S.S.; Tauber, A.L.; Sherry, M.E.; Levonis, S.M. Structure, Function and Inhibition of Poly(ADP-ribose)polymerase, Member 14 (PARP14). *Mini Rev. Med. Chem.* **2018**, *18*, 1659–1669. [CrossRef]
34. Palazzo, L.; Mikolcevic, P.; Mikoc, A.; Ahel, I. ADP-ribosylation signalling and human disease. *Open Biol.* **2019**, *9*, 190041. [CrossRef] [PubMed]

35. Hassa, P.O.; Haenni, S.S.; Elser, M.; Hottiger, M.O. Nuclear ADP-ribosylation reactions in mammalian cells: Where are we today and where are we going? *Microbiology and Molecular Biology Reviews* **2006**, *70*, 789–+. [CrossRef] [PubMed]
36. Morales, J.C.; Li, L.S.; Fattah, F.J.; Dong, Y.; Bey, E.A.; Patel, M.; Geo, J.M.; Boothman, D.A. Review of Poly (ADP-ribose) Polymerase (PARP) Mechanisms of Action and Rationale for Targeting in Cancer and Other Diseases. *Crit. Rev. Eukaryot. Gene Expr.* **2014**, *24*, 15–28. [CrossRef]
37. Watroba, M.; Dudek, I.; Skoda, M.; Stangret, A.; Rzodkiewicz, P.; Szukiewicz, D. Sirtuins, epigenetics and longevity. *Ageing Res. Rev.* **2017**, *40*, 11–19. [CrossRef]
38. Klein, M.A.; Denu, J.M. Biological and catalytic functions of sirtuin 6 as targets for small-molecule modulators. *J. Biol. Chem.* **2020**, *295*, 11021–11041. [CrossRef]
39. Chang, H.C.; Guarente, L. SIRT1 and other sirtuins in metabolism. *Trends Endocrinol. Metab.* **2014**, *25*, 138–145. [CrossRef] [PubMed]
40. Kar, A.; Mehrotra, S.; Chatterjee, S. CD38: T Cell Immuno-Metabolic Modulator. *Cells* **2020**, *9*, 1716. [CrossRef]
41. Aarhus, R.; Graeff, R.M.; Dickey, D.M.; Walseth, T.F.; Lee, H.C. ADP-ribosyl cyclase and CD38 catalyze the synthesis of a calcium-mobilizing metabolite from NADP$^+$. *J. Biol. Chem.* **1995**, *270*, 30327–30333. [CrossRef] [PubMed]
42. Nam, T.S.; Park, D.R.; Rah, S.Y.; Woo, T.G.; Chung, H.T.; Brenner, C.; Kim, U.H. Interleukin-8 drives CD38 to form NAADP from NADP$^+$ and NAAD in the endolysosomes to mobilize Ca^{2+} and effect cell migration. *FASEB J.* **2020**, *34*, 12565–12576. [CrossRef]
43. Yu, P.L.; Cai, X.B.; Liang, Y.; Wang, M.X.; Yang, W. Roles of NAD$^+$ and Its Metabolites Regulated Calcium Channels in Cancer. *Molecules* **2020**, *25*, 4826. [CrossRef]
44. Gul, R.; Park, D.R.; Shawl, A.I.; Im, S.Y.; Nam, T.S.; Lee, S.H.; Ko, J.K.; Jang, K.Y.; Kim, D.; Kim, U.H. Nicotinic Acid Adenine Dinucleotide Phosphate (NAADP) and Cyclic ADP-Ribose (cADPR) Mediate Ca^{2+} Signaling in Cardiac Hypertrophy Induced by beta-Adrenergic Stimulation. *PLoS ONE* **2016**, *11*, e0149515. [CrossRef]
45. Pissios, P. Nicotinamide N-Methyltransferase: More Than a Vitamin B3 Clearance Enzyme. *Trends Endocrinol. Metab.* **2017**, *28*, 340–353. [CrossRef]
46. Felsted, R.L.; Chaykin, S. N1-methylnicotinamide oxidation in a number of mammals. *J. Biol. Chem.* **1967**, *242*, 1274–1279. [CrossRef]
47. Real, A.M.; Hong, S.Y.; Pissios, P. Nicotinamide N-Oxidation by CYP2E1 in Human Liver Microsomes. *Drug Metab. Dispos.* **2013**, *41*, 550–553. [CrossRef]
48. Nadzhimutdinov, K.N.; Mavlianov, I.R.; Umarov, E.F.; Mutalov, N.K. The effect of alpha-tocopherol and nicotinamide on lipid peroxidation and the activity of the antioxidant system in the lung tissue of premature rat pups. *Eksp. Klin. Farmakol.* **1993**, *56*, 28–30.
49. Legon'kova, L.F.; Bushma, M.I.; Zverinskii, I.V.; Abakumov, G.Z.; Zavodnik, L.V. The effect of nicotinamide, methionine and alpha-tocopherol on the liver conjugating and mono-oxygenase systems and on lipid peroxidation in hepatosis-hepatitis in rats. *Eksp. Klin. Farmakol.* **1997**, *60*, 68–71.
50. Velykyi, M.M.; Burda, V.A.; Biront, N.V.; Oliiarnyk, O.D.; Velykyi, A.M. The effect of nicotinamide on the enzymatic activity of the antioxidant defense in experimental diabetes. *Ukr. Biokhimicheskii Zhurnal (1978)* **1996**, *68*, 109–114.
51. Kamat, J.P.; Devasagayam, T.P. Methylene blue plus light-induced lipid peroxidation in rat liver microsomes: Inhibition by nicotinamide (vitamin B3) and other antioxidants. *Chem. Biol. Interact.* **1996**, *99*, 1–16. [CrossRef]
52. Kamat, J.P.; Devasagayam, T.P.A. Nicotinamide (vitamin B-3) as an effective antioxidant against oxidative damage in rat brain mitochondria. *Redox Rep.* **1999**, *4*, 179–184. [CrossRef]
53. Izdebska, M.; Halas-Wisniewska, M.; Adamczyk, I.; Lewandowska, I.; Kwiatkowska, I.; Gagat, M.; Grzanka, A. The protective effect of niacinamide on CHO AA8 cell line against ultraviolet radiation in the context of main cytoskeletal proteins. *Adv. Clin. Exp. Med.* **2018**, *27*, 367–378. [CrossRef]
54. Chhabra, G.; Garvey, D.R.; Singh, C.K.; Mintie, C.A.; Ahmad, N. Effects and Mechanism of Nicotinamide Against UVA- and/or UVB-mediated DNA Damages in Normal Melanocytes. *Photochem. Photobiol.* **2019**, *95*, 331–337. [CrossRef] [PubMed]
55. Zhen, A.X.; Piao, M.J.; Kang, K.A.; Fernando, P.D.S.M.; Kang, H.K.; Koh, Y.S.; Yi, J.M.; Hyun, J.W. Niacinamide Protects Skin Cells from Oxidative Stress Induced by Particulate Matter. *Biomol. Ther.* **2019**, *27*, 562–569. [CrossRef] [PubMed]
56. Mi, T.Y.; Dong, Y.Y.; Santhanam, U.; Huang, N. Niacinamide and 12-hydroxystearic acid prevented benzo(a)pyrene and squalene peroxides induced hyperpigmentation in skin equivalent. *Exp. Dermatol.* **2019**, *28*, 742–746. [CrossRef]
57. Grange, P.A.; Raingeaud, J.; Calvez, V.; Dupin, N. Nicotinamide inhibits Propionibacterium acnes-induced IL-8 production in keratinocytes through the NF-kappaB and MAPK pathways. *J. Dermatol. Sci.* **2009**, *56*, 106–112. [CrossRef]
58. Monfrecola, G.; Gaudiello, F.; Cirillo, T.; Fabbrocini, G.; Balato, A.; Lembo, S. Nicotinamide downregulates gene expression of interleukin-6, interleukin-10, monocyte chemoattractant protein-1, and tumour necrosis factor-alpha gene expression in HaCaT keratinocytes after ultraviolet B irradiation. *Clin. Exp. Dermatol.* **2013**, *38*, 185–188. [CrossRef] [PubMed]
59. Bierman, J.C.; Laughlin, T.; Tamura, M.; Hulette, B.; Mack, C.E.; Sherrill, J.D.; Tan, C.Y.R.; Morenc, M.; Bellanger, S.; Oblong, J.E. Niacinamide mitigates SASP-related inflammation induced by environmental stressors in human epidermal keratinocytes and skin. *Int. J. Cosmet. Sci.* **2020**, *42*, 501–511. [CrossRef]
60. Bryniarski, K.; Biedron, R.; Jakubowski, A.; Chlopicki, S.; Marcinkiewicz, J. Anti-inflammatory effect of 1-methylnicotinamide in contact hypersensitivity to oxazolone in mice; involvement of prostacyclin. *Eur. J. Pharmacol.* **2008**, *578*, 332–338. [CrossRef]

61. Biedron, R.; Ciszek, M.; Tokarczyk, M.; Bobek, M.; Kurnyta, M.; Slominska, E.M.; Smolenski, R.T.; Marcinkiewicz, J. 1-Methylnicotinamide and nicotinamide: Two related anti-inflammatory agents that differentially affect the functions of activated macrophages. *Arch. Immunol. Ther. Exp.* **2008**, *56*, 127–134. [CrossRef]
62. Wozniacka, A.; Wieczorkowska, M.; Gebicki, J.; Sysa-Jedrzejowska, A. Topical application of 1-methylnicotinamide in the treatment of rosacea: A pilot study. *Clin. Exp. Dermatol.* **2005**, *30*, 632–635. [CrossRef] [PubMed]
63. Pietrzak, L.; Mogielnicki, A.; Buczko, W. Nicotinamide and its metabolite N-methylnicotinamide increase skin vascular permeability in rats. *Clin. Exp. Dermatol.* **2009**, *34*, 380–384. [CrossRef]
64. Jiang, N.; Wang, M.; Song, J.Y.; Liu, Y.G.; Chen, H.; Mu, D.; Xia, M. N-methylnicotinamide protects against endothelial dysfunction and attenuates atherogenesis in apolipoprotein E-deficient mice. *Mol. Nutr. Food Res.* **2016**, *60*, 1625–1636. [CrossRef] [PubMed]
65. Huynh, P.K.; Wilder, J.; Hiller, S.; Hagaman, J.; Takahashi, N.; Maeda-Smithies, N.; Li, F. Beneficial effects of nicotinamide on hypertensive mice with impaired endothelial nitric oxide function. *J. Exp. Nephrol.* **2020**, *1*, 1–8. [PubMed]
66. Zhou, X.R.; Du, H.H.; Ni, L.Y.; Ran, J.; Hu, J.; Yu, J.J.; Zhao, X. Nicotinamide Mononucleotide Combined with Lactobacillus fermentum TKSN041 Reduces the Photoaging Damage in Murine Skin by Activating AMPK Signaling Pathway. *Front. Pharmacol.* **2021**, *12*, 643089. [CrossRef] [PubMed]
67. Anderson, R.M.; Bitterman, K.J.; Wood, J.G.; Medvedik, O.; Sinclair, D.A. Nicotinamide and PNC1 govern lifespan extension by calorie restriction in Saccharomyces cerevisiae. *Nature* **2003**, *423*, 181–185. [CrossRef] [PubMed]
68. Matuoka, K.; Chen, K.Y.; Takenawa, T. Rapid reversion of aging phenotypes by nicotinamide through possible modulation of histone acetylation. *Cell. Mol. Life Sci.* **2001**, *58*, 2108–2116. [CrossRef]
69. Lim, C.S.; Potts, M.; Helm, R.E. Nicotinamide extends the replicative life span of primary human cells. *Mech. Ageing Dev.* **2006**, *127*, 511–514. [CrossRef]
70. Porcu, M.; Chiarugi, A. The emerging therapeutic potential of sirtuin-interacting drugs: From cell death to lifespan extension. *Trends Pharmacol. Sci.* **2005**, *26*, 94–103. [CrossRef]
71. Adams, J.D.; Klaidman, L.K. Sirtuins, nicotinamide and aging: A critical review. *Lett. Drug Des. Discov.* **2007**, *4*, 44–48. [CrossRef]
72. Massudi, H.; Grant, R.; Braidy, N.; Guest, J.; Farnsworth, B.; Guillemin, G.J. Age-Associated Changes In Oxidative Stress and NAD^+ Metabolism In Human Tissue. *PLoS ONE* **2012**, *7*, e42357. [CrossRef]
73. Oblong, J.E. The evolving role of the NAD plus/nicotinamide metabolome in skin homeostasis, cellular bioenergetics, and aging. *DNA Repair* **2014**, *23*, 59–63. [CrossRef]
74. Kang, H.T.; Il Lee, H.; Hwang, E.S. Nicotinamide extends replicative lifespan of human cells. *Aging Cell* **2006**, *5*, 423–436. [CrossRef] [PubMed]
75. Kwak, J.Y.; Ham, H.J.; Kim, C.M.; Hwang, E.S. Nicotinamide exerts antioxidative effects on senescent cells. *Mol. Cells* **2015**, *38*, 229–235. [CrossRef]
76. Oblong, J.E.; Bowman, A.; Rovito, H.A.; Jarrold, B.B.; Sherrill, J.D.; Black, M.R.; Nelson, G.; Kimball, A.B.; Birch-Machin, M.A. Metabolic dysfunction in human skin: Restoration of mitochondrial integrity and metabolic output by nicotinamide (niacinamide) in primary dermal fibroblasts from older aged donors. *Aging Cell* **2020**, *19*, e13248. [CrossRef]
77. Borradaile, N.M.; Pickering, J.G. Nicotinamide phosphoribosyltransferase imparts human endothelial cells with extended replicative lifespan and enhanced angiogenic capacity in a high glucose environment. *Aging Cell* **2009**, *8*, 100–112. [CrossRef] [PubMed]
78. Rovito, H.A.; Oblong, J.E. Nicotinamide preferentially protects glycolysis in dermal fibroblasts under oxidative stress conditions. *Br. J. Dermatol.* **2013**, *169*, 15–24. [CrossRef] [PubMed]
79. Khaidizar, F.D.; Nakahata, Y.; Kume, A.; Sumizawa, K.; Kohno, K.; Matsui, T.; Bessho, Y. Nicotinamide phosphoribosyltransferase delays cellular senescence by upregulating SIRT1 activity and antioxidant gene expression in mouse cells. *Genes Cells* **2017**, *22*, 982–992. [CrossRef]
80. Tan, C.L.; Chin, T.; Tan, C.Y.R.; Rovito, H.A.; Quek, L.S.; Oblong, J.E.; Bellanger, S. Nicotinamide Metabolism Modulates the Proliferation/Differentiation Balance and Senescence of Human Primary Keratinocytes. *J. Investig. Dermatol.* **2019**, *139*, 1638–1647.e3. [CrossRef] [PubMed]
81. Taub, A.F.; Pham, K. Stem Cells in Dermatology and Anti-aging Care of the Skin. *Facial Plast. Surg. Clin. N. Am.* **2018**, *26*, 425–437. [CrossRef] [PubMed]
82. Zouboulis, C.C.; Adjaye, J.; Akamatsu, H.; Moe-Behrens, G.; Niemann, C. Human skin stem cells and the ageing process. *Exp. Gerontol.* **2008**, *43*, 986–997. [CrossRef] [PubMed]
83. Liu, N.; Matsumura, H.; Kato, T.; Ichinose, S.; Takada, A.; Namiki, T.; Asakawa, K.; Morinaga, H.; Mohri, Y.; De Arcangelis, A.; et al. Stem cell competition orchestrates skin homeostasis and ageing. *Nature* **2019**, *568*, 344–350. [CrossRef] [PubMed]
84. Gannon, H.S.; Donehower, L.A.; Lyle, S.; Jones, S.N. Mdm2-p53 signaling regulates epidermal stem cell senescence and premature aging phenotypes in mouse skin. *Dev. Biol.* **2011**, *353*, 1–9. [CrossRef]
85. Chu, G.Y.; Chen, Y.F.; Chen, H.Y.; Chan, M.H.; Gau, C.S.; Weng, S.M. Stem cell therapy on skin: Mechanisms, recent advances and drug reviewing issues. *J. Food Drug Anal.* **2018**, *26*, 14–20. [CrossRef] [PubMed]
86. Grabowska, W.; Sikora, E.; Bielak-Zmijewska, A. Sirtuins, a promising target in slowing down the ageing process. *Biogerontology* **2017**, *18*, 447–476. [CrossRef]
87. Mayack, B.K.; Sippl, W.; Ntie-Kang, F. Natural Products as Modulators of Sirtuins. *Molecules* **2020**, *25*, 3287. [CrossRef]

88. Meng, Y.; Ren, Z.; Xu, F.; Zhou, X.; Song, C.; Wang, V.Y.; Liu, W.; Lu, L.; Thomson, J.A.; Chen, G. Nicotinamide Promotes Cell Survival and Differentiation as Kinase Inhibitor in Human Pluripotent Stem Cells. *Stem Cell Rep.* **2018**, *11*, 1347–1356. [CrossRef]
89. Cole, M.A.; Quan, T.; Voorhees, J.J.; Fisher, G.J. Extracellular matrix regulation of fibroblast function: Redefining our perspective on skin aging. *J. Cell Commun. Signal.* **2018**, *12*, 35–43. [CrossRef]
90. Shin, J.W.; Kwon, S.H.; Choi, J.Y.; Na, J.I.; Huh, C.H.; Choi, H.R.; Park, K.C. Molecular Mechanisms of Dermal Aging and Antiaging Approaches. *Int. J. Mol. Sci.* **2019**, *20*, 2126. [CrossRef]
91. Quan, T.H.; Fisher, G.J. Role of Age-Associated Alterations of the Dermal Extracellular Matrix Microenvironment in Human Skin Aging: A Mini-Review. *Gerontology* **2015**, *61*, 427–434. [CrossRef] [PubMed]
92. Imokawa, G.; Ishida, K. Biological mechanisms underlying the ultraviolet radiation-induced formation of skin wrinkling and sagging I: Reduced skin elasticity, highly associated with enhanced dermal elastase activity, triggers wrinkling and sagging. *Int. J. Mol. Sci.* **2015**, *16*, 7753–7775. [CrossRef] [PubMed]
93. Ghahary, A.; Marcoux, Y.; Karimi-Busheri, F.; Li, Y.; Tredget, E.E.; Kilani, R.T.; Lam, E.; Weinfeld, M. Differentiated keratinocyte-releasable stratifin (14-3-3 sigma) stimulates MMP-1 expression in dermal fibroblasts. *J. Investig. Dermatol.* **2005**, *124*, 170–177. [CrossRef]
94. Lam, E.; Kilani, R.T.; Li, Y.; Tredget, E.E.; Ghahary, A. Stratifin-induced matrix metalloproteinase-1 in fibroblast is mediated by c-fos and p38 mitogen-activated protein kinase activation. *J. Investig. Dermatol.* **2005**, *125*, 230–238. [CrossRef] [PubMed]
95. Adachi, H.; Murakami, Y.; Tanaka, H.; Nakata, S. Increase of stratifin triggered by ultraviolet irradiation is possibly related to premature aging of human skin. *Exp. Dermatol.* **2014**, *23* (Suppl. S1), 32–36. [CrossRef]
96. Seok, J.K.; Boo, Y.C. p-Coumaric Acid Attenuates UVB-Induced Release of Stratifin from Keratinocytes and Indirectly Regulates Matrix Metalloproteinase 1 Release from Fibroblasts. *Korean J. Physiol. Pharmacol.* **2015**, *19*, 241–247. [CrossRef]
97. Taylor, K.R.; Gallo, R.L. Glycosaminoglycans and their proteoglycans: Host-associated molecular patterns for initiation and modulation of inflammation. *FASEB J.* **2006**, *20*, 9–22. [CrossRef]
98. Frantz, C.; Stewart, K.M.; Weaver, V.M. The extracellular matrix at a glance. *J. Cell Sci.* **2010**, *123*, 4195–4200. [CrossRef] [PubMed]
99. Lee, D.H.; Oh, J.H.; Chung, J.H. Glycosaminoglycan and proteoglycan in skin aging. *J. Dermatol. Sci.* **2016**, *83*, 174–181. [CrossRef]
100. Ratcliffe, D.R.; Iqbal, J.; Hussain, M.M.; Cramer, E.B. Fibrillar collagen type I stimulation of apolipoprotein B secretion in Caco-2 cells is mediated by beta1 integrin. *Biochim. Biophys. Acta* **2009**, *1791*, 1144–1154. [CrossRef]
101. Philips, N.; Chalensouk-Khaosaat, J.; Gonzalez, S. Simulation of the Elastin and Fibrillin in Non-Irradiated or UVA Radiated Fibroblasts, and Direct Inhibition of Elastase or Matrix Metalloptoteinases Activity by Nicotinamide or Its Derivatives. *J. Cosmet. Sci.* **2018**, *69*, 47–56.
102. Wessels, Q.; Pretorius, E.; Smith, C.M.; Nel, H. The potential of a niacinamide dominated cosmeceutical formulation on fibroblast activity and wound healing in vitro. *Int. Wound J.* **2014**, *11*, 152–158. [CrossRef]
103. Ashkani Esfahani, S.; Khoshnevisadeh, M.; Namazi, M.R.; Noorafshan, A.; Geramizadeh, B.; Nadimi, E.; Razavipour, S.T. Topical Nicotinamide Improves Tissue Regeneration in Excisional Full-Thickness Skin Wounds: A Stereological and Pathological Study. *Trauma Mon.* **2015**, *20*, e18193. [CrossRef]
104. Choi, E.H. Aging of the skin barrier. *Clin. Dermatol.* **2019**, *37*, 336–345. [CrossRef]
105. Tanno, O.; Ota, Y.; Kitamura, N.; Katsube, T.; Inoue, S. Nicotinamide increases biosynthesis of ceramides as well as other stratum corneum lipids to improve the epidermal permeability barrier. *Br. J. Dermatol.* **2000**, *143*, 524–531. [CrossRef] [PubMed]
106. Bissett, D. Topical niacinamide and barrier enhancement. *Cutis* **2002**, *70*, 8–12; discussion 21–23. [PubMed]
107. Draelos, Z.D.; Ertel, K.; Berge, C. Niacinamide-containing facial moisturizer improves skin barrier and benefits subjects with rosacea. *Cutis* **2005**, *76*, 135–141.
108. Jacobson, E.L.; Kim, H.; Kim, M.; Williams, J.D.; Coyle, D.L.; Coyle, W.R.; Grove, G.; Rizer, R.L.; Stratton, M.S.; Jacobson, M.K. A topical lipophilic niacin derivative increases NAD, epidermal differentiation and barrier function in photodamaged skin. *Exp. Dermatol.* **2007**, *16*, 490–499. [CrossRef]
109. Virador, V.M.; Kobayashi, N.; Matsunaga, J.; Hearing, V.J. A standardized protocol for assessing regulators of pigmentation. *Anal. Biochem.* **1999**, *270*, 207–219. [CrossRef]
110. Lei, T.C.; Virador, V.M.; Vieira, W.D.; Hearing, V.J. A melanocyte-keratinocyte coculture model to assess regulators of pigmentation in vitro. *Anal. Biochem.* **2002**, *305*, 260–268. [CrossRef] [PubMed]
111. Greatens, A.; Hakozaki, T.; Koshoffer, A.; Epstein, H.; Schwemberger, S.; Babcock, G.; Bissett, D.; Takiwaki, H.; Arase, S.; Wickett, R.R.; et al. Effective inhibition of melanosome transfer to keratinocytes by lectins and niacinamide is reversible. *Exp. Dermatol.* **2005**, *14*, 498–508. [CrossRef] [PubMed]
112. Seiberg, M. Keratinocyte-melanocyte interactions during melanosome transfer. *Pigment Cell Res.* **2001**, *14*, 236–242. [CrossRef]
113. Boissy, R.E. Melanosome transfer to and translocation in the keratinocyte. *Exp. Dermatol.* **2003**, *12*, 5–12. [CrossRef]
114. Hearing, V.J. Regulating melanosome transfer: Who's driving the bus? *Pigment Cell Res.* **2007**, *20*, 334–335. [CrossRef]
115. Wu, X.F.; Hammer, J.A. Melanosome transfer: It is best to give and receive. *Curr. Opin. Cell Biol.* **2014**, *29*, 1–7. [CrossRef]
116. Scott, G.; Leopardi, S.; Printup, S.; Madden, B.C. Filopodia are conduits for melanosome transfer to keratinocytes. *J. Cell Sci.* **2002**, *115*, 1441–1451. [CrossRef]
117. Ando, H.; Niki, Y.; Ito, M.; Akiyama, K.; Matsui, M.S.; Yarosh, D.B.; Ichihashi, M. Melanosomes Are Transferred from Melanocytes to Keratinocytes through the Processes of Packaging, Release, Uptake, and Dispersion. *J. Investig. Dermatol.* **2012**, *132*, 1222–1229. [CrossRef]

118. Wu, X.F.S.; Masedunskas, A.; Weigert, R.; Copeland, N.G.; Jenkins, N.A.; Hammer, J.A. Melanoregulin regulates a shedding mechanism that drives melanosome transfer from melanocytes to keratinocytes. *Proc. Natl. Acad. Sci. USA* **2012**, *109*, E2101–E2109. [CrossRef]
119. Tarafder, A.K.; Bolasco, G.; Correia, M.S.; Pereira, F.J.C.; Iannone, L.; Hume, A.N.; Kirkpatrick, N.; Picardo, M.; Torrisi, M.R.; Rodrigues, I.P.; et al. Rab11b Mediates Melanin Transfer between Donor Melanocytes and Acceptor Keratinocytes via Coupled Exo/Endocytosis. *J. Investig. Dermatol.* **2014**, *134*, 1056–1066. [CrossRef]
120. Santulli, R.J.; Derian, C.K.; Darrow, A.L.; Tomko, K.A.; Eckardt, A.J.; Seiberg, M.; Scarborough, R.M.; Andradegordon, P. Evidence for the Presence of a Protease-Activated Receptor Distinct from the Thrombin Receptor in Human Keratinocytes. *Proc. Natl. Acad. Sci. USA* **1995**, *92*, 9151–9155. [CrossRef]
121. Derian, C.K.; Eckardt, A.J.; Andrade-Gordon, P. Differential regulation of human keratinocyte growth and differentiation by a novel family of protease-activated receptors. *Cell Growth Differ.* **1997**, *8*, 743–749.
122. Seiberg, M.; Paine, C.; Sharlow, E.; Andrade-Gordon, P.; Costanzo, M.; Eisinger, M.; Shapiro, S.S. The protease-activated receptor 2 regulates pigmentation via keratinocyte-melanocyte interactions. *Exp. Cell Res.* **2000**, *254*, 25–32. [CrossRef]
123. Seiberg, M.; Paine, C.; Sharlow, E.; Andrade-Gordon, P.; Costanzo, M.; Eisinger, M.; Shapiro, S.S. Inhibition of melanosome transfer results in skin lightening. *J. Investig. Dermatol.* **2000**, *115*, 162–167. [CrossRef]
124. Scott, G.; Deng, A.; Rodriguez-Burford, C.; Seiberg, M.; Han, R.J.; Babiarz, L.; Grizzle, W.; Bell, W.; Pentland, A. Protease-activated receptor 2, a receptor involved in melanosome transfer, is upregulated in human skin by ultraviolet irradiation. *J. Investig. Dermatol.* **2001**, *117*, 1412–1420. [CrossRef]
125. Tang, L.Y.; Li, J.; Lin, X.; Wu, W.Y.; Kang, K.F.; Fu, W.W. Oxidation Levels Differentially Impact Melanocytes: Low versus High Concentration of Hydrogen Peroxide Promotes Melanin Synthesis and Melanosome Transfer. *Dermatology* **2012**, *224*, 145–153. [CrossRef]
126. Scott, G.; Leopardi, S.; Printup, S.; Malhi, N.; Seiberg, M.; Lapoint, R. Proteinase-activated receptor-2 stimulates prostaglandin production in keratinocytes: Analysis of prostaglandin receptors on human melanocytes and effects of PGE2 and PGF2alpha on melanocyte dendricity. *J. Investig. Dermatol.* **2004**, *122*, 1214–1224. [CrossRef]
127. Ma, H.J.; Ma, H.Y.; Yang, Y.; Li, P.C.; Zi, S.X.; Jia, C.Y.; Chen, R. alpha-Melanocyte stimulating hormone (MSH) and prostaglandin E2 (PGE2) drive melanosome transfer by promoting filopodia delivery and shedding spheroid granules: Evidences from atomic force microscopy observation. *J. Dermatol. Sci.* **2014**, *76*, 222–230. [CrossRef]
128. Choi, E.J.; Kang, Y.G.; Kim, J.; Hwang, J.K. Macelignan Inhibits Melanosome Transfer Mediated by Protease-Activated Receptor-2 in Keratinocytes. *Biol. Pharm. Bull.* **2011**, *34*, 748–754. [CrossRef]
129. Ni, J.; Wang, N.; Gao, L.L.; Li, L.L.; Zheng, S.W.; Liu, Y.J.; Ozukum, M.; Nikiforova, A.; Zhao, G.M.; Song, Z.Q. The effect of the NMDA receptor-dependent signaling pathway on cell morphology and melanosome transfer in melanocytes. *J. Dermatol. Sci.* **2016**, *84*, 296–304. [CrossRef]
130. Hu, Q.M.; Yi, W.J.; Su, M.Y.; Jiang, S.; Xu, S.Z.; Lei, T.C. Induction of retinal-dependent calcium influx in human melanocytes by UVA or UVB radiation contributes to the stimulation of melanosome transfer. *Cell Prolif.* **2017**, *50*, e12372. [CrossRef]
131. Koike, S.; Yamasaki, K.; Yamauchi, T.; Inoue, M.; Shimada-Ohmori, R.; Tsuchiyama, K.; Aiba, S. Toll-like receptors 2 and 3 enhance melanogenesis and melanosome transport in human melanocytes. *Pigment Cell Melanoma Res.* **2018**, *31*, 570–584. [CrossRef]
132. Pillaiyar, T.; Manickam, M.; Jung, S.H. Recent development of signaling pathways inhibitors of melanogenesis. *Cell. Signal.* **2017**, *40*, 99–115. [CrossRef]
133. Chiu, P.C.; Chan, C.C.; Lin, H.M.; Chiu, H.C. The clinical anti-aging effects of topical kinetin and niacinamide in Asians: A randomized, double-blind, placebo-controlled, split-face comparative trial. *J. Cosmet. Dermatol.* **2007**, *6*, 243–249. [CrossRef]
134. Kawada, A.; Konishi, N.; Oiso, N.; Kawara, S.; Date, A. Evaluation of anti-wrinkle effects of a novel cosmetic containing niacinamide. *J. Dermatol.* **2008**, *35*, 637–642. [CrossRef] [PubMed]
135. Fu, J.J.J.; Hillebrand, G.G.; Raleigh, P.; Li, J.; Marmor, M.J.; Bertucci, V.; Grimes, P.E.; Mandy, S.H.; Perez, M.I.; Weinkle, S.H.; et al. A randomized, controlled comparative study of the wrinkle reduction benefits of a cosmetic niacinamide/peptide/retinyl propionate product regimen vs. a prescription 0.02% tretinoin product regimen. *Br. J. Dermatol.* **2010**, *162*, 647–654. [CrossRef] [PubMed]
136. Berardesca, E.; Ardigo, M.; Cameli, N.; Mariano, M.; Agozzino, M.; Matts, P.J. Randomized, double-blinded, vehicle-controlled, split-face study to evaluate the effects of topical application of a Gold Silk Sericin/Niacinamide/Signaline complex on biophysical parameters related to skin ageing. *Int. J. Cosmet. Sci.* **2015**, *37*, 606–612. [CrossRef]
137. Farris, P.; Zeichner, J.; Berson, D. Efficacy and Tolerability of a Skin Brightening/Anti-Aging Cosmeceutical Containing Retinol 0.5%, Niacinamide, Hexylresorcinol, and Resveratrol. *J. Drugs Dermatol.* **2016**, *15*, 863–868. [PubMed]
138. Lee, Y.I.; Kim, S.; Kim, J.; Kim, J.; Chung, K.B.; Lee, J.H. Randomized controlled study for the anti-aging effect of human adipocyte-derived mesenchymal stem cell media combined with niacinamide after laser therapy. *J. Cosmet. Dermatol.* **2021**, *20*, 1774–1781. [CrossRef] [PubMed]
139. Navarrete-Solis, J.; Castanedo-Cazares, J.P.; Torres-Alvarez, B.; Oros-Ovalle, C.; Fuentes-Ahumada, C.; Gonzalez, F.J.; Martinez-Ramirez, J.D.; Moncada, B. A Double-Blind, Randomized Clinical Trial of Niacinamide 4% versus Hydroquinone 4% in the Treatment of Melasma. *Dermatol. Res. Pract.* **2011**, *2011*, 379173. [CrossRef]

140. Castanedo-Cazares, J.P.; Larraga-Pinones, G.; Ehnis-Perez, A.; Fuentes-Ahumada, C.; Oros-Ovalle, C.; Smoller, B.R.; Torres-Alvarez, B. Topical niacinamide 4% and desonide 0.05% for treatment of axillary hyperpigmentation: A randomized, double-blind, placebo-controlled study. *Clin. Cosmet. Investig. Dermatol.* **2013**, *6*, 29–36. [CrossRef]
141. Pierard, G.E. EEMCO guidance for the assessment of skin colour. *J Eur Acad Dermatol Venereol* **1998**, *10*, 1–11. [CrossRef]
142. Hakozaki, T.; Takiwaki, H.; Miyamoto, K.; Sato, Y.; Arase, S. Ultrasound enhanced skin-lightening effect of vitamin C and niacinamide. *Skin Res. Technol.* **2006**, *12*, 105–113. [CrossRef]
143. Bissett, D.L.; Robinson, L.R.; Raleigh, P.S.; Miyamoto, K.; Hakozaki, T.; Li, J.; Kelm, G.R. Reduction in the appearance of facial hyperpigmentation by topical N-undecyl-10-enoyl-L-phenylalanine and its combination with niacinamide. *J. Cosmet. Dermatol.* **2009**, *8*, 260–266. [CrossRef] [PubMed]
144. Kimball, A.B.; Kaczvinsky, J.R.; Li, J.; Robinson, L.R.; Matts, P.J.; Berge, C.A.; Miyamoto, K.; Bissett, D.L. Reduction in the appearance of facial hyperpigmentation after use of moisturizers with a combination of topical niacinamide and N-acetyl glucosamine: Results of a randomized, double-blind, vehicle-controlled trial. *Br. J. Dermatol.* **2010**, *162*, 435–441. [CrossRef] [PubMed]
145. Viyoch, J.; Tengamnuay, I.; Phetdee, K.; Tuntijarukorn, P.; Waranuch, N. Effects of Trans-4-(Aminomethyl) Cyclohexanecarboxylic Acid/Potassium Azeloyl Diglycinate/Niacinamide Topical Emulsion in Thai Adults With Melasma: A Single-Center, Randomized, Double-Blind, Controlled Study. *Curr. Ther. Res. Clin. Exp.* **2010**, *71*, 345–359. [CrossRef]
146. Lee, D.H.; Oh, I.Y.; Koo, K.T.; Suk, J.M.; Jung, S.W.; Park, J.O.; Kim, B.J.; Choi, Y.M. Reduction in facial hyperpigmentation after treatment with a combination of topical niacinamide and tranexamic acid: A randomized, double-blind, vehicle-controlled trial. *Skin Res. Technol.* **2014**, *20*, 208–212. [CrossRef]
147. Desai, S.; Ayres, E.; Bak, H.; Manco, M.; Lynch, S.; Raab, S.; Du, A.; Green, D.; Skobowiat, C.; Wangari-Talbot, J.; et al. Effect of a Tranexamic Acid, Kojic Acid, and Niacinamide Containing Serum on Facial Dyschromia: A Clinical Evaluation. *J. Drugs Dermatol.* **2019**, *18*, 454–459.
148. Kalasho, B.D.; Minokadeh, A.; Zhang-Nunes, S.; Zoumalan, R.A.; Shemirani, N.L.; Waldman, A.R.; Pletzer, V.; Zoumalan, C.I. Evaluating the Safety and Efficacy of a Topical Formulation Containing Epidermal Growth Factor, Tranexamic Acid, Vitamin C, Arbutin, Niacinamide and Other Ingredients as Hydroquinone 4% Alternatives to Improve Hyperpigmentation: A Prospective, Randomized, Controlled Split Face Study. *J. Cosmet. Sci.* **2020**, *71*, 263–290.
149. Kim, J.H.; Seok, J.K.; Kim, Y.M.; Boo, Y.C. Identification of small peptides and glycinamide that inhibit melanin synthesis using a positional scanning synthetic peptide combinatorial library. *Br. J. Dermatol.* **2019**, *181*, 128–137. [CrossRef]
150. Boo, Y.C. Up- or Downregulation of Melanin Synthesis Using Amino Acids, Peptides, and Their Analogs. *Biomedicines* **2020**, *8*, 322. [CrossRef]
151. Boo, Y.C. p-Coumaric Acid as An Active Ingredient in Cosmetics: A Review Focusing on its Antimelanogenic Effects. *Antioxidants* **2019**, *8*, 275. [CrossRef]
152. Boo, Y.C. Human Skin Lightening Efficacy of Resveratrol and Its Analogs: From in Vitro Studies to Cosmetic Applications. *Antioxidants* **2019**, *8*, 332. [CrossRef]
153. Boo, Y.C. Arbutin as a Skin Depigmenting Agent with Antimelanogenic and Antioxidant Properties. *Antioxidants* **2021**, *10*, 1129. [CrossRef] [PubMed]
154. Chung, B.Y.; Choi, S.R.; Moon, I.J.; Park, C.W.; Kim, Y.H.; Chang, S.E. The Glutathione Derivative, GSH Monoethyl Ester, May Effectively Whiten Skin but GSH Does Not. *Int. J. Mol. Sci.* **2016**, *17*, 629. [CrossRef]
155. Lee, H.K.; Ha, J.W.; Hwang, Y.J.; Boo, Y.C. Identification of L-Cysteinamide as a Potent Inhibitor of Tyrosinase-Mediated Dopachrome Formation and Eumelanin Synthesis. *Antioxidants* **2021**, *10*, 1202. [CrossRef]
156. Hwang, E.S.; Song, S.B. Possible Adverse Effects of High-Dose Nicotinamide: Mechanisms and Safety Assessment. *Biomolecules* **2020**, *10*, 687. [CrossRef] [PubMed]
157. Li, D.; Tian, Y.J.; Guo, J.; Sun, W.P.; Lun, Y.Z.; Guo, M.; Luo, N.; Cao, Y.; Cao, J.M.; Gong, X.J.; et al. Nicotinamide supplementation induces detrimental metabolic and epigenetic changes in developing rats. *Br. J. Nutr.* **2013**, *110*, 2156–2164. [CrossRef] [PubMed]
158. Cosmetic Ingredient Review Expert Panel. Final report of the safety assessment of niacinamide and niacin. *Int. J. Toxicol.* **2005**, *24* (Suppl. 5), 1–31.
159. Wohlrab, J.; Kreft, D. Niacinamide—Mechanisms of Action and Its Topical Use in Dermatology. *Skin Pharmacol. Physiol.* **2014**, *27*, 311–315. [CrossRef] [PubMed]
160. Guan, X.Y.; Lin, P.; Knoll, E.; Chakrabarti, R. Mechanism of Inhibition of the Human Sirtuin Enzyme SIRT3 by Nicotinamide: Computational and Experimental Studies. *PLoS ONE* **2014**, *9*, e107729. [CrossRef] [PubMed]
161. Banasik, M.; Stedeford, T.; Strosznajder, R.P. Natural Inhibitors of Poly(ADP-ribose) Polymerase-1. *Mol. Neurobiol.* **2012**, *46*, 55–63. [CrossRef] [PubMed]
162. Mathialagan, S.; Bi, Y.A.; Costales, C.; Kalgutkar, A.S.; Rodrigues, A.D.; Varma, M.V.S. Nicotinic acid transport into human liver involves organic anion transporter 2 (SLC22A7). *Biochem. Pharmacol.* **2020**, *174*, 113829. [CrossRef] [PubMed]
163. Grolla, A.A.; Torretta, S.; Gnemmi, I.; Amoruso, A.; Orsomando, G.; Gatti, M.; Caldarelli, A.; Lim, D.; Penengo, L.; Brunelleschi, S.; et al. Nicotinamide phosphoribosyltransferase (NAMPT/PBEF/visfatin) is a tumoural cytokine released from melanoma. *Pigment Cell Melanoma Res.* **2015**, *28*, 718–729. [CrossRef]
164. Grozio, A.; Mills, K.F.; Yoshino, J.; Bruzzone, S.; Sociali, G.; Tokizane, K.; Lei, H.C.; Cunningham, R.; Sasaki, Y.; Migaud, M.E.; et al. Slc12a8 is a nicotinamide mononucleotide transporter. *Nat. Metab.* **2019**, *1*, 47–57. [CrossRef]

165. Khaidizar, F.D.; Bessho, Y.; Nakahata, Y. Nicotinamide Phosphoribosyltransferase as a Key Molecule of the Aging/Senescence Process. *Int. J. Mol. Sci.* **2021**, *22*, 3709. [CrossRef]
166. Kim, H.J.; Kazi, J.U.; Lee, Y.R.; Nguyen, D.H.; Lee, H.B.; Shin, J.H.; Soh, J.W.; Kim, E.K. Visualization of the melanosome transfer-inhibition in a mouse epidermal cell co-culture model. *Int. J. Mol. Med.* **2010**, *25*, 249–253. [CrossRef] [PubMed]
167. Kim, B.; Hwang, J.S.; Kim, H.S. N-Nicotinoyl dopamine inhibits skin pigmentation by suppressing of melanosome transfer. *Eur. J. Pharmacol.* **2015**, *769*, 250–256. [CrossRef] [PubMed]
168. Allouche, J.; Rachmin, I.; Adhikari, K.; Pardo, L.M.; Lee, J.H.; McConnell, A.M.; Kato, S.; Fan, S.; Kawakami, A.; Suita, Y.; et al. NNT mediates redox-dependent pigmentation via a UVB- and MITF-independent mechanism. *Cell* **2021**, *184*, 4268–4283.e4220. [CrossRef]

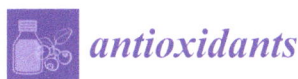

Review

The Role of Vitamin K in Humans: Implication in Aging and Age-Associated Diseases

Daniela-Saveta Popa [1],*, Galya Bigman [2] and Marius Emil Rusu [3]

[1] Department of Toxicology, Faculty of Pharmacy, Iuliu Hatieganu University of Medicine and Pharmacy, 8 Victor Babes, 400012 Cluj-Napoca, Romania
[2] The Baltimore Geriatric Research, Education and Clinical Center, Veterans Affairs Maryland Health Care System, Baltimore, MD 21201, USA; galya.bigman@va.gov
[3] Department of Pharmaceutical Technology and Biopharmaceutics, Faculty of Pharmacy, Iuliu Hatieganu University of Medicine and Pharmacy, 8 Victor Babes, 400012 Cluj-Napoca, Romania; rusu.marius@umfcluj.ro
* Correspondence: dpopa@umfcluj.ro; Tel.: +40-264-450-555

Abstract: As human life expectancy is rising, the incidence of age-associated diseases will also increase. Scientific evidence has revealed that healthy diets, including good fats, vitamins, minerals, or polyphenolics, could have antioxidant and anti-inflammatory activities, with antiaging effects. Recent studies demonstrated that vitamin K is a vital cofactor in activating several proteins, which act against age-related syndromes. Thus, vitamin K can carboxylate osteocalcin (a protein capable of transporting and fixing calcium in bone), activate matrix Gla protein (an inhibitor of vascular calcification and cardiovascular events) and carboxylate Gas6 protein (involved in brain physiology and a cognitive decline and neurodegenerative disease inhibitor). By improving insulin sensitivity, vitamin K lowers diabetes risk. It also exerts antiproliferative, proapoptotic, autophagic effects and has been associated with a reduced risk of cancer. Recent research shows that protein S, another vitamin K-dependent protein, can prevent the cytokine storm observed in COVID-19 cases. The reduced activation of protein S due to the pneumonia-induced vitamin K depletion was correlated with higher thrombogenicity and possibly fatal outcomes in COVID-19 patients. Our review aimed to present the latest scientific evidence about vitamin K and its role in preventing age-associated diseases and/or improving the effectiveness of medical treatments in mature adults >50 years old.

Keywords: vitamin K; phylloquinone; menaquinone; menadione; osteocalcin; matrix Gla protein; bone health; COVID-19; osteoporosis; vascular calcification

Citation: Popa, D.-S.; Bigman, G.; Rusu, M.E. The Role of Vitamin K in Humans: Implication in Aging and Age-Associated Diseases. *Antioxidants* **2021**, *10*, 566. https://doi.org/10.3390/antiox10040566

Academic Editor: Francesca Giampieri

Received: 28 February 2021
Accepted: 2 April 2021
Published: 6 April 2021

Publisher's Note: MDPI stays neutral with regard to jurisdictional claims in published maps and institutional affiliations.

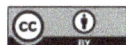

Copyright: © 2021 by the authors. Licensee MDPI, Basel, Switzerland. This article is an open access article distributed under the terms and conditions of the Creative Commons Attribution (CC BY) license (https://creativecommons.org/licenses/by/4.0/).

1. Introduction

Aging is a multifactorial process that gradually deteriorates the physiological functions of various organs, including the brain, musculoskeletal, cardiovascular, metabolic, and immune system leading to numerous pathological conditions with high rates of morbidity and mortality. Oxidative stress (OS) and chronic inflammation are fundamental pathophysiological mechanisms in the aging progression [1–3].

As human life expectancy is rising, age-related diseases will increase as well. Recent studies validated the importance of modifiable lifestyle factors, diet included, in the attenuation of pathological changes in mature adults [4]. Healthy fats, vitamins, minerals, polyphenolics, with antioxidant and anti-inflammatory activity, can increase the quality of life and influence the aging process, and among these factors, vitamin K (VK) has an important part [5].

VK is known for its role in synthesizing some blood-clotting proteins (K for koagulation in German). VK represents a fat-soluble family of compounds with a common chemical structure, a 2-methyl-1,4-naphthoquinone ring and a variable aliphatic side-chain. The variable aliphatic chain differentiates two isoforms: vitamin K1 (VK1) or phylloquinone

(PK) and vitamin K2 (VK2), usually designated as menaquinone (MK). MK exists in multiple structures, which are distinguished by the number of isoprenyl units and saturation in the side-chain (MK-n, where n is the number of isoprenyl units) [6]. These acronyms were used interchangeably throughout this article. The most common subtypes in humans are the short-chain MK-4, which is the only MK produced by systemic conversion of phylloquinone to menaquinone, and MK-7 through MK-10, which are synthesized by bacteria. VK3 (menadione), without side-chain and classified as a pro-vitamin, is a synthetic form of this vitamin (Figure 1).

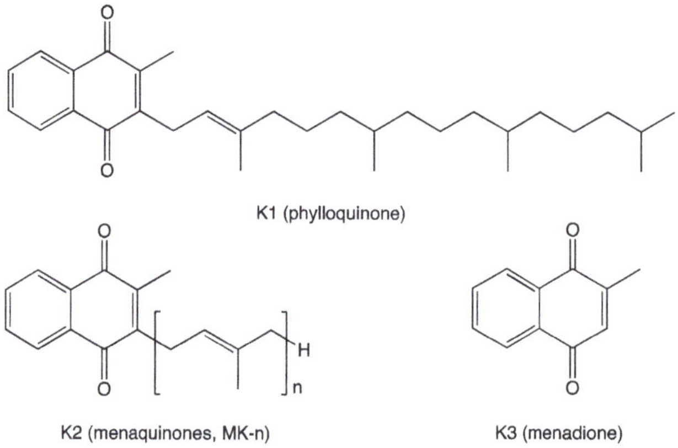

Figure 1. Vitamin K chemical structures. Vitamins K1 (VK1), K2 (VK2), and K3 (VK3) share the naphthoquinone ring; VK1 has a phytyl side-chain; VK2 has a side-chain with a varying number of isoprenyl units; VK3 has no side-chain.

Dark green leafy vegetables are the main sources for dietary PK (e.g., collards, turnip, broccoli, spinach, kale), 70–700 µg/100 g, as well as several fruits (e.g., dried prunes, kiwifruit, avocado, blueberries, blackberries, grapes), 15–70 µg/100 g, and some nuts (pine nuts, cashews, pistachios), 10–75 µg/100 g [7,8]. In contrast, the main sources of VK2 are fermented foods, cheeses, eggs, and meats (Table 1) [9,10].

Table 1. Vitamin K2: food category, sources, and amount.

Food Category	Food Source	VK2 *
Fermented foods	Natto	850–1000 (90% MK-7, 8% MK-8)
	Sauerkraut	5.5 (31% MK-6, 23% MK-9, 17% MK-5 and -8)
Hard cheeses		50–80 (15–67% MK-9, 6–22% MK-4, 6–22% MK-8)
Soft cheeses		30–60 (20–70% MK-9, 6–20% MK-4, 6–20% MK-8)
Eggs	Yolk	15–30 (MK-4)
Meats	Pork, beef, chicken	1.4 10 (MK-4)

*—µg/100 g food sample; MK-*n*—menaquinone.

Although dietary PK in vegetables is the major source of the VK intake (80–90%), only 5–10% is absorbed, whereas MKs from dairy products are almost completely absorbed. PK, tightly bound to plant chloroplasts, as well as PK digested with some phytochemicals (e.g., saponins, tannins, fibers, phytates) found in pulses, is less bioavailable to human. Though, PK from collards and broccoli is more bioavailable than PK from spinach [11,12].

Both VK1 and VK2 are recognized as cofactors for enzyme γ-glutamyl carboxylase (GGCX), which converts glutamic acid (Glu) to a new amino acid γ-carboxyglutamic acid (Gla), in VK-dependent proteins (VKDPs) during their biosynthesis [13]. These

VKDPs require carboxylation to become biologically active, and the negatively charged γ-carboxyglutamic acid residues have a high affinity for positively charged calcium ions [14].

VKDPs can be classified as hepatic and extrahepatic. The hepatic VKDPs are largely involved in blood coagulation. Extrahepatic VKDPs perform different tasks: osteocalcin (OC) regulates the bone formation and mineralization, the matrix Gla protein (MGP) is a potent inhibitor of vascular calcification, nephrocalcin is involved in kidney functions, the growth arrest-specific protein 6 (Gas6) in the development and differentiation of nervous system [15]. Additionally, some extrahepatic VKDPs (proteins C and S) inhibit coagulation by inactivating specific coagulation factors necessary to form blood clots [16].

Recent findings revealed the novel role of VK as an antioxidant and implicitly anti-inflammatory agent independent of its GGCX cofactor activity [17]. The antioxidant properties of VK are based on a protective action against oxidative cellular damage and cell death by (1) direct reactive oxygen species (ROS) uptake [17]; (2) the limiting of free radical intracellular accumulation [18], and (3) inhibition of the activation of 12-lipoxygenase [19].

Scientific evidence suggests that VK also has anti-inflammatory activity, a vital component against various chronic aging diseases [20]. VK inhibits the activation of the nuclear factor kappa B (NF-κB) and thus decreases the production of proinflammatory cytokines [17]. VK is significantly and inversely related to individual inflammatory biomarkers and inflammatory processes due to its anti-inflammatory effects [21].

The daily reference intake of VK is based mostly on bleeding-associated studies, and it varies between countries. US dietary guidelines recommend daily intakes of 90 and 120 μg for women and men, respectively, while the guidelines in the United Kingdom are set at 1 μg/kg body weight/day [11]. However, these recommendations are insufficient to induce complete carboxylation of all VKDPs. Only MK-7, having higher bioavailability and longer half-life, proved to promote γ-carboxylation of extrahepatic VKDPs at the current recommended levels, while the recommended levels of both PK and MK-4 have been shown to decrease γ-carboxylation of VKDPs [22].

Based on estimated dietary consumption, PK accounts for 50%, MK-4 makes up 10%, and MK-7, -8, and -9 represent 40% of total absorbed VK [23]. Being a fat-soluble vitamin, VK is taken up in the small intestine in the presence of dietary fat. A key mediator of intestinal VK absorption is Niemann–Pick C1-like 1 (NPC1L1) protein, a cholesterol and phytosterol transporter found in enterocytes and hepatocytes [24,25]. After absorption, PK is delivered to the liver and other tissues. It can be used unchanged, or it may be metabolized by certain types of microbiota into VK2 or into menadione in the human intestinal cells. A portion of menadione is transformed to MK-4, the dominant MK form in animal tissues [26]. However, there are tissue-specific VK distribution patterns. PK was found in all tissues with relatively high levels in the liver and heart but lower levels in the brain, lung and kidney. Compared to PK, MKs seem to be more important for extrahepatic tissues [27]. MK-4 levels were high in the brain and kidney and low in the liver, heart and lungs. The increased quantities of MK-4 in the brain suggest that this K vitamin is the active form of VK in this region [28]. Growing evidence advocates that MK-4 has a number of biological functions, including promoting growth factor of neuron-like cells, mediating apoptosis in several cancer cells, controlling glucose homeostasis [29]. In the central nervous system (CNS), MK-4 controls the activity of proteins involved in tissue renewal and cell growth control, myelination, mitogenesis, chemotaxis, neuroprotection [30]. The medium and long side-chain MKs were recovered mostly in the liver samples [31]. MK-7 and MK-4 converted from MK-7 increase collagen production and bone mineral density, promoting bone quality and strength [17]. As VK1, MK-4, and MK-7 have distinct bioavailability and biological activities, their recommended levels should be established based on their relative activities [32].

As present dietary intake recommendations are based on the dose required to prevent bleeding, novel data suggest that higher recommendations for VK consumption should be formulated [33]. Since both the bioavailability of VK from food as well as the endogenously produced VK are low, supplementation of VK should be considered for a number of chronic conditions, especially among elderly people [34].

Several scientific papers attested to the beneficial effects of VK in various chronic diseases, but supplement recommendations are difficult to outline. Nevertheless, a number of preclinical and clinical studies confirmed the safety of VK consumption. Several times higher dose levels than the estimated dietary intake for MK-7 did not show any toxicity in experimental animals [35]. In clinical studies, very high doses of MK-4 were used in the treatment of osteoporosis with no side effects [36].

The aim of this review was to summarize the recent scientific evidence on VK and its effect in preventing age-related diseases and/or improving the efficacy of some medical treatments in mature adults over 50 years old. To the best of our knowledge, it is the first study to concentrate on the effects of VK in this age group and to emphasize the role VK can play in the prevention of COVID-19.

2. Vitamin K in Bone Health

The musculoskeletal system, comprised primarily of muscle and bone, and the adipose tissue are connected through biological mechanisms underlying the physiological and pathophysiological crosstalk among muscle, bone, and fat [17]. Thus, several myokines (interleukin-6 (IL-6), myostatin) secreted by muscle have been identified as having effects on bone. Osteokines, especially OC, has been shown to have an endocrine impact on muscle, while adipokines (leptin, adiponectin, resistin) could act on either muscle or bone [37]. An in vitro study revealed that both carboxylated OC (cOC) and undercarboxylated OC (ucOC) increased secretion of adiponectin and the anti-inflammatory cytokine IL-10 and also inhibited secretion of tumor necrosis factor-α (TNF-α), but only cOC suppressed inflammatory IL-6 cytokine [38].

Thus, modifiable risk factors, such as healthy diets and physical activity, can positively affect these tissues. The role of calcium and vitamin D (vitD) in preventing osteoporosis is well established. However, more recent evidence suggests that other foods, such as fruit and vegetable, may have an essential role in bone health. Physical activity contributes to bone health by increasing serum total OC (tOC) and adiponectin, reducing leptin, and lowering insulin resistance [39].

Bone strength is determined by bone mineral content (BMC) and its quality and is associated with biological senescence and vitamin (B, D, K) deficiencies. As VK activates tissue-specific VKDPs, such as prothrombin, OC, or MGP, via the γ-carboxylation of Glu to Gla molecules, insufficient VKDPs γ-carboxylation is a sensitive, tissue-specific marker of VK deficiency [40]. Several studies revealed that VK is involved in bone metabolism and inhibits bone resorption in a dose-dependent manner. Binkley et al. showed that more than 250 μg/d VK intake is required for γ-carboxylation of OC [41].

Circulation OC is a marker of bone turnover. Of the total amount of OC that is released into the circulation, 40 to 60% is ucOC. This fraction of OC, being sensitive to VK intake, is a marker for VK status, usually revealing a lower VK availability [42]. Low dietary VK consumption and a high proportion of ucOC are independent risk factors for bone fractures in mature populations [43–47].

Table 2 summarizes the studies that showed an association between VK intake and bone parameters in mature subjects.

Table 2. The effect of VK intake on bone outcome parameters.

Author, Year, Country [Ref.]	Subjects (W:M) Age (Mean ± SD)	Design (Length)	Intervention Exposure	Findings
Shiraki et al. 2000 Japan [44]	241 PMO 67.2 y	prospective 2 y	45 mg/d MK-4 vs. control	↓ ucOC ($p < 0.0001$) ↑ cOC ($p = 0.0081$) ↓ fracture risk ($p = 0.0273$)
Iwamoto et al. 2001 Japan [48]	72 PMO 65.3 y	prospective 2 y	45 mg/d MK-4 + Ca vs. Ca	↓ vertebral fractures ($p < 0.0001$) ↑ BMD (forearm) ($p < 0.0001$)
Purwosunu et al. 2006 Indonesia [49]	63 PMO 60.8 y	RCT 48 w	45 mg/d MK-4 + Ca vs. Ca	↓ ucOC ($p < 0.01$) ↑ BMD (lumbar) ($p < 0.05$)
Bolton-Smith et al. 2007 UK [45]	244 healthy W 68.2 y	RCT 2 y	200 µg/d VK1 + 10 µg/d vitD3 + Ca vs. placebo	↓ ucOC ($p < 0.001$) ↑ BMD (ultradistal radius) ($p < 0.01$)
Knapen et al. 2007 Netherlands [50]	325 PMW 66.0 y	RCT 3 y	45 mg/d MK-4 vs. placebo	↑ BMC ($p < 0.05$) and bone strength (femoral neck)
Booth et al. 2008 USA [51]	452 (267:185) 68.4 y	RCT 3 y	500 µg/d PK vs. control	↓ ucOC ($p < 0.0001$)
Cheung et al. 2008 Canada [52]	400 PMOa 59.1 y	RCT 2–4 y	5 mg/d VK1 vs. placebo	↓ fracture risk ($p = 0.04$)
Hirao et al. 2008 Japan [53]	44 PMW 68.4 y	prospective 1 y	45 mg/d VK2 + 5 mg/d alendronate vs. 5 mg/d alendronate	↓ ucOC ($p = 0.014$) ↓ ucOC:cOC ($p = 0.007$) ↑ BMD (femoral neck) ($p = 0.03$)
Tsugawa et al. 2008 Japan [54]	379 W 63.0 y	prospective 3 y	high VK1 vs. low VK1	↓ vertebral fracture risk ($p < 0.001$)
Binkley et al. 2009 USA [46]	381 PMW 62.5 y	RCT 1 y	1 mg/d VK1 or 45 mg/d MK-4 vs. placebo	↓ ucOC ($p < 0.001$) for both VK1 and MK-4 groups
Yamauchi et al. 2010 Japan [55]	221 healthy W 60.8 ± 9.5 y	cross-sectional	260±85 µg/d VK	↓ ucOC ($p < 0.0001$) ↑ BMD (lumbar) ($p = 0.015$)
Je et al. 2011 Korea [56]	78 PMW 67.8 y	RCT 6 mo	45 mg/d MK-4 + vitD + Ca vs. vitD + Ca	↓ ucOC ($p = 0.008$) ↑ BMD (lumbar) ($p = 0.049$)
Kanellakis et al. 2012 Greece [57]	173 PMW 62.0 y	RCT 12 mo	100 µg PK or MK-7 + vitD + Ca vs. control	↓ ucOC ($p = 0.001$) * ↑ BMD (lumbar) ($p < 0.05$) *
Knapen et al. 2013 Netherlands [58]	244 PMW 60.0 y	RCT 3 y	180 µg/d MK-7 vs. placebo	↓ ucOC ($p < 0.001$) ↑ BMD (lumbar spine, femoral neck), bone strength ($p < 0.05$)
Jiang et al. 2014 China [59]	213 PMW 64.4 y	RCT 1 y	45 mg/d MK-4 + Ca vs. Ca	↓ ucOC ($p < 0.001$) ↑ BMD (lumbar) ($p < 0.001$)
Rønn et al. 2016 Denmark [47]	148 PMOa 67.5 y	RCT 1 y	375 µg/d MK-7 vs. placebo	↓ ucOC ($p < 0.05$) ↓ ucOC:cOC ($p < 0.05$) ↑ bone structure (tibia) ($p < 0.05$)
Bultynck et al. 2020 UK [60]	62 (42:20) 80.0 ± 9.6 y	Prospective	↑ serum VK	↓ hip fracture risk
Moore et al. 2020 UK [61]	374 PMO 68.7 y	cross-sectional	↑ serum VK1	↓ fracture risk ($p = 0.04$)
Sim et al. 2020 Australia [62]	30 (10:20) 61.8 ± 9.9 y	RCT 12 w	136.7 µg/d VK	↓ ucOC and ucOC:tOC ($p \leq 0.01$)

BMC—bone mineral content; BMD—bone mineral density; cOC—carboxylated osteocalcin; M—men; PMW—postmenopausal women; PMO—postmenopausal osteoporosis; PMOa—postmenopausal osteopenia; RCT—randomized controlled trial; SD—standard deviation; tOC—total osteocalcin; ucOC—undercarboxylated osteocalcin; W—women; ↑—increase; ↓—decrease. * for both VK1 and MK-4 groups.

In a study including 221 healthy women, VK intake was significantly and negatively correlated with ucOC [55]. Correspondingly, higher VK consumption was associated with beneficial effects on fracture risk and bone health. Following an increased dietary green leafy vegetable intake by consuming approximately 200 g/d, 30 healthy individuals substantially reduced serum tOC, ucOC, and ucOC:tOC levels, suggesting increased entry of OC into the bone matrix, improvement of bone quality and lower fracture risk [62].

Moore et al. investigated the association between circulating VK1 with fracture risk in a study, including osteoporosis, in postmenopausal women. The results showed that serum VK1 concentrations were significantly higher in the group with fewer fractures and negatively associated with fracture risk [61]. The results of a 3-year study had the same conclusions: subjects with low plasma VK1 concentration had significantly higher susceptibility for vertebral fracture, independently of BMD, compared to the high VK1 group [54].

Postmenopausal women with osteopenia who received 5 mg of VK1 supplementation daily for 4 years had a significantly lower rate of fractures ($p = 0.04$) [52].

Besides leafy vegetables, dried plums (*Prunus domestica* L.), a rich source of VK1, demonstrated bone-protective effects. In a study of 84 osteopenic, postmenopausal women, 65–79 years of age, daily consumption of 50 g of dried plums for 6 months revealed less total body, hip, and lumbar bone mineral density (BMD) loss compared with that of the control group ($p < 0.05$), which can be explained by the ability of dried plums to suppress bone turnover and inhibit bone resorption [63]. Dried plums are rich in VK, potassium and minerals that are important to bone metabolism [64]. Booth et al. assessed the spine and hip BMD change in healthy elderly subjects, and after three years of follow-up, the daily PK supplementation did not present any additional benefit to BMD. However, the level of ucOC, associated with increased risk of bone fracture in older adults, significantly decreased [51]. Similar to the previous study, Emaus et al. observed that the daily intake of 360 μg MK-7 for one year increased cOC and decreased ucOC serum levels ($p < 0.001$) [65]. Feskanich et al. showed that women aged 38–74 years with higher daily VK intake had lower serum concentrations of ucOC and a 30% reduction in the risk of hip fracture compared to women with an intake of less than 109 μg VK per day [66]. Equally, the prevalence of VK deficiency was found to be higher in older patients (mean age 80.0) with hip fractures than those without [60].

In an intervention study, the use of 150 μg VK1 per day, in combination with physiological relevant doses of genistein, an important isoflavone [67], vitD, and polyunsaturated fatty acids (eicosapentaenoic and docosahexaenoic acids), could reduce fracture risk, at least at the hip, and prevent osteoporosis in postmenopausal women [68]. On one hand, VK2 supplementation might enhance the efficacy of vitD in bone and muscle health, improve bone quality, and reduce fracture risk in osteoporotic patients. On the other hand, vitD enhanced the carboxylation of OC, thus promoting the incorporation of calcium into the bone matrix and supporting bone metabolism [69]. Increased vitD intake should be accompanied by VK and magnesium supplementation to prevent long-term health risks, including hypercalcemia, a calcium buildup leading to calcification of the blood vessels and eventually osteoporosis. Hypercalcemia is not a vitD hypervitaminosis but rather a VK deficiency and higher serum concentrations of ucOC that inhibit calcium absorption in the bones [70].

In clinical studies, combined administration of VK and vitD, plus calcium, improved BMD, bone quality and decrease fracture risk, demonstrating a positive synergistic effect on bone health [57,71]. In a group of 181 healthy postmenopausal women, between 50 and 60 years, after 3 years of daily treatment with VK1, in addition to vitD, calcium, magnesium, and zinc, the bone loss at the site of the femoral neck was significantly reduced compared to the placebo group [72]. Furthermore, the results of clinical studies involving osteoporotic women of different ethnicity suggested that MK-4 in combination with calcium may be a safe approach in the treatment of osteoporosis [48,49,56,73].

Cockayne et al. investigated the effect of VK1 (1–10 mg/day) or MK-4 (15–45 mg/day) supplementations and showed that daily supplementation of MK-4 (45 mg/day) reduced vertebral fractures (odds ratio (OR) = 0.40; 95% CI: 0.25–0.65), nonvertebral fractures (OR = 0.19; 95% CI: 0.11–0.35), and hip fractures (OR = 0.23; 95% CI: 0.12–0.47) compared to placebo and that MK-4 is a more effective antiosteoporotic agent than VK1 [74]. Hirao et al. observed that among postmenopausal women, who received osteoporosis monotherapy (alendronate, 5 mg/day) combined with 45 mg/day MK-4, over a period of one year, had a significant decrease in ucOC and ucOC:tOC ratio and reduced fracture rate compared with women, who received only alendronate monotherapy, suggesting that osteoporosis therapy could be improved with MK-4 supplements [53].

In another intervention study among healthy, non-osteoporotic women, the intervention group received 45 mg/day of MK-4 for three years and was compared to placebo. BMD did not change in the treatment group, though serum concentrations of tOC, cOC, and BMC significantly increased, maintaining bone strength at the site of the femoral neck. However, bone strength decreased significantly in the placebo group. Even at the very high doses of MK-4 used the adverse side effects [50].

The MK-7 isoform revealed the same benefits on bone health. In a 3-year randomized study, including healthy postmenopausal women, a daily supplement of MK-7 lowered circulating ucOC by ~50% and led to a significant improvement in bone density and bone strength [58].

Recent evidence showed that VK2 controls osteoblastogenesis and osteoclastogenesis via the NF-κB signal transduction pathway [75]. NF-κB signaling could, on one hand, inhibit osteoblastic differentiation and activity and, on the other hand, stimulate osteoclastic bone resorption. VK2 presented pro-osteoblastic and anti-osteoclastogenic actions, accomplished by downregulating inflammatory cytokines (e.g., TNF-α, IL-1) and inhibiting the activation of NF-κB [76]. This new mechanism explains the dual pro-anabolic and anti-catabolic activities of VK2 on bone. However, as no anti-NF-κB activity was associated with VK1 in this study, other mechanisms of action may be involved in the VK1 activity [75].

Liang et al. showed that BMD was significantly negatively associated with homeostatic model assessment for insulin resistance (HOMA-IR) and positively related with fasting glucose in the elderly population, suggesting that bone mass could be a predictor of glucose metabolism [77].

Several biological mechanisms may be involved in the prevention and treatment of aging-associated musculoskeletal disorders, including sarcopenia, osteoporosis, and osteoarthritis (OA). Clinical studies and animal experiments suggested an association between plasma VK status with muscle mass and strength, the link between the GGCX activity and bone protection, or the association between the steroid and xenobiotic receptor (SXR), a putative receptor for vitamin K, and cartilage protective effect [78]. Since VKDPs, including MGP, Gla-rich protein (GRP), periostin, and OC, were detected in cartilage and bone, VK may have a protective role in OA and joint health [79]. Thus, sufficient dietary VK intake and/or supplementation seemed to protect the population from age-related musculoskeletal diseases [80].

3. Vitamin K in the Prevention and Therapy of Vascular Calcification and Cardiovascular Diseases

Aging and several pathologic states, such as obesity, diabetes, or chronic kidney disease (CKD), cause degenerative changes of the vascular walls, including inflammation and vascular calcification (VC), leading to arterial stiffening and increased cardiovascular (CV) morbidity and mortality [81].

Ample evidence has shown that VK deficiency is related to the pathogenesis of VC [81–84]. VK has been suggested to inhibit VC and protect against cardiovascular disease (CVD) through the activation of VKDPs, such as MGP. To accomplish its potent calcification inhibitory function, MGP, secreted in the inactive form, needs activation (carboxylation), which takes place in the presence of VK. Upon activation, MGP binds calcium with high affinity, thereby inhibiting the VC process [82].

VC, a hallmark of senescence and a strong predictor of CV events, is another chronic inflammatory state induced via the generation of proinflammatory cytokines and mediated by the NF-κB signaling pathway. A high VK status may exert anti-inflammatory effects and prevent VC through antagonizing NF-κB signaling [83]. Growing evidence shows that VK as well as nuclear factor erythroid 2–related factor 2 (Nrf2) signaling could play a vital role in blocking ROS generation, cellular senescence, DNA damage, and inflammaging [84].

In CKD, a pathological condition characterized by osteoporosis, sarcopenia, and increase CVD events [85], VC is widespread even at early stages. Besides careful attention to calcium and phosphate balance, no particular therapy enabling regression or inhibiting the progression of VC existed [86]. Accumulating evidence describes the VC mechanism as an active process involving calcification promoters and inhibitors. The biologically active MGP, highly dependent on VK status, is viewed as a strong inhibitor of vascular elastic fiber damage and VC [87] and also the only factor that can actually reverse the process [88]. The inactive, uncarboxylated form of this protein reflected the deficiency of VK status and has been linked with VC and CV events. Growing scientific data show that VK-dependent MGP could offset age-related wear and tear on the arteries, VC, and CVD development [89].

To date, a number of experiments and observational studies examined the effects of VK supplementation and dietary intake on vascular calcification and CVD (Table 3) in mature populations.

Table 3. The effects of VK supplementation on vascular calcification.

Author, Year, Country (Ref.)	Subjects (W:M) Age (Mean ± SD)	Design (Length)	Intervention Exposure	Findings
Geleijnse et al. 2004 Netherlands [90]	4807 (2971:1836) 67.5 y	7 y	Q1 < 21.6 µg/d VK2 Q2 21.6–32.7 µg/d VK2 Q3 > 32.7 µg/d VK2	↓ CHD mortality: RR = 0.43 (95% CI: 0.24–0.77, p = 0.005) Q3 vs. Q1 ↓ AC: OR = 0.48 95% CI: 0.32–0.71, p < 0.001) Q3 vs. Q1
Gast et al. 2009 Netherlands [91]	16,057 W 57.0 ± 6.0 y	Longitudinal 8.1 y	211.7 µg/d VK1 29.1 µg/d VK2	↓ CHD risk for 10 µg VK2: HR = 0.91 (95% CI: 0.85–1.00, p = 0.04)
Shea et al. 2009 USA [92]	388 (235:153) 68 y	RCT 3 y	500 µg/d VK1 vs. control	↓progression of CAC
Schurgers et al. 2010 France [93]	107 (43:64) 67 ± 13 y	18 mo	VK levels dp-ucMGP	↓ VK levels ↑ dp-ucMGP levels with CKD stage
Ueland et al. 2010 Norway [94]	147 (66:81) 74.0 ± 10 y	20 mo	VK levels dp-ucMGP	↓ VK levels ↑ dp-ucMGP in symptomatic AS
Schlieper et al. 2011 Serbia [95]	188 (89:99) 58 ± 15 y	Follow-up, 1104 days	VK levels dp-ucMGP dp-cMGP	↓ dp-cMGP ↑ CV: HR = 2.7 (95% CI: 1.2–6.2, p = 0.015) ↑ All-cause: HR = 2.16 (95% CI: 1.1–4.3, p = 0.027)
Ueland et al. 2011 Norway [96]	179 (39:140) 56 y	2.9 y	VK levels dp-ucMGP	↓ VK levels; ↑ dp-ucMGP ↑ heart failure: HR = 5.62 (95% CI: 2.05–15.46, p = 0.001)
Westenfeld et al. 2011 Germany [97]	103 (48:55) >60.5 y	RCT 6 w	G1–45 µg/d MK-7 G2–135 µg/d MK-7 G3–360 µg/d MK-7	↓ dp-ucMGP by 77–93% G2 and G3 vs. control
Dalmeijer et al. 2012 Netherlands [98]	60 (36:24) 59.5 y	RCT 12 w	G1–180 µg/d MK-7 G2–360 µg/d MK-7	↓ dp-ucMGP by 31% G1 and 46% G2 vs. placebo
van den Heuvel et al. 2013 Netherlands [99]	577 (322:255) 59.9 ± 2.9 y	Follow-up 5.6 y	VK levels dp-ucMGP	↓ VK levels; ↑ dp-ucMGP ↑ CVD: HR = 2.69 (95% CI: 1.09–6.62, p = 0.032)

Table 3. Cont.

r, Year, Country (Ref.)	Subjects (W:M) Age (Mean ± SD)	Design (Length)	Intervention Exposure	Findings
Caluwé et al. 2014 Norway [100]	165 (83:82) 70.8 y	RCT 8 w	360, 720 or 1080 μg MK-7 thrice weekly	↓ dp-ucMGP by 17–33–46%
Liabeuf et al. 2014 France [101]	198 (40:158) 64 ± 8 y	Cross-sectional	VK levels dp-ucMGP	↓ VK levels; ↑ dp-ucMGP ↑ PAC: OR = 1.88 (95% CI: 1.14–3.11, $p = 0.014$)
Cheung et al. 2015 USA [102]	3401 (2245:1156) 61.9 y	Follow-up 13.3 y	↑ VK daily intake	↓ CVD mortality: HR = 0.78 (95% CI: 0.64–0.95, $p = 0.016$)
Knapen et al. 2015 Norway [103]	244 PMW 59.5 ± 3.3 y	RCT 3 y	180 μg/d MK-7 vs. placebo	↓ Stiffness Index β: −0.67 ± 2.78 vs. +0.15 ± 2.51, $p = 0.018$ ↓ cfPWV: −0.36 ± 1.48 m/s vs. +0.021 ± 1.22 m/s, $p = 0.040$
Kurnatowska et al. 2015 Poland [104]	42 (20:22) 58 y	RCT 270 days	90 μg/d MK-7 + 10 μg/d vitD vs. control	↑ CAC ↓dp-ucMGP
Asemi et al. 2016 Iran [105]	66 (31:35) 65.5 y	RCT 12 w	180 μg/d MK-7 + 10 μg/d vitD + 1 g/d Ca vs. placebo	↓ levels of left CIMT ($p = 0.02$) ↓ insulin (−0.9 vs. +2.6, $p = 0.01$) ↓ HOMA-IR (−0.4 vs. +0.7, $p = 0.01$)
Fulton et al. 2016 UK [106]	80 (36:44) 77 ± 5 y	RCT 6 mo	100 μg MK-7 vs. placebo	↓dp-ucMGP ($p < 0.001$)
Kurnatowska et al. 2016 Poland [107]	38 (17:21) 58.6 y	RCT 9 mo	90 μg/d MK-7 + 10 μg/d vitD vs. control	↓dp-ucMGP by 10.7%
Sardana et al. 2016 USA [108]	66 (6:60) T2D 62 ± 2 y	Cross-sectional	VK levels dp-ucMGP	↓ VK levels; ↑ dp-ucMGP ↑ cfPWV ($\beta = 0.40$, $p = 0.011$)
Aoun et al. 2017 Lebanon [109]	50 (20:30) 71.5 y	RCT 4 w	360 μg/d MK-7	↓ dp-ucMGP by 86%
Brandenburg et al. 2017 Germany [110]	99 (18:81) 69.1 y	RCT 1 y	2 mg/d VK1 vs. placebo	↓ progression of AVC (10.0% vs. 22.0%)
Shea et al. 2017 USA [111]	1061 (615:446) 74 ± 5 y	Follow-up 12.1 y	VK1 levels dp-ucMGP	↑ CVD risk in HBP patients ($n = 489$): HR = 2.94 (95% CI: 1.4–6.13, $p < 0.01$)
Puzantian et al. 2018 USA [112]	137 (8:129) 59.6 y		VK levels dp-ucMGP	↓ VK levels; ↑ dp-ucMGP ↑ cfPWV ($\beta = 0.21$; $p = 0.019$)
Dal Canto et al. 2020 Netherlands [113]	601 (303:298) 70 ± 6 y	Follow-up 7 and 17 y	↓ VK levels ↓ vitD levels	↑ LVMI: $\beta = 5.9$ g/m$^{2.7}$ (95% CI: 1.8–10.0 g/$^{2.7}$) ↑ All-cause mortality: HR = 1.64 (95% CI: 1.12–2.39, $p = 0.011$)
Roumeliotis et al. 2020 Greece [114]	66 (31:35) diabetic CKD 68.5 ± 8.6 y	Follow-up 7 y	VK levels dp-ucMGP	↓ VK levels; ↑ dp-ucMGP ↑ CVD mortality: HR = 2.82 (95% CI: 1.07–7.49, $p = 0.037$)
Shea et al. 2020 USA [115]	3891 (2154:1737) 65 ± 11 y	Follow-up 13 y	↓ VK1 levels	↑ CVD risk: HR = 1.12 (95% CI, 0.94–1.33) ↑ All-cause mortality
Wessinger et al. 2020 USA [116]	60 (11:49) chronic stroke 61.7 ± 7.2 y	Cross-sectional	VK dietary intake	Among stroke survivors, 82% reported consuming below the Dietary Reference Intake for VK

AC—aortic calcification; AS—aortic stenosis; AVC—aortic valve calcification; CAC—coronary artery calcification; cfPWV—carotid-femoral pulse wave velocity; CHD—coronary heart disease; CIMT—carotid intima-media thickness; CKD—chronic kidney disease; dp-ucMGP—dephosphorylated—undercarboxylated matrix gla protein; CVD—cardiovascular diseases; HF—heart failure; HR—hazard ratio; LVMI—left ventricular mass index; M—men; MK—menaquinone; OR—odds ratio; PAC—peripheral arterial calcification; PMW—postmenopausal women; PMO—postmenopausal osteoporosis; PMOa—postmenopausal osteopenia; RCT—randomized controlled trial; RR—relative risk; SD—standard deviation; W—women; ↑—increase; ↓—decrease.

Several studies demonstrated that higher dietary consumption of VK2 significantly reduced the incidence of VC and coronary heart disease (CHD) [90,91]. In these studies, no association between VK1 intake and CHD was detected while controlling for confounders. After monitoring 2987 participants during a median follow-up time of 11 years, only dietary MKs, but not VK1 intake, were significantly associated with a lower risk of CHD [117]. Scientific evidence specified that VK1 mainly carboxylate VK-dependent factors in the liver, while VK2 is responsible for the carboxylation of VKDPs in the extrahepatic tissues [118]. Nonetheless, it was demonstrated that higher doses of VK1, namely 2 mg/d, can also act in extrahepatic tissues and delay the progression of VC [110]. Furthermore, low plasma VK1 status was linked with higher all-cause mortality risk [115] and with an increased risk for CVD in older patients treated for hypertension [111].

VK intake slowed the progression of preexisting coronary artery calcification (CAC), a well-known independent predictor of CVD risk, in asymptomatic older men and women [92]. Moreover, adequate consumption of VK-rich foods has been suggested as both preventing action and prospective adjuvant therapy against atherosclerosis and stroke [116].

A combination of low VK and vitD status is associated with the increased left ventricular mass index, a parameter for cardiac structure, which has been shown to predict higher mortality, as well as the augmented risk of all-cause mortality in older populations [113]. In diabetic patients with stable CHD, combined supplementation with MK-7, vitD, and Ca was associated with a significant reduction in maximum levels of left carotid intima-media thickness (a parameter positively linked with diabetes, blood pressures, lipid profiles, inflammatory cytokines), C-reactive protein (CRP) and malondialdehyde (MDA) levels, and a significant increase in high-density lipoprotein (HDL)-cholesterol levels [105].

A functional VK deficiency is strongly associated with an increase in uncarboxylated VK-dependent protein levels, the hepatic protein induced by vitamin K absence-II (PIVKA-II) and extrahepatic dephosphorylated-uncarboxylated matrix Gla protein (dp-ucMGP) [99]. Scientific findings reported that VK could modulate dp-ucMGP levels and that plasma dp-ucMGP levels decline after VK intake in a dose-dependent manner [97,100]. Circulating plasma dp-ucMGP levels augmented progressively in many diseases and were directly correlated with the severity of VC, cardiac function and long-term mortality [93–96]. Equally, in a study involving 2318 subjects, elevated dp-ucMGP increased the risk of CV ($p = 0.027$) and all-cause ($p \leq 0.008$) mortality [119]. Similarly, in diabetes patients with high CV risk, elevated levels of dp-ucMGP and lower levels of total ucMGP (t-ucMGP) are independently related to the severity of peripheral artery calcification [101]. Moreover, higher dp-ucMGP values were independently associated with carotid-femoral pulse wave velocity (cfPWV) in diabetes and CKD patients and may lead to large arterial stiffening [108,112].

Adequate dietary intake of VK may be essential in reducing atherosclerosis progression, CV risk, or CVD and all-cause mortality in CKD patients [102,104,107]. CKD and hemodialysis patients could often present vascular VK deficiency due to significantly low VK intake, resulting in an elevated risk of VC and bone fractures [120]. After three years of 180 μg MK-7 daily intake, dp-ucMGP levels decreased by 50% compared to placebo [103]. Even after a shorter 12 week-period, ucMGP, an independent risk factor for arteriosclerosis and CVD, significantly decreased in the MK-7 supplementation groups compared to placebo [98]. Other interventions with different amounts of MK-7 (100 μg/d and 360 μg/d) provided significant effects on dp-ucMGP [106,109].

Diabetic CKD patients with plasma dp-ucMGP levels above the median (≥ 656 pM) had a significantly higher risk for CV events, CV mortality, and all-cause mortality compared to the low dp-ucMGP group [114]. High levels of dp-ucMGP were significantly associated with higher triglycerides ($p = 0.03$) and C-reactive protein ($p = 0.03$) levels, CV mortality ($p = 0.037$), all-cause mortality ($p = 0.02$), and progression of CKD ($p = 0.024$) [114]. Likewise, a prospective study investigating 4275 people (aged 53 ± 12 years, 46.0% male) for 10 years, concluded that plasma dp-ucMGP was associated with total (hazard ratio (HR) = 1.14; 95% CI: 1.10–1.17, $p \leq 0.001$) and CV (HR = 1.17; 95% CI: 1.11–1.23, $p \leq 0.001$) mortality [121].

Recent data indicated that dp-ucMGP levels might be associated with high-risk for CV mortality and all-cause mortality. One meta-analysis, which included 11 studies and 33,289 patients, revealed that high circulating dp-ucMGP was associated with increased risk of all-cause and CV mortality [122]. Correspondingly, another large meta-analysis comprising 21 articles and 222,592 subjects exposed that elevated plasma dp-ucMGP levels were correlated with higher risk of all-cause mortality (HR = 1.84; 95% CI: 1.48–2.28, $p < 0.001$), CVD mortality (HR = 1.96; 95% CI: 1.47–2.61, $p < 0.001$), as well as increased total CVD risk (HR = 1.57; 95% CI: 1.19–2.06, $p < 0.001$) [123]. This study also found a significant association between dietary VK1 and MKs with total CHD (HR = 0.92 and 0.70, respectively), but no correlation was noticed between dietary VK and all-cause or CVD mortality [123].

In conclusion, as no toxicity or serious side-effects of VK intake have been described, even for higher doses, patients with CVD risk could benefit from VK supplementation, a safe therapy, which can present significant clinical impact.

4. The Effects of Vitamin K on Metabolic Disorders

Obesity and type 2 diabetes (T2D) are metabolic disorders affecting the world population with serious health and economic complications. Obesity, as well as overweight, is a risk factor for deficiency of fat-soluble vitamins. Data reported that VK supplementation reduced OS, insulin resistance, and lowered progression of metabolic risk biomarkers for T2D. There was a clear association between circulating VK and dependent-OC concentration, obesity and T2D risk [124]. Scientific evidence suggests that OC, an osteoblast-derived hormone, is involved in glucose and energy metabolism through multiple mechanisms. It regulates secretion and insulin sensitivity through increase β-cell function and increases adiponectin expression in adipocytes. Metabolic disorders, including obesity or diabetes, can affect the synthesis and action of OC, causing a disruption of the bone–energy metabolism axis [125].

Dietary patterns stressing plant food consumption may be effective in both preventing T2D and improving diabetes management. VK may play an imperative role in the regulation of glycemic status by improvement of insulin sensitivity, which may decrease the risk for T2D [126].

The synergistic effect exerted by the bioactive molecules (e.g., lipophilic vitamins, such as VK) found in plant or animal source foods can improve insulin sensitivity through a number of signaling pathways in the prediabetic and diabetic population [127]. VK may regulate glucose levels through controlling OC levels and inflammation and exert beneficial effects in T2D [128].

The design and outcomes of studies assessing the effects of VK supplementation on metabolic disorders are shown in Table 4.

Table 4. The effect of VK intake on metabolic disorders.

Author, Year, Country [Ref.]	Subjects (W:M) Age (Mean ± SD)	Design (Length)	Intervention Investigations	Findings
Im et al. 2008 South Korea [129]	339 PMW T2D 57.2 y		Biochemical and hormonal parameters for (1) NG; (2) IGF; (3) T2D groups	↓ OC in (3) vs. (1) ($p < 0.005$) OC levels—inversely correlated with FG ($r = -0.195$, $p < 0.001$), HbA1c ($r = -0.219$, $p < 0.001$), FI ($r = -0.131$, $p < 0.016$), HOMA-IR ($r = -0.163$, $p < 0.003$)
Yoshida et al. 2008 USA [130]	355 (213:142) 68 y	RCT 36 mo	500 μg/d PK vs. control	↓ HOMA-IR (p-adjusted < 0.01) and ↓ plasma insulin (p-adjusted < 0.04)—only for men ↓% ucOC ($p < 0.001$) for both men and women
Kanazawa et al. 2009 Japan [131]	329 (149:179) 65.8 y		Biochemical and hormonal parameters	Negative correlation between OC and FG and HbA1c (for all: $p < 0.05$), % fat, baPWV and IMT in men ($p < 0.05$) Positive correlation between OC and total adiponectin in PMF ($p < 0.001$)

Table 4. Cont.

Author, Year, Country [Ref.]	Subjects (W:M) Age (Mean ± SD)	Design (Length)	Intervention Investigations	Findings
Kindblom et al. 2009 Sweden [132]	1010 M 857 non-T2D 153 T2D 75.3 ± 3.2 y	MrOS Sweden study	Biochemical and hormonal parameters	↓ OC in T2D (−21.7%, $p < 0.001$) vs. non-T2D Plasma OC—inversely correlated with BMI, fat mass, and plasma glucose ($p < 0.001$)
Shea et al. 2009 USA [133]	348 (206:142) non-T2D 68 y	Cross sectional 3 y	OC levels (tOC, ucOC, cOC) and HOMA-IR	↑ cOC and tOC were associated with ↓ HOMA-IR ($p = 0.006$ and $p = 0.02$, respectively)
Bao et al. 2011 China [134]	181 M 76 non-metS 105 metS 64.9 ± 10.7 y		Biochemical and hormonal parameters	↓ OC in MetS vs. non-MetS ($p < 0.001$); OC was independently associated with metS (OR = 0.060, 95% CI: 0.005–0.651)
Alfadda et al. 2013 Saudi Arabia [135]	203 T2D ± MetS 52.5 ± 9.6 y	Cross-sectional	Biochemical and hormonal parameters	↓ tOC ($p = 0.01$) and ucOC ($p = 0.03$) in metS vs. non-metS. Positive correlation between ucOC and HDL-C ($p = 0.023$). Negative correlation between tOC and HbA1c ($p = 0.01$) and serum TGs ($p = 0.049$).
Confraveux et al. 2014 France [136]	798 M 65.3 ± 7 y	MINOS study	Biochemical and hormonal parameters	Negative correlation between OC and glycemia ($p < 0.0001$)
Shea et al. 2017 USA [137]	401 (237:164) 69 ± 6 y	RCT 3 y	500 µg/d PK (+Ca and vitD) vs. control (Ca and vitD)	↓ ucOC ($p < 0.001$)
Knapen et al. 2018 Netherlands [138]	214 PMW 60 y	RCT 3 y	180 µg/d MK-7 vs. placebo	↑ cOC ($p < 0.0001$) ↓ ucOC ($p < 0.0001$)
Dumitru et al. 2019 Romania [139]	146 PMW T2D 62.1 y	Cross sectional 30 mo	Biochemical and hormonal parameters in T2D group vs. control	↓ tOC ($p < 0.05$) in T2D group Negative correlation between tOC and HbA1c, BMI, TGs (for all: $p < 0.05$), and HDL-C ($p = 0.001$)
Guney et al. 2019 Turkey [140]	191 PMW metS 56 y	cross-sectional	Biochemical and hormonal parameters in metS group vs. control	↓ OC ($p < 0.001$) in metS group Positive correlation between vitD and OC ($r = 0.198$; $p = 0.008$) Negative correlation between OC and hs-CRP ($p = 0.003$), HOMA-IR ($p = 0.048$), and HbA1c ($p = 0.001$)
Aguayo-Ruiz et al. 2020 Mexico [141]	40 (24:16) T2D 56 y	RCT 3 mo	(1) 100 µg/d K2 (2) 100 µg/d K2+vit D3 (3) vit D3	(1): ↓ glycemia ($p = 0.002$) ↑ cOC ($p < 0.041$) (2): ↓ glycemia ($p = 0.002$)
Jeannin et al. 2020 France [142]	198 (40:158) T2D 64 ± 8.4 y	Cohort	NDS, dp-ucMGP in plasma	↑ peripheral NDS (15.7%) correlated with dp-ucMGP ($r = 0.51$, $p < 0.0001$)
Sakak et al. 2020 Iran [143]	68 (42:26) T2D 57.6 y	RCT 12 w	360 µg MK-7 vs. placebo	↓ FPG (p-adjusted = 0.031) ↓ HbA1c (p-adjusted = 0.004) ↓ HOMA-IR ($p = 0.019$) vs. baseline

BMI—body mass index; cOC—carboxylated osteocalcin; dp-ucMGP—dephospho-uncarboxylated matrix-gla-protein; FG—fasting glucose; FI—fasting insulin; FPG—fasting plasma glucose; FPβC—functional pancreatic β cells; HbA1c—glycosylated hemoglobin; HDL-C—high—density lipoprotein cholesterol; HOMA-IR—homeostatic model assessment of insulin resistance; hs-CRP—high sensitive C—reactive protein; IFG—impaired fasting glucose; M—men; metS—metabolic syndrome; NDS—neuropathy disability score; NG—normal glucose; OC—total carboxylated osteocalcin; PMO—postmenopausal osteoporosis; PMW—postmenopausal women; RCT—randomized controlled trial; SD—standard deviation; tOC—total osteocalcin; ucOC—undercarboxylated osteocalcin; T2D—type 2 diabetes; TGs—triglycerides; W—women; ↑—increase; ↓—decrease.

The relation between OC and energetic metabolism was assessed in a cross-sectional study, including 146 postmenopausal women with and without T2D. Diabetic women presented lower levels of serum tOC ($p < 0.05$). There were significant negative correlations between OC concentration and glycated hemoglobin (HbA1c), serum triglycerides, and body mass index (p for all < 0.05), independent of the presence of T2D [139].

Similarly, in a study carried out in postmenopausal non-osteoporotic women, OC was found to be significantly lower in women with metabolic syndrome (metS) compared to control ($p < 0.001$). In this study, a significant positive correlation ($p = 0.008$) was detected between vitD and OC [140]. Supplementation of vitD, vitD3 metabolite more than vitD2, revealed to have favorable effects on metabolic profile measurements and depressive symptoms in T2D patients [144].

Apparently, VK supplementation had no significant consequences on glycemic control in healthy subjects [145]. However, studies performed on prediabetic and diabetic patients to determine the VK effect had different results. Rasekhi et al. studied 82 premenopausal and prediabetic women (40.17 ± 4.9 years), who were randomized to consume either 1000 µg PK supplement or placebo in a randomized controlled trial. After 4 weeks, the PK intake increased the serum levels of cOC and decreased ucOC compared with placebo (for both: $p < 0.001$) and improved the insulin sensitivity. A statistical significant association between changes of ucOC and 2 h post-oral glucose tolerance test (OGTT) glucose was found ($r = 0.308$, $p = 0.028$) [146].

Among patients with metS and T2D, both VK forms were beneficial. However, the risk reduction occurred at higher levels of PK intake compared to MK, suggesting that MK could be more effective than PK in reducing T2D risk [147]. It seemed that MK improved insulin sensitivity through the contribution of OC, anti-inflammatory activity, and lipid-lowering effect [148].

In a 12 week-trial involving T2D patients, the intake of 200 µg MK-7 daily supplements significantly decreased fasting blood sugar ($p = 0.02$) and HbA1c ($p = 0.01$) compared to the placebo group. Although MK-7 supplementation improved glycemic indices, the lipid profile did not significantly change within or between groups [149]. The same parameters were investigated in another randomized controlled trial (RCT), with a higher intake of MK-7, 180 µg twice daily. After 12-weeks, the T2D patients in the MK-7 group had significantly lower levels of fasting plasma glucose and HbA1c compared with the placebo group, while again, no significant changes were noticed in the lipid profiles. Fasting insulin and HOMA-IR significantly decreased in the MK-7 group compared to baseline, suggesting a decrease in insulin resistance [143].

The MK-7 isoform intake was yet again analyzed in another trial for eight weeks. A number of 84 polycystic ovary syndrome (PCOS) patients were randomly assigned into the 90 µg MK-7 daily treatment group and placebo. At the end of the study, MK-7 supplementation significantly decreased serum fasting insulin ($p = 0.002$) and HOMA-IR ($p = 0.002$) compared to the placebo group. Furthermore, MK-7 intake led to significantly lower serum triglyceride level ($p = 0.003$), waist circumference ($p = 0.03$), and body fat mass ($p < 0.001$). In this study, MK-7 intake showed beneficial effects on glycemic indices but also on lipid and anthropometric profiles in PCOS patients [150].

Knapen et al. assessed fat mass and body composition in postmenopausal women. The group that received 180 µg MK-7 per day revealed higher levels of circulating cOC. In subjects with an above-median response in cOC, a significant increase in adiponectin level and a decrease in abdominal fat mass and visceral adipose tissue area were observed compared with the placebo group and the subjects with low cOC level. Thus, MK-7 intake could reduce body weight or abdominal and visceral fat in subjects showing a strong increase in cOC [138].

A study, which evaluated the effect of vitD3 and VK2 supplements alone or in combination on OC levels and metabolic parameters was conducted in 40 diabetic patients. Diabetic patients are characterized by bone demineralization and changes in OC levels. In the vitD3 plus VK2 group, a significant decrease in glycemia ($p = 0.002$), percentage of pancreatic β-cells ($p = 0.004$), and in the uOC/cOC index ($p = 0.023$) were noticed. In the VK2 group, again a significant decrease in glycemia ($p = 0.002$), percentage of pancreatic β-cells ($p = 0.002$), and HOMA-IR ($p = 0.041$), and a statistically significant increase of cOC concentrations were observed. The increase in the cOC concentration could be explained by the action VK2 as a cofactor of carboxylases during activation of OC [141].

Yoshida et al. analyzed PK supplementation in an RCT comprising 355 nondiabetic men and women (mean age 68 years). After 36 months, HOMA-IR was significantly lower among men in the 500 μg PK daily supplement group compared to the control group, but no statistically significant result differences were noticed in women. Thus, PK supplementation for three years decreased the levels of ucOC and had a protective effect against the insulin resistance progression in older men [151]. In older humans, serum cOC and not ucOC concentration was associated with lower insulin resistance [133], which supports a potential link between bone physiology and insulin resistance in humans.

Jeannin et al. explored the association between VK status and diabetic peripheral neuropathy. The levels of dp-ucMGP, an inverse marker for VK status, were significantly higher in patients with neuropathy versus patients without neuropathy ($p = 0.009$). Since dp-ucMGP is a VK-dependent protein, reduced VK status is an independent risk factor for diabetic peripheral neuropathy. Hence, treatment with VK supplements may be a preventive measure in diabetic patients at risk of peripheral neuropathy [142].

VK consumption was linked with increased cOC, in addition to improved glycemic status, dyslipidemia, serum insulin, OS, and inflammation in T2D [152]. Possible mechanisms of these effects could be reduced hepatocyte gluconeogenesis and lipogenesis, decreased production of inflammatory cytokines and higher levels of adiponectin, inactivation of NF-κB pathway, or increased gene expression levels of AMP-activated protein kinase (AMPK) and sirtuin-1 (SIRT-1), important signaling molecules in the regulation of glucose hemostasis, lipid metabolism, and insulin sensitivity [152,153].

In animal studies, ucOC was found to be the active hormonal form that conferred beneficial glucose control and the only molecule involved in the production of insulin by the pancreatic β-cells [154]. Opposite to what was proposed in mouse models, in humans, the association between ucOC and insulin resistance may differ [155]. Higher VK intakes and increase cOC were associated with a low percentage of ucOC but also with reduced blood glucose, insulin resistance, and T2D risk [130,156,157]. The outcomes in these human studies assumed that a low percentage of ucOC actually improves glucose metabolism. Moreover, both cOC and ucOC levels could increase glucose transport in adipocytes and muscle cells and improve insulin sensitivity [38]. Although the in vivo experiments could have remarkable value in human pathology studies, some animal models cannot be extrapolated directly to humans [158].

Based on the current literature, healthier dietary habits and lifestyle, such as consumption of green leafy vegetables and fermented foods, major sources of VK, may independently contribute to reducing metabolic disorder risks.

5. The Effect of Vitamin K on Neurodegenerative Diseases

Age-related neurodegenerative diseases, such as Alzheimer's disease (AD) or Parkinson's disease (PD), lead to one of the most unfavorable health problems, cognitive impairment. It is a legitimate age-related health concern potentially affecting the wellbeing and independence of mature and old adults [159]. The dysregulations in these pathologies are mainly associated with OS, neuroinflammation, abnormal protein aggregation, or mitochondrial dysfunction. Recent animal and human studies showed that bioactive compounds could diminish the risk or delay the onset or progression of inflammation processes, cognitive impairment, or age-related syndromes [160–162].

Healthy nutritional diets, modifiable lifestyle factors may prevent or delay these diseases. Increased consumption of vegetables, fruits, nuts, seeds, with proven antioxidant and anti-inflammatory activities, is the principal dietary recommendation, with an important reminder that the beneficial effects may come from wholesome, healthy diets rather than from a particular nutrient [163].

AD, described by the existence of intracellular neurofibrillary tangles containing the microtubule-associated protein tau and extracellular aggregated amyloid-β (Aβ) peptides, is the most common cause of dementia in the old population. These modifications induce a chronic inflammatory state, leading to the neuronal damage observed in AD [164].

New findings suggest the participation of VK in brain physiology through the carboxylation of Gas6, a VKDP, which could defend against neuronal apoptosis induced by OS and Aβ [165]. Moreover, VK is implicated in neuron development and survival, which are mediated by protein S and sphingolipids. Sphingolipids are a class of lipids extensively present in brain cell membranes with important cell roles. They are active in neuroprotection and myelination, a critically important process for healthy CNS functioning [166]. VK may reduce cognitive decline and the risk of AD through modulating sphingolipid metabolism, which leads to enhanced Aβ clearance [166]. Altered sphingolipid profiles have been linked to neuroinflammation and neurodegeneration [167].

Recent evidence has shown that during remyelination, VK enhances the production of brain galactosyl ceramides, cerebrosides with a major role in nerve cell membranes. Furthermore, VK appears to have a survival-supporting effect on neurons [142].

Fat-soluble vitamins (A, D, E, and K) or water-soluble vitamin C are powerful antioxidant and anti-inflammatory agents [168]. Inadequate concentrations of vitamins have been linked with brain aging and cognitive decline in AD patients and the elderly [169]. VK has been shown to influence AD risk and cognitive functions, positively impact the mechanisms involved in AD pathogenesis, including OS, inflammation, Aβ-aggregation and Aβ-induced neurotoxicity [170].

Low plasma VK concentration was correlated with a greater degree of frailty, common in patients with neurodegenerative diseases. The relationship between VK status and frailty was assessed in a longitudinal study with 644 (54% women) community-dwelling adults, mean age 59.9 years over 13 years. After measuring dp-ucMGP as a marker of VK status, compared with the lowest tertile, the medium (1.40; 95% CI: 0.01–2.81, p for trend = 0.03) and highest (1.62; 95% CI: 0.18–3.06, p for trend = 0.03) tertiles were associated with higher degree of frailty [171].

Data reported low serum VK concentrations in AD patients and disclosed that patients with early-stage AD consumed lower VK per day than cognitively intact control subjects, which consumed around 139 μg VK daily [172]. Likewise, results from a mature population, 65 years and older, revealed a direct correlation between low VK dietary intake and low serum VK concentration, as well as declined cognitive performances [173]. Some MK isoforms, mainly the longer chains, produced by the gut microbiota were positively associated with cognition, as demonstrated by McCann et al. in a study on 74 old individuals at different cognitive ability levels [174].

The concentration of circulating PK is positively correlated with the intake, as it was demonstrated in a representative sample population aged over 65 years [175]. Tanprasertsuk et al. showed that in a group of nondemented centenarians, only circulating PK levels were significantly linked with a wide range of cognitive performance. Despite the fact that MK-4 was the predominant isomer in both the frontal and temporal cortex, cerebral MK-4 levels were not associated with cognitive measures. VK-rich food intake containing other bioactive molecules may act in synergy to cognitive health [176]. In a cross-sectional study, which comprised 320 old participants aged 70 to 85 years and without cognitive impairment, higher serum levels of PK were significantly connected with better verbal episodic memory performances (p = 0.048), exposing better cognition during aging [177].

The results of a prospective study that included 960 subjects (mean age 80 years) revealed that the intake of at least one serving of PK-rich foods daily, including green leafy vegetables, was linked with slower cognitive deterioration, corresponding to 11 years younger in age for the subjects in the highest quintile of PK intake (median 1.3 servings/d) [178]. Similarly, Chouet et al. indicated a statistically significant association between increased dietary PK intake and better cognition and behavior [179]. In a group of 192 participants (mean age 83 years), cognition was assessed with the mini-mental state examination (MMSE) and behavior with the frontotemporal behavioral rating scale (FBRS). Compared to lower intake, participants with higher PK intake had greater (i.e., better) mean MMSE score (22.0 ± 5.7 vs. 19.9 ± 6.2, $p = 0.024$) and lower (i.e., better) FBRS score (1.5 ± 1.2 vs. 1.9 ± 1.3, $p = 0.042$) [179].

Evaluating MS patients, Lasemi et al. showed that MK levels in this population were decreased compared to controls and suggested that MK supplementation might inhibit the disease's evolution [180]. Indeed, Sanchez et al. observed that prophylactic MK supplementation could suppress experimental autoimmune encephalomyelitis, an animal model of brain inflammation used to study human CNS demyelinating diseases, including MS [181].

A relationship between PD and serum VK2 levels was examined by Yu et al. in a study involving 93 PD patients and 95 healthy controls (age over 66) [182]. The results indicated that the serum VK2 level of PD patients was significantly lower (3.49 ± 1.68 ng/mL) than that of healthy controls (5.77 ± 2.71 ng/mL). Since inflammation is important pathogenesis of PD, and VK has anti-inflammatory action, deficiency of VK may lead to occurrence and aggravation of inflammatory state, and eventually the incidence of PD [182].

Significantly lower dietary VK consumption was associated as well with serious subjective memory complaints in 160 studied patients (mean age 82 y). Patients with serious subjective memory complaint had lower mean dietary VK intake compared to participants without serious subjective memory complaint (298.0 ± 191.8 μg/day vs. 393.8 ± 215.2 μg/day, $p = 0.005$). Increased VK intake was linked with fewer and less severe subjective memory disorders in participants taking no VK antagonists (VKAs) [183]. The use of VKAs as anticoagulant medications lowered the VK bioavailability, thus reducing the VK concentration and increasing the altered cognitive performance risk and the frequency of cognitive impairment in the elderly [184,185].

Scientific evidence confirmed that OC is involved in multiple biological processes, including energy metabolism, cognition, stress response, CV health. These physiological functions have been documented to be regulated by both OC forms, cOC and ucOC [186]. OC can bind to neurons of the hippocampus, brainstem, or midbrain, and enhance the production of monoamine neurotransmitters, prevent anxiety and depression, and support learning and memory. During aging, a decline in bone mass may cause a decrease in cognitive functions because of a drop in OC synthesis and/or activation [187]. As bone function and cognitive features deteriorate in parallel with OC levels during aging, this molecule could be defined as an antiaging tool with the potential to be used against age-related disorders, including cognitive alterations. Improving bone health during aging may have favorable effects on cognition [188].

Since pharmacological interventions have been unsuccessful in the prevention of dementia and evolution of AD or PD, other approaches, such as lifestyle changes and dietary therapies, may impact the prevention and evolution of dementia, AD, or PD. Thus, nutritional interventions could favorably modulate the epigenetic mechanisms through regulating DNA acetylation and methylation or altering the expression of miRNAs [189]. Foods, including green leafy vegetables, berries, or nuts, high in VK and other vitamins, minerals, polyphenols with powerful antioxidant properties, should be encouraged in older adults for the prevention or management of age-associated neurodegenerative diseases [190].

Moreover, VK, especially VK2, prevents an excess vascular calcification of retinal blood vessels and thus the age-related stiffness and atherosclerotic plaque of blood vessels. It can stop the evolution of an age-related macular degeneration (AMD) and, for better results, should be used in combination with magnesium, zinc, and/or vitamin D [191].

6. The Effect of Vitamin K on Cancer

The basic chemical structure of VK and the functional unit in several cancer chemotherapeutic drugs is a quinone, which partially explains the research involving VK use in the prevention and treatment of cancer [192].

Quinones can be converted into reduced forms, first into intermediate semiquinones (one-electron reduction), then hydroquinones (two-electron reduction). These reactions consume superoxide radicals, generally accepted as oncogenic, and also consume reducing equivalents (NADH, NADPH, glutathione), essential for cancer cell homeostasis [193], hence creating an intracellular setting proper for induction of apoptosis. The VK-modulated redox-cycle may partially explain VK anticancer activity [194].

Further research suggests that increased VK intake (e.g., MK) may have potent anticancer properties since it has shown an inverse association with overall cancer incidence. Although the exact anticancer activity of dietary VK is still unclear, there are several suggested mechanisms that may explain its effect on preventing carcinogenesis, such as scavenging oxygen free radicals, inhibiting polyamine metabolism, induction of apoptosis, production of reactive oxygen species (ROS), cell cycle arrest and activation of antimetastasis genes [195,196].

Both VK1 and VK2 have demonstrated antiproliferative, proapoptotic, autophagic activities, resulting in anticancer activity [195]. Moreover, VK3 and its analogs are potent inhibitors of cell proliferation on many cancer cell lines. They act as cellular redox mediators generating ROS and inducing apoptosis by mitochondrial pathway [197]. Combining VK3 with other molecules sharing structural similarity, such as plumbagin and juglone, naturally occurring naphthoquinones found in polyphenol-rich *Juglans regia* [198], or with vitamins or drugs that also function through modulation of intracellular redox states could potentiate the antitumor effects [199,200].

Cancer cell death induced by VK2 appears to vary among the type of cancers. In triple-negative breast cancer cell lines, VK2-induced non-apoptotic cell death along with autophagy [201]. In prostate cancer cell lines, VK2-induced cell death through ROS-mediated cell cycle arrest and mitochondrial-mediated apoptosis, as well as metastasis-inhibiting signaling molecules [202]. Moreover, in prostate cancer cells, VK2 showed anti-inflammatory activity as several inflammatory genes were downregulated after treatment with VK2. Additionally, VK2-reduced proliferation, induced apoptosis and lowered the angiogenic potential of prostate cancer cells. The proposed mechanisms for the potential anticancer effects were caspase-3 induction, inhibition of NF-κB pathway, downregulation of phosphorylated protein kinase B (AKT), and reduction of androgen receptor expression [203]. Moreover, certain essential proteins, such as Bak and Cx43, several protein kinases, such as PKA and PKC, and transcription factors, such as AP-2, are involved in the mechanism of VK2 activity against cancer cells [204].

In different cancer cell lines, VK2 can inhibit cancer cells' growth by the initiation of autophagy, a natural mechanism that removes damaged or dysfunctional cellular organelles and prevents diseases, such as cancer, diabetes, or neurodegeneration [205]. Yokoyama et al. demonstrated that MK-4 could simultaneously stimulate autophagy and apoptosis in leukemic cells, but rather autophagy was dominant in the presence of B-cell lymphoma 2 (Bcl-2) protein that inhibited apoptosis [206]. Similarly, MK-4 treatment-induced antitumor effects on cholangiocellular carcinoma (CCC) cells via autophagy. The apoptosis induction effect of MK-4 in CCC cells was relatively small compared to other cancer cells, a possible reason being, as in the previous experiment, the over-expression of the anti-apoptotic Bcl-2 protein in CCC cells [207]. Tokita et al. examined the growth inhibitory action by MK-4 on gastric cancer cell lines. The results established that MK-4-treatment-induced antitumor effects through apoptosis and cell cycle arrest in a dose-dependent manner [208].

In another study, MK-4 again inhibited the growth and invasion of hepatocellular carcinoma (HCC) cells via activation of protein kinase A. MK-4 reduced the ability of liver cancer cells to invade and spread via the portal venous system [209]. However, the beneficial effects of VK treatment alone were not enough to avoid or treat HCC in clinical settings. Thus, VK administration combined with other anticancer reagents could achieve satisfactory therapeutic effects against HCC [210]. Yoshiji et al. administered MK-4 (45 mg/d) and angiotensin-converting enzyme inhibitor (ACE-I) (4 mg/d) after curative therapy for HCC. After 48 months, the combination treatment with VK and ACE-I inhibited the cumulative recurrence of HCC, at least partly through suppression of the vascular endothelial growth factor (VEGF), an angiogenic factor [211].

Duan et al. examined the anticancer activity of VK2 in bladder cancer cells and investigated the underlying mechanism. VK2-induced apoptosis in bladder cancer cells through the phosphorylation of c-Jun N-terminal kinase and p38 mitogen-activated protein kinase (JNK/p38 MAPK), as well as through mitochondrial pathways, including loss of membrane potential, cytochrome C release, and caspase-3 cascade [212]. Furthermore, VK2 can upregulate glycolysis in bladder cancer cells, mediated by phosphatidylinositide-3-kinase and AKT (PI3K/AKT) and hypoxia-inducible factor-1α (HIF-1α), induce metabolic stress, along with increased phosphorylation of AMPK and reduced phosphorylation of mammalian target of rapamycin complex 1 (mTORC1). Thus, in response to metabolic stress, VK2 could activate AMPK and suppress the mTORC1 pathway, consequently causing AMPK-dependent autophagic cancer cell death. Upon glucose limitation, the increased glycolysis would result in metabolic stress and cell death. Hence, VK2 could induce metabolic stress and trigger AMPK-dependent autophagic cell death in bladder cancer cells by PI3K/AKT/HIF-1α-mediated glycolysis elevation, this being one of the VK2-induced anticancer mechanism [213].

Dietary polyamines are involved in various biological processes, including cell proliferation and differentiation, which can increase life span and be beneficial against aging and age-related disorders [214,215]. However, polyamines are detrimental in disease progression and are a target for anticancer agents [215]. PK proved to be a potential anticancer agent. Following PK administration to colon cancer cell lines, significant antiproliferative and proapoptotic effects were noticed, in addition to a significant decrease in the polyamine biosynthesis [216].

The association between dietary intake of PK and MKs and total and advanced prostate cancer was evaluated in 11,319 men during a mean follow-up time of 8.6 years. MKs intake presented a nonsignificant inverse association for total prostate cancer (RR = 0.65; 95% CI: 0.39–1.06) and a significant association for advanced prostate cancer (RR = 0.37; 95% CI: 0.16–0.88, p for trend = 0.03). The association was stronger for MKs from dairy products compared with MKs from meat. The PK intake did not correlate with prostate cancer incidence [192].

VK has been reported to have antiproliferative and proapoptotic activity in human melanoma cells. VK3 has been identified as a specific inhibitor of the E3 ubiquitin ligase Siah-2, an enzyme implicated through several mechanisms in melanoma development and progression [217].

Beaudin et al. reported distinct effects on breast cancer cells for the two forms of VK, as VK1 promoted γ-carboxylation and stem cell features, while VK2 presented antiproliferative or proapoptotic effects. The authors hypothesized that in normal breast, VK1 is converted to VK3, which is then prenylated by the enzyme UbiA prenyltransferase domain containing 1 (UBIAD1) to VK2, favoring tumor suppression. However, loss of UBIAD1 in tumors abrogates VK2 formation, leading to accumulation of VK1, which promotes aggressive phenotypes via γ-carboxylation if tumors express the enzyme GGCX. Future studies could clarify the function of UBIAD1 and the action of cellular VK1 and VK2 in breast cancer cells [218].

Contrary to the previous hypothetical opinion, the data from a large prospective cohort study showed that dietary VK2 was linked with breast cancer incidence and mortality. After adjustment for confounders, total VK and dietary VK1 were not associated with breast cancer incidence and mortality. However, total VK2 intake was significantly associated with 26% elevated breast cancer risk, and 71% increased risk of death from breast cancer [219]. In the general population, VK2 intake is mainly from cheese and meat and, based on recent scientific evidence, meat consumption and not VK2 was associated with increased breast cancer risk [220]. Other prospective studies found an association between better diet quality and higher consumption of salad vegetables, rich sources of VK1, and lower risk of breast cancer, offering indirect evidence for the antioncogenic effect of VK1 [221,222].

In the prospective European Prospective Investigation into Cancer and Nutrition—Heidelberg cohort study, 24,340 participants were followed for more than 10 years to estimate an association between VK intake and overall cancer incidence and mortality. Dietary intake of VK2, highly determined by cheese consumption, was significantly inversely associated with cancer mortality (HR = 0.72; 95% CI: 0.53–0.98, p for trend = 0.03) and nonsignificantly linked with overall cancer incidence (HR = 0.86; 95% CI: 0.73–1.01, p for trend = 0.08) for the highest compared with the lowest quartile. Cancer risk reduction after VK2 intake was more evident in men than in women, mostly driven by significant inverse associations with lung (p for trend = 0.002) and prostate (p for trend = 0.03) cancer. In women, almost 50% of all cancer cases were breast cancer, nonsignificantly associated with VK2 intake [223]. Dietary VK2 intake was more strongly inversely associated with cancer mortality than with cancer incidence because likely, factors having a role in apoptosis and cell cycle arrest appear later in carcinogenesis. In addition, the suggested VK2 inhibitory role in angiogenesis is strongly linked to metastasis development [224].

Another prospective cohort, the PREDIMED study, which enrolled 7216 participants with high CVD risk, means age 67 years, followed up for a median of 4.8 years, analyzed the link between dietary VK intake and cancer risk, among other parameters. After adjustment for potential confounders, the outcomes indicated that dietary VK1 intake was associated with a significantly reduced risk of cancer (HR = 0.54; 95% CI; 0.30–0.96). In longitudinal analyses, individuals who increased their intake of PK or MK during follow-up had a significantly lower risk of cancer (HR = 0.64; 95% CI; 0.43–0.95; and HR = 0.41; 95% CI; 0.26–0.64, respectively) compared to individuals, who diminished or did not change the VK intake. Thus, dietary intake of both PK and MK forms was associated with a reduced risk of cancer, besides a lower risk of CV and all-cause mortality [225]. Although in this study PK was positively correlated with cancer risk, in other studies, dietary PK intake was not associated with cancer. Considering that PK is converted to menadione and MK-4, it can be proposed that dietary PK exerts cancer inhibitory effects as part of the total VK concentration [223].

The universal agreement is that a healthy vegetable-rich diet could prevent cancer and its development. Thus, the protective effects of a high PK consumption on carcinogenesis may come from healthy diets with beneficial synergistic effects rather than from VK per se.

7. Correlation between Vitamin K and Pulmonary Disease

The most common chronic respiratory disease is a chronic obstructive pulmonary disease (COPD) involving chronic bronchitis and emphysema. In a cross-sectional study, the association of dark green vegetables with emphysema status was assessed among US adults. The consumption of recommended amounts of VK was associated with a 39% decrease in odds of emphysema. VK showed that it might slow the emphysematous process and, together with vitamin A are important in lung health [226].

VK can activate intrahepatic and extrahepatic procoagulant or anticoagulant factors, such as protein S. This protein, a VK-dependent plasma glycoprotein, has a role in the anti-coagulation pathway, where it functions as a cofactor to protein C [227]. Besides this action, protein S can prevent the production of inflammatory cytokines associated with the cytokine storm observed in acute lung injury [228]. Alterations in the serum levels of protein S can relate to the progression of fibrosis and inflammatory diseases in the lung, liver, or heart [229]. Low protein S levels were correlated lately with higher thrombogenicity, clinical severity, and fatal outcome in COVID-19 patients, independently of age or even Inflammatory biomarkers [230]. In COVID-19 cases, the reduced activation of MGP and protein S due to the pneumonia-induced VK depletion can lead to an escalation in pulmonary injury and thrombosis [231].

8. Conclusions

The latest scientific evidence summarized in this review indicated that VK has a significant role in mitigating aging and preventing age-related diseases and has the potential to improve the efficacy of some medical treatments among adults over the age of 50 years. The novel role of VK on aging and age-associated diseases is mainly due to its antioxidant and anti-inflammatory effects. The review focused on the most prevalent age-related diseases, including osteoporosis and bone fractures, neurodegenerative diseases, VC, CVD, and cancer, as well as metabolic disorders, mainly T2D and obesity. In addition, we presented the most recent findings on the association between VK and COVID-19 and its potential effect on reducing fatal outcomes in such cases. Specifically, the scientific data showed that VK has an integral role in bone metabolism through the carboxylation of OC, which is an important protein capable of transporting and depositing calcium in bone. MK-4 was revealed to be a more effective antiosteoporotic agent than VK1, with increased pro-osteoblastic and anti-osteoclastogenic actions achieved by inhibiting the NF-κB pathway. VitD improves OC carboxylation and, along with VK and magnesium supplementations, can be a better strategy for reducing bone fractures, a highly public health concern among the elderly. In addition, the review concluded that VK supplement could be a safe approach for reducing CVD morbidity and mortality. By activating matrix Gla protein, VK keeps calcium from accumulating in the walls of blood vessels, thus making VK a potential treatment for patients at risk for either VC or CVD. Furthermore, VK may reduce the risk for metabolic disorders, such as T2D, by improving insulin sensitivity and anti-inflammatory activity, as well as obesity, through a lipid-lowering effect. The review also showed the influence VK has on age-related neurodegenerative diseases, such as AD and PD. VK is involved in the brain's physiology and can reduce its cognitive decline by carboxylation of Gas6 protein, a VKDP that could defend against neuronal apoptosis induced by OS and Aβ. The anticancer potential of VK was summarized by reviewing several in vitro and epidemiological studies. There are multiple mechanisms where the potential anticancer agent of VK can react, including the modulation of various transcription factors, which induced antiproliferative, proapoptotic, and autophagic effects, which were found to be associated with a reduced risk of cancer. The latest evidence on VK and pulmonary disease stem from the fact that VK can activate protein S, which was recently shown to prevent the generation of inflammatory cytokines and cytokine storms detected in COVID-19 cases. Low levels of protein S, due to pneumonia-induced VK depletion, were correlated with higher thrombogenicity and possibly fatal outcomes in COVID-19 patients.

Consuming a healthy diet is vital throughout the aging process to maintain and promote wellbeing. The aging population may be at risk for many suboptimal nutrient intakes, including VK, which have been shown to be associated with adverse health outcomes highly prevalent in this age group. Thus, the intake of VK-rich diets or VK supplements could prevent age-related diseases and/or support the effectiveness of medical treatments. However, more studies are needed to formulate the exactly recommended intakes of VK, including VK1, MK-4, and MK-7, due to their distinct bioavailability and biological activities. According to this review, higher values of VK intakes are needed, especially among the elderly and people who have comorbidities conditions that are most likely to be VK deficient.

Author Contributions: Conceptualization, D.-S.P., M.E.R.; methodology, D.-S.P., M.E.R.; investigation, D.-S.P., G.B., M.E.R.; writing original draft preparation, D.-S.P., M.E.R.; writing, reviewing, and editing, D.-S.P., G.B., M.E.R. All authors have read and agreed to the published version of the manuscript.

Funding: This research received no external funding.

Conflicts of Interest: The authors declare no conflict of interest.

Abbreviations

ACE-I   Angiotensin-converting enzyme inhibitor
AD   Alzheimer's disease
AKT   Protein kinase B

AMPK	Adenosine monophosphate-activated protein kinase
Bcl-2	B-cell lymphoma 2
BMC	Bone mineral content
BMD	Bone mineral density
CCC	Cholangiocellular carcinoma
CHD	Coronary heart disease
CKD	Chronic kidney disease
CNS	Central nervous system
cOC	Carboxylated osteocalcin
CRP	C-reactive protein
CV	Cardiovascular
CVD	Cardiovascular disease
dp-ucMGP	Dephosphorylated-uncarboxylated matrix Gla protein
Gas6	Growth arrest-specific protein 6
GGCX	Gamma-glutamyl carboxylase
Gla	γ-carboxylated glutamic acid
Glu	Glutamic acid
GRP	Gla-rich protein
HbA1c	Glycated hemoglobin
HCC	Hepatocellular carcinoma
HDL	High-density lipoprotein
HIF-1α	Hypoxia-inducible factor-1α
HOMA-IR	Homeostatic model assessment for insulin resistance
HR	Hazard ratio
IL	Interleukin
JNK	C-Jun N-terminal kinase
metS	Metabolic syndrome
MGP	Matrix Gla protein
MK	Menaquinone
mTORC	Mammalian target of rapamycin complex
NF-κB	Nuclear factor kappa-light-chain-enhancer of activated B cells
Nrf2	Nuclear factor erythroid 2–related factor 2
OA	Osteoarthritis
OC	Osteocalcin
OR	Odds ratio
OS	Oxidative stress
PCOS	Polycystic ovary syndrome
PD	Parkinson's disease
PI3K	Phosphatidylinositide-3-kinase
PK	Phylloquinone
RCT	Randomized controlled trial
ROS	Reactive oxygen species
SIRT	Sirtuin
T2D	Type 2 diabetes
TNF-α	Tumor necrosis factor-alpha
tOC	Total osteocalcin
UBIAD1	UbiA prenyltransferase domain containing 1
ucMGP	Uncarboxylated matrix Gla protein
ucOC	Undercarboxylated osteocalcin
VC	Vascular calcification
vitD	Vitamin D
VK	Vitamin K
VKAs	Vitamin K antagonists
VKDP	Vitamin K-dependent protein

References

1. Franco, R.; Navarro, G.; Martínez-Pinilla, E. Hormetic and Mitochondria-Related Mechanisms of Antioxidant Action of Phytochemicals. *Antioxidants* **2019**, *8*, 373. [CrossRef]

2. Bjørklund, G.; Chirumbolo, S. Role of oxidative stress and antioxidants in daily nutrition and human health. *Nutrition* **2017**, *33*, 311–321. [CrossRef] [PubMed]
3. Maurya, P.K.; Kumar, P.; Chandra, P. Biomarkers of oxidative stress in erythrocytes as a function of human age. *World J. Methodol.* **2015**, *5*, 216–222. [CrossRef]
4. Rusu, M.E.; Gheldiu, A.-M.; Mocan, A.; Vlase, L.; Popa, D.-S. Anti-aging potential of tree nuts with a focus on phytochemical composition, molecular mechanisms and thermal stability of major bioactive compounds. *Food Funct.* **2018**, *9*, 2554–2575. [CrossRef] [PubMed]
5. Harshman, S.; Shea, M. The Role of Vitamin K in Chronic Aging Diseases: Inflammation, Cardiovascular Disease, and Osteoarthritis. *Curr. Nutr. Rep.* **2016**, *5*, 90–98. [CrossRef] [PubMed]
6. Braasch-Turi, M.; Crans, D.C. Synthesis of Naphthoquinone Derivatives: Menaquinones, Lipoquinones and Other Vitamin K Derivatives. *Molecules* **2020**, *25*, 4377. [CrossRef]
7. Schurgers, L.; Vermeer, C. Determination of phylloquinone and menaquinones in food. Effect of food matrix on circulating vitamin K concentrations. *Haemostasis* **2000**, *30*, 298–307. [CrossRef] [PubMed]
8. Turck, D.; Bresson, J.-L.; Burlingame, B.; Dean, T.; Fairweather-Tait, S.; Heinonen, M.; Hirsch-Ernst, K.I.; Mangelsdorf, I.; McArdle, H.; Naska, A.; et al. Dietary reference values for vitamin K. *EFSA J.* **2017**, *15*, e04780. [CrossRef]
9. Elder, S.J.; Haytowitz, D.B.; Howe, J.; Peterson, J.W.; Booth, S.L. Vitamin K Contents of Meat, Dairy, and Fast Food in the U.S. Diet. *J. Agric. Food Chem.* **2006**, *54*, 463–467. [CrossRef]
10. Melse-Boonstra, A. Bioavailability of Micronutrients from Nutrient-Dense Whole Foods: Zooming in on Dairy, Vegetables, and Fruits. *Front. Nutr.* **2020**, *7*, 101. [CrossRef] [PubMed]
11. Booth, S.L. Vitamin K: Food composition and dietary intakes. *Food Nutr. Res.* **2012**, *56*, 5505. [CrossRef] [PubMed]
12. Margier, M.; Antoine, T.; Siriaco, A.; Nowicki, M.; Halimi, C.; Maillot, M.; Georgé, S.; Reboul, E. The Presence of Pulses within a Meal can Alter Fat-Soluble Vitamin Bioavailability. *Mol. Nutr. Food Res.* **2019**, *63*, e1801323. [CrossRef]
13. Halder, M.; Petsophonsakul, P.; Akbulut, A.C.; Pavlic, A.; Bohan, F.; Anderson, E.; Maresz, K.; Kramann, R.; Schurgers, L. Vitamin K: Double Bonds beyond Coagulation Insights into Differences between Vitamin K1 and K2 in Health and Disease. *Int. J. Mol. Sci.* **2019**, *20*, 896. [CrossRef] [PubMed]
14. Wei, F.-F.; Trenson, S.; Verhamme, P.; Vermeer, C.; Staessen, J.A. Vitamin K-Dependent Matrix Gla Protein as Multifaceted Protector of Vascular and Tissue Integrity. *Hypertension* **2019**, *73*, 1160–1169. [CrossRef]
15. Gröber, U.; Reichrath, J.; Holick, M.F.; Kisters, K. Vitamin K: An old vitamin in a new perspective. *Dermato Endocrinol.* **2015**, *6*, e968490. [CrossRef] [PubMed]
16. Bender, D.; Vitamin, K. *Nutritional Biochemistry of the Vitamins*; Cambridge University Press: Cambridge, UK, 2003; pp. 131–147; ISBN 9780521803885.
17. Simes, D.; Viegas, C.; Araújo, N.; Marreiros, C. Vitamin K as a Diet Supplement with Impact in Human Health: Current Evidence in Age-Related Diseases. *Nutrients* **2020**, *12*, 138. [CrossRef]
18. Li, J.; Lin, J.C.; Wang, H.; Peterson, J.W.; Furie, B.C.; Furie, B.; Booth, S.L.; Volpe, J.J.; Rosenberg, P.A. Novel Role of Vitamin K in Preventing Oxidative Injury to Developing Oligodendrocytes and Neurons. *J. Neurosci.* **2003**, *23*, 5816–5826. [CrossRef]
19. Sinbad, O.O.; Folorunsho, A.A.; Olabisi, O.L.; Ayoola, A.O.; Temitope, J. Vitamins as Antioxidants. *J. Food Sci. Nutr. Res.* **2019**, *2*, 214–235. [CrossRef]
20. Rusu, M.E.; Simedrea, R.; Gheldiu, A.-M.; Mocan, A.; Vlase, L.; Popa, D.-S.; Ferreira, I.C.F.R. Benefits of tree nut consumption on aging and age-related diseases: Mechanisms of actions. *Trends Food Sci. Technol.* **2019**, *88*, 104–120. [CrossRef]
21. Fusaro, M.; Gallieni, M.; Rizzo, M.A.; Stucchi, A.; Delanaye, P.; Cavalier, E.; Moysés, R.M.A.; Jorgetti, V.; Iervasi, G.; Giannini, S.; et al. Vitamin K plasma levels determination in human health. *Clin. Chem. Lab. Med.* **2017**, *55*, 789–799. [CrossRef] [PubMed]
22. DiNicolantonio, J.J.; Bhutani, J.; O'Keefe, J.H. The health benefits of vitamin K. *Open Hear* **2015**, *2*, e000300. [CrossRef]
23. Akbulut, A.; Pavlic, A.; Petsophonsakul, P.; Halder, M.; Maresz, K.; Kramann, R.; Schurgers, L. Vitamin K2 Needs an RDI Separate from Vitamin K1. *Nutrients* **2020**, *12*, 1852. [CrossRef] [PubMed]
24. Louka, M.; Fawzy, A.; Naiem, A.; Elseknedy, M.; Abdelhalim, A.; Abdelghany, M. Vitamin D and K signaling pathways in hepatocellular carcinoma. *Gene* **2017**, *629*, 108–116. [CrossRef]
25. Kim, Y.; Keogh, J.; Clifton, P. Benefits of nut consumption on insulin resistance and cardiovascular risk factors: Multiple potential mechanisms of actions. *Nutrients* **2017**, *9*, 1271. [CrossRef] [PubMed]
26. Paul, C.I.; Vitamin, K. *Textbook of Natural Medicine*, 5th ed.; Pizzorno, J.E., Murray, M.T., Eds.; Churchill Livingstone: St. Louis, MO, USA, 2020; pp. 919–947.e5; ISBN 978-0-323-52342-4.
27. Vermeer, C.; Raes, J.; van't Hoofd, C.; Knapen, M.H.J.; Xanthoulea, S. Menaquinone Content of Cheese. *Nutrients* **2018**, *10*, 446. [CrossRef]
28. Ferland, G. Vitamin K and brain function. *Semin Thromb Hemost.* **2013**, *39*, 849–855. [CrossRef]
29. Beulens, J.W.J.; Booth, S.L.; van den Heuvel, E.G.; Stoecklin, E.; Baka, A.; Vermeer, C. The role of menaquinones (vitamin K_2) in human health. *Br. J. Nutr.* **2013**, *110*, 1357–1368. [CrossRef]
30. Ferland, G.; Vitamin, K. An emerging nutrient in brain function. *Biofactors* **2012**, *38*, 151–157. [CrossRef] [PubMed]
31. Thijssen, H.; Drittij-Reijnders, M. Vitamin K status in human tissues: Tissue-specific accumulation of phylloquinone and menaquinone-4. *Br. J. Nutr.* **1996**, *75*, 121–127. [CrossRef]

32. Sato, T.; Inaba, N.; Yamashita, T. MK-7 and Its Effects on Bone Quality and Strength. *Nutrients* **2020**, *12*, 965. [CrossRef] [PubMed]
33. Vermeer, C. Vitamin K: The effect on health beyond coagulation—An overview. *Food Nutr. Res.* **2012**, *56*. [CrossRef]
34. Schwalfenberg, G.K. Vitamins K1 and K2: The Emerging Group of Vitamins Required for Human Health. *J. Nutr. Metab.* **2017**, *2017*, 6254836. [CrossRef]
35. Ravishankar, B.; Dound, Y.A.; Mehta, D.S.; Ashok, B.K.; de Souza, A.; Pan, M.-H.; Ho, C.-T.; Badmaev, V.; Vaidya, A.D.B. Safety assessment of menaquinone-7 for use in human Nutrition. *J. Food Drug Anal.* **2015**, *23*, 99–108. [CrossRef]
36. Huang, Z.; Wan, S.; Lu, Y.; Ning, L.; Liu, C.; Fan, S. Does vitamin K2 play a role in the prevention and treatment of osteoporosis for postmenopausal women: A meta-analysis of randomized controlled trials. *Osteoporos Int.* **2015**, *26*, 1175–1186. [CrossRef] [PubMed]
37. Kirk, B.; Feehan, J.; Lombardi, G.; Duque, G. Muscle, Bone, and Fat Crosstalk: The Biological Role of Myokines, Osteokines, and Adipokines. *Curr. Osteoporos Rep.* **2020**, *18*, 388–400. [CrossRef] [PubMed]
38. Hill, H.S.; Grams, J.; Walton, R.G.; Liu, J.; Moellering, D.R.; Garvey, W.T. Carboxylated and uncarboxylated forms of osteocalcin directly modulate the glucose transport system and inflammation in adipocytes. *Horm. Metab. Res.* **2014**, *46*, 341–347. [CrossRef] [PubMed]
39. Mohammad Rahimi, G.R.; Niyazi, A.; Alaee, S. The effect of exercise training on osteocalcin, adipocytokines, and insulin resistance: A systematic review and meta-analysis of randomized controlled trials. *Osteoporos Int.* **2021**, *32*, 213–224. [CrossRef]
40. Tsugawa, N.; Shiraki, M. Vitamin K Nutrition and Bone Health. *Nutrients* **2020**, *12*, 1909. [CrossRef]
41. Binkley, N.C.; Krueger, D.C.; Kawahara, T.N.; Engelke, J.A.; Chappell, R.J.; Suttie, J.W. A high phylloquinone intake is required to achieve maximal osteocalcin gamma-carboxylation. *Am. J. Clin. Nutr.* **2002**, *76*, 1055–1060. [CrossRef]
42. Lin, X.; Brennan-Speranza, T.C.; Levinger, I.; Yeap, B.B. Undercarboxylated Osteocalcin: Experimental and Human Evidence for a Role in Glucose Homeostasis and Muscle Regulation of Insulin Sensitivity. *Nutrients* **2018**, *10*, 847. [CrossRef]
43. Fusaro, M.; Cianciolo, G.; Brandi, M.L.; Ferrari, S.; Nickolas, T.L.; Tripepi, G.; Plebani, M.; Zaninotto, M.; Iervasi, G.; La Manna, G.; et al. Vitamin K and Osteoporosis. *Nutrients* **2020**, *12*, 3625. [CrossRef]
44. Shiraki, M.; Shiraki, Y.; Aoki, C.; Miura, M. Vitamin K2 (menatetrenone) effectively prevents fractuRes. and sustains lumbar bone mineral density in osteoporosis. *J. Bone Min. Res.* **2000**, *15*, 515–521. [CrossRef] [PubMed]
45. Bolton-Smith, C.; McMurdo, M.E.; Paterson, C.R.; Mole, P.A.; Harvey, J.M.; Fenton, S.T.; Prynne, C.J.; Mishra, G.D.; Shearer, M.J. Two-year randomized controlled trial of vitamin K1 (phylloquinone) and vitamin D3 plus calcium on the bone health of older women. *J. Bone Min. Res.* **2007**, *22*, 509–519. [CrossRef]
46. Binkley, N.; Harke, J.; Krueger, D.; Engelke, J.; Vallarta-Ast, N.; Gemar, D.; Checovich, M.; Chappell, R.; Suttie, J. Vitamin K Treatment Reduces Undercarboxylated Osteocalcin but Does Not Alter Bone Turnover, Density, or Geometry in Healthy Postmenopausal North American Women. *J. Bone Min. Res.* **2009**, *24*, 983–991. [CrossRef] [PubMed]
47. Rønn, S.; Harsløf, T.; Pedersen, S.; Langdahl, B. Vitamin K2 (menaquinone-7) prevents age-related deterioration of trabecular bone microarchitecture at the tibia in postmenopausal women. *Eur. J. Endocrinol.* **2016**, *175*, 541–549. [CrossRef]
48. Iwamoto, J.; Takeda, T.; Ichimura, S. Effect of menatetrenone on bone mineral density and incidence of vertebral fractuRes. in postmenopausal women with osteoporosis: A comparison with the effect of etidronate. *J. Orthop. Sci.* **2001**, *6*, 487–492. [CrossRef]
49. Purwosunu, Y.; Muharram; Rachman, I.A.; Reksoprodjo, S.; Sekizawa, A. Vitamin K 2 treatment for postmenopausal osteoporosis in Indonesia. *J. Obs. Gynaecol. Res.* **2006**, *32*, 230–234. [CrossRef]
50. Knapen, M.; Schurgers, L.; Vermeer, C. Vitamin K 2 supplementation improves hip bone geometry and bone strength indices in postmenopausal women. *Osteoporos Int.* **2007**, *18*, 963–972. [CrossRef] [PubMed]
51. Booth, S.L.; Dallal, G.; Shea, M.K.; Gundberg, C.; Peterson, J.W.; Dawson-Hughes, B. Effect of Vitamin K Supplementation on Bone Loss in Elderly Men and Women. *J. Clin. Endocrinol. Metab.* **2008**, *93*, 1217–1223. [CrossRef] [PubMed]
52. Cheung, A.M.; Tile, L.; Lee, Y.; Tomlinson, G.; Hawker, G.; Scher, J.; Hu, H.; Vieth, R.; Thompson, L.; Jamal, S.; et al. Vitamin K supplementation in postmenopausal women with osteopenia (ECKO trial): A randomized controlled trial. *PLoS Med.* **2008**, *5*, e196. [CrossRef]
53. Hirao, M.; Hashimoto, J.; Ando, W.; Ono, T.; Yoshikawa, H. Response of serum carboxylated and undercarboxylated osteocalcin to alendronate monotherapy and combined therapy with vitamin K2 in postmenopausal women. *J. Bone Min. Metab.* **2008**, *26*, 260–264. [CrossRef]
54. Tsugawa, N.; Shiraki, M.; Suhara, Y.; Kamao, M.; Ozaki, R.; Tanaka, K.; Okano, T. Low plasma phylloquinone concentration is associated with high incidence of vertebral fracture in Japanese women. *J. Bone Min. Metab.* **2008**, *26*, 79–85. [CrossRef]
55. Yamauchi, M.; Yamaguchi, T.; Nawata, K.; Takaoka, S.; Sugimoto, T. Relationships between undercarboxylated osteocalcin and vitamin K intakes, bone turnover, and bone mineral density in healthy women. *Clin. Nutr.* **2010**, *29*, 761–765. [CrossRef]
56. Je, S.H.; Joo, N.-S.; Choi, B.-H.; Kim, K.-M.; Kim, B.-T.; Park, S.-B.; Cho, D.-Y.; Kim, K.-N.; Lee, D.-J. Vitamin K Supplement Along with Vitamin D and Calcium Reduced Serum Concentration of Undercarboxylated Osteocalcin While Increasing Bone Mineral Density in Korean Postmenopausal Women over Sixty-Years-Old. *J. Korean Med. Sci.* **2011**, *26*, 1093–1098. [CrossRef]
57. Kanellakis, S.; Moschonis, G.; Tenta, R.; Schaafsma, A.; van den Heuvel, E.; Papaioannou, N.; Lyritis, G.; Manios, Y. Changes in parameters of bone metabolism in postmenopausal women following a 12-month intervention period using dairy products enriched with calcium, vitamin D, and phylloquinone (vitamin K(1)) or menaquinone-7 (vitamin K (2)): The Postmenopausal Health Study II. *Calcif. Tissue Int.* **2012**, *90*, 251–262. [CrossRef]

58. Knapen, M.; Drummen, N.; Smit, E.; Vermeer, C.; Theuwissen, E. Three-year low-dose menaquinone-7 supplementation helps decrease bone loss in healthy postmenopausal women. *Osteoporos Int.* **2013**, *24*, 2499–2507. [CrossRef] [PubMed]
59. Jiang, Y.; Zhang, Z.-L.; Zhang, Z.-L.; Zhu, H.-M.; Wu, Y.-Y.; Cheng, Q.; Wu, F.-L.; Xing, X.-P.; Liu, J.-L.; Yu, W.; et al. Menatetrenone versus alfacalcidol in the treatment of Chinese postmenopausal women with osteoporosis: A multicenter, randomized, double-blinded, double-dummy, positive drug-controlled clinical trial. *Clin. Interv. Aging* **2014**, *9*, 121–127. [CrossRef] [PubMed]
60. Bultynck, C.; Munim, N.; Harrington, D.; Judd, L.; Ataklte, F.; Shah, Z.; Dockery, F. Prevalence of vitamin K deficiency in older people with hip fracture. *Acta Clin. Belg.* **2020**, *75*, 136–140. [CrossRef] [PubMed]
61. Moore, A.E.; Kim, E.; Dulnoan, D.; Dolan, A.L.; Voong, K.; Ahmad, I.; Gorska, R.; Harrington, D.J.; Hampson, G. Serum vitamin K 1 (phylloquinone) is associated with fracture risk and hip strength in post-menopausal osteoporosis: A cross-sectional study. *Bone* **2020**, *141*, 115630. [CrossRef]
62. Sim, M.; Lewis, J.R.; Prince, R.L.; Levinger, I.; Brennan-Speranza, T.C.; Palmer, C.; Bondonno, C.P.; Bondonno, N.P.; Devine, A.; Ward, N.C.; et al. The effects of vitamin K-rich green leafy vegetables on bone metabolism: A 4-week randomised controlled trial in middle-aged and older individuals. *Bone Rep.* **2020**, *12*, 100274. [CrossRef]
63. Hooshmand, S.; Kern, M.; Metti, D.; Shamloufard, P.; Chai, S.C.; Johnson, S.A.; Payton, M.E.; Arjmandi, B.H. The effect of two doses of dried plum on bone density and bone biomarkers in osteopenic postmenopausal women: A randomized, controlled trial. *Osteoporos Int.* **2016**, *27*, 2271–2279. [CrossRef]
64. Higgs, J.; Derbyshire, E.; Styles, K. Nutrition and osteoporosis prevention for the orthopaedic surgeon: A wholefoods approach. *EFORT Open Rev.* **2017**, *2*, 300–308. [CrossRef]
65. Emaus, N.; Gjesdal, C.G.; Almås, B.; Christensen, M.; Grimsgaard, A.; Berntsen, G.; Salomonsen, L.; Fønnebø, V. Vitamin K2 supplementation does not influence bone loss in early menopausal women: A randomised double-blind placebo-controlled trial. *Osteoporos Int.* **2010**, *21*, 1731–1740. [CrossRef] [PubMed]
66. Feskanich, D.; Weber, P.; Willett, W.C.; Rockett, H.; Booth, S.L.; Colditz, G.A. Vitamin K intake and hip fractuRes. in women: A prospective study. *Am. J. Clin. Nutr.* **1999**, *69*, 74–79. [CrossRef]
67. Popa, D.-S.; Rusu, M.E. Isoflavones: Vegetable Sources, Biological Activity, and Analytical Methods for Their Assessment. In *Superfood and Functional Food—The Development of Superfoods and Their Roles as Medicine*; Shiomi, N., Waisundara, V., Eds.; InTech: London, UK, 2017; ISBN 978-953-51-2942-4. [CrossRef]
68. Lappe, J.; Kunz, I.; Bendik, I.; Prudence, K.; Weber, P.; Recker, R.; Heaney, R.P. Effect of a combination of genistein, polyunsaturated fatty acids and vitamins D3 and K1 on bone mineral density in postmenopausal women: A randomized, placebo-controlled, double-blind pilot study. *Eur. J. Nutr.* **2013**, *52*, 203–215. [CrossRef]
69. Capozzi, A.; Scambia, G.; Lello, S. Calcium, vitamin D, vitamin K2, and magnesium supplementation and skeletal health. *Maturitas* **2020**, *140*, 55–63. [CrossRef]
70. Goddek, S. Vitamin D3 and K2 and their potential contribution to reducing the COVID-19 mortality rate. *Int. J. Infect. Dis.* **2020**, *99*, 286–290. [CrossRef] [PubMed]
71. Schröder, M.; Riksen, E.A.; He, J.; Skallerud, B.H.; Møller, M.E.; Lian, A.; Syversen, U.; Reseland, J.E. Vitamin K2 Modulates Vitamin D-Induced Mechanical Properties of Human 3D Bone Spheroids In Vitro. *JBMR Plus* **2020**, *4*, e10394. [CrossRef]
72. Braam, L.; Knapen, M.; Geusens, P.; Brouns, F.; Hamulyák, K.; Gerichhausen, M.; Vermeer, C. Vitamin K1 Supplementation Retards Bone Loss in Postmenopausal Women Between 50 and 60 Years of Age. *Calcif. Tissue Int.* **2003**, *73*, 21–26. [CrossRef] [PubMed]
73. Inoue, T.; Fujita, T.; Kishimoto, H.; Makino, T.; Nakamura, T.; Nakamura, T.; Sato, T.; Yamazaki, K. Randomized controlled study on the prevention of osteoporotic fractuRes. (OF study): A phase IV clinical study of 15-mg menatetrenone capsules. *J. Bone Min. Metab.* **2009**, *27*, 66–75. [CrossRef]
74. Cockayne, S.; Adamson, J.; Lanham-New, S.; Shearer, M.J.; Gilbody, S.; Torgerson, D.J. Vitamin K and the Prevention of Fractures. *Arch Int. Med.* **2006**, *166*, 1256–1261. [CrossRef] [PubMed]
75. Yamaguchi, M.; Weitzmann, M.N. Vitamin K2 stimulates osteoblastogenesis and suppresses osteoclastogenesis by suppressing NF-κB activation. *Int. J. Mol. Med.* **2011**, *27*, 3–14. [CrossRef]
76. Falcone, T.D.; Kim, S.S.W.; Cortazzo, M.H. Vitamin K: Fracture Prevention and Beyond. *PM&R* **2011**, *3*, S82–S87. [CrossRef]
77. Liang, J.; Lian, S.; Qian, X.; Wang, N.; Huang, H.; Yao, J.; Tang, K.; Chen, L.; Li, L.; Lin, W.; et al. Association Between Bone Mineral Density and Pancreatic β-Cell Function in Elderly Men and Postmenopausal Women. *J. Endocr. Soc.* **2017**, *1*, 1085–1094. [CrossRef] [PubMed]
78. Azuma, K.; Inoue, S. Multiple Modes of Vitamin K Actions in Aging-Related Musculoskeletal Disorders. *Int. J. Mol. Sci.* **2019**, *20*, 2844. [CrossRef] [PubMed]
79. Shea, M.K.; Kritchevsky, S.B.; Hsu, F.-C.; Nevitt, M.; Booth, S.L.; Kwoh, C.K.; McAlindon, T.E.; Vermeer, C.; Drummen, N.; Harris, T.B.; et al. The association between vitamin K status and knee osteoarthritis featuRes. in older adults: The Health, Aging and Body Composition Study. *Osteoarth. Cart.* **2015**, *23*, 370–378. [CrossRef] [PubMed]
80. Chin, K.-Y. The Relationship between Vitamin K and Osteoarthritis: A Review of Current Evidence. *Nutrients* **2020**, *12*, 1208. [CrossRef]
81. Mozos, I.; Stoian, D.; Luca, C.T. Crosstalk between Vitamins A, B12, D, K, C, and E Status and Arterial Stiffness. *Dis. Markers.* **2017**, *2017*, 8784971. [CrossRef]

82. Jaminon, A.M.G.; Dai, L.; Qureshi, A.R.; Evenepoel, P.; Ripsweden, J.; Söderberg, M.; Witasp, A.; Olauson, H.; Schurgers, L.J.; Stenvinkel, P. Matrix Gla protein is an independent predictor of both intimal and me*Dial*. vascular calcification in chronic kidney disease. *Sci. Rep.* **2020**, *10*, 6586. [CrossRef] [PubMed]
83. Shioi, A.; Morioka, T.; Shoji, T.; Emoto, M. The Inhibitory Roles of Vitamin K in Progression of Vascular Calcification. *Nutrients* **2020**, *12*, 583. [CrossRef] [PubMed]
84. Dai, L.; Schurgers, L.J.; Shiels, P.G.; Stenvinkel, P. Early vascular ageing in chronic kidney disease: Impact of inflammation, vitamin K, senescence and genomic damage. *Nephrol. Dial. Transplant.* **2020**, *35*, ii31–ii37. [CrossRef]
85. Simes, D.C.; Viegas, C.S.B.; Araújo, N.; Marreiros, C. Vitamin K as a Powerful Micronutrient in Aging and Age-Related Diseases: Pros and Cons from Clinical Studies. *Int. J. Mol. Sci.* **2019**, *20*, 4150. [CrossRef] [PubMed]
86. Cozzolino, M.; Fusaro, M.; Ciceri, P.; Gasperoni, L.; Cianciolo, G. The Role of Vitamin K in Vascular Calcification. *Adv. Chronic Kidney Dis.* **2019**, *26*, 437–444. [CrossRef] [PubMed]
87. Dofferhoff, A.S.M.; Piscaer, I.; Schurgers, L.J.; Visser, M.P.J.; van den Ouweland, J.; de Jong, P.; Gosens, R.; Hackeng, T.; van Daal, H.; Lux, P.; et al. Reduced vitamin K status as a potentially modifiable risk factor of severe COVID-19. *Clin. Infect. Dis.* **2020**, ciaa1258. [CrossRef] [PubMed]
88. Roumeliotis, S.; Dounousi, E.; Salmas, M.; Eleftheriadis, T.; Liakopoulos, V. Vascular Calcification in Chronic Kidney Disease: The Role of Vitamin K- Dependent Matrix Gla Protein. *Front. Med.* **2020**, *7*, 154. [CrossRef]
89. Shea, M.K.; Booth, S.L. Vitamin K, Vascular Calcification, and Chronic Kidney Disease: Current Evidence and Unanswered Questions. *Curr. Dev. Nutr.* **2019**, *3*, nzz077. [CrossRef]
90. Geleijnse, J.M.; Vermeer, C.; Grobbee, D.E.; Schurgers, L.J.; Knapen, M.H.J.; van der Meer, I.M.; Hofman, A.; Witteman, J.C.M. Dietary Intake of Menaquinone Is Associated with a Reduced Risk of Coronary Heart Disease: The Rotterd. *Am. Study J. Nutr.* **2004**, *134*, 3100–3105. [CrossRef] [PubMed]
91. Gast, G.C.M.; De Roos, N.M.; Sluijs, I.; Bots, M.L.; Beulens, J.W.J.; Geleijnse, J.M.; Witteman, J.C.; Grobbee, D.E.; Peeters, P.H.M.; Van Der Schouw, Y.T. A high menaquinone intake reduces the incidence of coronary heart disease. *Nutr. Metab. Cardiovasc. Dis.* **2009**, *19*, 504–510. [CrossRef]
92. Shea, M.K.; O'Donnell, C.J.; Hoffmann, U.; Dallal, G.E.; Dawson-Hughes, B.; Ordovas, J.; Price, P.A.; Williamson, M.K.; Booth, S.L. Vitamin K supplementation and progression of coronary artery calcium in older men and women. *Am. J. Clin. Nutr.* **2009**, *89*, 1799–1807. [CrossRef]
93. Schurgers, L.J.; Barreto, D.V.; Barreto, F.C.; Liabeuf, S.; Renard, C.; Magdeleyns, E.; Vermeer, C.; Choukroun, G.; Massy, Z. The circulating inactive form of matrix gla protein is a surrogate marker for vascular calcification in chronic kidney disease: A preliminary report. *Clin. J. Am. Soc. Nephrol.* **2010**, *5*, 568–575. [CrossRef]
94. Ueland, T.; Gullestad, L.; Dahl, C.P.; Aukrust, P.; Aakhus, S.; Solberg, O.G.; Vermeer, C.; Schurgers, L.J. Undercarboxylated matrix Gla protein is associated with indices of heart failure and mortality in symptomatic aortic stenosis. *J. Int. Med.* **2010**, *268*, 483–492. [CrossRef] [PubMed]
95. Schlieper, G.; Westenfeld, R.; Krüger, T.; Cranenburg, E.C.; Magdeleyns, E.J.; Brandenburg, V.M.; Djuric, Z.; Damjanovic, T.; Ketteler, M.; Vermeer, C.; et al. Circulating Nonphosphorylated Carboxylated Matrix Gla Protein Predicts Survival in ESRD. *J. Am. Soc. Nephrol.* **2011**, *22*, 387–395. [CrossRef] [PubMed]
96. Ueland, T.; Dahl, P.; Gullestad, L.; Aakhus, S.; Broch, K.; Skårdal, R.; Vermeer, C.; Aukrust, P.; Schurgers, L. Circulating levels of non-phosphorylated undercarboxylated matrix Gla protein are associated with disease severity in patients with chronic heart failure. *Clin. Sci. (Lond.)* **2011**, *121*, 119–127. [CrossRef]
97. Westenfeld, R.; Krueger, T.; Schlieper, G.; Cranenburg, E.C.M.; Magdeleyns, E.J.; Heidenreich, S.; Holzmann, S.; Vermeer, C.; Jahnen-Dechent, W.; Ketteler, M.; et al. Effect of vitamin K2 supplementation on functional vitamin K deficiency in hemodialysis patients: A randomized trial. *Am. J. Kidney Dis.* **2012**, *59*, 186–195. [CrossRef] [PubMed]
98. Dalmeijer, G.W.; van der Schouw, Y.T.; Magdeleyns, E.; Ahmed, N.; Vermeer, C.; Beulens, J.W.J. The effect of menaquinone-7 supplementation on circulating species of matrix Gla protein. *Atherosclerosis* **2012**, *225*, 397–402. [CrossRef]
99. Van Den Heuvel, E.G.H.M.; Van Schoor, N.M.; Lips, P.; Magdeleyns, E.J.P.; Deeg, D.J.H.; Vermeer, C.; Den Heijer, M. Circulating uncarboxylated matrix Gla protein, a marker of vitamin K status, as a risk factor of cardiovascular disease. *Maturitas* **2014**, *77*, 137–141. [CrossRef]
100. Caluwé, R.; Vandecasteele, S.; Van Vlem, B.; Vermeer, C.; De Vriese, A.S. Vitamin K2 supplementation in haemodialysis patients: A randomized dose-finding study. *Nephrol. Dial. Transplant.* **2014**, *29*, 1385–1390. [CrossRef] [PubMed]
101. Liabeuf, S.; Bourron, O.; Vemeer, C.; Theuwissen, E.; Magdeleyns, E.; Aubert, C.E.; Brazier, M.; Mentaverri, R.; Hartemann, A.; Massy, Z.A. Vascular calcification in patients with type 2 diabetes: The involvement of matrix Gla protein. *Cardiovasc. Diabetol.* **2014**, *13*, 85. [CrossRef]
102. Cheung, C.-L.; Sahni, S.; Cheung, B.M.Y.; Sing, C.-W.; Wong, I.C.K. Vitamin K intake and mortality in people with chronic kidney disease from NHANES III. *Clin. Nutr.* **2015**, *34*, 235–240. [CrossRef]
103. Knapen, M.H.J.; Braam, L.A.J.L.M.; Drummen, N.E.; Bekers, O.; Hoeks, A.P.G.; Vermeer, C. Menaquinone-7 supplementation improves arterial stiffness in healthy postmenopausal women. A double-blind randomised clinical trial. *Thromb.Haemost.* **2015**, *113*, 1135–1144. [CrossRef]

104. Kurnatowska, I.; Grzelak, P.; Masajtis-Zagajewska, A.; Kaczmarska, M.; Stefańczyk, L.; Vermeer, C.; Maresz, K.; Nowicki, M. Effect of vitamin K2 on progression of atherosclerosis and vascular calcification in nondialyzed patients with chronic kidney disease stages 3-5. *Pol. Arch. Med. Wewn.* **2015**, *125*, 631–640. [CrossRef]
105. Asemi, Z.; Raygan, F.; Bahmani, F.; Rezavandi, Z.; Talari, H.R.; Rafiee, M.; Poladchang, S.; Mofrad, M.D.; Taheri, S.; Mohammadi, A.A.; et al. The effects of vitamin D, K and calcium co-supplementation on carotid intima-media thickness and metabolic status in overweight type 2 diabetic patients with CHD. *Br. J. Nutr.* **2016**, *116*, 286–293. [CrossRef]
106. Fulton, R.L.; McMurdo, M.E.T.; Hill, A.; Abboud, R.J.; Arnold, G.P.; Struthers, A.D.; Khan, F.; Vermeer, C.; Knappen, M.H.J.; Drummen, N.E.A.; et al. Effect of Vitamin K on Vascular Health and Physical Function in Older People with Vascular DiseaseA Randomised Controlled Trial. *J. Nutr. Heal Aging* **2016**, *20*, 325–333. [CrossRef]
107. Kurnatowska, I.; Grzelak, P.; Masajtis-Zagajewska, A.; Kaczmarska, M.; Stefańczyk, L.; Vermeer, C.; Maresz, K.; Nowicki, M. Plasma Desphospho-Uncarboxylated Matrix Gla Protein as a Marker of Kidney Damage and Cardiovascular Risk in Advanced Stage of Chronic Kidney Disease. *Kidney Blood Press Res.* **2016**, *41*, 231–239. [CrossRef] [PubMed]
108. Sardana, M.; Vasim, I.; Varakantam, S.; Kewan, U.; Tariq, A.; Koppula, M.R.; Syed, A.A.; Beraun, M.; Drummen, N.E.A.; Vermeer, C.; et al. Inactive Matrix Gla-Protein and Arterial Stiffness in Type 2 Diabetes Mellitus. *Am. J. Hypertens.* **2016**, *30*, 196–201. [CrossRef]
109. Aoun, M.; Makki, M.; Azar, H.; Matta, H.; Chelala, D.N. High Dephosphorylated-Uncarboxylated MGP in Hemodialysis patients: Risk factors and response to vitamin K2, A pre-post intervention clinical trial. *BMC Nephrol.* **2017**, *18*, 191. [CrossRef]
110. Brandenburg, V.; Reinartz, S.; Kaesler, N.; Krüger, T.; Dirrichs, T.; Kramann, R.; Peeters, F.; Floege, J.; Keszei, A.; Marx, N.; et al. Slower Progress of Aortic Valve Calcification With Vitamin K Supplementation: Results From a Prospective Interventional Proof-of-Concept Study. *Circulation* **2017**, *135*, 2081–2084. [CrossRef]
111. Shea, M.K.; Booth, S.L.; Weiner, D.E.; Brinkley, T.E.; Kanaya, A.M.; Murphy, R.A.; Simonsick, E.M.; Wassel, C.L.; Vermeer, C.; Kritchevsky, S.B. Circulating Vitamin K Is Inversely Associated with Incident Cardiovascular Disease Risk among Those Treated for Hypertension in the Health, Aging, and Body Composition Study (Health ABC). *J. Nutr.* **2017**, *147*, 888–895. [CrossRef] [PubMed]
112. Puzantian, H.; Akers, S.R.; Oldland, G.; Javaid, K.; Miller, R.; Ge, Y.; Ansari, B.; Lee, J.; Suri, A.; Hasmath, Z.; et al. Circulating Dephospho-Uncarboxylated Matrix Gla-Protein Is Associated With Kidney Dysfunction and Arterial Stiffness. *Am. J. Hypertens.* **2018**, *31*, 988–994. [CrossRef] [PubMed]
113. Dal Canto, E.; Beulens, J.W.J.; Elders, P.; Rutters, F.; Stehouwer, C.D.A.; Van Der Heijden, A.A.; Van Ballegooijen, A.J. The Association of Vitamin D and Vitamin K Status with Subclinical MeasuRes. of Cardiovascular Health and All-Cause Mortality in Older Adults: The Hoorn Study. *J. Nutr.* **2020**, *150*, 3171–3179. [CrossRef]
114. Roumeliotis, S.; Roumeliotis, A.; Stamou, A.; Leivaditis, K.; Kantartzi, K.; Panagoutsos, S.; Liakopoulos, V. The Association of dp-ucMGP with Cardiovascular Morbidity and Decreased Renal Function in Diabetic Chronic Kidney Disease. *Int. J. Mol. Sci.* **2020**, *21*, 6035. [CrossRef]
115. Shea, M.K.; Barger, K.; Booth, S.L.; Matuszek, G.; Cushman, M.; Benjamin, E.J.; Kritchevsky, S.B.; Weiner, D.E. Vitamin K status, cardiovascular disease, and all-cause mortality: A participant-level meta-analysis of 3 US cohorts. *Am. J. Clin. Nutr.* **2020**, *111*, 1170–1177. [CrossRef]
116. Wessinger, C.; Hafer-Macko, C.; Ryan, A.S. Vitamin K Intake in Chronic Stroke: Implications for Dietary Recommendations. *Nutrients* **2020**, *12*, 3059. [CrossRef] [PubMed]
117. Haugsgjerd, T.R.; Egeland, G.M.; Nygård, O.K.; Vinknes, K.J.; Sulo, G.; Lysne, V.; Igland, J.; Tell, G.S. Association of dietary vitamin K and risk of coronary heart disease in middle-age adults: The Hordaland Health Study Cohort. *BMJ Open* **2020**, *10*, e035953. [CrossRef] [PubMed]
118. Caluwé, R.; Verbeke, F.; De Vriese, A.S. Evaluation of vitamin K status and rationale for vitamin K supplementation in dialysis patients. *Nephrol. Dial. Transplant.* **2020**, *35*, 23–33. [CrossRef]
119. Liu, Y.-P.; Gu, Y.-M.; Thijs, L.; Knapen, M.H.J.; Salvi, E.; Citterio, L.; Petit, T.; Carpini, S.D.; Zhang, Z.; Jacobs, L.; et al. Inactive Matrix Gla Protein Is Causally Related to Adverse Health Outcomes: A Mendelian Randomization Study in a Flemish Population. *Hypertension* **2015**, *65*, 463–470. [CrossRef] [PubMed]
120. Fusaro, M.; D'Alessandro, C.; Noale, M.; Tripepi, G.; Plebani, M.; Veronese, N.; Iervasi, G.; Giannini, S.; Rossini, M.; Tarroni, G.; et al. Low vitamin K1 intake in haemodialysis patients. *Clin. Nutr.* **2017**, *36*, 601–607. [CrossRef]
121. Riphagen, I.J.; Keyzer, C.A.; Drummen, N.E.A.; de Borst, M.H.; Beulens, J.W.J.; Gansevoort, R.T.; Geleijnse, J.M.; Muskiet, F.A.J.; Navis, G.; Visser, S.T.; et al. Prevalence and Effects of Functional Vitamin K Insufficiency: The PREVEND Study. *Nutrients* **2017**, *9*, 1334. [CrossRef] [PubMed]
122. Zhang, S.; Guo, L.; Bu, C. Vitamin K status and cardiovascular events or mortality: A meta-analysis. *Eur. J. Prev. Cardiol.* **2019**, *26*, 549–553. [CrossRef] [PubMed]
123. Chen, H.; Sheng, L.; Zhang, Y.; Cao, A.; Lai, Y.; Kunutsor, S.; Jiang, L.; Pan, A. Association of vitamin K with cardiovascular events and all-cause mortality: A systematic review and meta-analysis. *Eur. J. Nutr.* **2019**, *58*, 2195–2205. [CrossRef]
124. Al-Suhaimi, E.; Al-Jafary, M. Endocrine roles of vitamin K-dependent- osteocalcin in the relation between bone metabolism and metabolic disorders. *Rev. Endocr. Metab. Disord.* **2020**, *21*, 117–125. [CrossRef]

125. Lacombe, J.; Al Rifai, O.; Loter, L.; Moran, T.; Turcotte, A.; Grenier-Larouche, T.; Tchernof, A.; Biertho, L.; Carpentier, A.; Prud'homme, D.; et al. Measurement of bioactive osteocalcin in humans using a novel immunoassay reveals association with glucose metabolism and β-cell function. *Am. J. Physiol Endocrinol. Metab.* **2020**, *318*, E381–E391. [CrossRef] [PubMed]
126. Ho, H.-J.; Komai, M.; Shirakawa, H. Beneficial Effects of Vitamin K Status on Glycemic Regulation and Diabetes Mellitus: A Mini-Review. *Nutrients* **2020**, *12*, 2485. [CrossRef]
127. Rusu, M.E.; Mocan, A.; Ferreira, I.C.F.R.; Popa, D.-S. Health Benefits of Nut Consumption in Middle-Aged and Elderly Population. *Antioxidants* **2019**, *8*, 302. [CrossRef] [PubMed]
128. Salas-Salvadó, J.; Becerra-Tomás, N.; Papandreou, C.; Bulló, M. Dietary Patterns Emphasizing the Consumption of Plant Foods in the Management of Type 2 Diabetes: A Narrative Review. *Adv. Nutr.* **2019**, *10*, S320–S331. [CrossRef] [PubMed]
129. Im, J.-A.; Yu, B.-P.; Jeon, J.Y.; Kim, S.-H. Relationship between osteocalcin and glucose metabolism in postmenopausal women. *Clin. Chim Acta* **2008**, *396*, 66–69. [CrossRef] [PubMed]
130. Yoshida, M.; Booth, S.L.; Meigs, J.B.; Saltzman, E.; Jacques, P.F. Phylloquinone intake, insulin sensitivity, and glycemic status in men and women. *Am. J. Clin. Nutr.* **2008**, *88*, 210–215. [CrossRef]
131. Kanazawa, I.; Yamaguchi, T.; Yamamoto, M.; Yamauchi, M.; Kurioka, S.; Yano, S.; Sugimoto, T. Serum Osteocalcin Level Is Associated with Glucose Metabolism and Atherosclerosis Parameters in Type 2 Diabetes Mellitus. *J. Clin. Endocrinol. Metab.* **2009**, *94*, 45–49. [CrossRef] [PubMed]
132. Kindblom, J.; Ohlsson, C.; Ljunggren, O.; Karlsson, M.; Tivesten, A.; Smith, U.; Mellström, D. Plasma osteocalcin is inversely related to fat mass and plasma glucose in elderly Swedish men. *J. Bone Min. Res.* **2009**, *24*, 785–791. [CrossRef]
133. Shea, M.K.; Gundberg, C.M.; Meigs, J.B.; Dallal, G.E.; Saltzman, E.; Yoshida, M.; Jacques, P.F.; Booth, S.L. Gamma-carboxylation of osteocalcin and insulin resistance in older men and women. *Am. J. Clin. Nutr.* **2009**, *90*, 1230–1235. [CrossRef]
134. Bao, Y.; Zhou, M.; Lu, Z.; Li, H.; Wang, Y.; Sun, L.; Gao, M.; Wei, M.; Jia, W. Serum levels of osteocalcin are inversely associated with the metabolic syndrome and the severity of coronary artery disease in Chinese men. *Clin. Endocrinol. (Oxf.)* **2011**, *75*, 196–201. [CrossRef] [PubMed]
135. Alfadda, A.A.; Masood, A.; Shaik, S.A.; Dekhil, H.; Goran, M. Association between Osteocalcin, Metabolic Syndrome, and Cardiovascular Risk Factors: Role of Total and Undercarboxylated Osteocalcin in Patients with Type 2 Diabetes Assim. *Int. J. Endocrinol.* **2013**, *2013*, 197519. [CrossRef]
136. Confavreux, C.B.; Szulc, P.; Casey, R.; Varennes, A.; Goudable, J.; Chapurlat, R.D. Lower serum osteocalcin is associated with more severe metabolic syndrome in elderly men from the MINOS cohort. *Eur. J. Endocrinol.* **2014**, *171*, 275–283. [CrossRef] [PubMed]
137. Shea, M.K.; Dawson-Hughes, B.; Gundberg, C.M.; Booth, S.L. Reducing Undercarboxylated Osteocalcin With Vitamin K Supplementation Does Not Promote Lean Tissue Loss or Fat Gain Over 3 Years in Older Women and Men: A Randomized Controlled Trial. *J. Bone Min. Res.* **2017**, *32*, 243–249. [CrossRef]
138. Knapen, M.H.J.; Jardon, K.M.; Vermeer, C. Vitamin K-induced effects on body fat and weight: Results from a 3-year vitamin K2 intervention study. *Eur. J. Clin. Nutr.* **2018**, *72*, 136–141. [CrossRef] [PubMed]
139. Dumitru, N.; Carsote, M.; Cocolos, A.; Petrova, E.; Olaru, M.; Dumitrache, C.; Ghemigian, A. The Link Between Bone Osteocalcin and Energy Metabolism in a Group of Postmenopausal Women. *Curr. Heal Sci. J.* **2019**, *45*, 47–51. [CrossRef]
140. Guney, G.; Sener-Simsek, B.; Tokmak, A.; Yucel, A.; Buyukkagnici, U.; Yilmaz, N.; Engin-Ustun, Y.; Ozgu-Erdinc, A.S. Assessment of the Relationship between Serum Vitamin D and Osteocalcin Levels with Metabolic Syndrome in Non-Osteoporotic Postmenopausal Women. *Geburtshilfe Frauenheilkd.* **2019**, *79*, 293–299. [CrossRef] [PubMed]
141. Aguayo-Ruiz, J.I.; García-Cobián, T.A.; Pascoe-González, S.; Sánchez-Enríquez, S.; Llamas-Covarrubias, I.M.; García-Iglesias, T.; López-Quintero, A.; Llamas-Covarrubias, M.A.; Trujillo-Quiroz, J.; Rivera-Leon, E.A. Effect of supplementation with vitamins D3 and K2 on undercarboxylated osteocalcin and insulin serum levels in patients with type 2 diabetes mellitus: A randomized, double-blind, clinical trial. *Diabetol. Metab. Syndr.* **2020**, *12*, 73. [CrossRef]
142. Jeannin, A.-C.; Salem, J.-E.; Massy, Z.; Aubert, C.E.; Vermeer, C.; Amouyal, C.; Phan, F.; Halbron, M.; Funck-Brentano, C.; Hartemann, A.; et al. Inactive matrix gla protein plasma levels are associated with peripheral neuropathy in Type 2 diabetes. *PLoS ONE* **2020**, *15*, e0229145. [CrossRef]
143. Sakak, F.; Moslehi, N.; Niroomand, M.; Mirmiran, P. Glycemic control improvement in individuals with type 2 diabetes with vitamin K 2 supplementation: A randomized controlled trial. *Eur. J. Nutr.* **2020**. [CrossRef]
144. Bigman, G. Vitamin D metabolites, D3 and D2, and their independent associations with depression symptoms among adults in the United States. *Nutr. Neurosci.* **2020**, 1–9. [CrossRef]
145. Shahdadian, F.; Mohammadi, H.; Rouhani, M.H. Effect of Vitamin K Supplementation on Glycemic Control: A Systematic Review and Meta-Analysis of Clinical Trials. *Horm. Metab. Res.* **2018**, *50*, 227–235. [CrossRef]
146. Rasekhi, H.; Karandish, M.; Jalali, M.T.; Mohammad-Shahi, M.; Zarei, M.; Saki, A.; Shahbazian, H. The effect of vitamin K1 supplementation on sensitivity and insulin resistance via osteocalcin in prediabetic women: A double-blind randomized controlled clinical trial. *Eur. J. Clin. Nutr.* **2015**, *69*, 891–895. [CrossRef]
147. Manna, P.; Kalita, J. Beneficial role of vitamin K supplementation on insulin sensitivity, glucose metabolism, and the reduced risk of type 2 diabetes: A review. *Nutrition* **2016**, *32*, 732–739. [CrossRef] [PubMed]
148. Li, Y.; Chen, J.; Duan, L.; Li, S. Effect of Vitamin K2 on Type 2 Diabetes Mellitus: A Review. *Diabetes Res. Clin. Pr.* **2018**, *136*, 39–51. [CrossRef] [PubMed]

149. Karamzad, N.; Faraji, E.; Adeli, S.; Carson-Chahhoud, K.; Azizi, S.; Gargari, P.B. Effects of MK-7 Supplementation on Glycemic Status, Anthropometric Indices and Lipid Profile in Patients with Type 2 Diabetes: A Randomized Controlled Trial. *Diabetes Metab. Syndr. Obes.* **2020**, *13*, 2239–2249. [CrossRef] [PubMed]
150. Tarkesh, F.; Jahromi, N.B.; Hejazi, N.; Tabatabaee, H. Beneficial health effects of Menaquinone-7 on body composition, glycemic indices, lipid profile, and endocrine markers in polycystic ovary syndrome patients. *Food Sci. Nutr.* **2020**, *8*, 5612–5621. [CrossRef]
151. Yoshida, M.; Jacques, P.; Meigs, J.; Saltzman, E.; Shea, M.; Gundberg, C.; Dawson-Hughes, B.; Dallal, G.; Booth, S. Effect of vitamin K supplementation on insulin resistance in older men and women. *Diabetes Care* **2008**, *31*, 2092–2096. [CrossRef] [PubMed]
152. Karamzad, N.; Maleki, V.; Carson-Chahhoud, K.; Azizi, S.; Sahebkar, A.; Gargari, B.P. A systematic review on the mechanisms of vitamin K effects on the complications of diabetes and pre-diabetes. *Biofactors* **2020**, *46*, 21–37. [CrossRef]
153. Dihingia, A.; Ozah, D.; Baruah, P.; Kalita, J.; Manna, P. Prophylactic role of vitamin K supplementation on vascular inflammation in type 2 diabetes by regulating the NF-κB/Nrf2 pathway via activating Gla proteins. *Food Funct.* **2018**, *9*, 450–462. [CrossRef]
154. Mera, P.; Ferron, M.; Mosialou, I. Regulation of Energy Metabolism by Bone-Derived Hormones. *Cold Spring Harb Perspect Med.* **2018**, *8*, a031666. [CrossRef]
155. O'Connor, E.M.; Durack, E. Osteocalcin: The extra-skeletal role of a vitamin K-dependent protein in glucose metabolism. *J. Nutr. Intermed Metab.* **2017**, *7*, 8–13. [CrossRef]
156. Gundberg, C.M.; Lian, J.B.; Booth, S.L. Vitamin K-Dependent Carboxylation of Osteocalcin: Friend or Foe? *Adv. Nutr.* **2012**, *3*, 149–157. [CrossRef] [PubMed]
157. Beulens, J.; van der, A.D.; Grobbee, D.; Sluijs, I.; Spijkerman, A.; van der Schouw, Y. Dietary Phylloquinone and Menaquinones Intakes and Risk of Type 2 Diabetes. *Diabetes Care* **2010**, *33*, 1699–1705. [CrossRef]
158. Booth, S.; Centi, A.; Smith, S.; Gundberg, C. The role of osteocalcin in human glucose metabolism: Marker or mediator? *Nat. Rev. Endocrinol.* **2013**, *9*, 43–55. [CrossRef]
159. Parra, M.A.; Butler, S.; McGeown, W.J.; Brown Nicholls, L.A.; Robertson, D.J. Globalising strategies to meet global challenges: The case of ageing and dementia. *J. Glob Heal* **2019**, *9*, 020310. [CrossRef] [PubMed]
160. Rusu, M.E.; Georgiu, C.; Pop, A.; Mocan, A.; Kiss, B.; Vostinaru, O.; Fizesan, I.; Stefan, M.-G.; Gheldiu, A.-M.; Mates, L.; et al. Antioxidant Effects of Walnut (Juglans regia L.) Kernel and Walnut Septum Extract in a D-Galactose-Induced Aging Model and in Naturally Aged Rats. *Antioxidants* **2020**, *9*, 424. [CrossRef]
161. Chauhan, A.; Chauhan, V. Beneficial Effects of Walnuts on Cognition and Brain Health. *Nutrients* **2020**, *12*, 550. [CrossRef]
162. Carrillo, J.Á.; Arcusa, R.; Zafrilla, M.P.; Marhuenda, J. Effects of Fruit and Vegetable-Based Nutraceutical on Cognitive Function in a Healthy Population: Placebo-Controlled, Double-Blind, and Randomized Clinical Trial. *Antioxidants* **2021**, *10*, 116. [CrossRef]
163. Opie, R.; Itsiopoulos, C.; Parletta, N.; Sanchez-Villegas, A.; Akbaraly, T.; Ruusunen, A.; Jacka, F. Dietary recommendations for the prevention of depression. *Nutr. Neurosci.* **2017**, *20*, 161–171. [CrossRef]
164. Fernández-Sanz, P.; Ruiz-Gabarre, D.; García-Escudero, V. Modulating Effect of Diet on Alzheimer's Disease. *Diseases* **2019**, *7*, 12. [CrossRef] [PubMed]
165. Fenech, M. Vitamins Associated with Brain Aging, Mild Cognitive Impairment, and Alzheimer Disease: Biomarkers, Epidemiological and Experimental Evidence, Plausible Mechanisms, and Knowledge Gaps. *Adv. Nutr.* **2017**, *8*, 958–970. [CrossRef]
166. Vasefi, M.; Hudson, M.; Ghaboolian-Zare, E. Diet Associated with Inflammation and Alzheimer's Disease. *J. Alzheimers Dis. Rep.* **2019**, *3*, 299–309. [CrossRef] [PubMed]
167. Tamadon-Nejad, S.; Ouliass, B.; Rochford, J.; Ferland, G. Vitamin K Deficiency Induced by Warfarin Is Associated With Cognitive and Behavioral Perturbations, and Alterations in Brain Sphingolipids in Rats. *Front. Aging Neurosci.* **2018**, *10*, 213. [CrossRef]
168. Rusu, M.E.; Fizesan, I.; Pop, A.; Mocan, A.; Gheldiu, A.-M.; Babota, M.; Vodnar, D.C.; Jurj, A.; Berindan-Neagoe, I.; Vlase, L.; et al. Walnut (Juglans regia L.) Septum: Assessment of Bioactive Molecules and In Vitro Biological Effects. *Molecules* **2020**, *25*, 2187. [CrossRef]
169. Mohajeri, M.; Troesch, B.; Weber, P. Inadequate supply of vitamins and DHA in the elderly: Implications for brain aging and Alzheimer-type dementia. *Nutrition* **2015**, *31*, 261–275. [CrossRef]
170. Grimm, M.O.W.; Mett, J.; Hartmann, T. The Impact of Vitamin E and Other Fat-Soluble Vitamins on Alzheimer's Disease. *Int. J. Mol. Sci.* **2016**, *17*, 1785. [CrossRef] [PubMed]
171. Machado-Fragua, M.; Hoogendijk, E.; Struijk, E.; Rodriguez-Artalejo, F.; Lopez-Garcia, E.; Beulens, J.; van Ballegooijen, A. High dephospho-uncarboxylated matrix Gla protein concentrations, a plasma biomarker of vitamin K, in relation to frailty: The Longitudinal Aging Study Amsterdam. *Eur. J. Nutr.* **2020**, *59*, 1243–1251. [CrossRef]
172. Presse, N.; Shatenstein, B.; Kergoat, M.; Ferland, G. Low Vitamin K Intakes in Community-Dwelling Elders at an Early Stage of Alzheimer's Disease. *J. Am. Diet. Assoc.* **2008**, *108*, 2095–2099. [CrossRef] [PubMed]
173. Alisi, L.; Cao, R.; De Angelis, C.; Cafolla, A.; Caramia, F.; Cartocci, G.; Librando, A.; Fiorelli, M. The Relationships Between Vitamin K and Cognition: A Review of Current Evidence. *Front. Neurol.* **2019**, *10*, 239. [CrossRef]
174. McCann, A.; Jeffery, I.B.; Ouliass, B.; Ferland, G.; Fu, X.; Booth, S.L.; Tran, T.T.; O'Toole, P.; O'Connor, E. Exploratory analysis of covariation of microbiota-derived vitamin K and cognition in older adults. *Am. J. Clin. Nutr.* **2019**, *110*, 1404–1415. [CrossRef]
175. Thane, C.W.; Bates, C.J.; Shearer, M.J.; Unadkat, N.; Harrington, D.J.; Paul, A.A.; Prentice, A.; Bolton-Smith, C. Plasma phylloquinone (vitamin K1) concentration and its relationship to intake in a national sample of British elderly people. *Br. J. Nutr.* **2002**, *87*, 615–622. [CrossRef]

176. Tanprasertsuk, J.; Ferland, G.; Johnson, M.A.; Poon, L.W.; Scott, T.M.; Barbey, K.; Barger, K.; Wang, X.-D.; Johnson, E.J. Concentrations of Circulating Phylloquinone, but Not Cerebral Menaquinone-4, Are Positively Correlated with a Wide Range of Cognitive Measures: Exploratory Findings in Centenarians. *J. Nutr.* **2020**, *150*, 82–90. [CrossRef]
177. Presse, N.; Belleville, S.; Gaudreau, P.; Greenwood, C.E.; Kergoat, M.-J.; Morais, J.A.; Payette, H.; Shatenstein, B.; Ferland, G. Vitamin K status and cognitive function in healthy older adults. *Neurobiol. Aging* **2013**, *34*, 2777–2783. [CrossRef]
178. Morris, M.C.; Wang, Y.; Barnes, L.L.; Bennett, D.A.; Dawson-Hughes, B.; Booth, S.L. Nutrients and bioactives in green leafy vegetables and cognitive decline. *Neurology* **2018**, *90*, e214–e222. [CrossRef] [PubMed]
179. Chouet, J.; Ferland, G.; Féart, C.; Rolland, Y.; Presse, N.; Boucher, K.; Barberger-Gateau, P.; Beauchet, O.; Annweiler, C. Dietary Vitamin K Intake Is Associated with Cognition and Behaviour among Geriatric Patients: The CLIP Study. *Nutrients* **2015**, *7*, 6739–6750. [CrossRef] [PubMed]
180. Lasemi, R.; Kundi, M.; Moghadam, N.B.; Moshammer, H.; Hainfellner, J.A. Vitamin K2 in multiple sclerosis patients. *Wien Klin Wochenschr.* **2018**, *130*, 307–313. [CrossRef]
181. Sanchez, J.M.S.; DePaula-Silva, A.B.; Libbey, J.E.; Fujinami, R.S. Role of diet in regulating the gut microbiota and multiple sclerosis. *Clin. Immunol.* **2020**, 108379. [CrossRef] [PubMed]
182. Yu, Y.-X.; Yu, X.-D.; Cheng, Q.-Z.; Tang, L.; Shen, M.-Q. The association of serum vitamin K2 levels with Parkinson's disease: From basic case-control study to big data mining analysis. *Aging (Albany NY)* **2020**, *12*, 16410–16419. [CrossRef]
183. Soutif-Veillon, A.; Ferland, G.; Rolland, Y.; Presse, N.; Boucher, K.; Féart, C.; Annweiler, C. Increased dietary vitamin K intake is associated with less severe subjective memory complaint among older adults. *Maturitas* **2016**, *93*, 131–136. [CrossRef]
184. Annweiler, C.; Denis, S.; Duval, G.; Ferland, G.; Bartha, R.; Beauchet, O. Use of Vitamin K Antagonists and Brain Volumetry in Older Adults: Preliminary Results From the GAIT Study. *J. Am. Geriatr. Soc.* **2015**, *63*, 2199–2202. [CrossRef]
185. Brangier, A.; Ferland, G.; Rolland, Y.; Gautier, J.; Féart, C.; Annweiler, C. Vitamin K Antagonists and Cognitive Decline in Older Adults: A 24-Month Follow-Up. *Nutrients* **2018**, *10*, 666. [CrossRef] [PubMed]
186. Lin, X.; Onda, D.-A.; Yang, C.-H.; Lewis, J.R.; Levinger, I.; Loh, K. Roles of bone-derived hormones in type 2 diabetes and cardiovascular pathophysiology. *Mol. Metab.* **2020**, *40*, 101040. [CrossRef]
187. Oury, F.; Khrimian, L.; Denny, C.A.; Gardin, A.; Chamouni, A.; Goeden, N.; Huang, Y.; Lee, H.; Srinivas, P.; Gao, X.-B.; et al. Maternal and Offspring Pools of Osteocalcin Influence Brain Development and Functions. *Cell* **2013**, *155*, 228–241. [CrossRef]
188. Battafarano, G.; Rossi, M.; Marampon, F.; Minisola, S.; Del Fattore, A. Bone Control of Muscle Function. *Int. J. Mol. Sci.* **2020**, *21*, 1178. [CrossRef]
189. Bhatti, G.K.; Reddy, A.P.; Reddy, P.H.; Bhatti, J. Lifestyle Modifications and Nutritional Interventions in Aging-Associated Cognitive Decline and Alzheimer's Disease. *Front. Aging Neurosci.* **2020**, *11*, 369. [CrossRef]
190. Sinyor, B.; Mineo, J.; Ochner, C. Alzheimer's Disease, Inflammation, and the Role of Antioxidants. *J. Alzheimers Dis. Rep.* **2020**, *4*, 175–183. [CrossRef]
191. Wagenaar, L.J. Vitamin K2 and Macular Degeneration. European Patent Application. EP 3 106 158 A1. Bulletin 2016; 51. Available online: https://patentimages.storage.googleapis.com/4d/f9/ab/0d84c163c6b0d4/EP3106158A1.pdf (accessed on 2 April 2021).
192. Nimptsch, K.; Rohrmann, S.; Linseisen, J. Dietary intake of vitamin K and risk of prostate cancer in the Heidelberg cohort of the European Prospective Investigation into Cancer and Nutrition (EPIC-Heidelberg). *Am. J. Clin. Nutr.* **2008**, *87*, 985–992. [CrossRef] [PubMed]
193. Chen, G.; Wang, F.; Trachootham, D.; Huang, P. Preferential killing of cancer cells with mitochondrial dysfunction by natural compounds. *Mitochondrion* **2010**, *10*, 614–625. [CrossRef]
194. Ivanova, D.; Zhelev, Z.; Getsov, P.; Nikolova, B.; Aoki, I.; Higashi, T.; Bakalova, R. Vitamin K: Redox-modulation, prevention of mitochondrial dysfunction and anticancer effect. *Redox Biol.* **2018**, *16*, 352–358. [CrossRef]
195. Dasari, S.; Ali, S.M.; Zheng, G.; Chen, A.; Dontaraju, S.; Bosland, M.C.; Kajdacsy-Balla, A.; Munirathinam, G. Vitamin K and its analogs: Potential avenues for prostate cancer management. *Oncotarget* **2017**, *8*, 57782–57799. [CrossRef] [PubMed]
196. Dahlberg, S.; Ede, J.; Schött, U. Vitamin K and cancer. *Scand. J. Clin. Lab. Invest.* **2017**, *77*, 555–567. [CrossRef] [PubMed]
197. Wellington, K.; Hlatshwayo, V.; Kolesnikova, N.; Saha, S.; Kaur, M.; Motadi, L. Anticancer activities of vitamin K3 analogues. *Invest. N. Drugs* **2020**, *38*, 378–391. [CrossRef]
198. Fizeșan, I.; Rusu, M.E.; Georgiu, C.; Pop, A.; Ștefan, M.-G.; Muntean, D.M.; Mirel, S.; Vostinaru, O.; Kiss, B.; Popa, D.-S. Antitussive, Antioxidant, and Anti-Inflammatory Effects of a Walnut (*Juglans regia* L.) Septum Extract Rich in Bioactive Compounds. *Antioxidants* **2021**, *10*, 119. [CrossRef]
199. Vita, M.F.; Nagachar, N.; Avramidis, D.; Delwar, Z.M.; Cruz, M.; Siden, A.; Paulsson, K.; Yakisich, J.S. Pankiller effect of prolonged exposure to menadione on glioma cells: Potentiation by vitamin C. *Invest. N. Drugs* **2011**, *29*, 1314–1320. [CrossRef]
200. He, T.; Hatem, E.; Vernis, L.; Lei, M.; Huang, M.-E. PRX1 knockdown potentiates vitamin K3 toxicity in cancer cells: A potential new therapeutic perspective for an old drug. *J. Exp Clin. Cancer Res.* **2015**, *34*, 152. [CrossRef] [PubMed]
201. Miyazawa, S.; Moriya, S.; Kokuba, H.; Hino, H.; Takano, N.; Miyazawa, K. Vitamin K 2 induces non-apoptotic cell death along with autophagosome formation in breast cancer cell lines. *Breast Cancer.* **2020**, *27*, 225–235. [CrossRef]
202. Dasari, S.; Samy, A.; Kajdacsy-Balla, A.; Bosland, M.; Munirathinam, G. Vitamin K2, a menaquinone present in dairy products targets castration-resistant prostate cancer cell-line by activating apoptosis signaling. *Food Chem. Toxicol.* **2018**, *115*, 218–227. [CrossRef]

203. Samykutty, A.; Shetty, A.V.; Dakshinamoorthy, G.; Kalyanasundaram, R.; Zheng, G.; Chen, A.; Bosland, M.C.; Kajdacsy-Balla, A.; Gnanasekar, M. Vitamin K2, a naturally occurring menaquinone, exerts therapeutic effects on both hormone-dependent and hormone-independent prostate cancer cells. *Evid. Based Complement. Altern. Med.* **2013**, *2013*, 287358. [CrossRef]
204. Xv, F.; Chen, J.; Duan, L.; Li, S. Research progress on the anticancer effects of vitamin K2 (Review). *Oncol. Lett.* **2018**, *15*, 8926–8934. [CrossRef] [PubMed]
205. Glick, D.; Barth, S.; Macleod, K.F. Autophagy: Cellular and molecular mechanisms. *J. Pathol.* **2010**, *221*, 3–12. [CrossRef]
206. Yokoyama, T.; Miyazawa, K.; Naito, M.; Toyotake, J.; Tauchi, T.; Itoh, M.; Yuo, A.; Hayashi, Y.; Georgescu, M.-M.; Kondo, Y.; et al. Vitamin K2 induces autophagy and apoptosis simultaneously in leukemia cells. *Autophagy* **2008**, *4*, 629–640. [CrossRef]
207. Enomoto, M.; Tsuchida, A.; Miyazawa, K.; Yokoyama, T.; Kawakita, H.; Tokita, H.; Naito, M.; Itoh, M.; Ohyashiki, K.; Aoki, T. Vitamin K2-induced cell growth inhibition via autophagy formation in cholangiocellular carcinoma cell lines. *Int. J. Mol. Med.* **2007**, *20*, 801–808. [CrossRef]
208. Tokita, H.; Tsuchida, A.; Miyazawa, K.; Ohyashiki, K.; Katayanagi, S.; Sudo, H.; Enomoto, M.; Takagi, Y.; Aoki, T. Vitamin K2-induced antitumor effects via cell-cycle arrest and apoptosis in gastric cancer cell lines. *Int. J. Mol. Med.* **2006**, *17*, 235–243. [CrossRef] [PubMed]
209. Otsuka, M.; Kato, N.; Shao, R.-X.; Hoshida, Y.; Ijichi, H.; Koike, Y.; Taniguchi, H.; Moriyama, M.; Shiratori, Y.; Kawabe, T.; et al. Vitamin K2 Inhibits the Growth and Invasiveness of Hepatocellular Carcinoma Cells via Protein Kinase a Activation. *Hepatology* **2004**, *40*, 243–251. [CrossRef] [PubMed]
210. Jinghe, X.; Mizuta, T.; Ozaki, I. Vitamin K and hepatocellular carcinoma: The basic and clinic. *World J. Clin. Cases.* **2015**, *3*, 757–764. [CrossRef] [PubMed]
211. Yoshiji, H.; Noguchi, R.; Toyohara, M.; Ikenaka, Y.; Kitade, M.; Kaji, K.; Yamazaki, M.; Yamao, J.; Mitoro, A.; Sawai, M.; et al. Combination of vitamin K2 and angiotensin-converting enzyme inhibitor ameliorates cumulative recurrence of hepatocellular carcinoma. *J. Hepatol.* **2009**, *51*, 315–321. [CrossRef] [PubMed]
212. Duan, F.; Yu, Y.; Guan, R.; Xu, Z.; Liang, H.; Hong, L. Vitamin K2 Induces Mitochondria-Related Apoptosis in Human Bladder Cancer Cells via ROS and JNK/p38 MAPK Signal Pathways. *PLoS ONE* **2016**, *11*, e0161886. [CrossRef]
213. Duan, F.; Mei, C.; Yang, L.; Zheng, J.; Lu, H.; Xia, Y.; Hsu, S.; Liang, H.; Hong, L. Vitamin K2 promotes PI3K/AKT/HIF-1α-mediated glycolysis that leads to AMPK-dependent autophagic cell death in bladder cancer cells. *Sci. Rep.* **2020**, *10*, 7714. [CrossRef]
214. Muñoz-Esparza, N.C.; Latorre-Moratalla, M.L.; Comas-Basté, O.; Toro-Funes, N.; Veciana-Nogués, M.T.; Vidal-Carou, M.C. Polyamines in Food. *Front. Nutr.* **2019**, *6*, 108. [CrossRef]
215. Minois, N.; Carmona-Gutierrez, D.; Madeo, F. Polyamines in aging and disease. *Aging (Albany NY)* **2011**, *3*, 716–732. [CrossRef] [PubMed]
216. Orlando, A.; Linsalata, M.; Tutino, V.; D'Attoma, B.; Notarnicola, M.; Russo, F. Vitamin K1 Exerts Antiproliferative Effects and Induces Apoptosis in Three Differently Graded Human Colon Cancer Cell Lines. *Biomed. Res. Int.* **2015**, *2015*, 296721. [CrossRef]
217. Russo, I.; Caroppo, F.; Alaibac, M. Vitamins and Melanoma. *Cancers* **2015**, *7*, 1371–1387. [CrossRef]
218. Beaudin, S.; Kokabee, L.; Welsh, J. Divergent effects of vitamins K1 and K2 on triple negative breast cancer cells. *Oncotarget* **2019**, *10*, 2292–2305. [CrossRef]
219. Wang, K.; Wu, Q.; Li, Z.; Reger, M.K.; Xiong, Y.; Zhong, G.; Li, Q.; Zhang, X.; Li, H.; Foukakis, T.; et al. Vitamin K intake and breast cancer incidence and death: Results from a prospective cohort study. *Clin. Nutr.* **2020**. [CrossRef]
220. Lo, J.; Park, Y.; Sinha, R.; Sandler, D. Association between meat consumption and risk of breast cancer: Findings from the Sister Study. *Int. J. Cancer.* **2019**, *146*, 2156–2165. [CrossRef]
221. Sant, M.; Allemani, C.; Sieri, S.; Krogh, V.; Menard, S.; Tagliabue, E.; Nardini, E.; Micheli, A.; Crosignani, P.; Muti, P.; et al. Salad vegetables dietary pattern protects against HER-2-positive breast cancer: A prospective Italian study. *Int. J. Cancer.* **2007**, *121*, 911–914. [CrossRef]
222. George, S.; Ballard-Barbash, R.; Shikany, J.; Caan, B.; Freudenheim, J.; Kroenke, C.; Vitolins, M.; Beresford, S.; Neuhouser, M. Better postdiagnosis diet quality is associated with reduced risk of death among postmenopausal women with invasive breast cancer in the Women's Health Initiative. *Cancer Epidemiol. Biomarkers Prev.* **2014**, *23*, 575–583. [CrossRef]
223. Nimptsch, K.; Rohrmann, S.; Kaaks, R.; Linseisen, J. Dietary vitamin K intake in relation to cancer incidence and mortality: Results from the Heidelberg cohort of the European Prospective Investigation into Cancer and Nutrition (EPIC-Heidelberg). *Am. J. Clin. Nutr.* **2010**, *91*, 1348–1358. [CrossRef]
224. Matsubara, K.; Kayashima, T.; Mori, M.; Yoshida, H.; Mizushina, Y. Inhibitory effects of vitamin K3 on DNA polymerase and angiogenesis. *Int. J. Mol. Med.* **2008**, *22*, 381–387. [CrossRef]
225. Juanola-Falgarona, M.; Salas-Salvadó, J.; Martínez-González, M.; Corella, D.; Estruch, R.; Ros, E.; Fitó, M.; Arós, F.; Gómez-Gracia, E.; Fiol, M.; et al. Dietary Intake of Vitamin K Is Inversely Associated with Mortality Risk. *J. Nutr.* **2014**, *144*, 743–750. [CrossRef] [PubMed]
226. Shen, T.; Bimali, M.; Faramawi, M.; Orloff, M.S. Consumption of Vitamin K and Vitamin A Are Associated With Reduced Risk of Developing Emphysema: NHANES 2007–2016. *Front. Nutr.* **2020**, *7*, 47. [CrossRef] [PubMed]
227. ten Kate, M.; van der Meer, J. Protein S deficiency: A clinical perspective. *Haemophilia* **2008**, *14*, 1222–1228. [CrossRef]
228. Zagórska, A.; Través, P.; Lew, E.; Dransfield, I.; Lemke, G. Diversification of TAM receptor function. *Nat. Immunol.* **2014**, *15*, 920–928. [CrossRef]

229. Tutusaus, A.; Marí, M.; Ortiz-Pérez, J.; Nicolaes, G.; Morales, A.; de Frutos, P. Role of Vitamin K-Dependent Factors Protein S and GAS6 and TAM. Receptors in SARS-CoV-2 Infection and COVID-19-Associated Immunothrombosis. *Cells* **2020**, *9*, 2186. [CrossRef]
230. Baicus, C.; Stoichitoiu, L.E.; Pinte, L.; Badea, C. Anticoagulant Protein S in COVID-19: The Low Activity Level Is Probably Secondary. *Am. J. Ther.* **2021**, *28*, e139–e140. [CrossRef] [PubMed]
231. Janssen, R.; Visser, M.P.J.; Dofferhoff, A.S.M.; Vermeer, C.; Janssens, W.; Walk, J. Vitamin K metabolism as the potential missing link between lung damage and thromboembolism in Coronavirus disease 2019. *Br. J. Nutr.* **2020**, 1–8. [CrossRef]

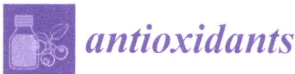 antioxidants

Review

Ginkgo biloba in the Aging Process: A Narrative Review

Sandra Maria Barbalho [1,2,3,*], Rosa Direito [4], Lucas Fornari Laurindo [2], Ledyane Taynara Marton [2], Elen Landgraf Guiguer [1,2,3], Ricardo de Alvares Goulart [1], Ricardo José Tofano [1,2], Antonely C. A. Carvalho [1], Uri Adrian Prync Flato [1,2], Viviane Alessandra Capelluppi Tofano [2], Cláudia Rucco Penteado Detregiachi [1], Patrícia C. Santos Bueno [1,5], Raul S. J. Girio [5] and Adriano Cressoni Araújo [1,2]

[1] Postgraduate Program in Structural and Functional Interactions in Rehabilitation, University of Marília (UNIMAR), Marília 17525-902, SP, Brazil; eleng@unimar.br (E.L.G.); rgoulart@unimar.br (R.d.A.G.); ricardo.tofano@unimar.br (R.J.T.); antonely.prefeito@ibaiti.pr.gov.br (A.C.A.C.); uriflato@unimar.br (U.A.P.F.); claudia.detregiachi@unimar.br (C.R.P.D.); patriciabueno@unimar.br (P.C.S.B.); araujo.01@unimar.br (A.C.A.)

[2] Department of Biochemistry and Pharmacology, School of Medicine, University of Marília (UNIMAR), Avenida Higino Muzzi Filho, 1001, Marília 17525-902, SP, Brazil; 1851730@unimar.br (L.F.L.); 1813975@unimar.br (L.T.M.); viviane.tofano@unimar.br (V.A.C.T.)

[3] School of Food and Technology of Marília (FATEC), Avenida Castro Alves, Marília 17500-000, SP, Brazil

[4] Laboratory of Systems Integration Pharmacology, Clinical & Regulatory Science, Research Institute for Medicines (iMed.ULisboa), Faculdade de Farmácia, Universidade de Lisboa, Av. Prof. Gama Pinto, 1649-003 Lisbon, Portugal; rdireito@ff.ulisboa.pt

[5] Department of Animal Sciences, School of Veterinary Medicine, University of Marília (UNIMAR), Avenida Higino Muzzi Filho 1001, Marília 17525-902, SP, Brazil; rgirio@unimar.br

* Correspondence: smbarbalho@gmail.com or sandra.barbalho@unimar.br; Tel.: +55-14-99655-3190

Abstract: Neurodegenerative diseases, cardiovascular disease (CVD), hypertension, insulin resistance, cancer, and other degenerative processes commonly appear with aging. *Ginkgo biloba* (GB) is associated with several health benefits, including memory and cognitive improvement, in Alzheimer's disease (AD), Parkinson's disease (PD), and cancer. Its antiapoptotic, antioxidant, and anti-inflammatory actions have effects on cognition and other conditions associated with aging-related processes, such as insulin resistance, hypertension, and cardiovascular conditions. The aim of this study was to perform a narrative review of the effects of GB in some age-related conditions, such as neurodegenerative diseases, CVD, and cancer. PubMed, Cochrane, and Embase databases were searched, and the PRISMA guidelines were applied. Fourteen clinical trials were selected; the studies showed that GB can improve memory, cognition, memory scores, psychopathology, and the quality of life of patients. Moreover, it can improve cerebral blood flow supply, executive function, attention/concentration, non-verbal memory, and mood, and decrease stress, fasting serum glucose, glycated hemoglobin, insulin levels, body mass index, waist circumference, biomarkers of oxidative stress, the stability and progression of atherosclerotic plaques, and inflammation. Therefore, it is possible to conclude that the use of GB can provide benefits in the prevention and treatment of aging-related conditions.

Keywords: *Ginkgo biloba*; aging; neurodegenerative diseases; Alzheimer's disease; metabolic syndrome; cardiovascular disease; cancer

1. Introduction

The medicine associated with basic sanitation and lifestyle modifications has benefited the world's population, and the repercussions are seen as an increase in longevity. On the other hand, the aging process is associated with physical and functional changes in different tissues and organs and is related to genetic factors, mutations, telomere loss, oxidative stress, mitochondrial dysfunction, inflammation, immune disorders, and other modifications that interfere with homeostasis. Neurodegenerative diseases, cardiovascular disease (CVD), hypertension, insulin resistance, cancer, osteoporosis, and other degenerative processes may commonly appear with aging, leading to a significant burden on health care systems [1–3].

Drug therapy can prevent age-related conditions or can be used in the therapeutic approach. However, the high cost of many medications, their side effects, and their response refractoriness in many patients makes other alternatives worth seeking. For these reasons, herbal medicine has been considered for maintaining health or as a therapeutic approach for aging people. Herbal therapies are relevant since they show few side effects, present cultural acceptability, and have reduced costs. These therapies can contribute to well-being and the prevention of several aging conditions and chronic illnesses. Among the medicinal plants that can improve age-related issues is *Gingko biloba* (GB) [4–6], a medicinal plant belonging to the *Ginkgoaceae* family in Ginkgoopsida that is considered to be the oldest tree alive in the world (*Ginkgo* species are from the Permian Period, around 286–248 million years ago). The gray-colored bark tree is native to China, Japan, and Korea; however, it is distributed in many regions of Europe, America, India, and New Zealand [7–9].

GB has been used for medicinal purposes for centuries. In traditional medicine, it is primarily used for respiratory and cardiovascular conditions; in Chinese medicine, it has been considered for treating pulmonary issues, bladder infections, and alcohol abuse. The therapeutic potential is attributed to its bioactive compounds that are mainly represented by terpenoids, flavonoids, polyphenols, and organic acids. The primary terpenoids are ginkgolides. GB standard extract contains 2.6 to 3.2% bilobalide, 2.8 to 3.4% ginkgolides (A, B, and C), and 24% flavone glycosides (quercetin, isorhamnetin, and kaempferol) [10–13]. Figure 1 summarizes the primary bioactive compounds of GB and its effects.

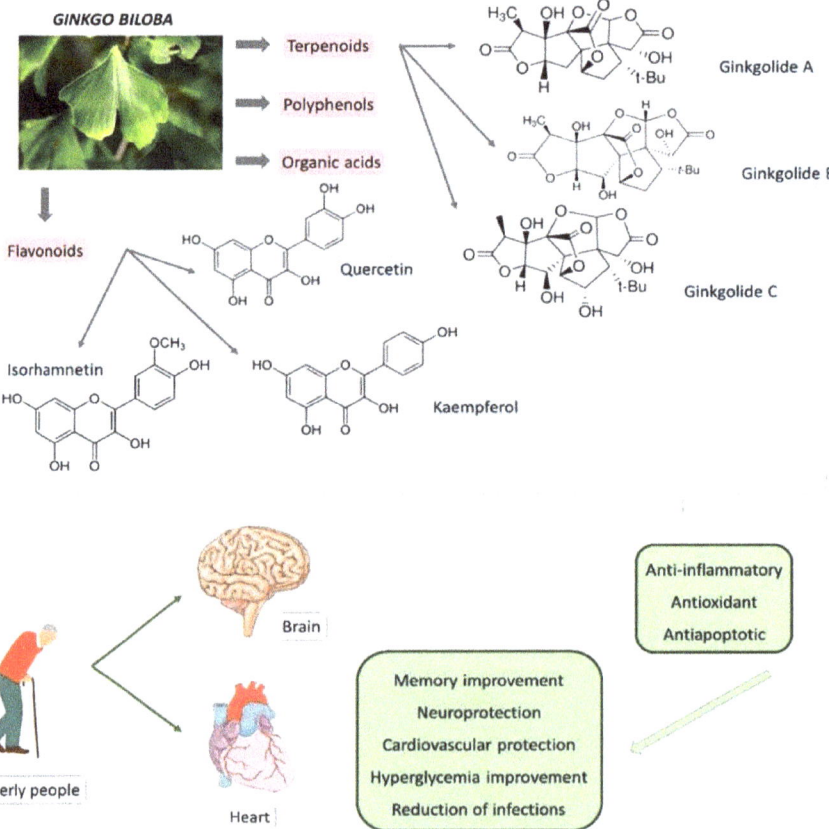

Figure 1. Primary bioactive compounds of *Ginkgo biloba* and its effects.

The leaves and the seeds of GB may represent one of the most common phytopharmaceutical products in the United States and Europe. GB is also commercialized as an extract (EGB 761®), producing several health benefits for memory, cognition, Alzheimer's disease (AD), Parkinson's disease (PD), and dementia. These pharmacological effects are attributed to the antiapoptotic, antioxidant, and anti-inflammatory actions that, in addition to having effects on cognition, also exert benefits in other conditions associated to aging-related processes, such as insulin resistance, hypertension, dyslipidemia, and cardiovascular disorders. In many European states, EGB 761® is the only drug therapy in the guideline for the treatment of mild cognitive impairment (MCI) [9,10,14–16].

Based on the above beneficial effects, this study aimed to perform a review on the effects of GB on some age-related conditions, such as neurodegenerative diseases, metabolic syndrome, and CVD.

2. Materials and Methods

2.1. Focused Question

The focal question of this review was: What are the effects of *Ginkgo biloba* on the aging process?

2.2. Language

Only studies in English were selected for this review.

2.3. Databases

The PubMed, Embase and Cochrane databases were searched. The descriptors used were *Ginkgo biloba* or *Ginkgo biloba* extract and neurodegenerative diseases, or memory, or Alzheimer's disease, or Parkinson's disease, or dementia, or hypertension, or insulin resistance, or metabolic syndrome, or cardiovascular diseases. These descriptors helped identify studies related to *Ginkgo biloba* and some aspects of the aging process. Although this is a narrative review, we followed the PRISMA (Preferred Reporting Items for a Systematic Review and Meta-Analysis) guidelines for improving the strategy of paper screening [17].

2.4. Study Selection

This review included studies that reported *Ginkgo biloba* or *Ginkgo biloba* extract to treat disorders associated with the aging process. The inclusion criteria comprised randomized clinical trials (RCTs), double-blind, and placebo-controlled studies that reported the use of GB in patients over the age of 45 years. We only included full texts. The PICO (population, intervention, comparison, and outcomes) format was followed to build this review.

The exclusion criteria were in vitro studies, studies with animals, clinical trials that associated different herb formulations, reviews, studies not in English, poster presentations, case reports, and editorials. Reviews were consulted to help in the discussion section but were not included in the systematization of the data.

2.5. Data Extraction

The search period for this review included the past ten years (January 2011 to May 2021). The selected studies are shown in Table 1.

2.6. Quality Assessment

The bias risk evaluation was performed by selecting the study, detection, and reporting bias of each clinical trial. Other risks of bias in the selection of patients, classification of interventions, evaluation of outcomes, and missing data were also considered. The Cochrane Handbook for Systematic Reviews of Interventions was used to perform the quality assessment [18].

Table 1. The effects of *Ginkgo biloba* on neurodegenerative diseases, diabetes, and metabolic syndrome.

Reference	Local	Model and Patients	Intervention	Outcomes	Adverse Effects (AEs)
		Neurodegenerative Diseases			
[19]	Germany	Randomized, double-blind, placebo-controlled, mono-center trial with 188 mentally healthy male and female subjects, 45–65 y, with higher secondary education.	Subjects received EGb 761 240 mg/day or placebo/6 w.	Subjects treated with EGb 761 significantly improved the number of appointments correctly recalled. The effects on qualitative recall performance (proportion of false to correct items) were similar. GB had no superiority in another routine memory test that required recognition of a driving route.	Seven AEs in the EGb 761 group (headache, n = 4; gastric complaints, n = 3) and five in the placebo group (gastric complaints, n = 3; conjunctivitis, nettle rash). No serious AEs occurred during the study.
[20]	Ukraine	Randomized, double-blind, placebo-controlled, multicenter trial with 410 outpatients (132 male and 272 female), 50 y or older with mild to moderate dementia (AD, vascular dementia, or mixed form) with scores between 9 and 23 on the SKT cognitive tests battery, at least 5 in the NPI and 3 or more in at least one item of the NPI.	Patients were allocated to receive 240 mg of EGb 761 or placebo once a day/24 w. Primary efficacy measures were the SKT, and the 12-item NPI.	EGb was found to be significantly superior to placebo in the treatment of patients with neuropsychiatric symptoms; significant improvement on the SKT and NPI total score (placebo showed deterioration on SKT).	AE rates were similar for both treatment groups (headache, respiratory tract infection, dizziness, angina pectoris, diarrhea, and tinnitus).
[21]	Republic of Belarus, Republic of Moldova, and Russian Federation	Multicenter, randomized, placebo-controlled study with 410 outpatients (279 female and 123 male) with mild to moderate dementia (AD or vascular dementia) related to neuropsychiatric symptoms. Participants scored 9–23 on the SKT cognitive battery and at least 6 on the NPI, with at least one of four items rated at minimum 4.	Patients were randomized to receive 240 mg of EGb 761 once a day/24 w.	Treatment with EGb 761 was safe and significantly improved functional measures, cognition, psychopathology, and quality of life of patients.	Lethal cardiac arrest due to chronic heart failure in a patient suffering from multiple illnesses; a lethal ischaemic infarction in the region of the terminal branches of the middle and posterior cerebral arteries in a patient with a history of DM, hypertension, atherosclerosis, myocardial infarction, and a previous stroke.
[22]	Iran	Randomized double-blind study with 56 patients (23 male and 28 female), 50–75 y, with a diagnosis of probable AD according to the DSM IV.	Patients were allocated into (1) GB (120 mg once a day) or (2) rivastigmine (4.5 mg once a day)/24 w. The SMT and the MMSE measured the severity of dementia.	There was a significant improvement of the MMSE scores in the rivastigmine group but not in the GB group. The same results were observed for the SMT.	AEs were not reported.

Table 1. *Cont.*

Reference	Local	Model and Patients	Intervention	Outcomes	Adverse Effects (AEs)
[23]	China	Randomized clinical trial with 80 patients with VCIND (60–75 y, 46 males and 34 females), disorder shown by revised mini-mental state examination.	Group 1 received 75 mg aspirin 3 times/d/3 m. Group 2 received 19.2 mg GBT 3 times/d/3 m with anti-platelet aggregation drugs. MoCA and TCD were used to observe changes in cognitive ability and cerebral blood flow in VCIND patients.	GBT can improve the therapeutic efficacy and enhance the cognitive ability and cerebral blood flow supply of patients with VCIND.	AEs were not reported.
[24]	EUA	Open-label phase II clinical trial with 34 patients (23 female and 11 male), symptomatic irradiated brain tumor survivors, life expectancy $\geq$ 30 w, partial or whole-brain radiation $\geq$ 6 m before enrollment, no imaging evidence of tumor progression in previous 3 m, or stable or decreasing steroid dose, and no brain tumor treatment planned while in the study.	The GB dose was 120 mg/day (40 mg t.i.d.) for 24 w, followed by a 6 w washout period.	There were significant improvements at 24 w in executive function, attention/concentration, and non-verbal memory and mood.	AEs included gastrointestinal toxicity and intracranial hemorrhage.
[25]	Russia	Double-blind randomized multicenter trial with 160 patients (124 female and 33 male, $\geq$55 y) with MCI who scored at least 6 on the 12-item NPI were enrolled.	Patients received 240 mg of EGb 761 daily or placebo/24 w. Effects on NPS were evaluated using the NPI, the state subscore of the State–Trait Anxiety Inventory and the Geriatric Depression Scale.	EGb 761 ameliorated NPS and cognitive performance in subjects with MCI. The drug was safe and well tolerated.	Headache, increased blood pressure, respiratory tract infection, and dyspepsia/epigastric discomfort.
[26]	China	Randomized clinical trial with 80 cerebral infarction patients (46 males and 34 females) 60–75 y.	Group 1 received aspirin 75 mg 3 times/d/3 m, and Group 2 received 40 m of GBT with aspirin 3 times/d/3 m.	GBT improved the therapeutic efficacy, cerebral blood flow supply, and cognitive ability of patients with VCIND.	AEs were not reported.

Table 1. Cont.

Reference	Local	Model and Patients	Intervention	Outcomes	Adverse Effects (AEs)
[27]	Germany	Randomized double-blind placebo-controlled trial with 75 volunteers (50–65 y) with subjective memory impairment evidenced by at least one answered item as "rather often" or "very often" or at least five questions answered "sometimes" in the Prospective and Retrospective Memory Questionnaire.	240 mg EGb 761® or placebo once a day in the morning as film coated tablet/56 ± 4 days.	Baseline fMRI data evidenced BOLD responses in regions commonly activated by the specific tasks. Task-switch costs reduced with EGb761®, suggesting improvement in cognitive flexibility. Go–NoGo task reaction times corrected for error rates showed a trend of improved response inhibition.	Headache.
[28]	Germany	Randomized, double-blind, placebo-controlled exploratory study with 50 patients (25 female and 25 males; 50–85 y) with MCI and associated dual task-related gait impairment.	Patients received GBE (Symfona® forte 120 mg) 2 times/d/6 m or placebo capsules. A 6 m open-label phase with identical GBE dosage followed. Gait was quantified at months 0, 3, 6, and 12.	After 6 m, dual task-related cadence increased in the intervention group compared to the control. GBE-associated numerical non-significant trends were found after 6 m for dual task-related gait velocity and stride time variability.	Seven SAEs in four patients in GB group and six SAEs in five patients of control group: nasal septum surgery, diverticula, suspected coronary heart disease, pancreatitis, symptomatic cholecystolithiasis, and transient ischemic attack.
			Gingko biloba and Diabetes Mellitus		
[29]	Lithuanian	Randomized double-blind placebo-controlled with 56 patients with T2DM (21 male and 35 females; 37–78 y) and followed up for diabetic retinopathy, nephropathy, or neuropathy.	Patients received standardized GB dry extract (80 mg) or placebo capsules. For the first 9 m, patients used one capsule 2 times/d, and for the second 9 m, one capsule 3 times/d.	The level of perceived stress was reduced significantly after 9 m and 18 m, and the psychological aspect of quality of life significantly improved after 18 m of GB use.	AEs were not reported.
[30]	Iraq	Randomized, placebo-controlled, double-blinded, multicenter trial with 60 T2DM patients, 25–65 y.	The patients currently using metformin were allocated to receive GB extract (120 mg/day) or placebo/3 m.	GBE significantly reduced HbA1c, glycemia and insulin levels, BMI, WC, and VAI. GB extract did not negatively impact the liver, kidneys, or hematopoietic functions.	No SAEs were observed.
			Gingko biloba and Metabolic Syndrome		
[31]	Bulgaria	Randomized preventive study with 11 patients (two male, nine female, 26–48 y) with MS, smokers, and Lp (a) concentration > 30 mg/dL.	The standard therapy was EGB 761 120 mg 2 times/d/2 m. No statins, no calcium antagonists, and no nitrate compounds were given.	There was a decrease in oxidative stress biomarkers, atherosclerotic plaque formation, plaque stability and progression, and inflammation.	No AEs occurred.

Table 1. Cont.

Reference	Local	Model and Patients	Intervention	Outcomes	Adverse Effects (AEs)
[32]	Bulgaria	Randomized preventive study with 11 patients (two male, nine female, 26–48 y) with MS, smokers, and Lp (a) concentration > 30 mg/dL.	The standard therapy was EGB 761 120 mg 2 times/d/2 m. No statins, no calcium antagonists, and no nitrate compounds were given.	Simultaneous decreases in hs-CRP and HOMA-IR, as well as a beneficial change in arteriosclerotic, inflammatory, and oxidative stress biomarkers, were observed. IL-6 and nano-plaque formation were additionally reduced.	No AEs occurred.

AD—Alzheimer's disease; BMI—body mass index; DSM IV—Diagnostic and Statistical Manual of Mental Disorders, 4th edition; GB—*Ginkgo biloba*; GBE—*Ginkgo* extract; EGb 761—extract of *Ginkgo biloba* leaves (drug extract ratio 35–67:1); GBT—*Ginkgo biloba* tablet; HbA1c—glycated hemoglobin; HOMA-IR—homeostasis model assessment of insulin resistance; hs-CRP—high-sensitivity C-reactive protein; IL-6—interleukin 6; Lp (a)—blood lipoprotein(a); MCI—mild cognitive impairment; MMSE—Mini-Mental State Examination; MoCA—Montreal Cognitive Assessment; NPI—Neuropsychiatric Inventory; NPS—neuropsychiatric symptoms; SAEs—serious adverse events; SKT—Short Cognitive Test; SMT—Seven Minute Test; TCD—transcranial Doppler; T2DM—type 2 diabetes mellitus; VAI—visceral adiposity index; VCIND—vascular cognitive impairment of none dementia; WC—waist circumference; d—day; w—week, y—year.

3. Results

Figure 2 represents the scheme of the search for studies. From the 14 articles selected, a total of 1681 participants were included: 188 mentally healthy, 410 with mild to moderate dementia, 410 with mild to moderate dementia and neuropsychiatric symptoms, 56 with AD, 80 with vascular cognitive impairment of none dementia, 34 symptomatic irradiated brain tumor survivors, 210 with mild cognitive impairment, 80 cerebral infarction patients, 75 with subjective memory impairment, 116 with type 2 diabetes mellitus, and 22 with metabolic syndrome. Nine hundred eleven participants were women and 472 were men. Two studies did not report the gender of the participants. The age range was over 25 years. No clinical trials that investigated the effects of GB on Parkinson's disease and cancer were found.

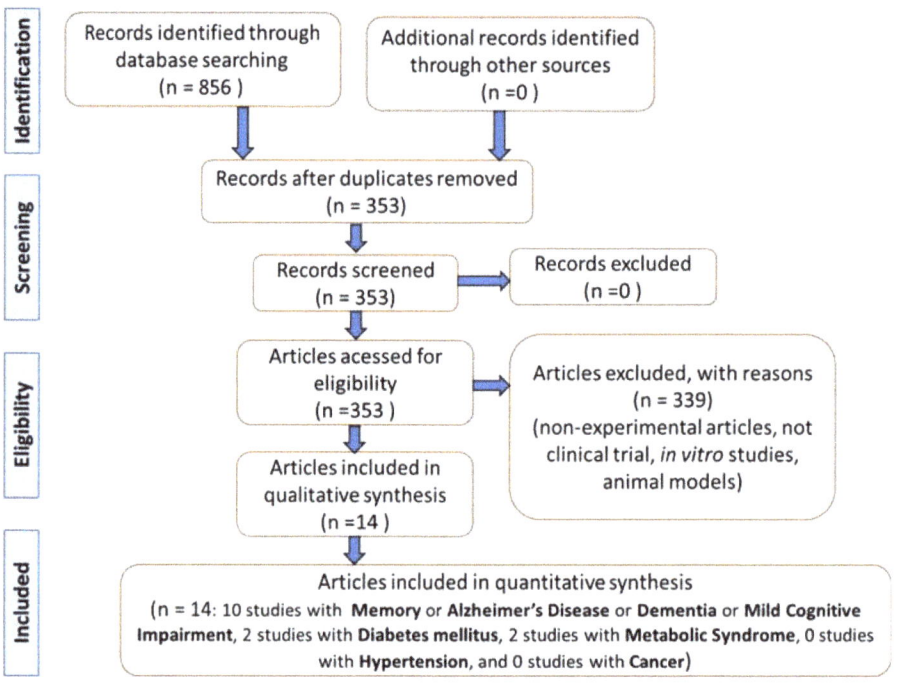

Figure 2. Flow diagram showing the study's selection criteria (based on PRISMA guidelines).

From the 14 articles (three from Germany (Kaschel et al., 2011 [19], Beck et al., 2016 [27], Gschwind et al., 2017 [28]); one from Ukraine (Ihl et al., 2011 [20]); one from the Republic of Belarus, Republic of Moldova, and Russian Federation (Herrschaft et al., 2012 [21]); one from Iran (Nasab, 2012 [22]; two from China (Zhang, 2012 [23], Wang, 2015 [26]); one from EUA (Attia et al., 2012 [24]); one from Russia (Gavrilova, 2015 [25]); one from Lithuania (Lasaite et al., 2015 [29]); one from Iraq [30]); and two from Bulgaria (Siegel et al., 2011 [31], Siegel et al., 2014 [32]), nine were randomized double-blind placebo-controlled clinical trials (Kaschel et al., 2011 [19], Beck et al., 2016 [27], Gschwind et al., 2017 [28], Ihl et al., 2011 [20], Herrschaft et al., 2012 [21], Nasab, 2012 [22], Gavrilova, 2015 [25], Lasaite et al., 2015 [29], Aziz et al., 2018 [30]); one was an open-label phase II clinical trial (Attia et al., 2012 [24]); and four were randomized placebo-controlled clinical trials (Zhang, 2012 [23], Wang, 2015 [26], Siegel et al., 2011 [31], Siegel et al., 2014 [32]).

Seven studies used GB 761 extract (Kaschel et al., 2011 [19], Beck et al., 2016 [27], Ihl et al., 2011 [20], Herrschaft et al., 2012 [21], Gavrilova, 2015 [25], Siegel et al., 2011 [31], Siegel et al., 2014 [32]), two used GB (Nasab, 2012 [22], Attia et al., 2012 [24]); two used

GB tablets (Zhang, 2012 [23], Wang, 2015 [26]); and three used GB extract (Gschwind et al., 2017 [28], Lasaite et al., 2015 [29], Aziz et al., 2018 [30]). The administered doses ranged from 40 mg per day to 240 mg per day, and the intervention period ranged from 6 weeks to 36 weeks. Two studies were associated with the use of aspirin (Zhang, 2012 [23], Wang, 2015 [26]) and one study was associated with the use of metformin (Aziz et al., 2018 [30]).

Studies have shown that the use of GB (in different formulations) can improve the memory, cognition, psychopathology, functional measures, and quality of life of patients, in addition to improving cerebral blood flow supply, executive function, attention/concentration, non-verbal memory, and mood and decreasing stress, HbA1c, fasting serum glucose and insulin levels, body mass index, waist circumference, visceral adipose index, biomarkers of oxidative stress, the stability and progression of atherosclerotic plaques, and inflammation. The main adverse effects reported were headache, respiratory tract infection, hypertension, and diarrhea (Table 1).

Table 2 shows the description of the bias in the included studies.

Table 2. Descriptive table showing the biases of the included randomized clinical trials.

Study	Question Focus	Appropriate Randomization	Allocation Blinding	Double-Blind	Losses (<20%)	Prognostics or Demographic Characteristics	Outcomes	Intention to Treat Analysis	Sample Calculation	Adequate Follow-Up
[19]	Yes	Yes	Yes	Yes	Yes	No	Yes	NR	Yes	Yes
[20]	Yes	Yes	Yes	Yes	Yes	Yes	Yes	Yes	Yes	Yes
[21]	Yes	Yes	Yes	Yes	Yes	Yes	Yes	Yes	Yes	Yes
[22]	Yes	NR	Yes	Yes	Yes	Yes	Yes	No	NR	Yes
[23]	Yes	NR	NR	No	NR	No	Yes	No	NR	Yes
[24]	Yes	NR	No	No	No	Yes	Yes	No	Yes	Yes
[25]	Yes	Yes	Yes	Yes	Yes	Yes	Yes	Yes	Yes	Yes
[26]	Yes	NR	NR	No	NR	No	Yes	No	NR	Yes
[27]	Yes	Yes	Yes	Yes	Yes	No	Yes	No	No	Yes
[28]	Yes	Yes	Yes	Yes	Yes	Yes	Yes	No	Yes	Yes

NR—not reported.

4. Discussion

The studies included in this review showed that GB generally and safely improved neuropsychiatric symptoms (SKT, NPI, and MMSE scores), cognition, mood, HbA1C, glycemia, waist circumference, BMI, atherosclerotic lesions formation, pro-inflammatory biomarkers (e.g., IL-6), and quality of life in healthy patients and subjects with mild cognitive impairment or vascular cognitive impairment.

4.1. Ginkgo biloba, Inflammation, and Oxidative Stress

Inflammation and oxidative stress are related to the aging process. As a result of the metabolism, several conditions, such as infections, stress, inflammation exposure, radiation, and smoke, produce reactive oxygen species (ROS). When the endogenous antioxidant system or the intake of exogenous antioxidants is insufficient, these molecules can lead to irreversible cell damage and are associated with various diseases, such as diabetes, obesity, hypertension, CVD, cataracts, neurodegenerative diseases, and cancer [33–36]. Several antioxidants can help to prevent the impact of the aging process. ROS are produced through endogenous and exogenous pathways and can be neutralized by enzymatic and non-enzymatic antioxidants. There are many defense systems, including glutathione peroxidase, catalase, thioredoxin, superoxide dismutase, coenzyme Q, cytochrome c oxidase (complex IV), vitamin E, ascorbic acid, and carotenes [37,38].

GB's bioactive compounds (Table 3) can act to minimize these conditions, mainly ginkgolide (diterpenoid) A, which is related to the suppression of the cyclo-oxygenase-2 (COX-2) and 5-lipo-oxygenase (5-LOX) enzymes. These molecules are responsible for the conversion of arachidonic acid to leukotrienes, diminishing the inflammatory process. They can reduce the production of malonaldehyde and increase the expression of glutathione (GSH) and superoxide dismutase (SOD). Furthermore, EGB 761® can reduce the effects of the lipopolysaccharide (LPS) and its action on transforming growth factor β (TGF-β), which results in the downregulation of interleukin-1 β (IL-1 β), IL-6, IL-8, and tumor necrosis factor alpha (TNF-α). On the other hand, ginkgolide B can inactivate platelet-activating factor, which plays a role in the inflammation of the pulmonary airways. In general, ginkgolides A, B, and C decrease ROS levels; the release of TNFα, IL-1β, and IL-6; and the expression of the gene c-fos and the gene c-jun mRNA. They may be related to the inhibition of platelet-activating factor and of the following signaling pathway: NF-kappa-B-inducing kinase (NIK), IκB kinase α (IKKα), nuclear factor kappa-B inhibitor (IκB), and nuclear factor kappa-B-inducing kinase. They are also associated with an increase in cellular proliferation; an increase in the activity of free radical scavengers; and the activation of extracellular signal-regulated kinases, mitogen-activated protein kinase (MAPK) pathways, and hypoxia-inducible factor 1-alpha (HIF-1α) [39–42].

Table 3. Bioactive compounds of *Gingko biloba* and their effects on aging-related conditions.

Bioactive Compound	Sources	Molecular Structure	Functions	References
Ginkgolide A (terpenoid)	Leaves, root, and bark.		- Anti-inflammatory (decreasing TNF-α, IL-1β, and NF-kB expression); - Antioxidant (reducing ROS and augmenting free radical capture by the cells); - Anxiolytic-like effects; - Neuroprotection (controlling neurodegeneration and inflammation); - Anti-atherosclerotic (prevention of OS to the endothelial cells/stimulation of NO); - Anti-thrombotic (inhibition of platelet aggregation by MMP-9 and controlling cAMP, inhibiting intracellular Ca^{2+} mobilization, and decreasing TXA2 activity); - Hepatoprotective (suppressing hepatocyte lipogenesis); - Antitumor (inhibition of cancer cell proliferation).	[12,42–44]
Ginkgolide B (terpenoid)	Leaves, root, and bark.		- Neuroprotective effects (protecting neurons from βA apoptotic events and in ischemia/reperfusion syndrome through the regulation of NF-kB pathways); - Anti-inflammatory (decreasing TNF-α, IL-1β, and NF-kB expressions); - Antioxidant (reducing ROS and augmenting free radical capture); - Protective effects of cardiomyocytes against ischemia/reperfusion syndrome; - Inhibition of cancer cell migration and invasion; - Induction of cancer cell apoptosis.	[12,43,45–51]

Table 3. Cont.

Bioactive Compound	Sources	Molecular Structure	Functions	References
Ginkgolide C (terpenoids)	Leaves, root, and bark.		- Anti-inflammatory (decrease in TNF-α, IL-1β, and NF-kB expression); - Antioxidant (reduces ROS and augments free radical capture); - Suppressor of adipogenesis via AMPK signaling pathways; - Hepatoprotective by protecting liver from lipid accumulation injuries; - Alleviation of ischemia/reperfusion syndrome in cardiomyocytes; - Antitumor effects (cancer cells apoptosis and inhibition of cancer cell growth).	[12,43,52–56]
Bilobalide (terpenoid)	Leaves and bark.		- Anti-inflammatory (decrease in TNF-α, IL-1β, and IL-6 levels); - Neuroprotective (reduction in neuroinflammation and protection against βA deposition in AD); - Hepatoprotective; - Antioxidant via multiple pathways; - Cardioprotective.	[12,43,57–59]
Ginkgolic acid (organic acid)	Leaves.		- Antibacterial and antiviral (suppression of gram-positive bacteria growth and fusion of enveloped viruses); - Antitumor effects (inhibiting invasion and migration of cancer cells).	[43,60–62]
Isorhamnetin (flavonoid)	Leaves.		- Anti-atherosclerosis and endothelium protective; - Neuroprotection (improvement of brain function and cognition); - Hypotensive effects; - Anti-ischemia and anti-fibrosis in myocardium; - Anti-inflammatory/antioxidant, - Antitumor effects (suppression of cancer growth and invasiveness).	[43,63–67]
Quercetin (flavonoid)	Leaves.		- Anti-inflammatory/antioxidant (decrease in lipid peroxidation and OS); - Increase in BDNF; - Reduces the degradation of serotonin by monoamine oxidases; - Antitumor (modulation of VEGF, P13K/Akt, apoptosis, mTOR, MAPK/ERK1-2, and Wnt/β-catenin signaling pathways); - Attenuation of atherosclerotic inflammation; - Cardioprotection (protection against OS/improvement of cardiomyocytes); - Antimicrobial.	[43,67–73]

Table 3. Cont.

Bioactive Compound	Sources	Molecular Structure	Functions	References
Kaempferol (flavonoid)	Leaves.		- Antitumor (inhibiting cancer cell proliferation and stimulating apoptosis); - Antioxidant (upregulation of GSH); - Anti-inflammatory (inhibiting NF-kB, COX-2, and iNOS expression); - Neuroprotection (suppression of oxidative and inflammatory damage to brain cells); - Protection against ischemia/reperfusion syndrome and myocardial injury; - Upregulation of BDNF; - Reduction of serotonin degradation.	[12,43,74–78]
Luteolin (flavonoid)	Leaves.		- Anti-inflammatory (suppressing TNF-α, IL-6, COX-2, and NF-kB expressions); - Antioxidant; - Antitumor (inhibiting cancer cell proliferation and stimulating cell cycle arrest and apoptosis); - Neuroprotective (limiting βA deposition, reducing neuroinflammation and brain OS); - Cardioprotective effects (stimulation of cardiomyocyte function through MAPKs); - Reduction of cardiomyocyte ischemic/reperfusion syndrome.	[43,79–81]

AD—Alzheimer's disease; AMPK—AMP (adenosine monophosphate)-activated protein kinase; βA—beta amyloid; BDNF—brain-derived neurotrophic factor; Ca—calcium; cAMP—cyclic adenosine monophosphate; COX-2—cyclooxygenase 2; GSH—glutathione; IL-1β—interleukin 1 beta; iNOS—nitric oxide synthase; IL-6—interleukin 6; MMP-9—matrix metallopeptidase 9; mTOR—mammalian target of rapamycin; MAPK/ERK1-2—mitogen activated protein kinase/extracellular signal-regulated kinase 1-2; NO—nitric oxide; NF-kB—nuclear factor kappa b; OS—oxidative stress; P13K/Akt—phosphatidyl inositol-3-kinase/protein-kinase b; ROS—reactive oxygen species; TXA2—thromboxane A2; VEGF—vascular endothelial growth factor.

Kaempferol is also present in GB, and its actions account for the upregulation in the expression of the glutamate-cysteine ligase catalytic subunit, brain-derived neurotrophic factor (BDNF), B-cell lymphoma protein 2 (BCL-2), and GSH; it also reduces serotonin breakdown by monoamine oxidase, the release of cytochrome C, the activity of caspase-3, the downregulation of NFkB, and apoptosis. Kaempferol is also related to the reduction of neurotoxicity induced by 3-nitropropionic acid and the increase in BCL-2-associated protein X through ROS [12,82,83].

Other relevant compounds found in GB are quercetin, bilobalide, and isorhamnetin [67], which also play an important role in inflammation and oxidative stress. Quercetin can promote the elevation of BDNF levels and reduce apoptosis, the transcription of TNFα, the degradation of serotonin by monoamine oxidases, phosphorylation, and the activation of c-Jun N-terminal kinase. Moreover, it can act as a free radical scavenger. Bilobalide has actions including the reduction of ROS induced through hydrogen peroxide. It is related to the upregulation of BCL-2 and the cytochrome c oxidase subunit III and increases the cellular proliferation of hippocampal neurons. Isorhamnetin is associated with the reduction of apoptosis and the fragmentation of DNA. Indeed, it also reduces the synthesis of pro-inflammatory cytokines and caspase-3. Some studies have shown that isorhamnetin has beneficial effects on the cardiovascular and cerebrovascular system and can have anti-inflammatory, antioxidant, and anti-tumor functions. These effects are associated with the regulation of NFkB, MAPK, PI3K, AKT, and PKB [13,84,85].

Although each bioactive compound has numerous effects on aging-related cellular and metabolic events, EGB 761® plays several critical effects in this process. It can decrease the levels of anion superoxide radical, hydrogen peroxide radicals, ROS and RNS (reactive nitrogen species), peroxyl radicals (ROO), and hydroxyl radicals (OH). In neurology, this plant extract can be used to improve circulation since it protects the cortical neurons from iron injuries and reduces the peroxide levels in cerebellar neurons. Moreover, it can upregulate the expression of antioxidant enzymes, such as glutathione peroxidase and superoxide dismutase [67,86–88].

4.2. Gingko biloba, Mitochondrial Dysfunction, and Apoptosis

Mitochondria are the organelle responsible for energy production in our cells and can use O_2 and glucose to produce ATP, CO_2, and H_2O. Mitochondrial dysfunction is associated with ROS production that triggers peroxidative reactions, culminating with harmful effects on mitochondrial biomolecules. This impairment in mitochondrial function can lead to neuronal cell death and augmented tissue loss. GB can reduce ROS levels in mitochondria, and EGB 761® can stabilize mitochondrial function. Furthermore, it can protect respiratory chain complexes I, IV, and V in mitochondria and improve mitochondrial membrane potential and morphology linked to aging in the liver and brain.

Interestingly, it can prevent mitochondrial dysfunction in both young and old mice. Still, the protective effect can only be observed in aged animals, possibly because of the increase in the permeability of the brain–blood barrier with aging. GB can also protect and upregulate mitochondrial DNA [89–92].

EGB 761® is also associated with the inhibition of cytochrome c oxidase activation and the reduction of mitochondrial ATP and GSH with aging. It also regulates the expression of Bas and pBcl-xL and their inhibition of the activation of caspase-9 to protect against mitochondrial dysfunction in rat cochlear tissue [92].

The increase in ROS production is associated with apoptosis, which has a critical role in the aging process, and bilobalide can prevent this process in aged animals. Some authors have demonstrated the use of hydrogen peroxide to induce apoptosis and the utilization of Aβ protein 1–42 to mimic impairments in age-related neurological functions. Bilobalide can inhibit hydrogen peroxide cell apoptosis due to the restriction of mitochondria-mediated caspase activation [89,93].

As already mentioned, EGB 761® can also inhibit the activation of NFκB stimulated by β-amyloid peptide, suppressing the expression of Toll-like receptors and, thus, reducing apoptosis in neuronal cells. NFκB is a critical regulator of cell death programming via apoptosis and necrosis. It is related to proapoptotic gene upregulation, for example, the death receptor Fas and TNF-α. In normal tissues, bilobalide suppresses apoptosis; however, it has an opposite action in cancer cells, inducing apoptosis [94,95].

4.3. Ginkgo biloba and Neurodegenerative Diseases

Neurodegenerative diseases are the leading cause of disabilities in the elderly. Many studies have shown that mitochondrial dysfunction, oxidative stress, neuroinflammation, and apoptosis accompanying the aging process are linked to neurodegenerative conditions [5]. GB possesses twenty-seven active compounds with multi-target synergistic actions for the therapeutic approach to neurodegenerative disorders. These compounds may interfere with biological events, such as the activation of transcription factor activities and oxidative reactions. Moreover, these active compounds can interfere with more than one hundred metabolic pathways [96]. Figure 3 shows the main effects of GB on neurodegenerative diseases.

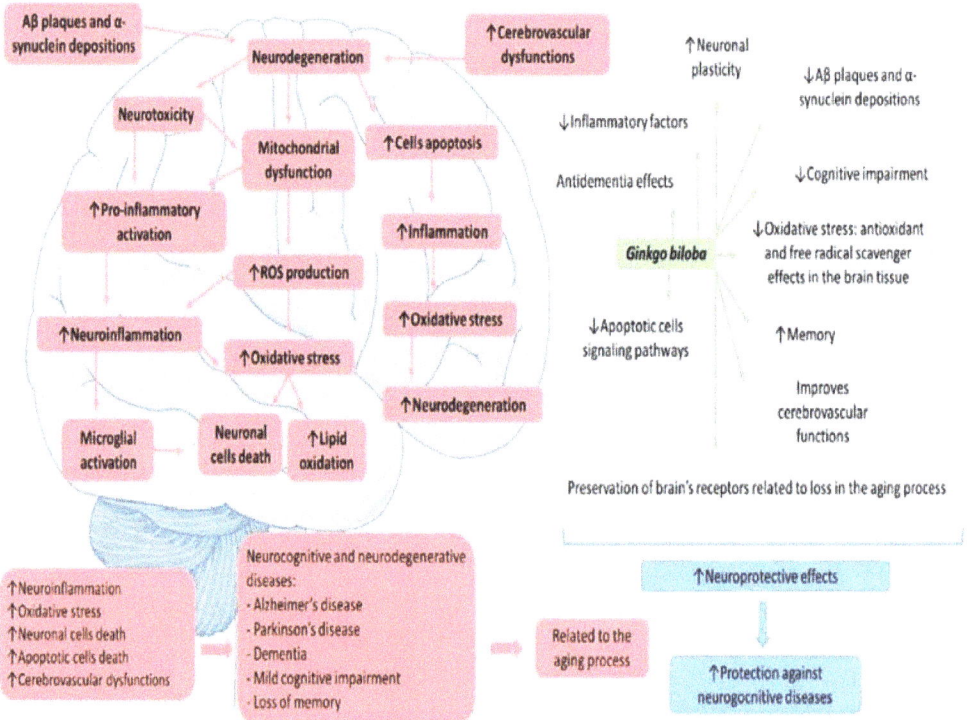

Figure 3. *Ginkgo biloba*: general effects against neurodegenerative diseases. ↑—increase; ↓—decrease; Aβ—beta amyloid.

4.3.1. *Ginkgo biloba* and Memory

The clinical concepts of memory divide this phenomenon into episodic, semantic, working, and procedural aspects. Loss of memory is one of the most common first symptoms of AD dementia, affecting 30 million people worldwide. Although AD is the most well-known type of memory impairment, many different neuro-pathologies can affect the neuronal networks of dissociable memory systems and cause memory loss (principally when the individual experiencing this loss belongs to a group with risk factors). GB extracts are related to the enhancement of cognitive functions, specifically memory, in addition to concentration. The extracts of this plant are the most related to memory improvements via their neuroprotective effects studied in human clinical trials. Since GB presents anti-inflammatory, antioxidant, and antiapoptotic actions, it leads to antidementia environments, together with the regulation of neurotransmitters (such as serotonin) and the expression of neurotransmitter receptors in the human brain. GB is also related to modulations of synaptic plasticity in humans and it regulates structural changes and neurogenesis in hippocampus circuity, affecting neuron excitability [97–99].

One study investigated the effects of EGb 761® on memory and the specificity of these effects on distinct memory functions. The results showed that EGb 761® (240 mg once daily) could significantly improve the number of appointments correctly remembered by healthy middle-aged people. This study adds to the evidence that GB can improve memory. However, we observed bias in this study; for example, no patient's predictive data or demographic characteristics were reported [19] (Table 1).

4.3.2. *Ginkgo biloba* and Dementia

Dementia is a neuronal condition that is increasing in prevalence in the aging population at a tremendous rate, such that 6% of people older than 65 years have some spectrum of dementia. It causes memory loss, followed by reduced executive functions, other cognitive deficits, and changes in the individual's personality. Initially, individuals with dementia present with a loss of recent events' memories, and over time, they start to become unable to make decisions and sequence complex tasks. There are many types of dementia, but the most common forms present one similar pathophysiological feature: cerebrovascular dysfunction. Many factors are involved in the dysfunction of the central nervous system's circulation and its relation to the pathophysiology of dementia. Cerebrovascular alterations and the apogee of dementia are associated with hypoxia, hypoperfusion, and dysfunctions in cerebrovascular hemodynamics [100–102].

Hypoxia and hypoperfusion lead principally to decreased cerebral blood flow and the occurrence of micro-infarcts and white matter abnormalities in brain tissue. More serious ischemic events in the brain tissue can also be associated with dementia. Alterations in the cerebrovascular hemodynamics are related to the impairment of cognitive functions that occur due to endothelial damage, changes in the neurovascular microvascular anatomy, modifications in vascular remodeling, neurovascular reactivity damage (blood vessel tortuosity and vessel-wall thickening), increases in oxidative stress, and increases in blood pressure. The emergence of dementia can be related to metabolic dysfunctions, such as impaired glucose metabolism and mitochondrial dysfunctions. The cerebrovascular and metabolic dysfunctions lead to neuroinflammation, and synaptic loss and neurodegeneration also occur. The brain's atrophy and the alterations in the permeability of the blood–brain barrier are related to the different causes of dementia [9,101,103].

GB can be used to treat and prevent dementia since it exhibits neuroprotective effects. It can protect against neuronal death by ischemic events and is associated with improvements in blood circulation by the reinforcement of capillary walls, preventing neuronal cell harm by hypoxia. GB extracts are also related to neuroprotection and improvements in neuronal plasticity. In vitro studies have demonstrated that they can protect neuron cultures against the harmful effects of hydrogen peroxide. GB can also improve memory implications and preserve the brain through the aging process, principally by protecting neuronal cells' receptors related to age loss in the aging process, which can be associated with the counteractions of cognitive impairments [9,28,101,102,104].

In a randomized, double-blind, multicenter study with a significant number of participants and an adequate follow-up, the authors showed that a once-daily formulation of EGb 761® in the treatment of dementia in patients with neuropsychiatric features was safe and superior to the use of a placebo in this population [20]. Another multicenter, double-blind, randomized, placebo-controlled trial was conducted to demonstrate the efficacy and safety of EGB 761® extract in patients with mild to moderate dementia associated with neuropsychiatric symptoms. The primary outcomes were changes from baseline to week 24 in SKT and NPI total scores. The Verbal Fluency Test, ADCS Clinical Global Impression of Change (ADCS-CGIC), International Activities of Daily Living Scale (ADL-IS), DEMQOL-Proxy quality of life scale, and 11-point box scales for tinnitus and dizziness were used as secondary outcome measures (Table 1) [21].

4.3.3. *Ginkgo biloba* and Mild Cognitive Impairment

MCI is characterized as a neurocognitive state of subjective complaints of impairments in an individual's cognitive performance. It is understood to be a mild cognitive state between normal cognitive aging and dementia. Although there are many diagnostic criteria for MCI, it is recognized that this neurocognitive condition corresponds to objective evidence in the lack of dementia diagnostic criteria in a subject. It is not related to a specific etiology. Still, it can be an early manifestation of AD (similar to a prodromal stage) or even a risk factor for this disease and other neurodegenerative conditions. The risk factors for this neurological condition include being of the male sex and older age. However, it is known that in older people, the principal risk factors for the development of MCI go beyond the traditional: depression, polypharmacy, and uncontrolled CVD. CVD has also been demonstrated to be a risk factor for the progression of MCI to AD. The prevalence of MCI increases by the age of 65 years, and it is known that the affected subjects can progress to dementia, remain at the MCI stage, or regress to normal. Although the identification and classification of MCI are considered to be a significant challenge, the diagnosis of this condition comprises neuroimaging, clinical assessments, and a neurophysiological evaluation. No medications are considered effective in combating dementia, mainly because MCI patients are only steps away from having dementia [105–107].

MCI subjects can demonstrate both neurocognitive and neuropsychiatric symptoms. The most common neurocognitive symptoms are impairments and alterations that lead to abnormalities in complex attention, social cognition, memory, learning, language function, perceptual-motor function, and executive function. Besides that, the neuropsychiatric symptoms may be summarized by changes in personality or usual conduct, depression, apathy, irritability, sleep and appetite disturbances, dysphoria, and hallucinations or delusions [25,107,108].

GB and its extracts show beneficial effects on cognitive dysfunctions, CVD, in the treatment of MCI by improving memory, learning abilities, and executive functions. GB and its derivatives enhance neuronal plasticity and mitochondrial function, promote neurogenesis, and improve neuronal energy metabolism. Besides that, GB can affect the neurotransmitter levels in the brain and has actions on the microcirculation and the brain's micro-perfusion. All of these effects can be associated with ameliorations in memory and, consequently, in MCI and MCI progression [25,108,109].

Gait instability in MCI patients, particularly in dual-task situations, has been associated with impaired executive function and an increased risk of falls. GB extract can be effective in improving gait stability [28]. In a study that associated 75 mg aspirin to 19.2 mg GB for the treatment of cognitive vascular impairment of non-dementia after three months, MoCA scores for executive ability, attention, abstract, delayed memory, and orientation were significantly increased compared to those before treatment and with the controls after treatment. Furthermore, the blood flow velocity of the anterior cerebral artery was significantly augmented. However, the study did not present demographic data, nor randomization or blinding data, nor the results on adverse effects; in addition, it used a small dose of GB when compared to other studies (Table 1) [23].

An open-label phase II study was conducted to assess the effects of GB in symptomatic irradiated brain tumor survivors. GB improved the patients' quality of life and cognitive function. However, a high dropout rate and a small sample may have interfered with the results in this study [24]. Another study showed the beneficial effects of EGB 761® on neuropsychiatric symptoms (NPS) and cognition in patients with MCI. It was observed to ameliorate NPS and cognitive performance in MCI patients, which are related to faster cognitive decline and an increased risk of developing AD. As EGb 761® is safe and well tolerated, it represents a promising treatment option for MCI as defined by international consensus criteria (Table 1) [25].

A study by Wang et al. also linked 75 mg aspirin to 40 mg GBT for the treatment of vascular cognitive impairment of non-dementia and demonstrated that, in general, GB could be used to improve cerebral blood flow and cognitive ability in patients with this condition. However, the study did not present diverse data, such as demographic data, randomization data, blinding data, or adverse effects. In addition to using a small dose of GB, the authors also specify in their abstract that they used 19.2 mg of GBT thrice a day; however, in the methods section, the authors indicate that 40 mg were used three times a day in the combined treatment group [26]. Moreover, this trial seems to be the same as Zhang et al. (2012), yet this study was not mentioned (Table 1).

One study found indications for improved cognitive flexibility without changes in brain activation, suggesting increased processing efficiency with EGb761®, along with a trend towards better response inhibition results compatible with a slight increase in prefrontal dopamine. Although these conclusions must be confirmed, EGb761® was shown to be safe and well tolerated. However, the study did not show demographic data, had a significant sample loss during the investigation, and did not perform a sample calculation (Table 1) [27].

4.3.4. *Ginkgo biloba* and Alzheimer's Disease

AD is a condition that accounts for one of the most distinguished global healthcare issues and is the third leading cause of death in the United States. The etiology of this disorder is not completely understood, but genetic factors are linked to approximately 10% of cases. The available therapies cannot cure AD and, in many cases, show limited effectiveness in the treatment of AD [110–112].

The pathophysiological processes triggered in this disease involve neuronal degeneration and the waste of synapses in the cortex, hippocampus, and subcortical areas, resulting in atrophy, loss of memory, executive dysfunction, mood swings, and an inability to learn new information and perform daily living activities [113,114]. The neurodegeneration that occurs in AD is associated with the elevation in the levels of Aβ42, an altered form of the amyloid-β peptide. This aberrant Aβ42 results in the production of extracellular oligomers and aggregates and leads to the hyperphosphorylation of the tau protein, culminating with deposition as insoluble neurofibrillary tangles. These processes interfere with synaptic function and neuronal survival. Moreover, glial cells also become abnormal, contributing to the pathophysiology of the disease [115,116].

When there is an accumulation of extracellular Aβ plaques, there is stimulation of astrocytes and microglia, resulting in the release of pro-inflammatory cytokines. The chronic release of these molecules leads to neuroinflammation, which is conducive to synapse loss and neuronal death. The imbalance in the functions of microglia and astrocytes is also related to the augmentation of extracellular glutamate, which is related to the neuron excitotoxicity resulting from the overactivation of the N-methyl-D-aspartate receptors (NMDA). Besides that, in the neuroinflammation scenario, astrocytes and microglia lose their capacity to release cytokines related to neuron survival and functioning [112,117–119].

The failure of available drugs targeting β-amyloid and tau proteins suggests a need for other preventative and therapeutic strategies for AD [120]. GB exhibits anti-inflammatory, antioxidant, and antiapoptotic actions; for these reasons, it can stimulate neurogenesis and cerebral blood flow, improve mitochondrial and neuronal function, and inhibit neural cell death. Beyond that, GB has anti-platelet-activating factor actions in vascular conditions, inhibits β-amyloid aggregation, and reduces the peripheral benzodiazepine receptor expression for stress relief. In vitro, it can reverse β-amyloid and NO-induced toxicity and diminish apoptosis. GB can also work as an iron-chelating compound that can also inhibit the formation of Aβ fibrils. It can also play a role as a cholinesterase inhibitor and delay the progression of the disease. Further, the use of GB is associated with mild or no side effects and can improve the quality of life in AD patients [10,93,121–124].

As mentioned before, the protective effects of GB against Aβ-induced neurotoxicity occur through the inhibition of Aβ-induced events, such as the accumulation of ROS; glucose uptake; mitochondrial dysfunction; the activation of JNK, ERK, and AKT pathways; and apoptosis. It can also inhibit the synthesis of Aβ in the brain by reducing circulating free cholesterol (amyloidogenesis); AβPP processing is potentially affected by the levels of free circulating and intracellular cholesterol [9,125–127].

Other properties of GB and GB extract reside in the improvement of blood circulation and the protection of the capillary walls and nerve cells from damage when oxygen is devoid. It can also be considered in the treatment of concentration disorders, memory impairment, and dementia. It shows positive effects on neurological and cognitive functions since it regulates vascular flow. Apart from its free radical scavenger property, GB also interferes in the transcription of many genes linked to oxidative stress, protecting the neuronal cells against the harmful effects of ROS [9,120,128].

Nasab et al. [22] compared rivastigmine, a cholinesterase inhibitor, with GB for dementia (AD type), and suggested that the drug is more effective than GB in treating Alzheimer's dementia (Table 1).

4.4. Ginkgo biloba, Metabolic Syndrome and Cardiovascular Diseases

Metabolic syndrome (MS) is one of the leading public health problems today for men and women (reaching almost 30% in some populations). It is defined for different diagnosis criteria, including cardiometabolic risk factors, such as insulin resistance, high triglycerides levels, low HDL-c levels, obesity (augmented waist circumference), and hypertension. An individual is considered to possess MS when presenting at least three of these risk factors. In this scenario, a pro-inflammatory state should also be considered in patients with MS, and chronic inflammatory conditions are related to the rise in the occurrence of CVD [129,130].

GB extract may have a significant antidiabetic effect. It can expand glycogen levels in the muscle and liver and thus can decrease plasma glucose levels. Moreover, it can reduce HbA1c, insulin levels, body weight, waist circumference, and visceral adiposity index. Priyanka et al. [131] and An et al. [132] have suggested that GB can improve insulin resistance and inflammation resulting from the increase in the secretion of adiponectin, reducing serine phosphorylation of IRS-1 receptors, reducing NFκB/JNK activation, and, consequently, reducing the release of inflammatory adipokines.

The use of GB has also been shown to be effective in the reduction of cholesterol absorption in rats; in the inhibition of 3-hydroxy-3-methylglutaryl–coenzyme A, an enzyme that is a center of regulation of cholesterol synthesis; and in the improvement of high-fat diet-induced hyperglycemia [133,134]. In rabbits, GB significantly diminished triglycerides and cholesterol levels and increased HDL-c. Besides that, GB increased the levels of antioxidant enzymes and decreased malonaldehyde levels [135]. GB extract can also reduce body weight and weight gain, and can upregulate the expression of IL-10 (and downregulate the expression of TNF-α and NFκB), insulin receptor (IR), and protein kinase B (Akt) phosphorylation, stimulating the insulin signaling cascade [136]. GB also has hypotensive actions related to its capacity for angiotensin-converting enzyme (ACE) inhibition and vasodilation, and its ability to increase the expression of endothelial nitric oxide synthase (eNOS) [8,137]. Figure 4 shows the effects of GB on MS.

GB was also associated with an improvement in cardiomyopathy, which is a common reason for heart failure and can lead to a higher risk of cardiac death. Due to its unclear pathogenesis, cardiomyopathy lacks an effective treatment, and new strategies are required. The beneficial effects of GB and its bioactive compounds in this pathological condition are linked to the improvement of blood circulation and other multi-pathways associated with the regulation of antiapoptotic, pro-survival, and anti-inflammatory actions via NFκB and PI3K-AKT signaling [138,139].

Aging-related vascular pathology is closely linked to endothelial dysfunction and arterial stiffening that culminate in CVD progression. As already mentioned in this paper, oxidative stress and inflammation lead to vascular impairment. The antioxidant and anti-inflammatory actions of GB extract are related to amelioration of aging-related vascular impairment. The main activities of this plant in aged vasculature are probably linked to the longevity signaling pathways and the slowing of vascular aging progression in diabetes owing to the regulation of glycemia and lipid metabolism [140,141].

Moreover, several studies have suggested that ginkgolide A plays a role as an antithrombotic agent and could be used for prevention and/or for controlling thrombosis. It can inhibit platelet aggregation and collagen-stimulated platelet aggregation due to the activation of MMP-9 and the intracellular production of cAMP and cGMP, which inhibits the mobilization of intracellular Ca^{2+} and reduces the release of thromboxane A2 by inhibiting COX-1 [142,143]. Figure 5 shows some effects of GB on CVD.

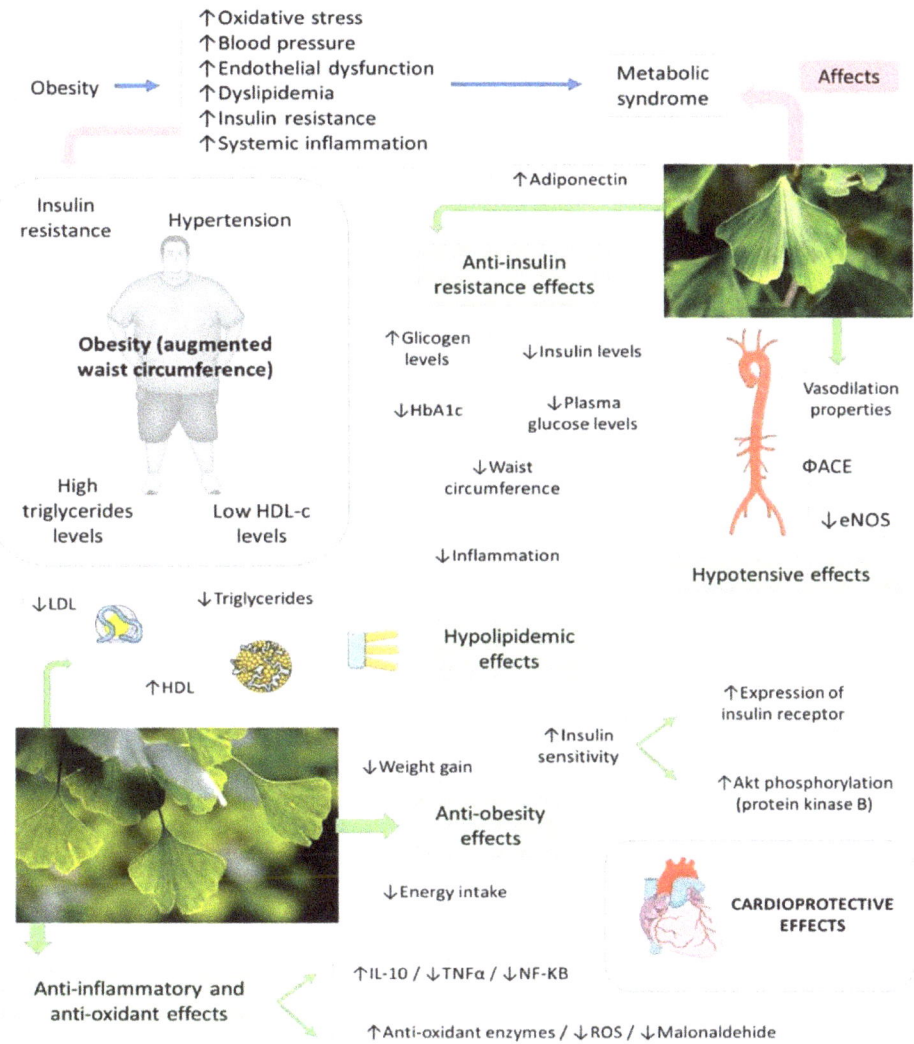

Figure 4. *Ginkgo biloba* and its extracts have many effects against cardiovascular risk factors that compound metabolic syndrome. ↑—increase; ↓—decrease; Φ—inhibition; ROS—reactive oxygen species; TNF-α—tumor necrosis factor; IL-10—interleukin 10; NK-KB—factor nuclear kappa B; ACE—angiotensin-converting enzyme; eNOS—nitric oxide synthase 3.

A survey in Lithuania aimed to assess the glycemic control and psychological status of patients' with type 2 diabetes mellitus (T2DM) after antioxidant plant preparations. Patients received a standardized dry extract of GB leaves, green tea dry extract, or placebo capsules. Glycemic control, HbA1c, antioxidant status, and psychological parameters were evaluated at baseline, and after nine and eighteen months of using antioxidant preparations or a placebo. GB leaf extract exhibited a moderate effect on psychological status and a tendency to improve glycemic control in patients with T2DM (Table 1).

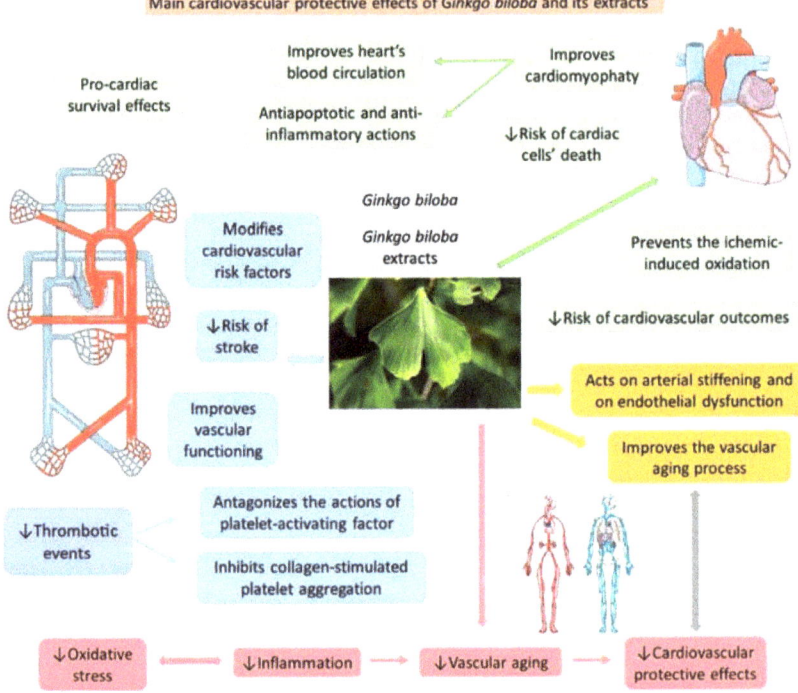

Figure 5. *Ginkgo biloba* and its extracts have cardiovascular protective effects that improve the functionality of the cardiovascular organs. ↓—decrease.

One study determined that GB extract as an adjuvant effectively improves metformin treatment outcomes in T2DM patients. However, the main limitations of this study include its small sample size, relatively short duration, and lack of dose-response data for GB extract as an adjuvant to the antidiabetic drug. For these reasons, further studies are necessary to determine the long-term effects of GB extract with a larger sample [30,42].

Siegel, Ermilov et al. [31] suggested that GB may be used as a complementary drug with a preventive character after a percutaneous intervention stent implantation and myocardial revascularization graft in patients with MS (Table 1). Moreover, in another publication with the same sample, Siegel et al. [32] showed that GB could reduce CVD risk factors since it reduces HOMA-IR, hs-C reactive protein, and IL-6.

4.5. Ginkgo biloba Bioavailability and Safety

A study investigating the absorption of radiolabeled GBE in animals showed a minimum absorption of 60%. Thus, GB extract is well tolerated and safe. Acute toxicity studies showed a lethal dose (LD50) of 1100, 1900, and 7700 mg/kg in mice and 1100, 2100, and over 10,000 mg/kg in rats when administered intravenously, intraperitoneal, and orally, respectively. The extensive use of GBE in the elderly population with T2DM, hypertension, or rheumatism, can interact with simultaneous drugs. Furthermore, GB supplements are associated with prolonged bleeding times in patients and are contraindicated during pregnancy or breastfeeding [20,21,144,145].

To the best of our knowledge, this is the first review showing the effects of *Ginkgo biloba* in the aging process.

4.6. Implication and Limitations

Most chronic degenerative diseases (including those related to aging) are related to oxidative stress and inflammatory aspects. Thus, GB could work as a complementary medicine in several aspects of these diseases.

On the other hand, this review has several limitations, such as the heterogeneity of the outcomes of the included studies, the different formulations of GB, doses used, and the age of the patients in the different studies. Moreover, only English studies were included, and the descriptive review had less evidence than systematic review.

5. Conclusions

This review showed that GB could be considered in the therapeutic and preventative approaches to aging-related conditions, such as neurodegenerative disorders, metabolic syndrome, and cardiovascular diseases. From this perspective, GB can be beneficial in chronic degenerative conditions associated with the aging process. Nevertheless, the existing clinical trials are heterogeneous since the different formulations, dosages, and administration times were variable. For these reasons, other studies are necessary to establish the doses, pharmaceutical form, and treatment time needed for preventive effects or therapeutic adjuvants in aging conditions.

Author Contributions: Conceptualization, S.M.B. and R.D.; methodology, L.T.M., L.F.L., A.C.A. and E.L.G.; software, L.T.M., L.F.L., A.C.A.C. and E.L.G.; validation, S.M.B., A.C.A.C., E.L.G., R.d.A.G. and R.J.T.; formal analysis, V.A.C.T., R.J.T. and R.d.A.G.; investigation, S.M.B., R.D., L.T.M., L.F.L., A.C.A.C. and E.L.G.; resources, all authors; data curation, A.C.A.C. and U.A.P.F.; writing—original draft preparation, S.M.B., R.D., L.T.M., L.F.L., A.C.A.C. and E.L.G.; writing—review and editing, S.M.B., R.D., L.T.M., L.F.L., A.C.A.C. and E.L.G.; visualization, C.R.P.D.; supervision, C.R.P.D. and P.C.S.B.; project administration, S.M.B., R.D. and R.S.J.G.; funding acquisition, S.M.B. All authors have read and agreed to the published version of the manuscript.

Funding: This research received no external funding.

Acknowledgments: The authors declare attribution to Smart Servier (https://smart.servier.com/ accessed on 21 December 2021) due to the provision of some scientific images that were used in this article under an attribution license of public copyrights (https://creativecommons.org/licenses/by/3.0/ accessed on 21 December 2021) and under a disclaimer of warranties. All of Smart Servier's images were not changed in the writing of this article, except the brain image in the Figure 3 of the article, which had its color changed to blue and clarified from the original (https://smart.servier.com/smart_image/brain-12/ accessed on 21 December 2021).

Conflicts of Interest: The authors declare no conflict of interest.

References

1. Wang, L.; Zuo, X.; Ouyang, Z.; Qiao, P.; Wang, F. A Systematic Review of Antiaging Effects of 23 Traditional Chinese Medicines. *Evid.-Based Complement. Altern. Med.* **2021**, *2021*, 5591573. [CrossRef] [PubMed]
2. Barbalho, S.M.; Flato, U.A.P.; Tofano, R.J.; Goulart, R.A.; Guiguer, E.L.; Detregiachi, C.R.P.; Buchaim, D.V.; Araújo, A.C.; Buchaim, R.L.; Reina, F.T.R.; et al. Physical Exercise and Myokines: Relationships with Sarcopenia and Cardiovascular Complications. *Int. J. Mol. Sci.* **2020**, *21*, 3607. [CrossRef] [PubMed]
3. Barbalho, S.M.; Tofano, R.J.; Chagas, E.F.B.; Detregiachi, C.R.P.; de Alvares Goulart, R.; Flato, U.A.P.J.E.G. Benchside to the bedside of frailty and cardiovascular aging: Main shared cellular and molecular mechanisms. *Exp. Gerontol.* **2021**, *148*, 111302. [CrossRef]
4. Morvaridzadeh, M.; Fazelian, S.; Agah, S.; Khazdouz, M.; Rahimlou, M.; Agh, F.; Potter, E.; Heshmati, S.; Heshmati, J.J.C. Effect of ginger (*Zingiber officinale*) on inflammatory markers: A systematic review and meta-analysis of randomized controlled trials. *Cytokine* **2020**, *135*, 155224. [CrossRef] [PubMed]
5. Grewal, A.K.; Singh, T.G.; Sharma, D.; Sharma, V.; Singh, M.; Rahman, M.H.; Najda, A.; Walasek-Janusz, M.; Kamel, M.; Albadrani, G.M.; et al. Mechanistic insights and perspectives involved in nfeuroprotective action of quercetin. *Biomed. Pharmacother. Biomed. Pharmacother.* **2021**, *140*, 111729. [CrossRef]
6. Soheili, M.; Karimian, M.; Hamidi, G.; Salami, M. Alzheimer's disease treatment: The share of herbal medicines. *Iran. J. Basic Med. Sci.* **2021**, *24*, 123–135. [CrossRef]

7. Banin, R.M.; Hirata, B.K.S.; Andrade, I.S.d.; Zemdegs, J.C.S.; Clemente, A.P.G.; Dornellas, A.P.S.; Boldarine, V.T.; Estadella, D.; Albuquerque, K.T.d.; Oyama, L.M.J.B.J.o.M.; et al. Beneficial effects of *Ginkgo biloba* extract on insulin signaling cascade, dyslipidemia, and body adiposity of diet-induced obese rats. *Braz. J. Med. Biol. Res.* **2014**, *47*, 780–788. [CrossRef]
8. Eisvand, F.; Razavi, B.M.; Hosseinzadeh, H. The effects of *Ginkgo biloba* on metabolic syndrome: A review. *Phytother. Res. PTR* **2020**, *34*, 1798–1811. [CrossRef]
9. Singh, S.K.; Srivastav, S.; Castellani, R.J.; Plascencia-Villa, G.; Perry, G. Neuroprotective and Antioxidant Effect of *Ginkgo biloba* Extract against AD and Other Neurological Disorders. *Neurother. J. Am. Soc. Exp. NeuroTher.* **2019**, *16*, 666–674. [CrossRef]
10. Tomino, C.; Ilari, S.; Solfrizzi, V.; Malafoglia, V.; Zilio, G.; Russo, P.; Proietti, S.; Marcolongo, F.; Scapagnini, G.; Muscoli, C.; et al. Mild Cognitive Impairment and Mild Dementia: The Role of *Ginkgo biloba* (EGb 761®). *Pharmaceuticals* **2021**, *14*, 305. [CrossRef]
11. Hirata, B.K.; Pedroso, A.P.; Machado, M.M.; Neto, N.I.; Perestrelo, B.O.; de Sá, R.D.; Alonso-Vale, M.I.C.; Nogueira, F.N.; Oyama, L.M.; Ribeiro, E.B. *Ginkgo biloba* extract modulates the retroperitoneal fat depot proteome and reduces oxidative stress in diet-induced obese rats. *Front. Pharmacol.* **2019**, *10*, 686. [CrossRef] [PubMed]
12. Achete de Souza, G.; de Marqui, S.V.; Matias, J.N.; Guiguer, E.L.; Barbalho, S.M. Effects of *Ginkgo biloba* on Diseases Related to Oxidative Stress. *Planta Med.* **2020**, *86*, 376–386. [CrossRef] [PubMed]
13. Unger, M. Pharmacokinetic drug interactions involving *Ginkgo biloba*. *Drug Metab. Rev.* **2013**, *45*, 353–385. [CrossRef] [PubMed]
14. Gauthier, S.; Schlaefke, S. Efficacy and tolerability of *Ginkgo biloba* extract EGb 761® in dementia: A systematic review and meta-analysis of randomized placebo-controlled trials. *Clin. Interv. Aging* **2014**, *9*, 2065. [CrossRef]
15. Meng, M.; Ai, D.; Sun, L.; Xu, X.; Cao, X. EGb 761 inhibits Aβ1–42-induced neuroinflammatory response by suppressing P38 MAPK signaling pathway in BV-2 microglial cells. *Neuroreport* **2019**, *30*, 434–440. [CrossRef]
16. Abdul-Latif, R.; Stupans, I.; Allahham, A.; Adhikari, B.; Thrimawithana, T. Natural antioxidants in the management of Parkinson's disease: Review of evidence from cell line and animal models. *J. Integr. Med.* **2021**, *19*, 300–310. [CrossRef]
17. Moher, D.; Liberati, A.; Tetzlaff, J.; Altman, D.G. Preferred reporting items for systematic reviews and meta-analyses: The PRISMA statement. *Ann. Intern. Med.* **2009**, *151*, 264–269. [CrossRef]
18. Higgins, J.P.; Thomas, J.; Chandler, J.; Cumpston, M.; Li, T.; Page, M.J.; Welch, V.A. *Cochrane Handbook for Systematic Reviews of Interventions*; John Wiley & Sons: Hoboken, NJ, USA, 2019.
19. Kaschel, R. Specific memory effects of *Ginkgo biloba* extract EGb 761 in middle-aged healthy volunteers. *Phytomed. Int. J. Phytother. Phytopharm.* **2011**, *18*, 1202–1207. [CrossRef]
20. Ihl, R.; Bachinskaya, N.; Korczyn, A.D.; Vakhapova, V.; Tribanek, M.; Hoerr, R.; Napryeyenko, O. Efficacy and safety of a once-daily formulation of *Ginkgo biloba* extract EGb 761 in dementia with neuropsychiatric features: A randomized controlled trial. *Int. J. Geriatr. Psychiatry* **2011**, *26*, 1186–1194. [CrossRef]
21. Herrschaft, H.; Nacu, A.; Likhachev, S.; Sholomov, I.; Hoerr, R.; Schlaefke, S. *Ginkgo biloba* extract EGb 761® in dementia with neuropsychiatric features: A randomised, placebo-controlled trial to confirm the efficacy and safety of a daily dose of 240 mg. *J. Psychiatr. Res.* **2012**, *46*, 716–723. [CrossRef]
22. Nasab, N.M.; Bahrammi, M.A.; Nikpour, M.R.; Rahim, F.; Naghibis, S.N. Efficacy of rivastigmine in comparison to ginkgo for treating Alzheimer's dementia. *J. Pak. Med. Assoc.* **2012**, *62*, 677–680. [PubMed]
23. Zhang, S.J.; Xue, Z.Y. Effect of Western medicine therapy assisted by *Ginkgo biloba* tablet on vascular cognitive impairment of none dementia. *Asian Pac. J. Trop. Med.* **2012**, *5*, 661–664. [CrossRef]
24. Attia, A.; Rapp, S.R.; Case, L.D.; D'Agostino, R.; Lesser, G.; Naughton, M.; McMullen, K.; Rosdhal, R.; Shaw, E.G. Phase II study of *Ginkgo biloba* in irradiated brain tumor patients: Effect on cognitive function, quality of life, and mood. *J. Neuro-Oncol.* **2012**, *109*, 357–363. [CrossRef] [PubMed]
25. Gavrilova, S.I.; Preuss, U.W.; Wong, J.W.; Hoerr, R.; Kaschel, R.; Bachinskaya, N. Efficacy and safety of *Ginkgo biloba* extract EGb 761 in mild cognitive impairment with neuropsychiatric symptoms: A randomized, placebo-controlled, double-blind, multi-center trial. *Int. J. Geriatr. Psychiatry* **2014**, *29*, 1087–1095. [CrossRef]
26. Wang, L.P.; Zhang, X.Y.; Liu, N.; Ma, Z.Z.; Fang, D.S. Comparison of integrated traditional Chinese and western medicine therapy on vascular cognitive impairment with no dementia. *Genet. Mol. Res. GMR* **2015**, *14*, 4896–4902. [CrossRef] [PubMed]
27. Beck, S.M.; Ruge, H.; Schindler, C.; Burkart, M.; Miller, R.; Kirschbaum, C.; Goschke, T. Effects of *Ginkgo biloba* extract EGb 761® on cognitive control functions, mental activity of the prefrontal cortex and stress reactivity in elderly adults with subjective memory impairment—A randomized double-blind placebo-controlled trial. *Hum. Psychopharmacol.* **2016**, *31*, 227–242. [CrossRef] [PubMed]
28. Gschwind, Y.J.; Bridenbaugh, S.A.; Reinhard, S.; Granacher, U.; Monsch, A.U.; Kressig, R.W. *Ginkgo biloba* special extract LI 1370 improves dual-task walking in patients with MCI: A randomised, double-blind, placebo-controlled exploratory study. *Aging Clin. Exp. Res.* **2017**, *29*, 609–619. [CrossRef]
29. Lasaite, L.; Spadiene, A.; Savickiene, N.; Skesters, A.; Silova, A. The effect of *Ginkgo biloba* and Camellia sinensis extracts on psychological state and glycemic control in patients with type 2 diabetes mellitus. *Nat. Prod. Commun.* **2014**, *9*, 1345–1350. [CrossRef]
30. Aziz, T.A.; Hussain, S.A.; Mahwi, T.O.; Ahmed, Z.A.; Rahman, H.S.; Rasedee, A. The efficacy and safety of *Ginkgo biloba* extract as an adjuvant in type 2 diabetes mellitus patients ineffectively managed with metformin: A double-blind, randomized, placebo-controlled trial. *Drug Des. Dev. Ther.* **2018**, *12*, 735–742. [CrossRef]
31. Siegel, G.; Ermilov, E. Hs-CRP may be associated with white blood cell count in metabolic syndrome patients treated with *Ginkgo biloba*. *Atherosclerosis* **2011**, *218*, 250–252. [CrossRef]

32. Siegel, G.; Ermilov, E.; Knes, O.; Rodríguez, M. Combined lowering of low grade systemic inflammation and insulin resistance in metabolic syndrome patients treated with *Ginkgo biloba*. *Atherosclerosis* **2014**, *237*, 584–588. [CrossRef] [PubMed]
33. Guimarães, G.R.; Almeida, P.P.; de Oliveira Santos, L.; Rodrigues, L.P.; de Carvalho, J.L.; Boroni, M. Hallmarks of Aging in Macrophages: Consequences to Skin Inflammaging. *Cells* **2021**, *10*, 1323. [CrossRef] [PubMed]
34. Baek, S.J.; Hammock, B.D.; Hwang, I.K.; Li, Q.; Moustaid-Moussa, N.; Park, Y.; Safe, S.; Suh, N.; Yi, S.S.; Zeldin, D.C.; et al. Natural Products in the Prevention of Metabolic Diseases: Lessons Learned from the 20th KAST Frontier Scientists Workshop. *Nutrients* **2021**, *13*, 1881. [CrossRef] [PubMed]
35. Edler, M.K.; Mhatre-Winters, I.; Richardson, J.R. Microglia in Aging and Alzheimer's Disease: A Comparative Species Review. *Cells* **2021**, *10*, 1138. [CrossRef]
36. Li, Z.; Zhao, H.; Wang, J. Metabolism and Chronic Inflammation: The Links between Chronic Heart Failure and Comorbidities. *Front. Cardiovasc. Med.* **2021**, *8*, 650278. [CrossRef] [PubMed]
37. Rabilloud, T.; Heller, M.; Rigobello, M.P.; Bindoli, A.; Aebersold, R.; Lunardi, J. The mitochondrial antioxidant defence system and its response to oxidative stress. *Proteomics* **2001**, *1*, 1105–1110. [CrossRef]
38. Hajam, Y.A.; Rani, R.; Ganie, S.Y.; Sheikh, T.A.; Javaid, D.; Qadri, S.S.; Pramodh, S.; Alsulimani, A.; Alkhanani, M.F.; Harakeh, S.; et al. Oxidative Stress in Human Pathology and Aging: Molecular Mechanisms and Perspectives. *Cells* **2022**, *11*, 552. [CrossRef]
39. Strømgaard, K.; Nakanishi, K. Chemistry and biology of terpene trilactones from *Ginkgo biloba*. *Angew. Chem. (Int. Ed.)* **2004**, *43*, 1640–1658. [CrossRef]
40. Tao, Z.; Jin, W.; Ao, M.; Zhai, S.; Xu, H.; Yu, L. Evaluation of the anti-inflammatory properties of the active constituents in *Ginkgo biloba* for the treatment of pulmonary diseases. *Food Funct.* **2019**, *10*, 2209–2220. [CrossRef]
41. Tian, J.; Liu, Y.; Liu, Y.; Chen, K.; Lyu, S. *Ginkgo biloba* leaf extract protects against myocardial injury via attenuation of endoplasmic reticulum stress in streptozotocin-induced diabetic ApoE$^{-/-}$ mice. *Oxid. Med. Cell. Longev.* **2018**, *2018*, 2370617. [CrossRef]
42. Sarkar, C.; Quispe, C.; Jamaddar, S.; Hossain, R.; Ray, P.; Mondal, M.; Abdulwanis Mohamed, Z.; Sani Jaafaru, M.; Salehi, B.; Islam, M.T.; et al. Therapeutic promises of ginkgolide A: A literature-based review. *Biomed. Pharmacother.* **2020**, *132*, 110908. [CrossRef] [PubMed]
43. Belwal, T.; Giri, L.; Bahukhandi, A.; Tariq, M.; Kewlani, P.; Bhatt, I.D.; Rawal, R.S. Chapter 3.19—*Ginkgo biloba*. In *Nonvitamin and Nonmineral Nutritional Supplements*; Nabavi, S.M., Silva, A.S., Eds.; Academic Press: Cambridge, MA, USA, 2019; pp. 241–250.
44. Kuribara, H.; Weintraub, S.T.; Yoshihama, T.; Maruyama, Y. An Anxiolytic-Like Effect of *Ginkgo biloba* Extract and Its Constituent, Ginkgolide-A, in Mice. *J. Nat. Prod.* **2003**, *66*, 1333–1337. [CrossRef] [PubMed]
45. Gu, J.-H.; Ge, J.-B.; Li, M.; Wu, F.; Zhang, W.; Qin, Z.-H. Inhibition of NF-κB activation is associated with anti-inflammatory and anti-apoptotic effects of Ginkgolide B in a mouse model of cerebral ischemia/reperfusion injury. *Eur. J. Pharm. Sci.* **2012**, *47*, 652–660. [CrossRef] [PubMed]
46. Xiao, Q.; Wang, C.; Li, J.; Hou, Q.; Li, J.; Ma, J.; Wang, W.; Wang, Z. Ginkgolide B protects hippocampal neurons from apoptosis induced by beta-amyloid 25-35 partly via up-regulation of brain-derived neurotrophic factor. *Eur. J. Pharmacol.* **2010**, *647*, 48–54. [CrossRef] [PubMed]
47. Zhang, R.; Xu, L.; Zhang, D.; Hu, B.; Luo, Q.; Han, D.; Li, J.; Shen, C. Cardioprotection of Ginkgolide B on Myocardial Ischemia/Reperfusion-Induced Inflammatory Injury via Regulation of A20-NF-κB Pathway. *Front. Immunol.* **2018**, *9*, 2844. [CrossRef]
48. Liu, J.; Wu, P.; Xu, Z.; Zhang, J.; Liu, J.; Yang, Z. Ginkgolide B inhibits hydrogen peroxide-induced apoptosis and attenuates cytotoxicity via activating the PI3K/Akt/mTOR signaling pathway in H9c2 cells. *Mol. Med. Rep.* **2020**, *22*, 310–316. [CrossRef]
49. Wang, X.; Shao, Q.-H.; Zhou, H.; Wu, J.-L.; Quan, W.-Q.; Ji, P.; Yao, Y.-W.; Li, D.; Sun, Z.-J. Ginkgolide B inhibits lung cancer cells promotion via beclin-1-dependent autophagy. *BMC Complement. Med. Ther.* **2020**, *20*, 194. [CrossRef]
50. Zhi, Y.; Pan, J.; Shen, W.; He, P.; Zheng, J.; Zhou, X.; Lu, G.; Chen, Z.; Zhou, Z. Ginkgolide B Inhibits Human Bladder Cancer Cell Migration and Invasion through MicroRNA-223-3p. *Cell. Physiol. Biochem.* **2016**, *39*, 1787–1794. [CrossRef]
51. Chan, W.-H. The Signaling Cascades of Ginkgolide B-Induced Apoptosis in MCF-7 Breast Cancer Cells. *Int. J. Mol. Sci.* **2007**, *8*, 1177–1195. [CrossRef]
52. Liou, C.-J.; Lai, X.-Y.; Chen, Y.-L.; Wang, C.-L.; Wei, C.-H.; Huang, W.-C. Ginkgolide C Suppresses Adipogenesis in 3T3-L1 Adipocytes via the AMPK Signaling Pathway. *Evid.-Based Complement. Altern. Med.* **2015**, *2015*, 298635. [CrossRef]
53. Huang, W.-C.; Chen, Y.-L.; Liu, H.-C.; Wu, S.-J.; Liou, C.-J. Ginkgolide C reduced oleic acid-induced lipid accumulation in HepG2 cells. *Saudi Pharm. J.* **2018**, *26*, 1178–1184. [CrossRef] [PubMed]
54. Zhang, R.; Han, D.; Li, Z.; Shen, C.; Zhang, Y.; Li, J.; Yan, G.; Li, S.; Hu, B.; Li, J.; et al. Ginkgolide C Alleviates Myocardial Ischemia/Reperfusion-Induced Inflammatory Injury via Inhibition of CD40-NF-κB Pathway. *Front. Pharmacol.* **2018**, *9*, 109. [CrossRef] [PubMed]
55. Yang, M.H.; Ha, I.J.; Lee, S.-G.; Lee, J.; Um, J.-Y.; Ahn, K.S. Ginkgolide C promotes apoptosis and abrogates metastasis of colorectal carcinoma cells by targeting Wnt/β-catenin signaling pathway. *IUBMB Life* **2021**, *73*, 1222–1234. [CrossRef] [PubMed]
56. Yang, M.H.; Baek, S.H.; Um, J.-Y.; Ahn, K.S. Anti-neoplastic Effect of Ginkgolide C through Modulating c-Met Phosphorylation in Hepatocellular Carcinoma Cells. *Int. J. Mol. Sci.* **2020**, *21*, 8303. [CrossRef] [PubMed]
57. Xiang, J.; Yang, F.; Zhu, W.; Cai, M.; Li, X.T.; Zhang, J.S.; Yu, Z.H.; Zhang, W.; Cai, D.F. Bilobalide inhibits inflammation and promotes the expression of Aβ degrading enzymes in astrocytes to rescue neuronal deficiency in AD models. *Transl. Psychiatry* **2021**, *11*, 542. [CrossRef] [PubMed]

58. Zhao, M.; Qin, J.; Shen, W.; Wu, A. Bilobalide Enhances AMPK Activity to Improve Liver Injury and Metabolic Disorders in STZ-Induced Diabetes in Immature Rats via Regulating HMGB1/TLR4/NF-κB Signaling Pathway. *BioMed Res. Int.* **2021**, *2021*, 8835408. [CrossRef]
59. Maerz, S.; Liu, C.-H.; Guo, W.; Zhu, Y.-Z. Anti-ischaemic effects of bilobalide on neonatal rat cardiomyocytes and the involvement of the platelet-activating factor receptor. *Biosci. Rep.* **2011**, *31*, 439–447. [CrossRef]
60. Hua, Z.; Wu, C.; Fan, G.; Tang, Z.; Cao, F. The antibacterial activity and mechanism of ginkgolic acid C15:1. *BMC Biotechnol.* **2017**, *17*, 5. [CrossRef]
61. Borenstein, R.; Hanson, B.A.; Markosyan, R.M.; Gallo, E.S.; Narasipura, S.D.; Bhutta, M.; Shechter, O.; Lurain, N.S.; Cohen, F.S.; Al-Harthi, L.; et al. Ginkgolic acid inhibits fusion of enveloped viruses. *Sci. Rep.* **2020**, *10*, 4746. [CrossRef]
62. Baek, S.H.; Ko, J.-H.; Lee, J.H.; Kim, C.; Lee, H.; Nam, D.; Lee, J.; Lee, S.-G.; Yang, W.M.; Um, J.-Y.; et al. Ginkgolic Acid Inhibits Invasion and Migration and TGF-β-Induced EMT of Lung Cancer Cells through PI3K/Akt/mTOR Inactivation. *J. Cell. Physiol.* **2017**, *232*, 346–354. [CrossRef]
63. Ku, S.-K.; Kim, T.H.; Bae, J.-S. Anticoagulant activities of persicarin and isorhamnetin. *Vasc. Pharmacol.* **2013**, *58*, 272–279. [CrossRef] [PubMed]
64. Jaramillo, S.; Lopez, S.; Varela, L.M.; Rodriguez-Arcos, R.; Jimenez, A.; Abia, R.; Guillen, R.; Muriana, F.J.G. The Flavonol Isorhamnetin Exhibits Cytotoxic Effects on Human Colon Cancer Cells. *J. Agric. Food Chem.* **2010**, *58*, 10869–10875. [CrossRef] [PubMed]
65. Teng, B.-s.; Lu, Y.-H.; Wang, Z.-T.; Tao, X.-Y.; Wei, D.-Z. In vitro anti-tumor activity of isorhamnetin isolated from *Hippophae rhamnoides* L. against BEL-7402 cells. *Pharmacol. Res.* **2006**, *54*, 186–194. [CrossRef] [PubMed]
66. Yang, J.H.; Shin, B.Y.; Han, J.Y.; Kim, M.G.; Wi, J.E.; Kim, Y.W.; Cho, I.J.; Kim, S.C.; Shin, S.M.; Ki, S.H. Isorhamnetin protects against oxidative stress by activating Nrf2 and inducing the expression of its target genes. *Toxicol. Appl. Pharmacol.* **2014**, *274*, 293–301. [CrossRef]
67. Gong, G.; Guan, Y.-Y.; Zhang, Z.-L.; Rahman, K.; Wang, S.-J.; Zhou, S.; Luan, X.; Zhang, H. Isorhamnetin: A review of pharmacological effects. *Biomed. Pharmacother.* **2020**, *128*, 110301. [CrossRef]
68. Milanezi, F.G.; Meireles, L.M.; de Christo Scherer, M.M.; de Oliveira, J.P.; da Silva, A.R.; de Araujo, M.L.; Endringer, D.C.; Fronza, M.; Guimarães, M.C.C.; Scherer, R. Antioxidant, antimicrobial and cytotoxic activities of gold nanoparticles capped with quercetin. *Saudi Pharm. J.* **2019**, *27*, 968–974. [CrossRef]
69. Ferenczyova, K.; Kalocayova, B.; Bartekova, M. Potential Implications of Quercetin and its Derivatives in Cardioprotection. *Int. J. Mol. Sci.* **2020**, *21*, 1585. [CrossRef]
70. Almatroodi, S.A.; Alsahli, M.A.; Almatroudi, A.; Verma, A.K.; Aloliqi, A.; Allemailem, K.S.; Khan, A.A.; Rahmani, A.H. Potential Therapeutic Targets of Quercetin, a Plant Flavonol, and Its Role in the Therapy of Various Types of Cancer through the Modulation of Various Cell Signaling Pathways. *Molecules* **2021**, *26*, 1315. [CrossRef]
71. Li, H.; Xiao, L.; He, H.; Zeng, H.; Liu, J.; Jiang, C.; Mei, G.; Yu, J.; Chen, H.; Yao, P.; et al. Quercetin Attenuates Atherosclerotic Inflammation by Inhibiting Galectin-3-NLRP3 Signaling Pathway. *Mol. Nutr. Food Res.* **2021**, *65*, 2000746. [CrossRef]
72. Boots, A.W.; Drent, M.; de Boer, V.C.J.; Bast, A.; Haenen, G.R.M.M. Quercetin reduces markers of oxidative stress and inflammation in sarcoidosis. *Clin. Nutr.* **2011**, *30*, 506–512. [CrossRef]
73. Chen, S.; Jiang, H.; Wu, X.; Fang, J. Therapeutic Effects of Quercetin on Inflammation, Obesity, and Type 2 Diabetes. *Mediat. Inflamm.* **2016**, *2016*, 9340637. [CrossRef] [PubMed]
74. Zhang, Y.; Chen, A.Y.; Li, M.; Chen, C.; Yao, Q. *Ginkgo biloba* Extract Kaempferol Inhibits Cell Proliferation and Induces Apoptosis in Pancreatic Cancer Cells. *J. Surg. Res.* **2008**, *148*, 17–23. [CrossRef] [PubMed]
75. García-Mediavilla, V.; Crespo, I.; Collado, P.S.; Esteller, A.; Sánchez-Campos, S.; Tuñón, M.J.; González-Gallego, J. The anti-inflammatory flavones quercetin and kaempferol cause inhibition of inducible nitric oxide synthase, cyclooxygenase-2 and reactive C-protein, and down-regulation of the nuclear factor kappaB pathway in Chang Liver cells. *Eur. J. Pharmacol.* **2007**, *557*, 221–229. [CrossRef] [PubMed]
76. Pan, X.; Liu, X.; Zhao, H.; Wu, B.; Liu, G. Antioxidant, anti-inflammatory and neuroprotective effect of kaempferol on rotenone-induced Parkinson's disease model of rats and SH-S5Y5 cells by preventing loss of tyrosine hydroxylase. *J. Funct. Foods* **2020**, *74*, 104140. [CrossRef]
77. Suchal, K.; Malik, S.; Khan, S.I.; Malhotra, R.K.; Goyal, S.N.; Bhatia, J.; Ojha, S.; Arya, D.S. Molecular Pathways Involved in the Amelioration of Myocardial Injury in Diabetic Rats by Kaempferol. *Int. J. Mol. Sci.* **2017**, *18*, 1001. [CrossRef] [PubMed]
78. Zhou, M.; Ren, H.; Han, J.; Wang, W.; Zheng, Q.; Wang, D. Protective Effects of Kaempferol against Myocardial Ischemia/Reperfusion Injury in Isolated Rat Heart via Antioxidant Activity and Inhibition of Glycogen Synthase Kinase-3. *Oxid. Med. Cell. Longev.* **2015**, *2015*, 481405. [CrossRef]
79. Shukla, R.; Pandey, V.; Vadnere, G.P.; Lodhi, S. Chapter 18—Role of Flavonoids in Management of Inflammatory Disorders. In *Bioactive Food as Dietary Interventions for Arthritis and Related Inflammatory Diseases*, 2nd ed.; Watson, R.R., Preedy, V.R., Eds.; Academic Press: Cambridge, MA, USA, 2019; pp. 293–322.
80. Sathya, S.; Pandima Devi, K. Chapter 15—The Use of Polyphenols for the Treatment of Alzheimer's Disease. In *Role of the Mediterranean Diet in the Brain and Neurodegenerative Diseases*; Farooqui, T., Farooqui, A.A., Eds.; Academic Press: Cambridge, MA, USA, 2018; pp. 239–252.

81. Luo, Y.; Shang, P.; Li, D. Luteolin: A Flavonoid that Has Multiple Cardio-Protective Effects and Its Molecular Mechanisms. *Front. Pharmacol.* **2017**, *8*, 692. [CrossRef]
82. Trebaticka, J.; Ďuračková, Z. Psychiatric disorders and polyphenols: Can they be helpful in therapy? *Oxid. Med. Cell. Longev.* **2015**, *2015*, 248529. [CrossRef]
83. Choudhary, S.; Kumar, P.; Malik, J.J.P.R. Plants and phytochemicals for Huntington's disease. *Pharmacogn. Rev.* **2013**, *7*, 81.
84. Saini, A.S.; Taliyan, R.; Sharma, P.L. Protective effect and mechanism of *Ginkgo biloba* extract-EGb 761 on STZ-induced diabetic cardiomyopathy in rats. *Pharmacogn. Mag.* **2014**, *10*, 172. [CrossRef]
85. Wang, L.; Bai, Y.; Wang, B.; Cui, H.; Wu, H.; Lv, J.-R.; Mei, Y.; Zhang, J.-S.; Liu, S.; Qi, L.-W. Suppression of experimental abdominal aortic aneurysms in the mice by treatment with *Ginkgo biloba* extract (EGb 761). *J. Ethnopharmacol.* **2013**, *150*, 308–315. [CrossRef] [PubMed]
86. Wang, A.; Yang, Q.; Li, Q.; Wang, X.; Hao, S.; Wang, J.; Ren, M. *Ginkgo biloba* L. extract reduces H_2O_2-induced bone marrow mesenchymal stem cells cytotoxicity by regulating mitogen-activated protein kinase (MAPK) signaling pathways and oxidative stress. *Med. Sci. Monit.* **2018**, *24*, 3159. [CrossRef] [PubMed]
87. Wang, C.; Wang, B. *Ginkgo biloba* extract attenuates oxidative stress and apoptosis in mouse cochlear neural stem cells. *Phytotherapy Res.* **2016**, *30*, 774–780. [CrossRef] [PubMed]
88. Kaur, S.; Sharma, N.; Nehru, B. Anti-inflammatory effects of *Ginkgo biloba* extract against trimethyltin-induced hippocampal neuronal injury. *Inflammopharmacology* **2018**, *26*, 87–104. [CrossRef]
89. Zuo, W.; Yan, F.; Zhang, B.; Li, J.; Mei, D. Advances in the Studies of *Ginkgo biloba* Leaves Extract on Aging-Related Diseases. *Aging Dis.* **2017**, *8*, 812–826. [CrossRef]
90. Rhein, V.; Giese, M.; Baysang, G.; Meier, F.; Rao, S.; Schulz, K.L.; Hamburger, M.; Eckert, A. *Ginkgo biloba* extract ameliorates oxidative phosphorylation performance and rescues Aβ-induced failure. *PLoS ONE* **2010**, *5*, e12359. [CrossRef]
91. Eckert, A.; Keil, U.; Scherping, I.; Hauptmann, S.; Müller, W.E. Stabilization of mitochondrial membrane potential and improvement of neuronal energy metabolism by *Ginkgo biloba* extract EGb 761. *Ann. N. Y. Acad. Sci.* **2005**, *1056*, 474–485. [CrossRef]
92. Shi, C.; Xiao, S.; Liu, J.; Guo, K.; Wu, F.; Yew, D.T.; Xu, J. *Ginkgo biloba* extract EGb761 protects against aging-associated mitochondrial dysfunction in platelets and hippocampi of SAMP8 mice. *Platelets* **2010**, *21*, 373–379. [CrossRef]
93. Schindowski, K.; Leutner, S.; Kressmann, S.; Eckert, A.; Müller, W.E. Age-related increase of oxidative stress-induced apoptosis in micePrevention by *Ginkgo biloba* extract (EGb761). *J. Neural Transm.* **2001**, *108*, 969–978. [CrossRef]
94. Longpré, F.; Garneau, P.; Ramassamy, C. Protection by EGb 761 against β-amyloid-induced neurotoxicity: Involvement of NF-κB, SIRT1, and MAPKs pathways and inhibition of amyloid fibril formation. *Free Radic. Biol. Med.* **2006**, *41*, 1781–1794. [CrossRef]
95. You, O.H.; Kim, S.-H.; Kim, B.; Sohn, E.J.; Lee, H.-J.; Shim, B.-S.; Yun, M.; Kwon, B.-M.; Kim, S.-H. Ginkgetin induces apoptosis via activation of caspase and inhibition of survival genes in PC-3 prostate cancer cells. *Bioorg. Med. Chem. Lett.* **2013**, *23*, 2692–2695. [CrossRef] [PubMed]
96. Wang, J.; Chen, X.; Bai, W.; Wang, Z.; Xiao, W.; Zhu, J. Study on Mechanism of *Ginkgo biloba* L. Leaves for the Treatment of Neurodegenerative Diseases Based on Network Pharmacology. *Neurochem. Res.* **2021**, *46*, 1881–1894. [CrossRef] [PubMed]
97. Suliman, N.A.; Mat Taib, C.N.; Mohd Moklas, M.A.; Adenan, M.I.; Hidayat Baharuldin, M.T.; Basir, R. Establishing Natural Nootropics: Recent Molecular Enhancement Influenced by Natural Nootropic. *Evid.-Based Complement. Altern. Med. Ecam* **2016**, *2016*, 4391375. [CrossRef]
98. Rendeiro, C.; Guerreiro, J.D.; Williams, C.M.; Spencer, J.P. Flavonoids as modulators of memory and learning: Molecular interactions resulting in behavioural effects. *Proc. Nutr. Soc.* **2012**, *71*, 246–262. [CrossRef] [PubMed]
99. Matthews, B.R. Memory dysfunction. *Continuum* **2015**, *21*, 613–626. [CrossRef] [PubMed]
100. Butler, R.; Radhakrishnan, R. Dementia. *BMJ Clin. Evid.* **2012**, *2012*, 1001.
101. Raz, L.; Knoefel, J.; Bhaskar, K. The neuropathology and cerebrovascular mechanisms of dementia. *J. Cereb. Blood Flow Metab. Off. J. Int. Soc. Cereb. Blood Flow Metab.* **2016**, *36*, 172–186. [CrossRef]
102. Weinmann, S.; Roll, S.; Schwarzbach, C.; Vauth, C.; Willich, S.N. Effects of *Ginkgo biloba* in dementia: Systematic review and meta-analysis. *BMC Geriatr.* **2010**, *10*, 14. [CrossRef]
103. Ton, A.M.M.; Campagnaro, B.P.; Alves, G.A.; Aires, R.; Côco, L.Z.; Arpini, C.M.; Guerra, E.O.T.; Campos-Toimil, M.; Meyrelles, S.S.; Pereira, T.M.C.; et al. Oxidative Stress and Dementia in Alzheimer's Patients: Effects of Synbiotic Supplementation. *Oxid. Med. Cell. Longev.* **2020**, *2020*, 2638703. [CrossRef]
104. Lopez, O.L.; Chang, Y.; Ives, D.G.; Snitz, B.E.; Fitzpatrick, A.L.; Carlson, M.C.; Rapp, S.R.; Williamson, J.D.; Tracy, R.P.; DeKosky, S.T.; et al. Blood amyloid levels and risk of dementia in the Ginkgo Evaluation of Memory Study (GEMS): A longitudinal analysis. *Alzheimer's Dement. J. Alzheimer's Assoc.* **2019**, *15*, 1029–1038. [CrossRef]
105. Li, F.; Harmer, P.; Voit, J.; Chou, L.S. Implementing an Online Virtual Falls Prevention Intervention during a Public Health Pandemic for Older Adults with Mild Cognitive Impairment: A Feasibility Trial. *Clin. Interv. Aging* **2021**, *16*, 973–983. [CrossRef] [PubMed]
106. do Rosario, V.A.; Fitzgerald, Z.; Broyd, S.; Paterson, A.; Roodenrys, S.; Thomas, S.; Bliokas, V.; Potter, J.; Walton, K.; Weston-Green, K.; et al. Food anthocyanins decrease concentrations of TNF-α in older adults with mild cognitive impairment: A randomized, controlled, double blind clinical trial. *Nutr. Metab. Cardiovasc. Dis. NMCD* **2021**, *31*, 950–960. [CrossRef] [PubMed]

107. Kandiah, N.; Ong, P.A.; Yuda, T.; Ng, L.L.; Mamun, K.; Merchant, R.A.; Chen, C.; Dominguez, J.; Marasigan, S.; Ampil, J.; et al. Treatment of dementia and mild cognitive impairment with or without cerebrovascular disease: Expert consensus on the use of *Ginkgo biloba* extract, EGb 761®. *CNS Neurosci. Ther.* **2019**, *25*, 288–298. [CrossRef] [PubMed]
108. Zhang, H.-F.; Huang, L.-B.; Zhong, Y.-B.; Zhou, Q.-H.; Wang, H.-L.; Zheng, G.-Q.; Lin, Y. An overview of systematic reviews of *Ginkgo biloba* extracts for mild cognitive impairment and dementia. *Front. Aging Neurosci.* **2016**, *8*, 276. [CrossRef]
109. Dong, Z.H.; Zhang, C.Y.; Pu, B.H. Effects of *Ginkgo biloba* tablet in treating mild cognitive impairment. *Zhongguo Zhong Xi Yi Jie He Za Zhi Zhongguo Zhongxiyi Jiehe Zazhi Chin. J. Integr. Tradit. West. Med.* **2012**, *32*, 1208–1211.
110. Gregory, J.; Vengalasetti, Y.V.; Bredesen, D.E.; Rao, R.V. Neuroprotective Herbs for the Management of Alzheimer's Disease. *Biomolecules* **2021**, *11*, 543. [CrossRef]
111. Liu, J.; Hlávka, J.; Hillestad, R.J.; Mattke, S. *Assessing the Preparedness of the US Health Care System Infrastructure for an Alzheimer's Treatment*; RAND: Santa Monica, CA, USA, 2017.
112. Kim, E.; Otgontenger, U.; Jamsranjav, A.; Kim, S.S. Deleterious Alteration of Glia in the Brain of Alzheimer's Disease. *Int. J. Mol. Sci.* **2020**, *21*, 6676. [CrossRef]
113. Zuin, M.; Cervellati, C.; Trentini, A.; Passaro, A.; Rosta, V.; Zimetti, F.; Zuliani, G. Association between Serum Concentrations of Apolipoprotein A-I (ApoA-I) and Alzheimer's Disease: Systematic Review and Meta-Analysis. *Diagnostics* **2021**, *11*, 984. [CrossRef]
114. Chen, X.; Drew, J.; Berney, W.; Lei, W. Neuroprotective Natural Products for Alzheimer's Disease. *Cells* **2021**, *10*, 1309. [CrossRef]
115. D'Mello, S.R. When Good Kinases Go Rogue: GSK3, p38 MAPK and CDKs as Therapeutic Targets for Alzheimer's and Huntington's Disease. *Int. J. Mol. Sci.* **2021**, *22*, 5911. [CrossRef]
116. Gallardo, G.; Holtzman, D.M. Amyloid-β and Tau at the Crossroads of Alzheimer's Disease. *Tau Biol.* **2019**, *1184*, 187–203.
117. De Strooper, B.; Karran, E. The cellular phase of Alzheimer's disease. *Cell* **2016**, *164*, 603–615. [CrossRef] [PubMed]
118. Giovannini, M.G.; Lana, D.; Traini, C.; Vannucchi, M.G. The Microbiota-Gut-Brain Axis and Alzheimer Disease. From Dysbiosis to Neurodegeneration: Focus on the Central Nervous System Glial Cells. *J. Clin. Med.* **2021**, *10*, 2358. [CrossRef]
119. Onyango, I.G.; Jauregui, G.V.; Čarná, M.; Bennett, J.P., Jr.; Stokin, G.B. Neuroinflammation in Alzheimer's Disease. *Biomedicines* **2021**, *9*, 524. [CrossRef] [PubMed]
120. Arslan, J.; Jamshed, H.; Qureshi, H. Early Detection and Prevention of Alzheimer's Disease: Role of Oxidative Markers and Natural Antioxidants. *Front. Aging Neurosci.* **2020**, *12*, 231. [CrossRef]
121. Smith, J.; Luo, Y. Studies on molecular mechanisms of *Ginkgo biloba* extract. *Appl. Microbiol. Biotechnol.* **2004**, *64*, 465–472.
122. Yao, Z.-x.; Drieu, K.; Papadopoulos, V. The *Ginkgo biloba* extract EGb 761 rescues the PC12 neuronal cells from β-amyloid-induced cell death by inhibiting the formation of β-amyloid-derived diffusible neurotoxic ligands. *Brain Res.* **2001**, *889*, 181–190. [CrossRef]
123. Gong, Q.-H.; Wu, Q.; Huang, X.-N.; Sun, A.-S.; Nie, J.; Shi, J.-S. Protective effect of *Ginkgo biloba* leaf extract on learning and memory deficit induced by aluminum in model rats. *Chin. J. Integr. Med.* **2006**, *12*, 37–41.
124. Liao, Z.; Cheng, L.; Li, X.; Zhang, M.; Wang, S.; Huo, R. Meta-analysis of *Ginkgo biloba* Preparation for the Treatment of Alzheimer's Disease. *Clin. Neuropharmacol.* **2020**, *43*, 93–99. [CrossRef]
125. Shi, C.; Zhao, L.; Zhu, B.; Li, Q.; Yew, D.T.; Yao, Z.; Xu, J. Protective effects of *Ginkgo biloba* extract (EGb761) and its constituents quercetin and ginkgolide B against β-amyloid peptide-induced toxicity in SH-SY5Y cells. *Chem. Interact.* **2009**, *181*, 115–123. [CrossRef]
126. Yao, Z.-X.; Han, Z.; Drieu, K.; Papadopoulos, V. *Ginkgo biloba* extract (Egb 761) inhibits β-amyloid production by lowering free cholesterol levels. *J. Nutr. Biochem.* **2004**, *15*, 749–756. [CrossRef] [PubMed]
127. Carrizzo, A.; Moltedo, O.; Damato, A.; Martinello, K.; Di Pietro, P.; Oliveti, M.; Acernese, F.; Giugliano, G.; Izzo, R.; Sommella, E.; et al. New Nutraceutical Combination Reduces Blood Pressure and Improves Exercise Capacity in Hypertensive Patients via a Nitric Oxide-Dependent Mechanism. *J. Am. Heart Assoc.* **2020**, *9*, e014923. [CrossRef] [PubMed]
128. Ramassamy, C. Emerging role of polyphenolic compounds in the treatment of neurodegenerative diseases: A review of their intracellular targets. *Eur. J. Pharmacol.* **2006**, *545*, 51–64. [CrossRef] [PubMed]
129. Tofano, R.J.; Pescinni-Salzedas, L.M.; Chagas, E.F.B.; Detregiachi, C.R.P.; Guiguer, E.L.; Araujo, A.C.; Bechara, M.D.; Rubira, C.J.; Barbalho, S.M. Association of Metabolic Syndrome and Hyperferritinemia in Patients at Cardiovascular Risk. *Diabetes Metab. Syndr. Obesity Targets Ther.* **2020**, *13*, 3239. [CrossRef] [PubMed]
130. Yarmohammadi, F.; Ghasemzadeh Rahbardar, M.; Hosseinzadeh, H. Effect of eggplant (*Solanum melongena*) on the metabolic syndrome: A review. *Iran. J. Basic Med. Sci.* **2021**, *24*, 420–427. [CrossRef]
131. Priyanka, A.; Sindhu, G.; Shyni, G.; Rani, M.P.; Nisha, V.; Raghu, K. Bilobalide abates inflammation, insulin resistance and secretion of angiogenic factors induced by hypoxia in 3T3-L1 adipocytes by controlling NF-κB and JNK activation. *Int. Immunopharmacol.* **2017**, *42*, 209–217. [CrossRef]
132. An, X.F.; Zhao, Y.; Yu, J.Y. Treatment of Early Diabetic Retinopathy by Liuwei Dihuang Pill Combined Ginkao Leaf Tablet. *Chin. J. Integr. Tradit. West. Med.* **2016**, *36*, 674–677.
133. Tanaka, S.; Han, L.-K.; Zheng, Y.-N.; Okuda, H. Effects of the flavonoid fraction from *Ginkgo biloba* extract on the postprandial blood glucose elevation in rats. *Yakugaku Zasshi* **2004**, *124*, 605–611. [CrossRef]
134. Hussein, A.A.; Assad, H.C.; Rabeea, I.S. Research. Antihyperlipidemic, Antioxidant and Anti-Inflammatory Effects of *Ginkgo biloba* in High Cholesterol Fed Rabbits. *J. Pharm. Sci. Res.* **2017**, *9*, 2163–2167.

135. Hirata, B.K.S.; Banin, R.M.; Dornellas, A.P.S.; de Andrade, I.S.; Zemdegs, J.C.S.; Caperuto, L.C.; Oyama, L.M.; Ribeiro, E.B.; Telles, M.M. *Ginkgo biloba* extract improves insulin signaling and attenuates inflammation in retroperitoneal adipose tissue depot of obese rats. *Mediat. Inflamm.* **2015**, *2015*, 419106. [CrossRef]
136. Shinozuka, K.; Umegaki, K.; Kubota, Y.; Tanaka, N.; Mizuno, H.; Yamauchi, J.; Nakamura, K.; Kunitomo, M. Feeding of *Ginkgo biloba* extract (GBE) enhances gene expression of hepatic cytochrome P-450 and attenuates the hypotensive effect of nicardipine in rats. *Life Sci.* **2002**, *70*, 2783–2792. [CrossRef]
137. Li, Y.; Xu, C.; Wang, H.; Liu, X.; Jiang, L.; Liang, S.; Wu, Z.; Wang, Z.; Zhou, J.; Xiao, W.; et al. Systems pharmacology reveals the multi-level synergetic mechanism of action of *Ginkgo biloba* L. leaves for cardiomyopathy treatment. *J. Ethnopharmacol.* **2021**, *264*, 113279. [CrossRef] [PubMed]
138. Tan, D.; Wu, J.; Duan, X.; Cui, Y.; Liu, S.; Jing, Z. Efficacy and safety of ginkgo injections in the treatment of angina pectoris caused by coronary heart disease in China: A network Meta-analysis and systematic review. *J. Tradit. Chin. Med. Chung I Tsa Chih Ying Wen Pan* **2019**, *39*, 285–296. [PubMed]
139. Li, X.; Lu, L.; Chen, J.; Zhang, C.; Chen, H.; Huang, H. New Insight into the Mechanisms of *Ginkgo biloba* Extract in Vascular Aging Prevention. *Curr. Vasc. Pharmacol.* **2020**, *18*, 334–345. [CrossRef] [PubMed]
140. Liu, Y.; Weng, W.; Gao, R.; Liu, Y. New Insights for Cellular and Molecular Mechanisms of Aging and Aging-Related Diseases: Herbal Medicine as Potential Therapeutic Approach. *Oxid. Med. Cell. Longev.* **2019**, *2019*, 4598167. [CrossRef]
141. Zhang, H.; Luo, Y.-P.; Cao, Z.-Y.; Zhang, X.-Z.; Cao, L.; Wang, Z.-Z.; Xiao, W. Effect of compatibility of ginkgolide A, ginkgolide B and ginkgolide K. *J. Pharm. Biomed. Anal.* **2018**, *43*, 1410–1415.
142. Lu, X.; Chen, L.; Liu, T.; Ke, H.; Gong, X.; Wang, Q.; Zhang, J.; Fan, X. Chemical analysis, pharmacological activity and process optimization of the proportion of bilobalide and ginkgolides in *Ginkgo biloba* extract. *J. Pharm. Biomed. Anal.* **2018**, *160*, 46–54.
143. Mei, N.; Guo, X.; Ren, Z.; Kobayashi, D.; Wada, K.; Guo, L. Review of *Ginkgo biloba*-induced toxicity, from experimental studies to human case reports. *J. Environ. Sci. Health Part C* **2017**, *35*, 1–28. [CrossRef]
144. Mahady, G.B. *Ginkgo biloba*: A review of quality, safety, and efficacy. *Nutr. Clin. Care* **2001**, *4*, 140–147. [CrossRef]
145. McKenna, D.J.; Jones, K.; Hughes, K. Efficacy, safety, and use of *Ginkgo biloba* in clinical and preclinical applications. *Altern. Ther. Health Med.* **2001**, *7*, 70.

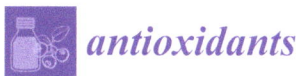

Systematic Review

Walnut Intake Interventions Targeting Biomarkers of Metabolic Syndrome and Inflammation in Middle-Aged and Older Adults: A Systematic Review and Meta-Analysis of Randomized Controlled Trials

Letiția Mateș [1], Daniela-Saveta Popa [1,*], Marius Emil Rusu [2,*], Ionel Fizeșan [1] and Daniel Leucuța [3]

[1] Department of Toxicology, Faculty of Pharmacy, Iuliu Hatieganu University of Medicine and Pharmacy, 8 Victor Babes, 400012 Cluj-Napoca, Romania; micu.letitia@umfcluj.ro (L.M.); ionel.fizesan@umfcluj.ro (I.F.)
[2] Department of Pharmaceutical Technology and Biopharmaceutics, Faculty of Pharmacy, Iuliu Hatieganu University of Medicine and Pharmacy, 8 Victor Babes, 400012 Cluj-Napoca, Romania
[3] Department of Medical Informatics and Biostatistics, Faculty of Medicine, Iuliu Hatieganu University of Medicine and Pharmacy, 8 Victor Babes, 400012 Cluj-Napoca, Romania; dleucuta@umfcluj.ro (D.L.)
* Correspondence: dpopa@umfcluj.ro (D.-S.P.); rusu.marius@umfcluj.ro (M.E.R.); Tel.: +40-264-450-555 (D.-S.P.)

Abstract: Biomarkers of metabolic syndrome and inflammation are pathophysiological predictors and factors of senescence and age-related diseases. Recent evidence showed that particular diet components, such as walnuts rich in antioxidant bioactive compounds and with a balanced lipid profile, could have positive outcomes on human health. A systematic search in PubMed, EMBASE, Cochrane Library, Scopus, and ClinicalTrials.gov databases was performed to retrieve randomized controlled trials published from the beginning of each database through November 2021, reporting on the outcomes of walnut consumption over 22 metabolic syndrome and inflammatory markers in middle-aged and older adults. The search strategy rendered 17 studies in the final selection, including 11 crossover and 6 parallel trials. The study revealed that walnut-enriched diets had statistically significant decreasing effects for triglyceride, total cholesterol, and LDL cholesterol concentrations on some inflammatory markers and presented no consequences on anthropometric and glycemic parameters. Although further studies and better-designed ones are needed to strengthen these findings, the results emphasize the benefits of including walnuts in the dietary plans of this age group.

Keywords: nuts; tree nuts; nut consumption; aging; age-related diseases; cardiometabolic markers; antioxidants; inflammation; lipid profile; diabetes

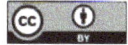

1. Introduction

Metabolic syndrome (MetS) conditions, chronic, low-grade inflammation, and oxidative stress are significant risk factors for morbidity and mortality with higher prevalence in the aging population [1]. These pathophysiological components increase the probability of age-associated diseases, including cardiovascular disease (CVD), type 2 diabetes (T2D), cognitive impairment, neurodegenerative disorders, or cancer [2,3]. Compelling evidence demonstrates that inflammatory markers, such as serum C-reactive protein (CRP), tumor necrosis factor-alpha (TNF-α), interleukin-1β (IL-1β), interleukin-6 (IL-6), intercellular adhesion molecule-1 (ICAM-1), and vascular cell adhesion molecule-1 (VCAM-1), are predictors and factors in cellular senescence and chronic inflammatory conditions [4].

Human and animal examinations suggested that plant matrices rich in antioxidant and anti-inflammatory compounds could prove efficient in protecting against oxidative stress and excessive inflammation [5–8]. Extensive research examined the effects of plant-based diets on various health outcomes [9,10]. Tree nuts, important plant nutrient sources, are rich in monounsaturated fatty acids (MUFAs) and polyunsaturated fatty acids (PUFAs), tocols, phytosterols, and polyphenols, essential bioactive phytochemicals with demonstrated antioxidant properties [11]. Several studies consistently showed the antioxidant activity and anti-inflammation potential of the active compounds from tree nut kernels or by-products and their association with a reduced risk for CVD, T2D, cancer, and all-cause mortality [12–15]. Of the different types of nuts, walnuts are especially rich in linoleic acid (18:2n–6), α-linolenic acid (ALA) (18:3n–3), polyphenols, L-arginine, and magnesium [16], a unique phytochemical profile responsible for many beneficial effects. It was suggested that walnuts might modulate neuroplasticity, neuroprotection, and vasodilation of brain arteries [17] or decrease cancer growth, reduce metastasis, and increase cancer cell death via altering tumor gene expression [18].

Several studies have previously linked walnut intake with lipid profile beneficial effects and lowering of reactive oxygen species (ROS) and inflammatory markers in different age groups [19–21].

Contrary to the above results, a recent meta-analysis found no associations between walnut consumption and glucose homeostasis as well as inflammation [22]. Moreover, increasing dietary ALA intake did not affect inflammatory markers [23].

Based on these conflicting conclusions, we aimed to perform a systematic review and meta-analysis of randomized controlled trials (RCTs) to thoroughly assess the data concerning the effects of walnut intake on selected markers of inflammation and metabolic syndrome in mature adults. As the exact etiology of chronic inflammation and its potential causal function in unfavorable health outcomes are mostly unknown, research on markers of inflammation and the identification of pathways to control age-associated inflammation is of great relevance for the prevention of inflammation and management of age-associated diseases. To the best of our knowledge, this is the first meta-analysis conducted on the impact of walnut consumption on markers of inflammation and metabolic syndrome in middle-aged and older adults.

2. Materials and Methods

The current meta-analysis was performed following the PRISMA criteria guidelines [24]. The registration code is INPLASY202260058, with DOI 10.37766/inplasy2022.6.0058, https://inplasy.com/inplasy-2022-6-0058/ (accessed on 13 June 2022).

2.1. Eligibility Criteria

Our systematic review included (1) randomized controlled parallel or crossover trial studies that compared the effect of (2) walnuts consumption, (3) with a minimum 3-week intervention period in (4) middle-aged and older adults ($\geq$40 years of age or mean age $\geq$ 50 years), (5.a) on MetS biomarkers, including waist circumference (WC), body weight (BW), body mass index (BMI), systolic blood pressure (SBP), diastolic blood pressure (DBP), triglyceride (TG), total cholesterol (TC), high-density lipoprotein (HDL) cholesterol (HDL-C), low-density lipoprotein (LDL) cholesterol (LDL-C), fasting blood glucose (FBG), and glycosylated hemoglobin A1c (HbA1c), as well as on the insulin resistance index (homeostatic model assessment for insulin resistance (HOMA-IR) and insulin), and on (5.b) inflammatory biomarkers, including C-reactive protein (CRP), high-sensitivity C-reactive protein (hs-CRP), interferon gamma (IFN-γ), E-selectin, VCAM-1, ICAM-1, TNF-α, and interleukins (IL-6 and IL-1β), as primary or secondary outcomes. We excluded: (1) abstracts, narrative reviews, comments, opinions, methodological papers, editorials, letters, observational studies, conference abstracts, case studies, in vitro studies, non-human, with a mechanistic, non-stochastic modeling, or any other publications lacking primary data and/or explicit method explanations; (2) irrelevant interventions (walnuts oil, walnut extract, nut mix); (3) irrelevant comparisons (compulsory comparison); (4) publications with full text not available; (5) duplicate studies or databases; and (6) publications in languages that were not known.

2.2. Information Sources

We performed a systematic literature search in PubMed, EMBASE, Cochrane Library, Scopus, and ClinicalTrials.gov databases for controlled trials describing the effects of walnut consumption on metabolic syndrome and inflammatory biomarkers in mature adults from the inception of each database through November 2021. The literature search had no language constraint. To ensure thorough research, the bibliographies of the included studies and current reviews were also screened.

2.3. Search Strategy

To search the databases, we used a combination of free-text words, along with their synonyms, singular and plural forms, thesaurus words (Medical Subject Headings for PubMed, and Emtree for EMBASE), and abbreviations concerning the following concepts: (1) walnuts; (2) inflammatory biomarkers, C-reactive protein, interleukins, tumor necrosis factor, vascular cell adhesion molecule, intercellular adhesion molecule, selectin, adiponectin, adhesion molecules; (3) metabolic syndrome, waist circumference, weight, body mass index, systolic and diastolic blood pressure, triglycerides, total, HDL-C and LDL-C, glycemia, HbA1c, insulin resistance, HOMA-IR, insulin; and (4) randomized controlled trial. The entire search strategy for each database is presented in Supplementary Table S1.

2.4. Selection Process

Three investigators (D.L., L.M., and D.-S.P.) independently checked the titles and abstracts for relevant articles. Following that, the full texts of those that looked to satisfy the selection criteria were retrieved for further selection. The same investigators independently checked each full text. In the event of a disagreement, the studies were debated until a consensus was reached. In the instance of multiple publications from the same trial, only the most recent or informative article was selected.

2.5. Data Items

Data regarding the outcomes were extracted in a spreadsheet Microsoft (Microsoft Office 365, MS, Redmond, WA, USA) Excel file: (1) inflammatory biomarkers, C-reactive protein, interleukins, tumor necrosis factor, vascular cell adhesion molecule, intercellular adhesion molecule, selectin, adiponectin, adhesion molecules; (2) metabolic syndrome, waist circumference, weight, body mass index, systolic and diastolic blood pressure, triglycerides, total, HDL and LDL cholesterol, glycemia, HbA1c, insulin resistance, HOMA-IR, insulin. For each variable, the baseline, final, and differences between baseline and final observations were extracted, as well as the differences between the interventions regarding the final values or the differences between baseline and final observations.

Furthermore, data regarding study characteristics were extracted in a spreadsheet file: country, study design, exposure period, washout period, participants number in each group, health status, age, female percentage, walnut intervention quantity and type, control intervention, and the outcome of interest.

Other investigators than those who extracted the initial full-text articles rechecked the extracted data.

2.6. Study Risk of Bias Assessment

The risk of bias was assessed for each selected article using the Risk of Bias 2 Tool from Cochrane [25] in duplicate, and the disagreements were resolved by discussion.

2.7. Effect Measures

For all the outcomes, we used the standardized mean difference in the synthesis and presentation of results.

2.8. Synthesis Methods

We calculated the means and standard deviations for each variable utilized in the meta-analysis. When the standard deviation (SD) was not known, it was calculated using the standard error (SE) or mean, medians and interquartile ranges (IQRs), confidence intervals (CIs), or *p*-values, according to Cochrane Handbook recommendations [26]. The differences between the intervention groups in terms of changes (baseline–final values) were the preferred values in analyses. Otherwise, we computed the differences between the final values if these data were unavailable for the changes. We calculated the mean difference (between changes or between final values) and the SE for each trial, either parallel or crossover, in order to be able to pool the results from both designs, as recommended by Elbourne et al. [27]. The meta software was used to perform meta-analyses on these mean differences and SE [28]. The standardized mean difference along with 95% CI was computed for each variable, using the random effects model due to clinical heterogeneity between the trials. The Paule–Mandel estimator was used to estimate the between-study variance within the inverse variance method. The statistical heterogeneity between the studies was assessed with χ^2-based Q-test and I^2. Next, high leverage studies were identified with the dmeta package [29]. Furthermore, subgroup analyses were performed for risk of bias, trial design, exposure duration, walnut quantity, health status, control group, and age, in case more than ten studies were available. To assess the robustness of the results, a leave-one-out sensitivity analysis was used. If the *p*-value was less than 0.05, statistical significance was assumed. For all analyses, the R environment for statistical computing and graphics (R Foundation for Statistical Computing, Vienna, Austria) version 4.1.2 [30] was used.

2.9. Quality Assessment

We used the Cochrane Collaboration's Risk of Bias Tool 2 to examine the selected studies: the parallel trial version for the parallel studies and the crossover trial version for the crossover studies.

2.10. Reporting Bias Assessment

In case there were more than ten studies available to analyze a variable of interest, a funnel plot and the Egger test were performed to assess the presence of publication bias.

3. Results

A total of 685 articles were considered from the systematic search and review of relevant reference lists. After applying exclusion criteria, 17 articles were included in the systematic review and meta-analysis. The procedure of study inclusion and exclusion is shown in Figure 1. The characteristics of the included studies are revealed in Table 1 and Supplementary Table S2.

3.1. Metabolic Syndrome Biomarkers

The effects of walnut-enriched diets on the biomarkers of MetS and inflammation are presented in Table 2.

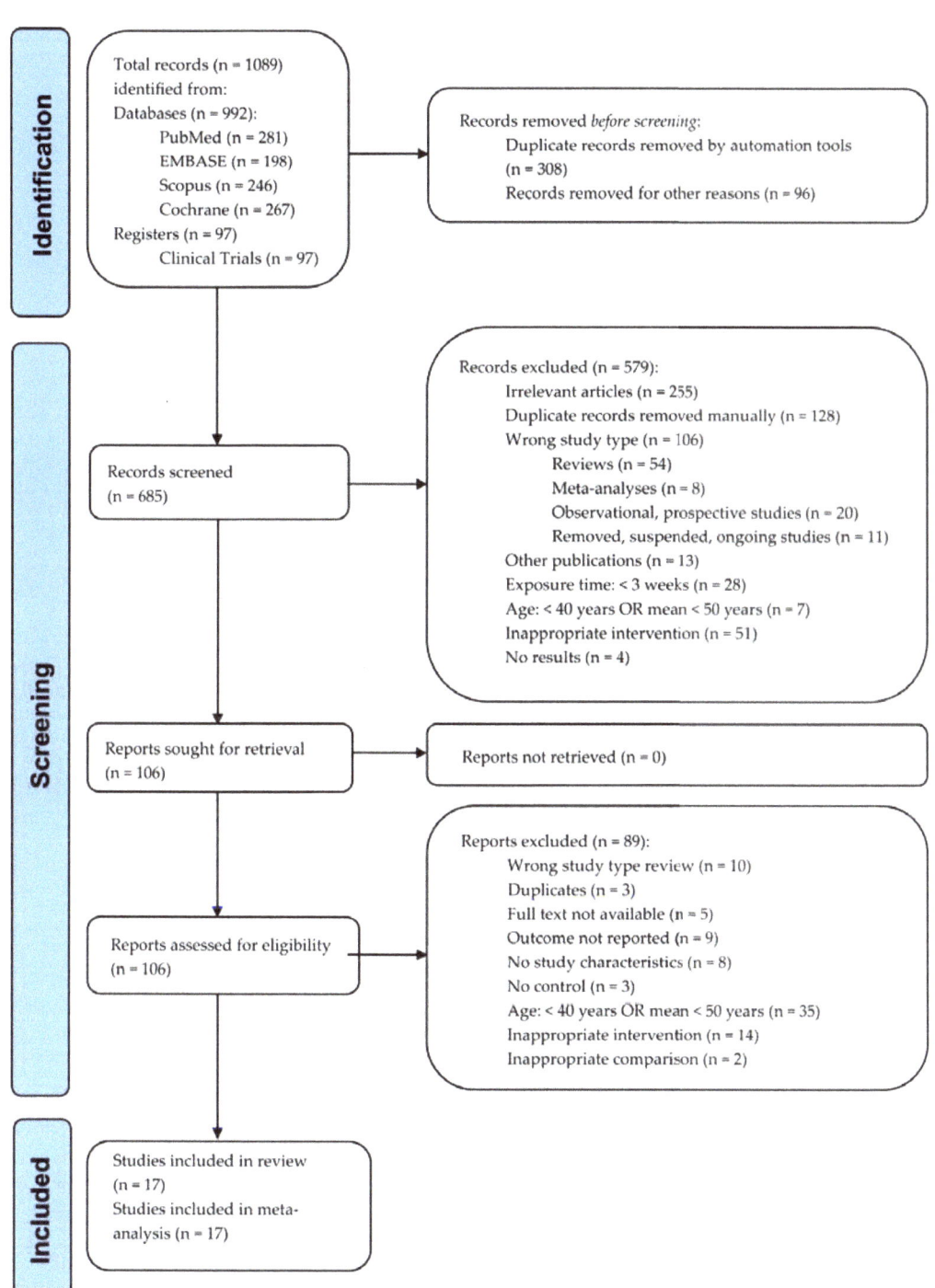

Figure 1. PRISMA flow diagram of study selection.

Table 1. Characteristics of the selected studies.

Reference	Country	Study (RCT) Design	Exposure Period	Washout Period	Participants (n), Health Status	Age (Years), (SD/IQR) (Range)	Female (%)	Walnut Intervention (g/d)	Control Intervention	Outcome of Interest
Zambón et al., 2000 [31]	Spain, USA	Crossover	6 weeks	0	49 polygenic hypercholesterolemia *	56 (±11)	47%	41–56 g/d (18% of the energy need)	MedD (no walnut)	BW, TC, LDL-C, HDL-C, TG
Ros et al., 2004 [32]	Spain	Crossover	4 weeks	0	20 healthy, non-smokers (hypercholesterolemia)	55 (±55.9)	60%	40–65 g/d (18% of energy need)	MedD (no walnut)	BW, SBP, DBP, TC, LDL-C, HDL-C, CRP,
Tapsell et al., 2004 [33]	Australia	Parallel	6 months	NA	58 T2D *	59.3 (±8.1)	41.37%	30 g/d—walnut-enriched modified low-fat diet	Modified low-fat diet (no walnuts)	BW, BMI, HbA1c, TC, LDL-C, HDL-C, TG
Olmedilla-Alonso et al., 2008 [34]	Spain	Crossover	5 weeks	1 month	25 CV risk, smokers	54.4 (±8.1)	40%	19.4 g/d (20% walnut-enriched meat products)	Restructured meat products (no walnut)	TC, HDL-C, LDL-C, TG, BW, SBP, DBP
Spaccarotella et al., 2008 [35]	USA	Crossover	8 weeks	2 weeks	21 healthy, non-smokers	65.9 (55–75)	0%	75 g/d (24% of energy need)	Western-type diet (no walnut)	SBP, DBP, TC, HDL-C, LDL-C
Tapsell et al., 2009 [36]	Australia	Parallel	1 year	NA	50 T2D *	54 (±8.7)	NI	30 g/d (walnut-enriched 2000 kcal diet, 30% fat)	2000 kcal diet, 30% fat (no walnut)	BW, FBG, TC, HDL-C, LDL-C, TG, HbA1c, insulin
Ma et al., 2010 [37]	USA	Crossover	8 weeks	8 weeks	21 T2D, non-smokers	58.1 (±9.2)	58.30%	56 g/d	Habitual diet (no walnut)	TC, HDL-C, LDL-C, TG, FPG, insulin, HOMA-IR, BW, BMI, WC, SBP, DBP
Torabian et al., 2010 [38]	USA	Crossover	6 months	0	87 healthy, non-smokers	54 (±10.2)	56%	28–64 g/d (12% of energy need)	Habitual diet (no walnut)	TC, LDL-C, HDL-C, TG
Canales et al., 2011 [39]	Spain	Crossover	5 weeks	4–6 weeks	22 CV risk, smokers	54.8 (±9.4)	40%	34–29 g/d (20% walnut-enriched meat)	Low-fat meat products (no walnut)	VCAM-1, ICAM-1, HDL-C
Katz et al., 2012 [40]	USA	Crossover	8 weeks	4 weeks	40 healthy, non-smokers (overweight, MetS risk)	57.4 (±11.9)	60.9%	56 g/d	Habitual diet (no walnut)	TC, HDL-C, LDL-C, TG, FPG, insulin, HOMA-IR, BW, BMI, WC, SBP, DBP
Wu et al., 2014 [41]	Germany, USA	Crossover	8 weeks	2 weeks	40 healthy *	60 (±6.32)	75%	43 g/d (replacing 30 g saturated fat in Western-type diet)	Western-type diet (no walnut)	TC, LDL-C, HDL-C, FBG, insulin, HOMA-IR, HbA1c, VCAM-1, ICAM-1
Bamberger et al., 2017 [42]	Germany	Crossover	8 weeks	4 weeks	194 healthy, non-smokers	63 (±7)	69%	43 g/d	Western-type diet (no walnut)	TC, LDL-C, HDL-C, TG
Bitok et al., 2018 [43]	USA, Spain	Parallel	2 years	NA	307 healthy *	69.4 (±3.9)	67%	28; 42; 56 g/d (15% of energy need)	Habitual diet (no walnut)	BW, WC
Domenech et al., 2019 [44]	USA, Spain	Parallel	2 years	NA	236 healthy * (60% mild hyper-tension)	68.8 (±3.3)	65%	30–60 g/d (15% of energy need)	Habitual diet (no walnut)	SBP, DBP

Table 1. Cont.

Reference	Country	Study (RCT) Design	Exposure Period	Washout Period	Participants (n), Health Status	Age (Years), (SD)/IQR (Range)	Female (%)	Walnut Intervention (g/d)	Control Intervention	Outcome of Interest
Sanchis et al., 2019 [45]	Spain	Crossover	30 days	30 days	13 CKD *	71 (±10.11)	46.20%	30 g/d (walnut-enriched CKD diet)	CKD patients' diet (no walnut)	BMI, TC, HDL-C, LDL-C, TG, FBG, HbA1c, CRP
Abdrabalnabi et al., 2020 [46]	USA, Spain	Parallel	2 years	NA	625 healthy *	69.1 (±3.6)	67%	30; 45; 60 g/d (15% of energy need)	Habitual diet (no walnut)	BMI, SBP, DBP, TG, HDL-C, FBG
Cofán et al., 2020 [47]	USA, Spain	Parallel	2 years	NA	634 healthy *	69.1 (±3.6)	66%	30; 45; 60 g/d (15% of energy need)	Western-type diet (no walnut)	VCAM-1, ICAM-1, IL-6, IFN-γ, IL-1β, TNF-α, E-selectin, hs-CRP

*—non-specified smoking status; RCT—randomized controlled trials; NA—not applicable; BMI—body mass index; BW—body weight; CKD—chronic kidney disease; CV—cardiovascular; CRP—C-reactive protein; hs-CRP—high-sensitivity C-reactive protein; DBP—diastolic blood pressure; FBG—fasting blood glucose; HbA1c—glycosylated hemoglobin A1c; HDL-C—high-density lipoprotein cholesterol; HOMA-IR—homeostatic model assessment for insulin resistance; ICAM—intercellular adhesion molecule; IFN-γ—interferon gamma; IL-1β—interleukin-1β; IL-6—interleukin-6; IQR—interquartile range; LDL-C—low-density lipoprotein cholesterol; MedD—Mediterranean diet; MetS—metabolic syndrome; NI—no information; SBP—systolic blood pressure; SD—standard deviation; T2D—type 2 diabetes; TC—total cholesterol; TG—triglycerides; TNF-α—tumor necrosis factor-alpha; VCAM—the vascular cell adhesion molecule; WC—waist circumference.

Table 2. Effects of walnut-enriched diets on inflammatory and metabolic syndrome biomarkers.

Characteristic, Effect Size Type, SMD	Effect Size (95% CI)	p-Value	I² (95% CI)	p-Value	Egger Test	Studies
CRP (mg/L)	−0.37 (−1.39–0.65)	0.478	NC		NC	[32,45]
hs-CRP (mg/L)	−0.01 (−0.12–0.11)	0.903	NC		NC	[47]
IFN-γ (pg/mL)	−1.26 (−2.01–−0.51)	<0.001	NC		NC	[47]
IL-6 (pg/mL)	−0.18 (−0.33–−0.03)	0.021	NC		NC	[47]
IL-1β (pg/mL)	−0.1 (−0.16–−0.04)	<0.001	NC		NC	[47]
TNF-α (pg/mL)	−0.31 (−0.54–−0.08)	0.009	NC		NC	[47]
E-selectin (ng/mL)	−2.57 (−4.09–−1.05)	<0.001	NC		NC	[47]
ICAM-1 (ng/mL)	−0.02 (−0.11–0.07) ANC	0.672	-	-	-	[39,41,47]
VCAM-1 (ng/mL)	−0.11 (−0.32–0.1) ANC	0.305	-	-	-	[39,41,47]
WC (cm)	−0.14 (−0.8–0.51)	0.671	0 (0–89.6)	0.71	0.572	[37,40,43]
BMI (kg/m²)	0.11 (−0.11–0.34)	0.326	63.1 (2.4–86)	0.028	0.683	[33,37,40,45,46]
BW (kg)	0 (−0.4–0.39)	0.987	22.2 (0–64.1)	0.253	0.537	[31–34,36,37,40,43]
SBP (mmHg)	−0.85 (−4.48–2.77)	0.644	64.4 (24–83.4)	0.006	0.699	[32,34,35,37,40,44–46]
DBP (mmHg)	−0.34 (−1.68–1)	0.62	35.3 (0–71.4)	0.146	0.551	[32,34,35,37,40,44–46]
FBG (mg/dL)	0.01 (0–0.02)	0.088	0 (0–74.6)	0.692	0.57	[36,37,40,41,45,46]
TG (mg/dL)	−7.41 (−10.89–−3.94)	<0.001	99.1 (99–99.3)	<0.001	0.264	[31–38,40–42,45,46]
TC (mg/dL)	−5.22 (−7.64–−2.8)	<0.001	97.4 (96.5–98.1)	<0.001	0.375	[31,32,34–38,40–42,45]
HDL-C (mg/dL)	−0.18 (−0.59–0.22)	0.375	47.4 (0–72.4)	0.029	0.507	[31–42,45,46]
LDL-C (mg/dL)	−5.93 (−7.77–−4.09)	<0.001	24.8 (0–61.8)	0.2	0.83	[31–38,40–42,45]
HbA1c (%)	0.08 (−0.04–0.2)	0.196	0 (0–84.7)	0.774	0.816	[33,36,41,45]
HOMA-IR	0.03 (−0.44–0.5)	0.891	57.1 (0–87.8)	0.097	0.95	[37,40,41]
Insulin (mIU/mL)	0.91 (−2.16–3.98)	0.561	65.4 (0–88.2)	0.034	0.505	[36,37,40,41]

ANC—algorithm did not converge (when study [39] was entered; thus, the result is based only on studies [41,47]); BMI—body mass index; BW—body weight; CI—confidence interval; CRP—C-reactive protein; hs-CRP—high-sensitivity C-reactive protein; DBP—diastolic blood pressure; FBG—fasting blood glucose; HbA1c—glycosylated hemoglobin A1c; HDL-C—high-density lipoprotein cholesterol; HOMA-IR—homeostatic model assessment for insulin resistance; ICAM—intercellular adhesion molecule; IFN-γ—interferon gamma; IL-1β—interleukin-1β; IL-6—interleukin-6; LDL-C—low-density lipoprotein cholesterol; NC—not computed for less than three studies; SBP—systolic blood pressure; SD—standard deviation; SMD—standardized mean change difference; TC—total cholesterol; TG—triglycerides; TNF-α—tumor necrosis factor-alpha; VCAM—vascular cell adhesion molecule; WC—waist circumference.

3.1.1. Triglycerides

From the selected studies, thirteen studies reported TG values. The meta-analysis found a higher reduction in TG values in the walnut group compared to the control group (SMD = −7.41 (95% CI: −10.89–−3.94), $p < 0.001$) (Figure 2). There was a significant heterogeneity between the studies, I^2 of 99.1% (95% CI: 99–99.3%), and the Q test for heterogeneity gave $p < 0.001$. The results remained statistically significant after performing a leave-one-out sensitivity analysis for each study. The studies that influenced the final result the most were Tapsell et al. (2009) [36] and Abdrabalnabi et al. [45]; their removal brought the I^2 to values lower than or equal to 7%. A subgroup analysis found that studies with a high risk of bias had higher reductions in TG values than studies with some concerns or low risk of bias, the pooled result remaining statistically significant only for high risk of bias studies (Figure 3). The subgroup analyses regarding treatment exposure duration, study population health, and diet showed statistically significant results for each subgroup (Supplementary Figures S1–S4). The subgroup exposed to walnut portions greater than 42 g/day had statistically significant results, but for those having lower portions, the pooled result lost its significance (Supplementary Figure S5). Finally, for the crossover studies subgroup, the final result was statistically significant, but not for the parallel studies subgroup (Supplementary Figure S6).

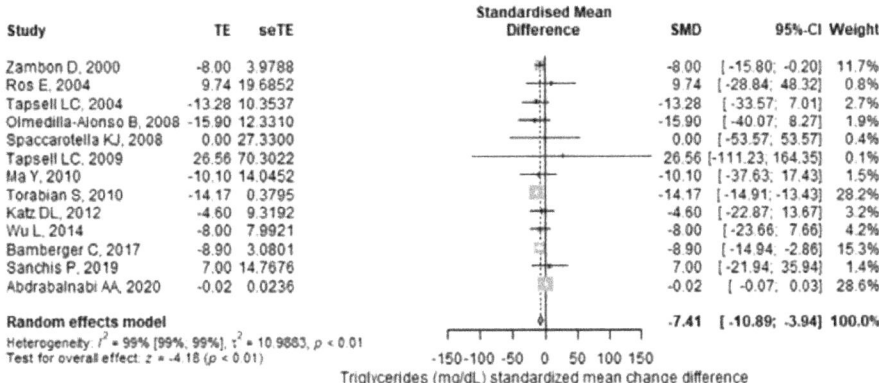

Figure 2. Forest plot for triglycerides (mg/dL) standardized mean change difference. TE—treatment effect; seTE—the standard error of the treatment effect; SMD—standardized mean difference; CI—confidence interval.

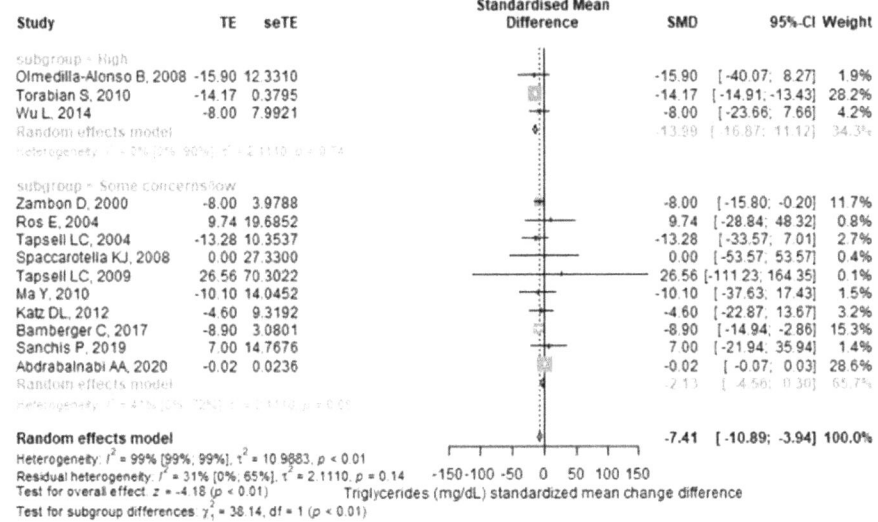

Figure 3. Forest plot for triglycerides (mg/dL) standardized mean change difference compared with subgroup analyses for risk of bias. TE—treatment effect; seTE—the standard error of the treatment effect; SMD—standardized mean difference; CI—confidence interval.

3.1.2. Total Cholesterol, LDL, and HDL Cholesterol

Results for mean differences in TC and LDL-C between intervention and control groups were reported in 12 trials (10 crossover and 2 parallel). We noticed significantly lower values for TC concentrations in walnut-enriched diets compared to control diets (SMD = −5.22, 95% CI: −7.64−−2.8), $p < 0.001$) (Figure 4), with significant heterogeneity between the experiments ($I^2 = 99.1\%$; 95% CI: 99–99.3%, p-heterogeneity < 0.001).

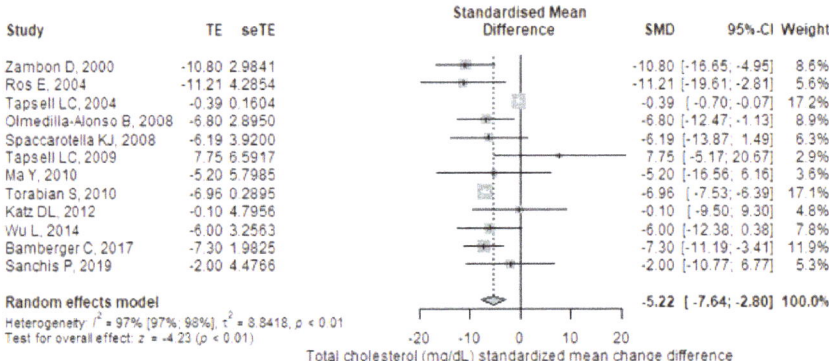

Figure 4. Forest plot for total cholesterol (mg/dL) standardized mean change difference. TE—treatment effect; seTE—the standard error of the treatment effect; SMD—standardized mean difference; CI—confidence interval.

Similarly, the meta-analyzed SMD displayed a significantly greater reduction in LDL-C concentrations with the walnut diets than with the control diets (SMD = −5.93; 95% CI: −7.77–−4.09, $p < 0.001$) (Figure 5), but without significant heterogeneity (I^2 = 24.8%; 95% CI: 0–61.8%, p-heterogeneity = 0.2).

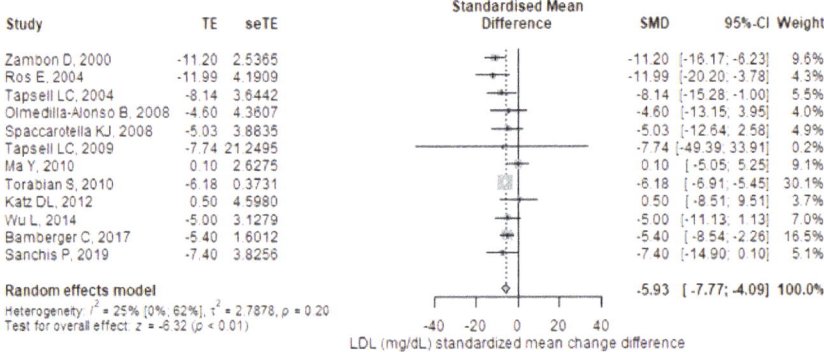

Figure 5. Forest plot for LDL cholesterol (mg/dL) standardized mean change difference. TE—treatment effect; seTE—the standard error of the treatment effect; SMD—standardized mean difference; CI—confidence interval.

Sensitivity analyses showed that the outcomes remained statistically significant after removing one study at a time for both parameters. The reports with the highest influence on the final effects were Tapsell et al. (2004) [33] and Tapsell et al. (2009) [36] for TC, while for LDL-C they were Torabian et al. [38] and Tapsell et al. (2009) [36].

In the subgroup analyses, for TC and LDL-C parameters, walnut diets had statistically significant effects in high risk and some concern studies for risk of bias, as well as for exposure duration, walnut quantity, population health, and diet in both study designs, parallel and crossover. The results remained significant for the participant subgroup with ages over 40 years (Supplementary Figures S7–S19).

Fourteen controlled trials documented results for HDL-C. There were no statistically significant changes in HDL-C concentrations between the walnut and the control diets (SMD = −0.18; 95% CI: −0.59–0.22, p = 0.375). However, a significant heterogeneity was reported (I^2 = 47.4%; 95% CI: 0–72.4%, p-heterogeneity = 0.029) (Supplementary Figure S20).

3.1.3. Anthropometric Markers

WC, BMI, and BW changes were reported in three, five, and eight trials, respectively. On these parameters, individual trials did not show significant differences compared to the control after following a walnut-enriched diet (WC SMD = −0.14; 95% CI: −0.8–0.51, p = 0.671; BMI SMD = 0.11; 95% CI: −0.11–0.34, p = 0.326; BW SMD = 0; 95% CI: −0.4–0.39, p = 0.987). A significant heterogeneity was observed only for BMI (p = 0.028) (Supplementary Figures S21–S23).

3.1.4. Blood Pressure

The effect on blood pressure was analyzed in eight studies (six crossover and two parallel). Walnut-enhanced diets did not significantly modify SBP (SMD = −0.85; 95% CI: −4.48–2.77, p = 0.644) or DBP (SMD = −0.34; 95% CI: −1.68–1, p = 0.62), with significant heterogeneity for SBP (I^2 = 64.4%; 95% CI: 24–83.4%, p-heterogeneity = 0.006) (Supplementary Figures S24 and S25).

3.1.5. Glycemic Biomarkers

Similarly, no significant reductions were detected for FBG, HbA1c, HOMA-IR, and insulin assessed in six, four, three, and four studies, respectively. Compared with control diets, walnut-enriched diets accounted for a non-significant decrease of these glycemic markers (FBG SMD = 0.01; 95% CI: 0–0.02, p = 0.088; HbA1c SMD = 0.08; 95% CI: −0.04–0.2, p = 0.196; HOMA-IR SMD = 0.03; 95% CI: −0.44–0.5, p = 0.891; insulin SMD = 0.91; 95% CI: −2.16–3.98, p = 0.561). The Q test for heterogeneity gave a significant value only for insulin (p = 0.034) (Supplementary Figures S26–S29).

3.2. Inflammatory Biomarkers

In the meta-analysis of the inflammatory markers, the walnut consumption revealed no significant influence on CRP (SMD = −0.37; 95% CI: −1.39–0.65, p = 0.478) and hs-CRP (SMD = −0.01; 95% CI: −0.12–0.11, p = 0.903) (Supplementary Figures S30 and S31).

For the other studied inflammatory biomarkers, the walnut diet showed significant changes (IFN-γ SMD = −1.26; 95% CI: −2.01–−0.51, p < 0.001; IL-6 SMD = −0.18; 95% CI: −0.00–−0.03, p < 0.001; IL-1β SMD = −0.1; 95% CI: −0.16–−0.04, p < 0.001; TNF-α SMD = −0.31; 95% CI: −0.54–−0.08, p = 0.009; E-selectin SMD = −2.57; 95% CI: −4.09–−1.05, p < 0.001), but the publication bias test and the heterogeneity could not be calculated since there was only one assessed study (Supplementary Figures S32–S36).

The endothelial adhesion molecules, ICAM-1 and VCAM-1, could not be computed since the algorithm did not converge when the study of Canales et al. [39] was included in the analysis. When we excluded this analysis, the results based on the studies of Wu et al. and Cofan et al. [41,47] were not statistically significant.

3.3. Quality Assessment

The results obtained after quality (risk of bias) assessment for the six parallel and eleven crossover studies are presented in the Supplementary Materials (Supplementary Figures S37 and S38). Several papers [43,44,46,47] analyzed data from the same study, Walnuts and Healthy Aging (WAHA), and for the quality assessment they were considered as only one.

Concerning the randomization process domain, eleven studies (79%) had some concerns of bias, and three were at low risk of bias. The randomization generation method was presented in five studies. Only one study mentioned allocation concealment. Only two studies (14%) explained how randomization was undertaken. For crossover studies, seven had no information to assess the start of clinical study baseline differences, and three probably did not have differences, while for parallel trials, all four probably did not have differences.

For crossover trials, we assessed the risk of bias arising from period and carryover effects. Four studies had some concerns of bias, and seven were at low risk of bias. Five studies had a similar number of subjects allocated to the interventions. Two studies probably did not have important differences in the number of subjects allocated to the interventions. The other studies reported no information. Five studies did not analyze whether the period effect was verified. All studies had sufficient time for the disappearance of any carryover effects before the outcome assessment in the second period.

Regarding deviations from the intended interventions, four studies were at high risk of bias, six had some concerns of bias, and four were at low risk of bias. Although not mentioned in all trials, participants, caregivers, and those administering interventions were likely all aware of the assigned intervention, except for one study where the investigator was blinded to the intervention. The studies did not mention whether deviations from the intended intervention arose due to trial context, except in one study where those deviations probably did not affect the outcome. Five studies mentioned or it could be deducted that they used an intention-to-treat analysis. Five studies gave no information about the use of an intention-to-treat analysis, and the other four stated or it could be deducted that they used a per-protocol analysis. Only one study was impacted by the lack of intention-to-treat analysis of the results.

Moreover, only one study had some concern of bias with respect to missing outcome data domain; the others had a low risk of bias. Seven studies probably had data for all or nearly all randomized participants. Six studies had important percentages of subjects that dropped out. One study did not report anything about missing data. No study provided missing data analysis or sensitivity analyses to demonstrate that missing data did not skew the results. In all the research, it is more likely to conclude that the missingness of the outcomes was unrelated to its genuine value.

Concerning the measuring of the outcome domain, all the studies were at low risk of bias. All of the studies used the same instruments and standard and exact measuring methods to test the outcomes at the same time points throughout their research (laboratory assays or anthropometric measurements). In the case of laboratory measurements, it is likely the measurement was blinded (only three studies reported it). It is unlikely that knowing the intervention would influence the measurement.

Considering the selection of the reported result domain, all the studies had a low risk of bias. Two studies had variables of interest for our review specified as the primary endpoint in the research protocol. Four studies had research protocols published before their study but with different primary endpoints compared to our review. Only one instrument and one statistical analysis approach were employed in all of the investigations for each variable of interest.

Overall, four studies were considered at high risk of bias, and the others showed some concerns of bias.

3.4. Reporting Bias Assessment

The Egger test yielded non-statistically significant findings for all of the outcomes of interest when it was used to examine the presence of publication bias. Moreover, funnel plots were not indicative of asymmetry either.

4. Discussion

To the best of our knowledge, the current study is the first systematic review and meta-analysis to focus on comprehensively analyzing the evidence to date regarding the effects of walnut-enriched diets on biomarkers of MetS and inflammation in middle-aged and older adults.

Walnut is considered a nutraceutical dietary source due to the high content of good fatty acids, such as MUFA and omega-3 PUFA, its nutritional value, the high antioxidant phytochemical content, and its beneficial effects on human health.

In the present meta-analysis, we assessed the results of seventeen randomized clinical trials that analyzed the impact of walnut-enriched diets. Our findings showed that walnut-enriched diets significantly decreased TG, TC, and LDL-C concentrations, while HDL-C level was not significantly affected. No significant changes were noticed on anthropometric, cardiometabolic, and glycemic indices after higher walnut consumption. Moreover, the inflammatory biomarkers did not record statistically significant results.

Considering the evidence from recent meta-analyses, nut consumption [48–50] and walnut-enriched diets [22,51] are negatively associated with specific biomarkers of MetS and inflammation in different age groups.

Regarding the duration of exposure to treatment (in a range between 4 weeks and 2 years), the health of the studied population (healthy people, hypertensive, hypercholesterolemic, or T2D patients), and the diet (mostly Western-type or habitual diet, without walnuts), each subgroup presented statistically significant results. Different doses of walnut showed that the subgroup exposed to walnut portions greater than 42 g per day had statistically significant results. This result reinforces the Food and Drug Administration (FDA) [52] recommendation for the inclusion of 42 g (1.5 ounces) of walnuts in the daily diet and differs from the conclusions of another meta-analysis, which states that the TG lowering effects reach a plateau at doses higher than 20 g [53].

Our meta-analysis identified a statistically significant reduction of TG values ($p < 0.001$) in walnut consumption groups compared to control groups in the thirteen trials analyzed for this marker. Furthermore, it showed statistically significant decreases in terms of TC and LDL-C levels. Analyzing the twelve studies reporting results for mean differences in TC and LDL-C, we noticed significantly lower values for TC concentrations in walnut-enriched diets ($p < 0.001$) compared to control diets. Similarly, we registered a significantly greater reduction in LDL-C concentrations with the walnut diets ($p < 0.001$) than with the control diets. The statistically significant beneficial effects in the lipid profile noticed after walnut-enriched diets have the potential of decreasing the age-related disease risks for the age category targeted in this meta-analysis.

Several observational studies obtained the same answers. A cross-sectional study analyzing data from three large US prospective cohort studies concluded that an increase of 0.5 servings (~14 g) per day in walnut consumption was significantly associated with 17% lower CVD risk and 20% lower stroke risk [54]. After assessing the same data but with slightly different covariates, another study found that consuming at least one serving (~28 g) of walnuts per week was linked with 19% lower CVD risk and 17% lower stroke risk, in addition to a 21% decrease in the risk of CHD [55]. Similarly, a recent systematic review and meta-analysis of prospective studies revealed that higher walnut intake was associated with lower risks of CVD and CHD incidence [56]. Moreover, data from two large prospective cohort studies associated higher walnut consumption with a lower CVD risk and mortality and a greater life expectancy among U.S. older adults [57]. The PREDIMED study also disclosed a significantly lower risk of stroke in participants who consumed 30 g of mixed nuts (including 15 g of walnuts) per day compared with a no-nut consumer group [58].

Based on our results, the improvement of the lipid profile and decrease of oxidative stress and inflammation are primary mechanisms of walnut intake against CVD. Furthermore, bioactive compounds found in walnuts, both hydrophilic and lipophilic, could protect against MetS complications and CVD [15].

Thereby, polyphenols, hydrosoluble micronutrients found in walnuts such as quercetin and its glycosides, ellagic acid and ellagitannins, and cyanidin and proanthocyanidins [59] exert their antioxidant action through multiple mechanisms, including the activation of the Nrf2/ARE (nuclear factor erythroid 2-related factor 2/antioxidant response element) pathway. By this pathway, polyphenols increase the activity of some antioxidant and detoxifying enzymatic systems and down-regulate the nuclear factor kappa B (NF-κB) pathway that is directly implicated in the inflammatory response. Tocopherols and tocotrienols, as well as n-3 PUFAs and n-6 PUFAs and other lipophilic antioxidants from walnuts, can also inhibit the NF-κB pathway by activation of Nrf2/ARE. By preventing oxidation of LDL, antioxidants improve the lipid profile, preventing and reducing the formation of atherosclerotic plaques and the risks for CVD [11]. Melatonin, found in minute quantities in walnuts (3.5 ± 1.0 ng/g), holds antioxidant and anti-inflammatory properties, with CV protection [16]. Moreover, phytosterols from walnuts can lower LDL-C levels. They are more hydrophobic than cholesterol and can dislocate cholesterol from intestinal micelles and reduce LDL-C absorption. In combination with n-3 PUFAs, phytosterols show both complementary and synergistic lipid-lowering effects [16].

In our study, the effect on blood pressure was analyzed in eight trials. Neither SBP nor DBP was significantly modified by walnut-enhanced diets, confirming the results of previous analyses [53,55,60]. Furthermore, our study did not show statistically significant changes in terms of glycemic markers, which also corroborated prior studies [22,51,53]. After following walnut-enriched diets, the anthropometric parameters did not show significant differences compared to the control. These results were consistent with those obtained in former works [49,61].

Low-grade chronic inflammation, referred to as inflammaging in the older population, plays a key role in atherosclerosis, while inflammation biomarker concentrations can predict future T2D or CVD events [62]. The results of our study showed no significant effects of walnut intake on inflammatory markers. These findings concur with recently published data showing that the hs-CRP level was not influenced by walnut consumption [53]. Moreover, our findings agree with a recently published meta-analysis of both interventional and observational studies, which established that walnut intake had no statistical significance on glucose homeostasis and inflammation [22]. In contrast, observational studies found that nut consumption was inversely associated with inflammatory markers [63]. These findings might point to other types of nuts being responsible for these positive effects. However, Cofán et al. (2020) [47] are the only researchers who have studied several biomarkers of inflammation in correlation with a walnut-diet and found statistically significant reduction for IL-6, IFN-γ, IL-1β, TNF-α, and E-selectin, but not for hs-CRP and adhesion molecules VCAM-1 and ICAM-1. These results are noteworthy, but further clinical trials are needed to confirm them.

The negative relationship between walnut intake and MetS pathophysiology may also be attributed to the antioxidant and anti-inflammatory activity of vitamin E [62] and other antioxidant phytochemicals found in walnuts [64].

Similar to other studies, our meta-analysis presents several limitations. The most important limitation concerns the risk of bias present in the selected studies. Blinding participants and personnel in the case of walnut eating is clearly challenging, particularly for participants, and was not performed in the studies. Nonetheless, because the majority of the outcomes of interest are objective laboratory measurements, this methodological shortcoming is less likely to impact the measurement of the findings. The absence of any declaration on allocation concealment (just one study mentioned it) and the randomization process (stated in five studies) is the most critical issue. The Cochrane Risk of Bias Tool 2 has a dose of subjectivity in the assessment, and we deemed most of the studies to have some concerns of bias. However, if there had been no allocation concealment, in reality, the trials would have been regarded as having a high risk of bias overall. This is more troublesome for parallel designs, although they only accounted for roughly a third of the total in our assessment. Nevertheless, we performed subgroup analyses for studies with high bias and some concerns of bias and the main results of our review remained statistically significant in both cases. Another disadvantage is the relatively small number of individuals per research; nevertheless, systematic inclusion of a large number of publications helps to increase overall power. We had a long list of potential outcomes, but only a few papers provided measurements for several of them. For some outcomes, there was an important heterogeneity, but after the sensitivity leave-one-out analysis, they seemed robust and remained statistically significant.

Additionally, our review has several strengths: (1) the publications' methodological flaws were assessed using the newest edition of the Cochrane Collaboration's Risk of Bias Tool, version 2, one of the most prestigious organizations that conducts systematic reviews and creates high-quality instruments for study validity evaluation; (2) a comprehensive search strategy was used; (3) many databases (PubMed, Embase, Scopus, Cochrane

Database) were searched; (4) only randomized controlled trials were included; (5) sensitivity and subgroup analyses were performed; and (6) twenty-two metabolic syndrome and inflammatory markers in middle-aged and older adults were assessed.

Future studies should focus more on inflammatory markers that were assessed in only a small number of studies, but with significant results. The value close to statistical significance level of fasting blood glucose suggests a need for further studies to check if this was a spurious result or a real useful signal. Furthermore, the quality of future randomized controlled trials on walnut diets should be improved, especially regarding allocation concealment, the randomization process, and intention to treat analyses.

5. Conclusions

In conclusion, despite some heterogeneity in the intervention outcomes, our meta-analysis found significant amelioration in the lipid profiles (TG, TC, and LDL-C levels) with walnut consumption compared with different control diets in the studied age category, middle-aged and older adults. Incipient data from a single study [47], which should be further investigated, suggest that long-term walnut consumption displayed potential benefits in lowering inflammation and indirectly on preventing several age-related diseases. Even though further and better-designed studies are needed to strengthen these findings, the results stress the importance of including walnuts in the dietary plans of middle-aged and older populations.

Supplementary Materials: The following supporting information can be downloaded at: https://www.mdpi.com/article/10.3390/antiox11071412/s1.

Author Contributions: Conceptualization, D.L., M.E.R., L.M. and D.-S.P.; methodology, D.L.; investigation, L.M., M.E.R., D.-S.P., D.L. and I.F.; writing—original draft preparation, D.L., M.E.R. and L.M.; writing—reviewing, and editing, L.M., M.E.R., D.L., D.-S.P. and I.F. All authors have read and agreed to the published version of the manuscript.

Funding: This research received no external funding.

Conflicts of Interest: The authors declare no conflict of interest.

Abbreviations

ALA	α-linolenic acid
apoB	apolipoprotein B
BMI	body mass index
BW	body weight
CI	confidence interval
CI	confidence interval
CRP	C-reactive protein
CVD	cardiovascular diseases
DBP	diastolic blood pressure
eTE	the standard error of the treatment effect
FBG	fasting blood glucose
HbA1c	glycosylated hemoglobin A1c
HDL-C	high density lipoprotein-cholesterol
HOMA-IR	homeostatic model assessment for insulin resistance
hs-CRP	high-sensitivity C-reactive protein
ICAM-1	intercellular adhesion molecule-1
IF	interferon gamma
IL-1β	interleukin-1β
IL-6	interleukin-6
IQR	interquartile ranges
LDL-C	low density lipoprotein-cholesterol
MedD	Mediterranean diet

MetS	metabolic syndrome
MUFAs	monounsaturated fatty acids
NF-κB	nuclear factor kappa B
Nrf2/ARE	nuclear factor erythroid 2-related factor 2/antioxidant response element
PUFAs	polyunsaturated fatty acids
RCT	randomized controlled trial
ROS	reactive oxygen species
SBP	systolic blood pressure
SD	standard deviation
SE	standard error
SMD	standardized mean difference
SMD	standardized mean change difference
T2D	type 2 diabetes
TC	total cholesterol
TE	treatment effect
TG	triglycerides
TNF-α	tumor necrosis factor-alpha
VCAM-1	vascular cell adhesion molecule-1
W	weight
WC	waist circumference

References

1. Rea, I.M.; Gibson, D.S.; McGilligan, V.; McNerlan, S.E.; Denis Alexander, H.; Ross, O.A. Age and Age-Related Diseases: Role of Inflammation Triggers and Cytokines. *Front. Immunol.* **2018**, *9*, 586. [CrossRef] [PubMed]
2. Franceschi, C.; Campisi, J. Chronic Inflammation (Inflammaging) and Its Potential Contribution to Age-Associated Diseases. *J. Gerontol. Ser. A Biol. Sci. Med. Sci.* **2014**, *69*, S4–S9. [CrossRef]
3. Furman, D.; Campisi, J.; Verdin, E.; Carrera-Bastos, P.; Targ, S.; Franceschi, C.; Ferrucci, L.; Gilroy, D.W.; Fasano, A.; Miller, G.W.; et al. Chronic Inflammation in the Etiology of Disease across the Life Span. *Nat. Med.* **2019**, *25*, 1822–1832. [CrossRef] [PubMed]
4. Kirkland, J.L.; Tchkonia, T. Cellular Senescence: A Translational Perspective. *EBioMedicine* **2017**, *21*, 21–28. [CrossRef] [PubMed]
5. Rapa, S.F.; di Iorio, B.R.; Campiglia, P.; Heidland, A.; Marzocco, S. Inflammation and Oxidative Stress in Chronic Kidney Disease—Potential Therapeutic Role of Minerals, Vitamins and Plant-Derived Metabolites. *Int. J. Mol. Sci.* **2020**, *21*, 263. [CrossRef]
6. Popa, D.S.; Bigman, G.; Rusu, M.E. The Role of Vitamin K in Humans: Implication in Aging and Age-Associated Diseases. *Antioxidants* **2021**, *10*, 566. [CrossRef]
7. Ajabnoor, S.M.; Thorpe, G.; Abdelhamid, A.; Hooper, L. Long-Term Effects of Increasing Omega-3, Omega-6 and Total Polyunsaturated Fats on Inflammatory Bowel Disease and Markers of Inflammation: A Systematic Review and Meta-Analysis of Randomized Controlled Trials. *Eur. J. Nutr.* **2021**, *60*, 2293–2316. [CrossRef]
8. Kiss, B.; Popa, D.-S.; Crişan, G.; Bojiţă, M.; Loghin, F. The Evaluation of Antioxidant Potential of Veronica Officinalis and Rosmarinus Officinalis Extracts by Monitoring Malondialdehide and Glutathione Levels in Rats. *Farmacia* **2009**, *57*, 432–441.
9. Trautwein, E.A.; McKay, S. The Role of Specific Components of a Plant-Based Diet in Management of Dyslipidemia and the Impact on Cardiovascular Risk. *Nutrients* **2020**, *12*, 2671. [CrossRef]
10. Fizeșan, I.; Rusu, M.E.; Georgiu, C.; Pop, A.; Ștefan, M.G.; Muntean, D.M.; Mirel, S.; Vostinaru, O.; Kiss, B.; Popa, D.S. Antitussive, Antioxidant, and Anti-Inflammatory Effects of a Walnut (*Juglans Regia* L.) Septum Extract Rich in Bioactive Compounds. *Antioxidants* **2021**, *10*, 119. [CrossRef]
11. Rusu, M.E.; Simedrea, R.; Gheldiu, A.M.; Mocan, A.; Vlase, L.; Popa, D.S.; Ferreira, I.C.F.R. Benefits of Tree Nut Consumption on Aging and Age-Related Diseases: Mechanisms of Actions. *Trends Food Sci. Technol.* **2019**, *88*, 104–120. [CrossRef]
12. de Souza, R.G.M.; Schincaglia, R.M.; Pimente, G.D.; Mota, J.F. Nuts and Human Health Outcomes: A Systematic Review. *Nutrients* **2017**, *9*, 1311. [CrossRef] [PubMed]
13. Pop, A.; Fizesan, I.; Vlase, L.; Rusu, M.E.; Cherfan, J.; Babota, M.; Gheldiu, A.-M.; Tomuta, I.; Popa, D.-S. Enhanced Recovery of Phenolic and Tocopherolic Compounds from Walnut (*Juglans Regia* L.) Male Flowers Based on Process Optimization of Ultrasonic Assisted-Extraction: Phytochemical Profile and Biological Activities. *Antioxidants* **2021**, *10*, 607. [CrossRef] [PubMed]
14. Ros, E.; Singh, A.; O'Keefe, J.H. Nuts: Natural Pleiotropic Nutraceuticals. *Nutrients* **2021**, *13*, 3269. [CrossRef] [PubMed]
15. Rusu, M.E.; Mocan, A.; Ferreira, I.C.F.R.; Popa, D.S. Health Benefits of Nut Consumption in Middle-Aged and Elderly Population. *Antioxidants* **2019**, *8*, 302. [CrossRef]
16. Ros, E.; Izquierdo-Pulido, M.; Sala-Vila, A. Beneficial Effects of Walnut Consumption on Human Health: Role of Micronutrients. *Curr. Opin. Clin. Nutr. Metab. Care* **2018**, *21*, 498–504. [CrossRef] [PubMed]
17. Blondeau, N.; Lipsky, R.H.; Bourourou, M.; Duncan, M.W.; Gorelick, P.B.; Marini, A.M. Alpha-Linolenic Acid: An Omega-3 Fatty Acid with Neuroprotective Properties—Ready for Use in the Stroke Clinic? *BioMed Res. Int.* **2015**, *2015*, 519830. [CrossRef]

18. Hardman, W.E.; Primerano, D.A.; Legenza, M.T.; Morgan, J.; Fan, J.; Denvir, J. Dietary Walnut Altered Gene Expressions Related to Tumor Growth, Survival, and Metastasis in Breast Cancer Patients: A Pilot Clinical Trial. *Nutr. Res.* **2019**, *66*, 82–94. [CrossRef]
19. Borkowski, K.; Yim, S.J.; Holt, R.R.; Hackman, R.M.; Keen, C.L.; Newman, J.W.; Shearer, G.C. Walnuts Change Lipoprotein Composition Suppressing TNFα-Stimulated Cytokine Production by Diabetic Adipocyte. *J. Nutr. Biochem.* **2019**, *68*, 51–58. [CrossRef]
20. Hwang, H.J.; Liu, Y.; Kim, H.S.; Lee, H.; Lim, Y.; Park, H. Daily Walnut Intake Improves Metabolic Syndrome Status and Increases Circulating Adiponectin Levels: Randomized Controlled Crossover Trial. *Nutr. Res. Pract.* **2019**, *13*, 105–114. [CrossRef]
21. Arab, L.; Dhaliwal, S.K.; Martin, C.J.; Larios, A.D.; Jackson, N.J.; Elashoff, D. Association between Walnut Consumption and Diabetes Risk in NHANES. *Diabetes/Metab. Res. Rev.* **2018**, *34*, e3031. [CrossRef] [PubMed]
22. Cahoon, D.; Shertukde, S.P.; Avendano, E.E.; Tanprasertsuk, J.; Scott, T.M.; Johnson, E.J.; Chung, M.; Nirmala, N. Walnut Intake, Cognitive Outcomes and Risk Factors: A Systematic Review and Meta-Analysis. *Ann. Med.* **2021**, *53*, 971–997. [CrossRef] [PubMed]
23. Su, H.; Liu, R.; Chang, M.; Huang, J.; Jin, Q.; Wang, X. Effect of Dietary Alpha-Linolenic Acid on Blood Inflammatory Markers: A Systematic Review and Meta-Analysis of Randomized Controlled Trials. *Eur. J. Nutr.* **2018**, *57*, 877–891. [CrossRef] [PubMed]
24. Page, M.J.; Moher, D.; Bossuyt, P.M.; Boutron, I.; Hoffmann, T.C.; Mulrow, C.D.; Shamseer, L.; Tetzlaff, J.M.; Akl, E.A.; Brennan, S.E.; et al. PRISMA 2020 Explanation and Elaboration: Updated Guidance and Exemplars for Reporting Systematic Reviews. *BMJ* **2021**, *372*, n160. [CrossRef]
25. Sterne, J.A.C.; Savović, J.; Page, M.J.; Elbers, R.G.; Blencowe, N.S.; Boutron, I.; Cates, C.J.; Cheng, H.Y.; Corbett, M.S.; Eldridge, S.M.; et al. RoB 2: A Revised Tool for Assessing Risk of Bias in Randomised Trials. *BMJ* **2019**, *366*, l4898. [CrossRef]
26. Higgins, J.P.T.; Thomas, J.; Chandler, J.; Cumpston, M.; Li, T.; Page, M.J.; Welch, V.A. (Eds.) *Cochrane Handbook for Systematic Reviews of Interventions*, 2nd ed.; John Wiley & Sons: Chichester, UK, 2019; ISBN 9781119536628.
27. Elbourne, D.R.; Altman, D.G.; Higgins, J.P.; Curtin, F.; Worthington, H.V.; Vail, A. Meta-Analyses Involving Cross-over Trials: Methodological Issues. *Int. J. Epidemiol.* **2002**, *31*, 140–149. [CrossRef]
28. Balduzzi, S.; Rücker, G.; Schwarzer, G. How to Perform a Meta-Analysis with R: A Practical Tutorial. *Evid. Based Ment. Health* **2019**, *22*, 153–160. [CrossRef]
29. Harrer, M.; Cuijpers, P.; Furukawa, T.A.; Ebert, D.D. *Doing Meta-Analysis with R: A Hands-On Guide*, 1st ed.; CRC Press: Boca Raton, FL, USA, 2021. [CrossRef]
30. R Core Team R: A Language and Environment for Statistical Computing. Available online: https://www.R_project.org/ (accessed on 4 June 2022).
31. Zambón, D.; Sabaté, J.; Muñoz, S.; Campero, B.; Casals, E.; Merlos, M.; Laguna, J.C.; Ros, E. Substituting Walnuts for Monounsaturated Fat Improves the Serum Lipid Profile of Hypercholesterolemic Men and Women A Randomized Crossover Trial. *Ann. Intern. Med.* **2000**, *132*, 538–546. [CrossRef]
32. Ros, E.; Núñez, I.; Pérez-Heras, A.; Serra, M.; Gilabert, R.; Casals, E.; Deulofeu, R. A Walnut Diet Improves Endothelial Function in Hypercholesterolemic Subjects: A Randomized Crossover Trial. *Circulation* **2004**, *109*, 1609–1614. [CrossRef]
33. Tapsell, L.C.; Gillen, L.J.; Patch, C.S.; Batterham, M.; Owen, A.; Baré, M.; Kennedy, M. Including Walnuts in a Low-Fat/Modified-Fat Diet Improves HDL Cholesterol-to-Total Cholesterol Ratios in Patients With Type 2 Diabetes. *Diabetes Care* **2004**, *27*, 2777–2783. [CrossRef]
34. Olmedilla-Alonso, B.; Granado-Lorencio, F.; Herrero-Barbudo, C.; Blanco-Navarro, I.; Blázquez-García, S.; Pérez-Sacristán, B. Consumption of Restructured Meat Products with Added Walnuts Has a Cholesterol-Lowering Effect in Subjects at High Cardiovascular Risk: A Randomised, Crossover, Placebo-Controlled Study. *J. Am. Coll. Nutr.* **2008**, *27*, 342–348. [CrossRef] [PubMed]
35. Spaccarotella, K.J.; Kris-Etherton, P.M.; Stone, W.L.; Bagshaw, D.M.; Fishell, V.K.; West, S.G.; Lawrence, F.R.; Hartman, T.J. The Effect of Walnut Intake on Factors Related to Prostate and Vascular Health in Older Men. *Nutr. J.* **2008**, *7*, 13. [CrossRef] [PubMed]
36. Tapsell, L.C.; Batterham, M.J.; Teuss, G.; Tan, S.Y.; Dalton, S.; Quick, C.J.; Gillen, L.J.; Charlton, K.E. Long-Term Effects of Increased Dietary Polyunsaturated Fat from Walnuts on Metabolic Parameters in Type II Diabetes. *Eur. J. Clin. Nutr.* **2009**, *63*, 1008–1015. [CrossRef] [PubMed]
37. Ma, Y.; Njike, V.Y.; Millet, J.; Dutta, S.; Doughty, K.; Treu, J.A.; Katz, D.L. Effects of Walnut Consumption on Endothelial Function in Type 2 Diabetic Subjects: A Randomized Controlled Crossover Trial. *Diabetes Care* **2010**, *33*, 227–232. [CrossRef] [PubMed]
38. Torabian, S.; Haddad, E.; Cordero-Macintyre, Z.; Tanzman, J.; Fernandez, M.L.; Sabate, J. Long-Term Walnut Supplementation without Dietary Advice Induces Favorable Serum Lipid Changes in Free-Living Individuals. *Eur. J. Clin. Nutr.* **2010**, *64*, 274–279. [CrossRef]
39. Canales, A.; Sánchez-Muniz, F.J.; Bastida, S.; Librelotto, J.; Nus, M.; Corella, D.; Guillen, M.; Benedi, J. Effect of Walnut-Enriched Meat on the Relationship between VCAM, ICAM, and LTB4 Levels and PON-1 Activity in ApoA4 360 and PON-1 Allele Carriers at Increased Cardiovascular Risk. *Eur. J. Clin. Nutr.* **2011**, *65*, 703–710. [CrossRef]
40. Katz, D.L.; Davidhi, A.; Ma, Y.; Kavak, Y.; Bifulco, L.; Njike, V.Y. Effects of Walnuts on Endothelial Function in Overweight Adults with Visceral Obesity: A Randomized, Controlled, Crossover Trial. *J. Am. Coll. Nutr.* **2012**, *6*, 415–423. [CrossRef]
41. Wu, L.; Piotrowski, K.; Rau, T.; Waldmann, E.; Broedl, U.C.; Demmelmair, H.; Koletzko, B.; Stark, R.G.; Nagel, J.M.; Mantzoros, C.S.; et al. Walnut-Enriched Diet Reduces Fasting Non-HDL-Cholesterol and Apolipoprotein B in Healthy Caucasian Subjects: A Randomized Controlled Cross-over Clinical Trial. *Metab. Clin. Exp.* **2014**, *63*, 382–391. [CrossRef]

42. Bamberger, C.; Rossmeier, A.; Lechner, K.; Wu, L.; Waldmann, E.; Stark, R.G.; Altenhofer, J.; Henze, K.; Parhofer, K.G. A Walnut-Enriched Diet Reduces Lipids in Healthy Caucasian Subjects, Independent of Recommended Macronutrient Replacement and Time Point of Consumption: A Prospective, Randomized, Controlled Trial. *Nutrients* **2017**, *9*, 1097. [CrossRef]
43. Bitok, E.; Rajaram, S.; Jaceldo-Siegl, K.; Oda, K.; Sala-Vila, A.; Serra-Mir, M.; Ros, E.; Sabaté, J. Effects of Long-Term Walnut Supplementation on Body Weight in Free-Living Elderly: Results of a Randomized Controlled Trial. *Nutrients* **2018**, *10*, 1317. [CrossRef]
44. Domènech, M.; Serra-Mir, M.; Roth, I.; Freitas-Simoes, T.; Valls-Pedret, C.; Cofán, M.; López, A.; Sala-Vila, A.; Calvo, C.; Rajaram, S.; et al. Effect of a Walnut Diet on Office and 24-Hour Ambulatory Blood Pressure in Elderly Individuals: Findings from the WAHA Randomized Trial. *Hypertension* **2019**, *73*, 1049–1057. [CrossRef] [PubMed]
45. Sanchis, P.; Molina, M.; Berga, F.; Muñoz, E.; Fortuny, R.; Costa-Bauzá, A.; Grases, F.; Buades, J.M. A Pilot Randomized Crossover Trial Assessing the Safety and Short-Term Effects of Walnut Consumption by Patients with Chronic Kidney Disease. *Nutrients* **2020**, *12*, 63. [CrossRef] [PubMed]
46. Abdrabalnabi, A.; Rajaram, S.; Bitok, E.; Oda, K.; Beeson, W.L.; Kaur, A.; Cofán, M.; Serra-Mir, M.; Roth, I.; Ros, E.; et al. Effects of Supplementing the Usual Diet with a Daily Dose of Walnuts for Two Years on Metabolic Syndrome and Its Components in an Elderly Cohort. *Nutrients* **2020**, *12*, 451. [CrossRef] [PubMed]
47. Cofán, M.; Rajaram, S.; Sala-Vila, A.; Valls-Pedret, C.; Serra-Mir, M.; Roth, I.; Freitas-Simoes, T.M.; Bitok, E.; Sabaté, J.; Ros, E. Effects of 2-Year Walnut-Supplemented Diet on Inflammatory Biomarkers. *J. Am. Coll. Cardiol.* **2020**, *76*, 2282–2284. [CrossRef]
48. Tindall, A.M.; Johnston, E.A.; Kris-Etherton, P.M.; Petersen, K.S. The Effect of Nuts on Markers of Glycemic Control: A Systematic Review and Meta-Analysis of Randomized Controlled Trials. *Am. J. Clin. Nutr.* **2019**, *109*, 297–314. [CrossRef]
49. Fernández-Rodríguez, R.; Mesas, A.E.; Garrido-Miguel, M.; Martínez-Ortega, I.A.; Jiménez-López, E.; Martínez-Vizcaíno, V. The Relationship of Tree Nuts and Peanuts with Adiposity Parameters: A Systematic Review and Network Meta-Analysis. *Nutrients* **2021**, *13*, 2251. [CrossRef]
50. Fernández-Rodríguez, R.; Martínez-Vizcaíno, V.; Garrido-Miguel, M.; Martínez-Ortega, I.A.; Álvarez-Bueno, C.; Eumann Mesas, A. Nut Consumption, Body Weight, and Adiposity in Patients with Type 2 Diabetes: A Systematic Review and Meta-Analysis of Randomized Controlled Trials. *Nutr. Rev.* **2022**, *80*, 645–655. [CrossRef]
51. Neale, E.P.; Guan, V.; Tapsell, L.C.; Probst, Y.C. Effect of Walnut Consumption on Markers of Blood Glucose Control: A Systematic Review and Meta-Analysis. *Br. J. Nutr.* **2020**, *124*, 641–653. [CrossRef]
52. Tarantino, L.M. *Qualified Health Claims: Letter of Enforcement Discretion-Walnuts and Coronary Heart Disease*; (Docket No 02P-0292); U.S. Food and Drug Administration: Washington, DC, USA, 2004.
53. Arabi, S.M.; Bahrami, L.S.; Milkarizi, N.; Nematy, M.; Kalmykov, V.; Sahebkar, A. Impact of Walnut Consumption on Cardio Metabolic and Anthropometric Parameters in Metabolic Syndrome Patients: GRADE-Assessed Systematic Review and Dose-Response Meta-Analysis of Data from Randomized Controlled Trials. *Pharmacol. Res.* **2022**, *178*, 106190. [CrossRef]
54. Liu, X.; Guasch-Ferré, M.; Drouin-Chartier, J.P.; Tobias, D.K.; Bhupathiraju, S.N.; Rexrode, K.M.; Willett, W.C.; Sun, Q.; Li, Y. Changes in Nut Consumption and Subsequent Cardiovascular Disease Risk Among US Men and Women: 3 Large Prospective Cohort Studies. *J. Am. Heart Assoc.* **2020**, *9*, e013877. [CrossRef]
55. Guasch-Ferré, M.; Li, J.; Hu, F.B.; Salas-Salvadó, J.; Tobias, D.K. Effects of Walnut Consumption on Blood Lipids and Other Cardiovascular Risk Factors: An Updated Meta-Analysis and Systematic Review of Controlled Trials. *Am. J. Clin. Nutr.* **2018**, *108*, 174–187. [CrossRef] [PubMed]
56. Becerra-Tomás, N.; Paz-Graniel, I.; Kendall, C.; Kahleova, H.; Rahelić, D.; Sievenpiper, J.L.; Salas-Salvadó, J. Nut Consumption and Incidence of Cardiovascular Diseases and Cardiovascular Disease Mortality: A Meta-Analysis of Prospective Cohort Studies. *Nutr. Rev.* **2019**, *77*, 691–709. [CrossRef] [PubMed]
57. Liu, X.; Guasch-Ferré, M.; Tobias, D.K.; Li, Y. Association of Walnut Consumption with Total and Cause-Specific Mortality and Life Expectancy in U.S. Adults. *Nutrients* **2021**, *13*, 2699. [CrossRef] [PubMed]
58. Estruch, R.; Ros, E.; Salas-Salvadó, J.; Covas, M.-I.; Corella, D.; Arós, F.; Gómez-Gracia, E.; Ruiz-Gutiérrez, V.; Fiol, M.; Lapetra, J.; et al. Primary Prevention of Cardiovascular Disease with a Mediterranean Diet Supplemented with Extra-Virgin Olive Oil or Nuts. *N. Engl. J. Med.* **2018**, *378*, e34. [CrossRef] [PubMed]
59. Rusu, M.E.; Gheldiu, A.M.; Mocan, A.; Vlase, L.; Popa, D.S. Anti-Aging Potential of Tree Nuts with a Focus on the Phytochemical Composition, Molecular Mechanisms and Thermal Stability of Major Bioactive Compounds. *Food Funct.* **2018**, *9*, 2554–2575. [CrossRef] [PubMed]
60. Li, J.; Jiang, B.; Santos, H.O.; Santos, D.; Singh, A.; Wang, L. Effects of Walnut Intake on Blood Pressure: A Systematic Review and Meta-Analysis of Randomized Controlled Trials. *Phytother. Res.* **2020**, *34*, 2921–2931. [CrossRef]
61. Banel, D.K.; Hu, F.B. Effects of Walnut Consumption on Blood Lipids and Other Cardiovascular Risk Factors: A Meta-Analysis and Systematic Review. *Am. J. Clin. Nutr.* **2009**, *90*, 56–63. [CrossRef]
62. Lopez-Garcia, E.; Schulze, M.B.; Fung, T.T.; Meigs, J.B.; Rifai, N.; Manson, J.E.; Hu, F.B. Major Dietary Patterns Are Related to Plasma Concentrations of Markers of Inflammation and Endothelial Dysfunction 1-3. *Am. J. Clin. Nutr.* **2004**, *80*, 1029–1064. [CrossRef]

63. Yu, Z.; Malik, V.S.; Keum, N.N.; Hu, F.B.; Giovannucci, E.L.; Stampfer, M.J.; Willett, W.C.; Fuchs, C.S.; Bao, Y. Associations between Nut Consumption and Inflammatory Biomarkers. *Am. J. Clin. Nutr.* **2016**, *104*, 722–728. [CrossRef]
64. Rusu, M.E.; Fizesan, I.; Pop, A.; Mocan, A.; Gheldiu, A.M.; Babota, M.; Vodnar, D.C.; Jurj, A.; Berindan-Neagoe, I.; Vlase, L.; et al. Walnut (*Juglans Regia* L.) Septum: Assessment of Bioactive Molecules and in Vitro Biological Effects. *Molecules* **2020**, *25*, 2187. [CrossRef]

MDPI
St. Alban-Anlage 66
4052 Basel
Switzerland
Tel. +41 61 683 77 34
Fax +41 61 302 89 18
www.mdpi.com

Antioxidants Editorial Office
E-mail: antioxidants@mdpi.com
www.mdpi.com/journal/antioxidants

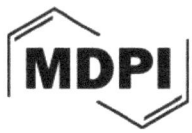